D1577246

MEDICINE FOR NURSES

First Edition	.	.	. 1953
Reprinted .	.	.	. 1954
Second Edition	.	.	. 1955
First Reprint	.	.	. 1956
Second Reprint	.	.	. 1956
Third Edition	.	.	. 1957
Reprinted .	.	.	. 1958
Fourth Edition	.	.	. 1959
Reprinted .	.	.	. 1959
Fifth Edition	.	.	. 1960
Reprinted .	.	.	. 1962

Made and Printed in Great Britain

MEDICINE FOR NURSES

by

M. TOOHEY
M.D., M.R.C.P., D.C.H.

Formerly Physician, New End Hospital, London

With a chapter on Psychological Medicine

by

HENRY R. ROLLIN, M.D., D.P.M.

Psychiatrist, Horton Hospital, Epsom,
and New End Hospital, London

FIFTH EDITION
(Reprint)

E. & S. LIVINGSTONE LTD.
EDINBURGH AND LONDON
1962

TO MY WIFE JOYCE
WITHOUT WHOM THIS BOOK WOULD
NEVER HAVE BEEN WRITTEN

PREFACE TO THE FIFTH EDITION

THIS new edition of "Medicine for Nurses" has again made it possible to bring the book fully up to date and to incorporate in it the most recent developments both in treatment and in the use of new drugs.

In addition, the two lists of drugs at the end of the book have been revised and enlarged and a new illustration has been included.

Once more I must express my gratitude to my wife and my publishers for their help in the preparation of this new edition. In particular I would wish to tender my sincerest thanks to Mr Charles Macmillan of E. & S. Livingstone Ltd., with whom, I should like to record, it has been a pleasure and a privilege to work.

M. TOOHEY.

1960.

PREFACE TO THE FIRST EDITION

IN writing this textbook of medicine for nurses I have tried to make it as comprehensive as possible so that it may not only help the nurse during her training but also serve as a reference book afterwards.

The basic physiological and pathological facts which are needed for the understanding of the various diseases and their treatment have accordingly been dealt with in some detail. Moreover, summaries of the more difficult chapters are included in order to stress the most significant points. In addition, other summaries have been given at the end of most chapters of the more important drugs and routine procedures used in the major diseases.

Perhaps a special word about the illustrations may be useful. Apart from the photographs, there are many original diagrams intended to emphasise in a simple and effective fashion the salient facts relating to the most important diseases.

Finally, a chapter on Psychosomatic Medicine has been contributed by Dr H. R. Rollin.

No attempt has, however, been made to deal with the purely nursing procedures which I consider are best learned from actual practice in the wards. Furthermore, there are many books which already cover this aspect of nursing.

I have received much help and advice from many people, and in particular I wish to thank Miss E. A. Calow, Miss D. K. Fisher, Miss B. A. Thorogood, Mr W. W. Davey, Dr F. D. Rosenthal and Mr J. Sayer. To Mr Charles Macmillan of E. & S. Livingstone Ltd. I owe a special debt of gratitude for his unfailing assistance at all times.

M. TOOHEY.

1953.

ACKNOWLEDGMENTS OF ILLUSTRATIONS

THE Author wishes to express his sincere thanks to the following for the use of illustrations and material from which illustrations were made :—

Dr B. BARLING (Fig. 83).

Dr A. B. BRATTON.

Dr C. C. BRYSON.

Dr J. H. BURKENSHAW (Figs. 158, 159, 160).

Mr W. W. DAVEY.

Dr A. GIBSON (Figs. 127, 131).

Dr R. GREENE (Fig. 151).

Dr A. KAHAN (Figs. 21, 150, 169).

Mr T. LEVITT.

Mr I. R. MCCAUL (Figs. 105, 106, 111, 112).

Dr J. F. MACMAHON (Figs. 120, 122, 123, 162).

PARKE, DAVIS & CO. LTD. (Figs. 15, 19).

Mr J. E. PIERCY (Figs. 124, 125, 152, 153, 154, 155, 156, 157).

Dr F. H. G. ROBINSON.

Mr T. HOLMES SELLORS (Fig. 24).

Mr N. TANNER (Fig. 71).

CLARKE, "Fundus of the Human Eye," Oxford University Press.

WHITBY and BRITTON, "Disorders of the Blood," J. & A. Churchill Ltd. (Fig. 130).

The publishers have also granted permission to use some illustrations from Low and Dodds, "Atlas of Bacteriology"; Percival, "Introduction to Dermatology"; and Bell, Davidson and Scarborough, "Textbook of Physiology."

CONTENTS

CHAPTER III

TUBERCULOSIS

CHAPTER IV

VENEREAL DISEASE

CHAPTER V

DISEASES OF THE CIRCULATORY SYSTEM

CHAPTER VI

DISEASES OF THE RESPIRATORY SYSTEM

CHAPTER VII

DISEASES OF THE ALIMENTARY SYSTEM

CHAPTER VIII

DISEASES OF THE LIVER AND BILIARY TRACT

CHAPTER IX

DISEASES OF THE CENTRAL NERVOUS SYSTEM

CHAPTER X

DISEASES OF THE BLOOD

CHAPTER XI

DISEASES OF THE SPLEEN AND LYMPH GLANDS

CHAPTER XII

DISEASES OF THE URINARY SYSTEM

CHAPTER XIII

DISEASES OF THE DUCTLESS GLANDS

CHAPTER XIV

METABOLISM AND ITS DISORDERS

CHAPTER XVIII

ON PAIN AND VOMITING

CHAPTER XIX

ON ACUTE POISONING AND COMA

CHAPTER XX

PSYCHOLOGICAL MEDICINE

CHAPTER XXI

IMPORTANT DRUGS

common to many different causes of disease, there are also individual specific changes in the different diseases :—

1. Inflammation :—
    (a) Acute.
    (b) Chronic.
2. Repair of Inflammation.
3. Vascular Changes and Effects :—
    (a) Thrombosis.
    (b) Embolism.
    (c) Ischæmia.
    (d) Hæmorrhage.
4. Degeneration.
5. Hypertrophy and Atrophy.
6. Tumour Formation.

1. INFLAMMATION

Inflammation is very common.   It mainly occurs in diseases due to infection with living agents (for example, bacteria, viruses, etc.), but is also seen as a result of injury.   There are two main forms of inflammation, acute and chronic.

(a) Acute.

The changes are usually very fully described in books on surgical diseases, as acute inflammation can be most readily observed in these diseases.   Only a brief description will be given here :—

    (i) Redness.
    (ii) Swelling.
    (iii) Heat.
    (iv) Pain.
    (v) Impairment or loss of function.

(b) Chronic.

In the acute stage dilatation of the vessels and, even more particularly, exudation of fluid are predominant.   In the chronic stage the main changes occur in the tissue cells of the area.   These tissue cells multiply, especially the small round cells (known as lymphocytes) and the fibrous tissue cells.   The latter form strands of dense tough tissue as a result of the chronic irritation set up by the disease, and also as part of the body's effort to ward off the infection. If the chronic inflammation is extensive, it can cause marked distortion and deformity of the area. Actual loss of tissue occurs when an ulcer forms.

Acute inflammation may subside without going on to the chronic stage. Chronic inflammation can also start without being preceded by acute inflammation. Whether acute or chronic inflammation occurs depends mainly on the type of organism or agent causing the inflammation and also on the severity and violence of the organism or agent. Some diseases, such as tuberculosis, tend to cause a chronic, as opposed to an acute, inflammation. Finally, in addition to differentiating between acute and chronic forms of inflammation, we can also distinguish several different varieties of both these forms :—

(i) SEROUS.—Here there is an exudation of clear yellowish fluid.
(ii) PURULENT.—The exudate is thick and creamy owing to the presence of pus. Pus is composed of masses of organisms, white blood cells, especially polymorphs, and debris of dead tissue cells.
(iii) HÆMORRHAGIC.—The exudation is bloodstained owing to the presence of large numbers of red cells.

The type of inflammation that occurs—serous, purulent, or hæmorrhagic—depends mainly on the infecting agent. Some organisms (pyogenic organisms) nearly always cause a purulent inflammation ; others only a serous and hardly ever, or never, a purulent one. Again, other diseases may particularly cause hæmorrhagic exudation ; this is very commonly so with malignant tumours (cancers).

2. REPAIR OF INFLAMMATION

If the inflammation is mild, then the protective forces of the body can overcome the disease and healing can occur with very little permanent change in the affected area. If it is more severe, permanent changes, principally fibrosis or scarring, may occur. It can be seen that if this scarring is extensive, owing to severe inflammation, then it can interfere with the proper function of the part. This may be a serious disability, perhaps with fatal results, if the part affected is a vital organ. For example, disease causing a chronic inflammation of the valves of the heart can give rise to scarring and deformity, with the result that the heart cannot function properly, so that after a period it fails and death occurs.

3. VASCULAR CHANGES AND EFFECTS

As the result of many different diseases which affect the arteries
and veins, certain typical changes occur.   As these can have serious
and widespread effects on the body generally, it is best at this stage
to describe these changes and their effects.   The common changes
are :—

(a) **Thrombosis.**

Thrombosis means clotting of the blood in a vessel.   When a
vessel is the seat of disease, from injury or other cause, certain
changes occur in the wall of the vessel and in the blood which may
result in thrombosis or clotting.   Certain cells normally present in
the blood, called platelets, adhere to the roughened, injured, or
diseased wall of the vessel.   The platelets and the injured tissues
give off a substance known as thromboplastin which acts on another
substance normally present in blood, called prothrombin, to convert
the prothrombin into thrombin.   Thrombin immediately converts
the fibrinogen in the blood into fibrin.   Fibrin is a solid, dense,
fibrous substance which binds the platelets, white cells and red cells
of the blood together to form a clot or thrombus.

Fibrinogen is present in blood, to be converted into fibrin or
clot, as a necessary protective measure to prevent excessive loss of
blood from the circulation when a vessel is damaged.

We can represent the above changes as follows :—

   (i) Artery or vein—damaged.
   (ii) Platelets in blood crowd to the area.
   (iii) Thromboplastin given off by the platelets and injured tissues.
   (iv) Thromboplastin converts prothrombin into thrombin.
   (v) Thrombin changes fibrinogen into
   (vi) Fibrin (clot).

Damage to the wall of a blood vessel is one cause of thrombosis ;
another most important cause is a slowing of the circulation of blood
in a blood vessel.   Thrombosis is therefore much more often seen in
veins than in arteries because the normally rapid flow in the arteries
usually prevents a clot forming.

EFFECTS OF THROMBOSIS.—These depend on the size of the clot
and also on the importance of the vessel affected.   If the vein
(arteries, as mentioned above, are less often involved) is completely
blocked, the result is swelling of the area drained by the vein owing

to the obstruction to the return of fluid from the area. *Œdema* is the name given to this swelling and means fluid in the tissues. Severe swelling or œdema occurs only if the vein involved is a main one, as there is so much intercommunication between the veins that the blocking of a small vein only shunts the blood through another part of the communicating network. The veins most commonly affected by thrombosis are the long veins in the legs. Inflammation of a vein is called phlebitis, and when, as is common, thrombosis occurs as well, the condition of thrombophlebitis results.

When thrombosis occurs in an artery the blood supply to the area is cut off, and if this is a main artery there may be no other source of supply of blood to the affected part. As tissue cannot live without blood, death of the tissue (**necrosis** or **gangrene**) occurs.

Apart from the interference with the blood supply mentioned above, there is one further important change that can occur with thrombosis of a vessel, whether it is a vein or an artery. The clot in the vessel can become dislodged by the force of the blood stream, and this detached clot (called an embolus) can then travel in the circulation.

(b) Embolism.

A detached thrombus or clot is, we have just seen, called an embolus. Apart from a detached clot, fat, or even air which remains undissolved in the circulation, can act as an embolus. The importance of an embolus is that if it is large enough it may become impacted in some part of the vascular tree and cut off the blood supply to the area or organ supplied by the affected vessel. When this happens, embolism is said to have occurred.

TYPES OF EMBOLISM.

(i) *Pulmonary Embolism.*—A detached thrombus from any vein in the body must travel through the venous system, through the right auricle and the right ventricle, and eventually arrive in the pulmonary artery. Up to this point the veins have been increasing in size so that a clot is unlikely to lodge in any of the veins or in the right side of the heart. The pulmonary artery divides, however, into smaller branches so that an embolus from a large vein, say in the leg, may become lodged in one of the branches of the pulmonary artery—pulmonary embolism has then occurred.

(ii) *Arterial Embolism.*—In arterial embolism the initial thrombus is in the arterial instead of the venous system. The most common site from which a thrombus becomes dislodged is the left side of the heart. An embolus which lodges in the brain (cerebral embolism) or in a peripheral artery of a limb is commonly seen in medicine owing to a clot being dislodged from the left side of the heart.

EFFECTS OF EMBOLISM.—As in the case of thrombosis, the effects depend on the size of the vessel occluded by the embolus and on whether there is any *collateral circulation* (that is, other vessels which can take the place of the blocked one to supply the necessary blood). If any major degree of obstruction affects an organ, the part deprived of its blood supply undergoes certain typical changes known as *infarction.* When, however, a limb is affected, the changes that occur as a result of the loss of blood supply are usually known as *gangrene.*

If an alternative blood supply to the affected organ or tissue is not quickly provided, death of the tissue results. If the embolus is sufficiently large to cut off the blood supply to the major part of a vital organ (*e.g.*, lungs, brain, or heart), then sudden death occurs.

When a limb is affected, the loss of blood supply causes the tissues to become cold and dead and the affected area turns black—gangrene.

Embolism, as it affects the individual vessels, is described further under Diseases of the Blood Vessels.

(*c*) **Ischæmia.**

The term *ischæmia* is used to denote a deficient (but not complete lack of) blood supply to an organ or tissue. The essential changes produced by a deficient blood supply are the same no matter what the cause of the deficiency may be, or, in general, what the part affected. There is a lack of oxygen supply to the tissue, and as a result inability to function fully. As can be understood, this inability is likely to be very important when it affects vital organs such as the heart, brain and kidneys. Many organs and tissues, however, are hardly ever the seat of ischæmic changes as they have a large and plentiful supply of blood vessels, or, as it is often put, they have a large collateral circulation.

As will be seen in discussing the diseases which cause ischæmia, the common result of all is diminished function of the part affected.

(*d*) **Hæmorrhage.**

When a vessel is the seat of disease a common result is for the wall of the vessel to give way, so that loss of blood or hæmorrhage occurs. How serious the loss of blood will be depends on how large a vessel is involved. We have already seen in discussing thrombosis how the body reacts to disease or injury of a vessel by causing a clot to form. This is an important protective mechanism to try and prevent loss of blood.

Serious loss of blood or hæmorrhage is seen most commonly in the following diseases :—

(i) Injury.

(ii) Ulceration of an artery due to inflammation. For example, tuberculosis, peptic ulcer in the stomach or duodenum, and typhoid fever, all commonly cause hæmorrhage.

(iii) Malignant tumours (cancers). Cancers, by destroying tissue as they grow, commonly ulcerate an artery to cause hæmorrhage.

(iv) Blood diseases. Hæmorrhage in blood diseases differs from the other forms in that here the hæmorrhage is not due to injury or ulceration but to a defect in the normal mechanism for blood clotting. Various types of defect exist and will be discussed under Blood Diseases.

Before leaving this brief general discussion of hæmorrhage it is important to realise that in addition to the thrombosis or clotting mechanism for stopping hæmorrhage an equally important factor in cases of a large hæmorrhage is contraction of the vessel wall to close the opening in the vessel. This is called *vasoconstriction*.

4. DEGENERATION

Many different diseases produce their pathological changes in the body neither by inflammation nor through their effects on the vascular tree but by causing changes in the individual cells of the tissues or organs. A common way for this to occur is through the formation of toxic (poisonous) substances, but in many diseases the exact way in which the changes in the cells are caused is unknown. The changes in the cells are usually spoken of as degenerative changes or lesions, and several different forms exist. It is not necessary at this stage to go further into the detailed changes occurring in degeneration. The main lesions present are, usually, swelling of the cells, loss of their normal appearance and loss of function.

5. HYPERTROPHY AND ATROPHY

One of the main results of certain diseases is enlargement of the affected organs or tissues. This enlargement is known as hypertrophy and is usually an effort on the part of the body to improve or restore the function lost owing to the disease. This change is frequently seen in heart disease.

The opposite effect, where the affected organs or tissues decrease in size, is spoken of as atrophy. For instance, muscles which are not being used soon become wasted ; the kidneys in chronic renal failure often become small and shrunken.

6. TUMOUR FORMATION

One very important group of diseases produces its effects in the body by growing abnormal cells which may invade or replace normal tissue. Tumours are the most important class of disease which produces this abnormal growing tissue. There are two main groups of tumours :—

(a) Benign or innocent.   (b) Malignant.

Benign tumours, which are often encapsulated, do not spread throughout the body but remain localised in one area. They cause symptoms mainly as a result of pressure on the tissues. Malignant tumours, on the other hand, are not surrounded by a capsule and therefore invasion of organs by the growing number of malignant cells occurs, causing destruction and ulceration of the normal tissues. A frequent development is ulceration of blood vessels leading to hæmorrhage ; hæmorrhage from organs such as the stomach, lungs, uterus, etc., is therefore often seen as a result of malignant tumours arising in these sites. The growing malignant tumour also often causes obstruction of a vital passage-way, such as the respiratory air passages or the intestinal tract.

Malignant tumours, unlike benign tumours, very often spread throughout the body, travelling via the blood stream or the lymphatic system. When the malignant tumour has spread from the primary site of growth to other parts of the body, metastases (secondary growths) are said to be present. Malignant tumours often cause death through destruction or obstruction of a vital organ or by hæmorrhage.

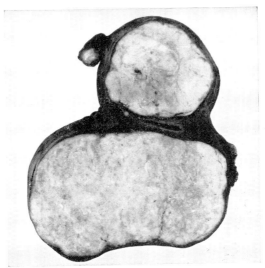

Fig. 1

Benign tumour (fibroid) of the uterus.

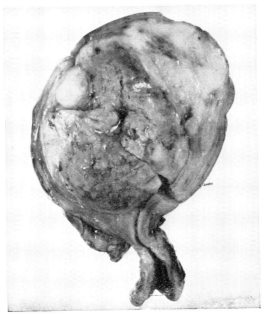

Fig. 2

Malignant tumour (carcinoma) of the uterus. It can be seen that, in contrast with Fig. 1, there is marked invasion and destruction of the walls of the uterus and gross ulceration. Severe hæmorrhage from the uterus occurred.

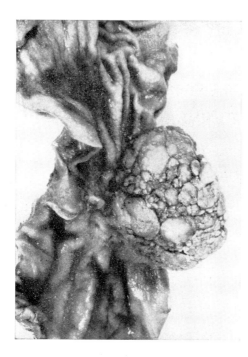

FIG. 3

Benign tumour (papilloma)
growing from the intestinal
mucous membrane.

FIG. 4

Malignant tumour (carcinoma) of
the rectum. When compared with
Fig. 3 it can be seen that there
is invasion of the intestinal wall
with ulceration of the tissues. In
addition it can be seen how the
growing tumour is causing obstruction of the intestinal canal.

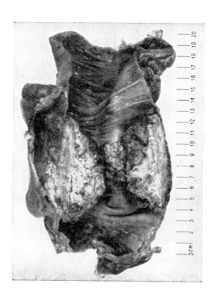

There are many different types of tumours and they derive their names from the type of cell from which they grow. The commonest of importance in medicine are :—

(*a*) Carcinoma—malignant tumour of epithelial cells.

(*b*) Adenoma—benign tumour of epithelial cells.

(*c*) Papilloma—benign tumour of lining epithelial cells.

(*d*) Sarcoma—malignant group affecting bones, muscles and fibrous tissue.

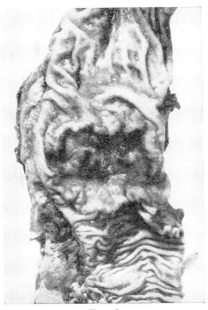

FIG. 5

Another example of a carcinoma of the intestine showing the marked ulceration of the tissues. Intestinal hæmorrhage was a feature of this case.

Carcinoma is the commonest and therefore the most important type of tumour in medicine. Carcinomas of the individual organs or tissues are described under the appropriate systems.

(B) GENERAL CAUSES OF DISEASE

The most common pathological changes which occur as a result of disease have now been briefly outlined and we can now discuss in a general manner the main causes of disease met with in medicine.

The term *ætiology* is used to denote causation of disease. As can be readily appreciated there are perhaps thousands of different causes which set up disease in the human body and it is impossible to give a complete list in a short space. The following classification gives only the main causes :—

1. LIVING ORGANISMS OR MICROBES.

    (*a*) Bacteria.
    (*b*) Viruses.
    (*c*) Parasites.
    (*d*) Fungi.

2. PHYSICAL AND CHEMICAL AGENTS.

    (*a*) Injury (trauma).
    (*b*) Excess of heat or cold.   } Physical.
    (*c*) Electricity, X-rays and radioactive substances.
    (*d*) Toxic drugs.   } Chemical.
    (*e*) Poisonous gases.

3. DEFICIENCY AND HORMONAL DISEASES.
Lack or disturbance of:

    (*a*) Vitamins.
    (*b*) Hormones.
    (*c*) Diet.

4. HEREDITY.

5. UNKNOWN (including causes of tumours).

GENERAL NOTES ON THE MORE COMMON AGENTS CAUSING DISEASE

1. Living Organisms or Microbes.

Living organisms are among the commonest causes of disease in man. They include an immense number and variety of small bodies which can be seen only under a microscope, called **bacteria**. Other organisms are even smaller so that an ordinary microscope will not show them, and they have to be identified by other special means. These organisms are called **viruses**. Yet other organisms, which are larger than bacteria and are conveyed from animals to man, are often called *parasites*. Lastly, there are the organisms known as *fungi*, which are fine branching hair-like structures, some of which resemble moulds.

So important are these bacteria, viruses, etc., in causing disease that a special study is usually made of them under the term *bacteriology*. This will be dealt with later.

2. Physical and Chemical Agents.

(*a*) INJURY OR TRAUMA usually causes disease through damage to tissues and bones (*e.g.*, wounds and fractures). These are often associated with hæmorrhage and a severe general upset to the body known as shock. Shock, which causes severe depression of the bodily functions, is discussed in more detail on page 368.

(*b*) EXCESS OF HEAT OR COLD.—The effects of excessive heat or cold are likewise fully described in textbooks on surgical diseases. Briefly, excess of heat can cause burns or scalds with loss of tissue substance and ulcers. Excess of cold (frost-bite) can damage tissues and even cause actual death of tissue (*i.e.*, gangrene).

(*c*) ELECTRICITY, X-RAYS AND RADIOACTIVE SUBSTANCES.—An excessive current of electricity passing through the body can cause death, usually by respiratory or cardiac failure. It can also cause local damage by burning the tissues. X-rays may also cause severe burns and, in addition, anæmia, by depressing the formation of the blood. Radium and other radioactive substances can cause changes similar to those caused by X-rays.

(*d*) TOXIC DRUGS OR CHEMICALS.—Certain drugs or chemicals are extremely poisonous to man whilst others, if used to excess, can also have a poisonous or toxic action on the body. The exact effect on the body varies, but is usually a depression of the function of cells in different organs or tissues, with in some cases death of the tissue. The liver, skin, kidneys and blood formation are particularly affected.

(*e*) POISONOUS GASES.—Poisonous gases can also cause serious or fatal damage through their effects on the lungs or on the blood.

(*f*) CIGARETTE SMOKING.—Heavy cigarette smoking predisposes to cancer of the lung and contributes to the development of chronic bronchitis and emphysema.

3. Deficiency and Hormonal Diseases.

Certain factors or substances are essential for the proper working of the bodily mechanism, and a lack or disturbance of these has well recognised effects on the body.

(*a*) VITAMINS.—These substances are usually found in different foods, and in the main deal with the proper growth of the body and its cells, bones, blood formation and nerve tissue. The effects of lack of vitamins are dealt with fully under the vitamin diseases.

(*b*) HORMONES.—Hormones are chemical substances manu-factured by various glands in the body and have many complicated actions which are not all as yet fully understood. Certain definite diseases are met with which are due to either deficiency of, or excess of, production of these hormones. These diseases are discussed under Diseases of the Ductless Glands.

(*c*) DIET.—An adequate diet containing all the important foods is essential for the maintenance of good health. Lack of any of the essential foods will set up disease in the body.

4. Heredity.

Many diseases have their origin or cause in some abnormal or peculiar factor passed on from the parent or parents. This may continue to be effective from generation to generation. These hereditary defects are more likely to be seen when there is any inbreeding in families, as when near cousins marry. The reason for this is that many of the defects passed on to the future generation are what are known as *recessive* (quiescent or dormant). Such a quiescent or recessive defect may only cause disease if it links up with a similar recessive defect. The mating of two recessive defects is much more likely to occur in marriage between people in the same family.

Other hereditary defects are known as *dominant* because they give rise to disease in future generations without having to link up with other similar defects. Certain hereditary defects in blood formation are fairly common, the disease known as hæmophilia and hæmolytic disease of the newborn (Rh factor) being linked up with heredity. Again, mental deficiency commonly runs in certain families owing to the inheritance of some defect. Mongolism, although not familial, is due to a chromosomal abnormality of the ovum at the time of conception.

5. Unknown Causes (including causes of tumours).

After considering all the above causes of disease we are left with a large number and variety of common diseases for the causes of which we have no very adequate explanation.

For instance, the cause of the common serious disease called malignant disease or " cancer " is still unknown. What causes hypertension (high blood pressure) ? To what is due the kidney disease called nephritis ? These and many more problems still await a proper explanation.

BACTERIOLOGY

The study of bacteria, viruses and parasites is so important for the proper understanding of many of the commonest and most important diseases met with in medicine that a special study is usually made of these organisms under the term *bacteriology*.

We know most about the bacteria, so that the longest discussion is taken up with these organisms. Viruses are almost of equal importance in causing disease, but as yet we know much less about them, and their study requires highly specialised techniques outside the scope of most hospitals.

Parasites and fungi cause disease to a much lesser extent than the bacteria or viruses, so less time will be spent on them.

A. BACTERIA

There are a large number of different types of bacteria, some of more importance than others in both the seriousness and the frequency with which they cause disease. Only the most common and important bacteria will be discussed here.

Bacteria are usually divided up into different groups or families, the chief being :—

1. Cocci.　　2. Bacilli.　　3. Spirochætes.

1. Cocci.

These are rounded organisms and, according to the manner in which they grow, they are divided up into different groups. When they grow in bunches or clusters they are spoken of as *staphylococci*. If they form chains as they grow they are called *streptococci*, and if they grow in pairs they are called *diplococci*.

These main groups are further divided into classes according to various factors. For example, certain important streptococci, when they grow in a special medium containing blood, cause the red cells to be destroyed, or, as it is said, the blood is hæmolysed. For this reason these are called *hæmolytic* streptococci, to distinguish them from other forms of streptococci which do not cause hæmolysis when they grow on blood.

Again, some cocci are called by the name of the disease they set up in the body. The common disease of the lungs known as pneumonia is usually due to a certain group of cocci which are given the name of *pneumococci*.

Some cocci and bacilli in causing disease usually set up an

inflammation with pus formation, and for this reason they are often classed together as **pyogenic** organisms. These include, especially, staphylococci, streptococci, pneumococci, meningococci and the coliform bacilli.

Table I gives the names, main types of lesion or pathological change, and finally the most common diseases caused by the more important cocci.

TABLE I.—THE COCCI

NAME.	PATHOLOGICAL EFFECTS.	DISEASES.
Staphylococci . .	Acute inflammation with pus formation. Lesions tend to remain localised with the development of abscesses.	Skin conditions : Boils, carbuncles, impetigo. Bone lesions : Osteomyelitis. Otitis media, meningitis, pneumonia, acute bacterial endocarditis, septicæmia.
Streptococci. (a) Hæmolytic .	Acute inflammation with pus. Lesions usually spread.	Skin conditions : Cellulitis, erysipelas and impetigo. Acute tonsillitis, scarlet fever, otitis media, meningitis, pneumonia, acute bacterial endocarditis, septicæmia.
(b) Non-hæmolytic	Subacute inflammation.	Subacute bacterial endocarditis.
Pneumococci . .	Acute inflammation with pus.	Pneumonia of both lobar and broncho types. Otitis media, meningitis, peritonitis.
Meningococci . .	Acute inflammation with pus.	Meningitis (cerebrospinal fever).
Gonococci . .	Acute and chronic inflammation with pus.	Gonorrhœa, causing acute urethritis, epididymo-orchitis and prostatitis in the male ; acute urethritis, vaginitis and salpingitis in the female. Ophthalmia in the newborn. Arthritis.

2. Bacilli.

Bacilli instead of being rounded bodies are rod-shaped, and are mainly classified according to the type of disease which they cause.

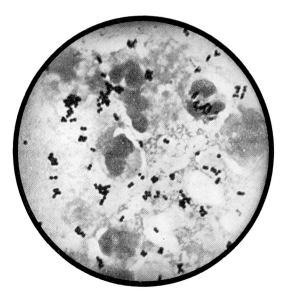

Fig. 6
Staphylococci after staining appear under the
microscope in clusters.

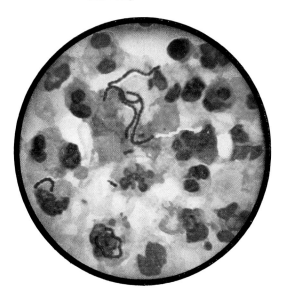

Fig. 7
Streptococci. Note the characteristic arrangement
in chains.

[To face page 16

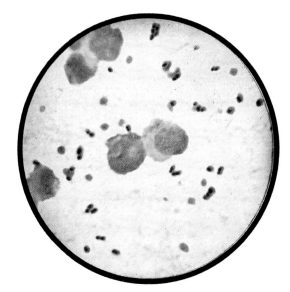

FIG. 8
Pneumococci are in pairs.

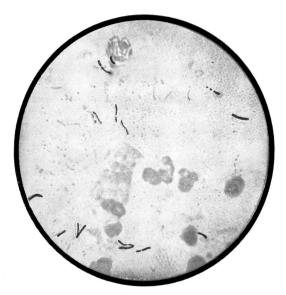

FIG. 9
Tubercle bacillus is slender, straight or curved with
rounded ends.

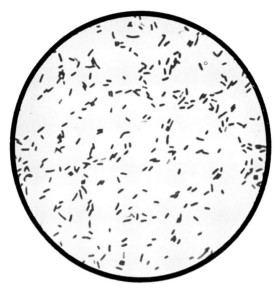

FIG. 10
Bacillus coli.

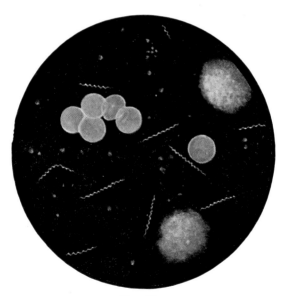

FIG. 11
The spirochæte of syphilis.

Table II gives the commonest bacilli and the diseases caused by them :—

TABLE II.—THE BACILLI

NAME.	PATHOLOGICAL EFFECTS.	DISEASES.
Tubercle bacilli	Specific type of subacute and chronic inflammation. Tubercles form which often break down to a cheesy material (caseation). Ulceration with cavity formation is also a feature. Healing by fibrosis.	Tuberculosis, which affects many organs and tissues. Especially important are: pulmonary tuberculosis, tuberculous meningitis, glandular tuberculosis, tuberculosis of the bones (N.B. spine), joints, kidneys and skin.
Coliform bacilli	Acute and chronic inflammation with pus.	Pyelitis, cystitis, peritonitis, cholecystitis, meningitis, puerperal sepsis.
Pertussis bacilli	Specific acute infectious fever mainly involving the lungs.	Whooping-cough.
Diphtheria bacilli	Specific localised lesion, the diphtheritic membrane, and a powerful toxin with widespread effects.	Diphtheria, with the membrane in the throat, nose, or larynx. Toxin causes albuminuria, acute myocarditis and neuritis.
Typhoid and paratyphoid bacilli	Specific infectious fevers with acute inflammation and ulceration. General invasion of the body including the blood stream, but marked local changes in the small intestine.	Typhoid and paratyphoid fever (enteric fever).
Dysentery bacilli	Specific acute inflammation with ulceration of the intestinal tract. Toxin also produced.	Acute bacillary dysentery.
Salmonella bacilli	Acute inflammation of the intestinal tract. Toxin.	Food poisoning.
Influenzal bacilli	Acute inflammation with pus.	Influenzal meningitis.
Abortus and melitensis bacilli	Specific inflammation of a subacute type mainly involving the joints, glands and spleen.	Undulant fever (brucellosis).
Tetanus bacilli	Powerful toxin produced which has a selective effect on the nerve cells.	Tetanus.

3. Spirochætes.

The last important group of bacteria is the spirochætal group. These organisms are larger than either cocci or bacilli and their bodies have several curves. Fewer diseases are caused by spirochætes than by the two preceding groups. The most important disease in man due to a spirochæte is syphilis.

Table III lists the few well-known diseases caused by the spirochætes :—

TABLE III.—THE SPIROCHÆTES

NAME.	PATHOLOGICAL EFFECTS.	DISEASES.
Treponema pallidum .	Chronic inflammation with fibrosis and ulceration. Widespread lesions, with the heart, arteries and nervous system particularly affected.	Syphilis.
Leptospira icterohæmorrhagica	Toxin which particularly affects the liver to cause a hepatitis and jaundice.	Weil's disease (spirochætal jaundice).
Spironema vincente .	Acute inflammation and ulceration of the throat and gums.	Vincent's angina.

B. VIRUSES

As mentioned earlier, we do not know so much about the characteristics of this important group as we know about bacteria. The main difference between viruses and bacteria is that viruses cannot be seen through an ordinary microscope, so that a highly specialised technique is needed to identify them. One means of identification is their ability to pass through a very fine filter which will hold back bacteria. For this reason they are often called *filter-passing viruses.*

Viruses are at present classified according to the disease they cause in man, and they are responsible for a large number of the diseases termed the *acute infectious fevers.*

The common virus diseases of importance are : measles, German measles (rubella), mumps, acute anterior poliomyelitis (infantile paralysis), smallpox, chickenpox, common cold, influenza and virus pneumonia.

C. PARASITES AND FUNGI

There remain a number of different living organisms which can be divided into several classes and which are responsible for some important diseases in man. For the sake of convenience, here they are grouped under the heading of parasites and fungi.

The commoner groups of these organisms or parasites causing disease are :—

1. PROTOZOA.
   - (a) Malarial parasites, causing malaria.
   - (b) Amœba (*Entamœba histolytica*), causing amœbic dysentery.

2. ANIMAL PARASITES.
   - (a) Pediculi (lice), causing skin diseases.
   - (b) *Acarus scabiei*, causing the skin disease scabies.

3. FUNGI.
   - (a) Ringworm fungi (disease of skin and hair).
   - (b) Thrush fungi (disease of the mouth).

SPECIMENS FOR BACTERIOLOGICAL EXAMINATION

The primary object of practical bacteriological methods is to find out what part a particular organism plays in causing a particular disease. Of course to do this it is essential to obtain the particular organism : therefore if a disease is suspected of being caused by bacteria, certain methods are adopted to try to obtain the organism. From experience it is known that in certain diseases the responsible organism can be found in specific excretions or tissues : these are accordingly examined for presence of the organism.

In general the common specimens or material examined for the presence of bacteria are as follows :—

1. Throat Swabs.

A swab is a piece of sterile cotton wool wrapped round the end of a stick. The sterile wool is rubbed over the surface or area from which the specimen is to be taken. Swabs are often taken from the throat, as in many diseases the causative organism is to be found in the throat.

Diseases in which throat swabs are normally taken are :—

- (a) Acute tonsillitis or any " sore throat."
- (b) Diphtheria.
- (c) Scarlet fever.
- (d) Rheumatic fever

2. Nasal Swabs.

These are less important than throat swabs but are taken in suspected nasal diphtheria.

3. Sputum.

In most diseases in which sputum is being coughed up it is sent for bacteriological examination, but this is of special importance in the following:—

     (a) Pulmonary tuberculosis.
     (b) Pneumonia.

Sputum examination for the presence of **tubercle bacilli,** the bacteria causing pulmonary tuberculosis, is of great importance. Firstly, it establishes the diagnosis of the case as one of active pulmonary tuberculosis; and secondly, it denotes that the case is infectious and should be treated with full isolation procedure. In pneumonia, examination of the sputum for bacteria is often carried out to determine what is the causative organism.

4. Fæces.

Many bacteria cause lesions in the intestinal tract and the organisms in these cases can often be found in the fæces. Diseases in which this examination of fæces for organisms is most commonly performed are:—

     (a) All cases of acute diarrhœa.
     (b) Dysentery.
     (c) Food poisoning.
     (d) Typhoid and paratyphoid fevers.
     (e) Tuberculosis of the intestinal tract.

5. Urine.

The urine is frequently examined for the presence of bacteria and, if sent for this examination, it must be obtained with aseptic precautions. A specimen is obtained after washing with soap and water and discarding the first urine passed (*mid-stream specimen*). Urine examination for bacteria is of importance in the following diseases:—

     (a) Acute pyelitis and cystitis.
     (b) Acute urethritis.
     (c) Tuberculosis of the renal tract.

6. Blood.

In cases where it is suspected that the bacteria may be actually growing in the blood stream (that is, in septicæmia) a small quantity of blood, usually 2 to 3 ml., is put into a special bottle known as a *blood culture* bottle. This bottle contains a special medium, usually glucose broth or cooked meat, which helps the organisms to grow. It is of the utmost importance that the blood should be collected under strict aseptic technique, as otherwise contaminating organisms will get into the blood culture bottle and confuse the result of the test. An all-glass syringe, specially sterilised in the laboratory, is generally used.

Blood cultures are usually taken in the following diseases :—

(*a*) All cases of suspected septicæmia.

(*b*) Bacterial endocarditis.

(*c*) Typhoid and paratyphoid fevers.

(*d*) All cases of prolonged undiagnosed fever.

7. Pleural and Cerebrospinal Fluid.

When fluid is present in the chest a sample is frequently aspirated in order to isolate any organism that may be present. Such organisms include pneumococci, streptococci, staphylococci and tubercle bacilli. All these organisms commonly cause disease of the lungs and pleura with resulting fluid in the pleural cavity.

Cerebrospinal fluid is withdrawn by doing a lumbar puncture. It is examined for bacteria in all cases of meningitis (inflammatory disease of the meninges). The bacteria often found include, in particular, meningococci, pneumococci, and tubercle bacilli.

8. Any Discharge of Pus from any Abscess, Sore, or other Lesion.

9. Swabs from the Genital Regions.

In all cases of a discharge from the vagina or urethra a swab is taken and an examination for the presence of organisms, particularly the gonococcus, made.

If there is a sore on the genital organs, a scraping from the sore is taken for examination for the presence of the spirochæte of syphilis.

10. Eye Swabs,

In many cases of inflammation of the eyes, and also before any operation on the eyes, swabs are taken. Before eye operations are performed it is essential that no organisms should be present in the conjunctiva.

METHODS OF IDENTIFICATION OF ORGANISMS

The usual way in which material is obtained for bacteriological examination has just been described. The material so obtained is treated in the laboratory by many different methods so that the organism may be identified.

1. Staining of Smears.

In some cases the material obtained is smeared on to a slide and various stains or dyes are applied to colour and show up the organisms. By means of these stains we can differentiate between certain organisms, as some turn one colour while others turn another. For example, one important and commonly used stain is known as **Gram's stain.** By means of this most of the common organisms can be divided into two groups :—

(a) Gram-positive organisms, which turn blue on application of the stain.

(b) Gram-negative organisms, which turn red.

The cocci (except for the meningococci and gonococci) are usually Gram-positive, whilst many of the more important bacilli (but not the tubercle bacilli or *B. diphtheriæ*) are Gram-negative.

Again, by washing out the stain with acid most organisms are distinguished from the tubercle bacillus which resists the action of acid and is thus called an *acid-fast bacillus*.

2. Cultures.

Most specimens taken are put on a special plate containing suitable material, such as blood, which will enable the organism to grow to the best advantage and, as far as possible, in a pure state. The plate is placed in a special box, known as an *incubator*, which is kept at a temperature of 37° C. (body temperature) ; most organisms grow best at body temperature. After twenty-four to forty-eight hours the plate is examined for growth of the organism. This method of examination is spoken of as a culture. Smears or films are then taken from the culture plate and stained for examination under the microscope as outlined above. The culture plate yields very useful information on the identity of the organisms, as in their growth certain characteristics are shown. For instance, the hæmolytic streptococcus, an important organism causing several diseases, can be distinguished from the non-hæmolytic streptococcus. As the names imply, the latter does not cause hæmolysis on a blood culture plate while the hæmolytic streptococcus does.

3. Agglutination Reactions.

To explain what is meant by an agglutination reaction it is best to take a particular example, *e.g.*, the **Widal reaction,** a typical agglutination reaction, which is used in the diagnosis of typhoid fever. If a patient is suffering from typhoid fever, antibodies are developed in the body against the typhoid bacilli as part of the body's protective mechanism to fight the disease. If serum from the patient is mixed with *known* typhoid bacilli in a test-tube the bacilli become clumped or agglutinated owing to the action of the antibodies on the bacilli. No agglutination would occur if serum and organisms other than typhoid bacilli were mixed together. In this way the agglutination reaction can be used for diagnosis in certain infections. This test is of value where it is difficult to isolate the actual organisms and is mostly used in cases of the enteric fevers. Agglutination reactions only become positive after the illness has lasted approximately a week, as it takes this time for the antibodies to form in the body.

ON HOW BACTERIA ENTER THE BODY

Organisms must enter the body if they are to set up a disease. The ways in which the organisms can do so are often referred to as the modes of spread.

1. **Droplet Infection.**—If organisms are present in the upper air passages they are expelled into the air on speaking and especially on sneezing and coughing, and they can then be readily inhaled by others. Infection can thus easily spread through close proximity to the infected person ; direct contact is not necessary. In some cases the infected droplets can contaminate dust, and inhalation of the dust can cause infection. Fortunately most organisms soon die outside the body, but an important exception is the tubercle bacillus which can remain alive in dust for many months.

The majority of the acute infectious diseases, such as measles, whooping-cough, diphtheria, etc., are contracted in this way through the respiratory tract.

2. Infection may spread through **handling articles** which have become infected with the organism, *e.g.*, clothes, bed-linen, toys, pencils, etc. Neglect in washing the hands thoroughly is very likely to spread infection from patient to patient.

3. The infecting organism may be present in the **fæces** and **urine** and, if the hands are not washed properly after visits to the toilet, food can become contaminated and the infection may thus

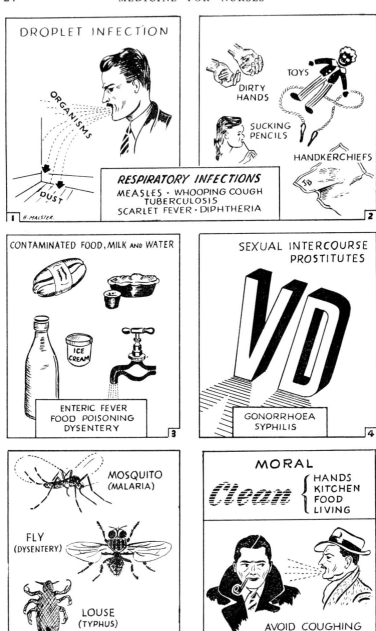

FIG. 12

Common ways by which infection is spread.

spread to others. Contamination of water supplies from leaking drains was also formerly a common cause of large epidemics. *Flies* which feed on excreta are another common means by which food can become contaminated.

The diseases which are spread through contamination of food, milk or water are the intestinal infections such as food poisoning, dysentery and typhoid fever.

4. Certain organisms, especially gonococci and the syphilitic spirochæte, require actual **direct contact** between the infected person and the one to be infected.

5. Infecting organisms may be conveyed by means of a **blood-sucking insect,** *e.g.*, by mosquitoes carrying the malarial parasites and lice carrying the typhus organisms.

6. Finally, infection may spread to man from contact with **animals,** *e.g.*, rabies from dogs and anthrax from sheep.

ON HOW BACTERIA CAUSE DISEASE

We have now seen how bacteria can enter the body. Before going further it must be realised that bacteria exist all around us but they do not necessarily cause disease. Why is this ? It is because to cause disease, even after entry of the organism into the body, certain conditions must prevail :—

1. The bacteria must be present in *sufficient* numbers.
2. The bacteria must be *virulent*, that is, of a sufficient degree of activity.
3. The organisms must have entered the body by the *proper pathway*, *e.g.*, gonococci, if swallowed, are destroyed and do not cause disease, while dysentery organisms cause disease only if swallowed.
4. The person infected must be *sensitive* to the organism, that is, must not be resistant (immune). This subject is discussed further under Immunity.

Given the above suitable conditions, the organisms entering the body will multiply and produce toxins, which are poisonous substances that react on tissues and cells. The nature of these reactions varies with different bacteria, some toxins causing inflammation, either acute or chronic, whilst others cause degeneration of cells. Many toxins tend to have specific selective action on particular tissues or cells, *e.g.*, diphtheria toxin on the nerves and heart. These specific actions will be described more fully under the individual diseases.

ON HOW THE BODY RESISTS AND OVERCOMES INFECTION (IMMUNITY)

So far in our discussion we have considered :—

1. The identification of bacteria causing disease.
2. How these bacteria get into the body.
3. The conditions necessary before these bacteria, having entered the body, can give rise to disease.
4. How these bacteria set up their toxic effects to cause disease.

In discussing the conditions necessary before bacteria can cause disease we saw that the person infected must be sensitive or susceptible to the organisms. In many cases the infected person is *not* susceptible and does not suffer from the disease even though he or she is harbouring the organism in the body. In these circumstances the person is said to be immune to the disease.

A person may be immune to a particular disease for a number of reasons, and to understand some very important diseases and their treatment it is necessary to discuss further the different types of immunity and how they arise.

Types of Immunity.—Immunity is a complex subject and it is proposed to give here only a broad outline. For this reason the following brief classification of immunity is used :—

(A) Naturally Acquired Immunity.

(B) Artificially Acquired Immunity.

(A) Naturally Acquired Immunity.

Natural immunity to a particular disease may be acquired in several different ways :—

1. *The Individual has an Actual Attack of the Disease.*—As a result of having had and recovered from the disease the body develops certain protective substances which can thereafter repel and prevent a similar infection. The exact mechanism adopted by the body to develop these protective substances will be discussed more fully later. At this stage it is only essential to emphasise that the body does not develop protective substances against all infections, so that it is possible—and indeed frequently happens—for the individual to suffer from repeated attacks of the same disease. One further point must also be stressed at this stage and that is that the efficiency of the development of these protective substances also varies with different infections, so that resistance or immunity to one disease may be complete, while to another it may be only partial.

2. *The individual is exposed to repeated infection in small doses,* so that an actual attack of the disease does not occur.

By repeated stimulation of the body's protective mechanisms by infections too small to cause an actual attack of the disease a

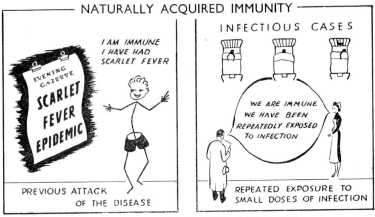

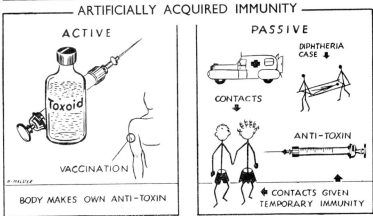

Fig. 13

Types of immunity.

complete development of protective substances can in the course of time occur. These can then resist a *full* dose of infection, which would normally set up an attack of the disease. This method of developing an immunity to a particular disease explains why some people are immune or resistant to a disease without ever having suffered from an actual attack.

3. *Resistance to a Disease is Inherited.*—For example, an infant may be immune for a short period owing to the passage of the mother's protective substances into its circulation by way of the placenta or through the mother's milk.

In addition to the above, there is the natural immunity of animals to such diseases as syphilis and gonorrhœa. Again, certain animals may be immune to a disease whilst others are highly susceptible, *e.g.*, sheep and cattle are very susceptible to the disease anthrax while dogs and rats are practically immune.

(B) Artificially Acquired Immunity (Active and Passive).

Artificial immunity is the result of a deliberate and successful attempt, by one means or another, to make the body develop protective substances against disease. For ease of understanding a short history of how this intentional effort was first thought of and developed may be useful.

Jenner (1798) observed that people who suffered from the mild disease known as cowpox, caught from cattle, rarely suffered from the much more serious and often fatal disease known as smallpox. If they did suffer from smallpox the attack was usually mild. From this he inferred that the cowpox attack developed in some way a resistance or immunity to smallpox in the person concerned. He also believed that probably the organism causing cowpox was almost identical with that causing smallpox, but of a milder nature. Jenner then proceeded to inoculate a boy with cowpox, and after the boy had overcome the disease, tried to infect him with smallpox but without success. This brilliant experiment of Jenner's has laid the whole foundation of vaccination.

The next advance in the creation of an immunity was that due to Pasteur (1885), who discovered that a particular organism could be modified by different methods so that it ceased to cause actual disease but nevertheless did not lose its effect of producing protective substances in the body. Thus infecting an individual with this modified type of organism created an immunity or resistance in the person without causing an attack of the disease. The means Pasteur adopted to modify the virulence or activity of an organism were heating the organism, adding an antiseptic, or passing it through an animal. Passage of an organism through an animal for some reason modifies it so that it is no longer capable of setting up active disease in man but can still create an immunity to infection by **active organisms**. The term *vaccine* is given to a suspension of modified avirulent organisms, and the procedure of inoculating is spoken of as vaccination or immunisation.

Instead of using modified avirulent organisms the toxins produced by organisms, suitably modified, may be used as an alternative in order to create an immunity. Modified toxin as used in immunisation is known as *toxoid*.

In addition to the above-mentioned type of artificial immunity, which is called **active immunity**, there is still a further form, known as passive immunity. Passive immunity will be discussed later.

Changes in the Body producing Immunity.—It is as well for the nurse to have some knowledge of the way in which the body reacts to produce the protective substances which set up immunity or resistance.

1. Most organisms, though not all, when they get into the body stimulate certain tissues and cells to produce substances which will act on the toxic invading organisms and destroy them. These substances are called **antibodies** and **antitoxins**. The organisms are said to act as *antigens* to produce antibodies.

2. The antibodies and antitoxins produced, *e.g.*, against the diphtheria organism, will have effect *only* against this organism and will have no effect against any other organism.

3. The antibodies produced vary in how long they last. Some last for many years, others only for a few weeks or months.

4. Antibodies and antitoxins are produced in a special group of cells, scattered throughout the body but particularly numerous in the spleen, lymphoid tissue and liver. (In the liver they are often called Kupffer cells to distinguish them from the ordinary hepatic or liver cells.) This special system of cells is known as the reticulo-endothelial system, and plays a very important role in the body's defensive mechanism against disease.

Clinical Use of Vaccination (Immunisation) and Serum Treatment.

Vaccination, to produce immunity to a disease, is a well recognised and frequently adopted measure to prevent certain diseases. As mentioned in the discussion on artificial immunity, however, not all organisms produce lasting antibodies in the body and so lasting immunity to the disease. Again, the antibody formation, and consequently the immunity, may be incomplete and therefore insufficient to prevent an actual attack of the disease although the disease may be made milder. For these reasons vaccination is of use only in certain diseases and not in all types of infection.

The type of immunity described so far is known as an active

immunity, because it depends on the activity of the vaccinated person's *own* tissues and cells in producing the antibodies and antitoxins necessary to form an immunity.

The individual who has acquired an active immunity, either artificial or natural (by having had an actual attack of the disease, etc.), has circulating in his blood the specific antibodies and antitoxins necessary to attack the organisms if infection should take place. If some serum from this person is withdrawn and inoculated into a second person who is not immune to the particular organism, then this person also becomes immune to the infecting organism, but only for a short period of a few weeks. This type of immunity is spoken of as a **passive immunity**—passive because it does not require the person's own tissues or cells to manufacture the antibodies or antitoxins. Serum containing the appropriate antitoxin or antibodies is often given to contacts of a case of infectious disease to prevent them from developing the disease. Giving antitoxic serum creates a temporary passive immunity in the contacts.

It will be realised that this blood (serum is generally used as it is more convenient to give than whole blood, and contains all the necessary antibodies and antitoxins), because it contains antibodies and antitoxins, might also be of use in treatment where actual disease has already occurred. Giving serum immediately supplies substances to act against the toxins of the invading organisms. This is known as *serum* or *antitoxin therapy*.

Serum or antitoxin therapy is, however, of value only in those cases where a potent active serum can be prepared, and for the reasons given when discussing the creation of an active immunity by vaccination, not all organisms produce in the body a potent antitoxin.

Diseases in which Preventive Vaccination (Immunisation) is of Value.

1. Smallpox.
2. Diphtheria.
3. Tuberculosis.
4. Typhoid.
5. Tetanus.
6. Whooping-cough.
7. Poliomyelitis.

The individual methods and the value of immunisation in each case will be discussed later in dealing with the individual diseases.

Diseases in which Serum or Antitoxin is used in Treatment.

1. Diphtheria.
2. Tetanus.
3. Measles.
4. Scarlet fever.

Potent serum or antitoxin is at present of value only in the above diseases. In practice the serum or antitoxin is usually manufactured by inoculating a suitable animal, such as a horse, with a vaccine, so as to stimulate the production of antibodies and antitoxins and thus create an active immunity in the horse's blood. The horse is then bled and the serum withdrawn and suitably sterilised for use in treatment. Measles serum is not produced in this way but taken from patients convalescing from the disease.

ANAPHYLAXIS, SERUM SICKNESS, HYPERSENSITIVENESS AND ALLERGY

All the above conditions are in some way allied to each other and the terms are often used in different senses by different people. This is especially so with the term *allergy*. To explain the above conditions, which are rather difficult to understand, it is best to describe how they are seen in clinical practice.

1. Anaphylaxis.

In some people who have been given an injection of serum a second injection, if it is given more than ten to fourteen days after the first, may be followed by a very severe and often fatal reaction known as anaphylaxis. The essential features of the reaction are a spasm of smooth muscle and a dilatation of small capillaries. This leads to collapse, extreme difficulty in breathing, convulsions and, in some cases, death. These effects are supposed to be due to the action of a foreign protein in the first serum injection which produces an excess of sensitive antibodies which, on the second serum injection, cause this violent reaction. If the second injection is given before ten days have elapsed, the anaphylactic reaction does not for some reason develop.

Anaphylaxis is very rare and in the treatment the immediate injection of adrenaline, 5 to 10 minims, is of great value. When injecting serum of any kind, adrenaline should always be readily available.

2. Serum Sickness.

About seven to fourteen days after an injection of serum (especially of large amounts) the person may develop an urticarial reaction in the skin, joint pains, fever and enlarged glands. These symptoms occur after the first injection of serum. As in anaphylaxis, they are due to a sensitisation of the body against a foreign protein in the serum. Serum sickness, however, unlike anaphylaxis, is never fatal.

The antihistamine drugs (phenergan, benadryl, etc.) will often relieve symptoms, and adrenaline is also helpful by injection. Should these measures fail, cortisone or its allies are usually prescribed.

3. Hypersensitiveness.

Anaphylaxis and serum sickness, just discussed, are of the nature of hypersensitive reactions, but these terms are usually reserved for sensitiveness following serum injections only. Many individuals, however, are sensitive to a great many different foreign proteins present in foods, dust, flowers, drugs, etc. When they come in contact with the offending substances by eating, inhaling or touching them, they develop certain characteristic reactions such as :—

(a) Laboured wheezing breathing (asthma).

(b) Wheals, like bites on the skin (urticaria).

(c) Vomiting and diarrhœa.

(d) Severe running from the nose and eyes (similar to hay fever).

(e) Fever.

These individuals are said to have an idiosyncrasy to the offending substance or to be " allergic." Certain diseases such as asthma, urticaria, hay fever and eczema are often due to a sensitiveness to a food, plant, or drug, etc., and are therefore called allergic diseases.

SUMMARY

1. Diseases are caused by many different agents ; especially important are :—

    (a) Infections with bacteria, viruses and parasites.

    (b) Lack of vitamins or proper food leading to deficiency diseases.

    (c) Alteration in the hormones of the ductless glands.

    (d) There remains a large group where the exact cause is as yet unknown, including the cause of carcinoma.

2. Most of these agents set up disease by causing changes in the tissues and organs and thereby interfering with their normal functions. These changes are usually referred to as pathological lesions. Pathology is the study of these lesions.

3. Some of these lesions are common to many different diseases and so are particularly important. They include :—

    (a) Inflammation—acute and chronic.

    (b) Lesions in the vessels—arteries and veins—

        (i) Thrombosis (clotting in a vessel).

        (ii) Embolism (detachment of a clot and its lodging in some other part of the circulation, thus cutting off the blood supply to an organ or tissue).

        (iii) Hæmorrhage (loss of blood from the body or rupture of blood into an organ or tissue).

        (iv) Gangrene (death or necrosis of tissue due to lack of blood supply).

(c) Degeneration or toxic changes—
Poisoning of tissue cells, often with death of cells, owing to toxic (poisonous) substances in the body.

4. In view of the frequency with which bacteria, viruses and parasites cause important diseases in man, a special study of these organisms, or microbes, is made under the term " bacteriology." Bacteria are divided into many different types including cocci, bacilli and spirochætes. The materials needed (specimens) to isolate the organism from the body are commonly throat swabs, sputum, fæces, urine, pus, fluids from serous cavities or a sample of blood itself. The material is examined by special methods in the laboratory (stains, cultures) to identify the organism.

5. Bacteria, viruses, etc., may enter the body through the respiratory tract, alimentary system, skin or genitals to set up disease. To do so they must be of sufficient strength or virulence and in sufficient numbers, otherwise the protective mechanisms of the body quickly destroy them.

In some cases, however, even if the organism enters the body in sufficient numbers and strength, actual disease may not occur because the individual is not susceptible. In these cases the person is said to be immune. Immunity to disease can occur owing to previous infection having produced protective substances in the body so that it can resist further attacks. These protective substances are called antibodies and antitoxins. Not all organisms causing disease produce antibodies or antitoxins of any permanence in the body. As a result such organisms can cause repeated attacks of disease in the same person, e.g., the common cold virus.

6. Immunity from certain diseases can be deliberately created in a person by inoculating him with small doses of killed bacteria or their toxins. This preventive inoculation or vaccination (a vaccine is a suspension of killed bacteria) against disease is widely used in medicine with great success (e.g., vaccination against smallpox, inoculation against diphtheria).

7. If an actual attack of certain infectious diseases occurs, antitoxin, specially prepared, can be used to help overcome the infection by its neutralising action on the toxins produced by the bacteria, especially those causing diphtheria and tetanus. Treatment with antitoxin is often known as serum treatment, as antitoxin is present in serum.

8. In some people, injection of serum produces severe symptoms owing to the reaction of the body against the presence of some foreign protein in the serum. Anaphylaxis is a very severe, often fatal, reaction which occurs in rare instances after a second injection of serum. Serum sickness is a less severe reaction, occurring seven to fourteen days after one or more injections of serum.

9. Certain people are sensitive and react to foreign proteins in foods, dust, plants or drugs. These people are said to be allergic to the offending substance. The reactions may take various forms, e.g., a spasm of the smooth muscles of the bronchioles in the lungs (asthma), œdema and inflammation of the skin (urticaria) and œdema of the mucous membranes of the eyes and nose (hay fever).

In all these sensitive and allergic reactions, injections of adrenaline are of the greatest value. The antihistamine group of drugs and cortisone are also helpful.

CHAPTER II

ACUTE INFECTIOUS FEVERS

VERY many of the diseases met with in medicine are acute, infectious to some degree, and accompanied by a rise in temperature (fever). For the sake of convenience many of these diseases are dealt with as diseases of the system in which the predominant signs develop (*e.g.*, pneumonia, an acute infection, is always classified as a respiratory disease because the signs are mainly in the lungs).

The term *acute infectious fever* is therefore usually reserved for those infections which tend to display the following characteristics :—

1. The disease is acute with fever.
2. Is caused by a specific bacterium or virus.
3. It tends to run a definite course and often occurs in epidemic form.
4. It is very infectious.
5. In many cases one attack confers immunity from second attacks. (Common important exceptions to this do occur, however.)

Certain terms are frequently used in discussing the infectious fevers and are best explained at the outset.

1. *Epidemic.*—When a large number of cases occur at the same time, to be followed by a period in which few or no cases occur.

2. *Endemic.*—Where the disease occurs at any time.

3. *Sporadic.*—Where scattered cases only of the disease arise.

4. *Pandemic.*—Where there is a world-wide distribution of the disease.

5. *Isolation and Period of Isolation.*—Most cases of infectious disease are isolated to prevent the disease spreading to other people. The period of isolation required varies with the different diseases, but in any case generally lasts until the patient no longer harbours the infecting organisms. With some people, however, the organisms may persist indefinitely, even when they themselves have fully recovered from the illness. Such people are called *carriers*, because they carry virulent organisms capable of spreading disease to others.

It should further be noted that these people can also carry virulent organisms without themselves ever having had an actual attack of the disease. This is because they have a natural resistance or immunity to the disease.

6. *Incubation Period.*—The incubation period is the length of time which elapses between the patient's becoming infected and the appearance of the first symptoms. The incubation period varies with the different diseases.

7. *Quarantine.*—Quarantine is the restriction of the activities of people who have been in contact with a case of infectious disease until such time as it is known whether they have acquired the disease or not. The period of quarantine is just longer than the incubation period. In practice, strict quarantine of contacts is not usually enforced except in cases of such serious infectious diseases as small-pox or typhus. Known contacts of most other infectious diseases are nowadays simply kept under medical observation so that they can be isolated as soon as any symptoms develop. Strict quarantine of all known contacts involves too much disruption of everyday life, and in most cases close observation, with prompt isolation if necessary, is just as effective in controlling the incidence of infectious diseases.

8. *Notifiable Diseases.*—Certain diseases, usually the infectious diseases, have to be notified to the public health authorities. This is to enable the authorities to take all necessary measures to prevent spread of the disease. Some diseases are notifiable only at certain times, *e.g.*, when they are especially prevalent or there is a large epidemic of the disease.

GENERAL SYMPTOMS AND SIGNS OF FEVER

With all acute feverish illnesses there is of course some fever, although the degree varies considerably. Fever, whatever its cause, is usually accompanied by certain symptoms and signs, and it is therefore convenient, before describing the individual infectious fevers, to consider what may be termed the general symptoms and signs of a fever.

1. Fever or Pyrexia.

(*a*) DEFINITION.—Fever or pyrexia is present when the body temperature is raised above the normal. In health the body temperature remains very constant around 98·4° F., although a slight swing of 0·5° F. above or below this figure may be normal in some people. The temperature taken in the mouth is usually half a degree higher than that taken in the axilla or groin, while the rectal temperature is usually one degree higher than the axillary temperature.

The temperature of the body is the balance between heat production by means of the general metabolism of the various bodily functions and heat loss through the skin, lungs and excretions. The heat regulating centre in the brain is responsible for the constant level of the body temperature in health.

In infection, fever is one of the most constant and reliable signs. It is probably caused by the toxic products produced by the infecting organism.

(b) GRADES OF FEVER.—According to the height of the fever, various grades are often spoken of, such as slight or moderate for 99° to 101° F. and severe for any fever between 102° and 104° F. A temperature of 105° F. or over is known as a hyperpyrexia.

(c) TYPES OF FEVER.

>   (i) *Continuous Fever.*—The temperature remains continuously above the normal.
>   (ii) *Remittent Fever.*—Considerable fluctuations occur, but the temperature is at all times above the normal.
>   (iii) *Intermittent Fever.* — Temperature fluctuates from normal to above normal from time to time.

The type of fever is sometimes of value in diagnosis, as some diseases tend to cause a specific type of fever.

(d) TERMINATION OF FEVER.

>   (i) *Crisis.*—This is a sudden abrupt termination of the fever accompanied by a marked improvement in the patient's condition.
>   (ii) *Lysis.*—Here the fever gradually subsides over a matter of days.

Some diseases generally terminate with a crisis (*e.g.*, lobar pneumonia), others with lysis. Nowadays the importance of crisis and lysis as clinical signs is much less because the whole course of so many acute infections with fever has been altered by the use of antibiotic drugs.

(e) FEVER IN THE YOUNG AND OLD.—Any rise in temperature in an infant or young child is likely to be much higher than would be the case in an adult. Children often have very high temperatures—102° to 104° F.—from trivial infections. In contrast, elderly people may have a fairly severe infection without much rise in temperature.

The presence of fever is so important and constant a finding in nearly all infections and many other diseases that the temperature is always taken in any patient no matter what the cause of the disease. Similarly the pulse is always taken and the urine examined.

2. Feeling of being off colour or general malaise.

3. Headache and vague pains in the muscles of the limbs and back.

4. Restlessness.

5. Diminution or loss of appetite, often with nausea (inclination to vomit).

6. Shivering feeling; in severe cases, rigors (see below).

7. The skin may be cold to the touch in the earliest stages, but later usually becomes hot and dry. As the fever progresses, sweating may be profuse.

8. The tongue is usually dry and furred.

9. The pulse rate is in most cases above the normal rate of seventy-two beats a minute. There are, however, a few exceptions to this normal rise in the pulse rate in fevers, notably in typhoid fever.

10. The respirations are usually slightly faster than the normal rate of eighteen a minute.

11. The output of urine is diminished, and as a result the urine passed is dark and concentrated. As sweating is usually present with a consequent loss of fluid, the diminished urinary output is a compensatory measure to conserve fluid in the body.

12. Constipation.

The above symptoms and signs are almost always present to some extent in most cases of fever. In very severe infections, however, other more serious symptoms may also develop.

13. **Rigors.**—A rigor is a severe shivering attack which is usually accompanied by a rise in temperature. Rigors are a characteristic feature of some diseases, *e.g.*, septicæmia, severe sepsis, pyelitis, lobar pneumonia and malaria. Recurrent rigors every day or on alternate days are a particular feature of malaria.

Rigors do not occur in infants or young children in whom convulsions or fits are the equivalent.

14. **Delirium.**—Delirium is the presence of mental confusion resulting in incoherence in speech and thought. Hallucinations

(*e.g.*, seeing imaginary objects), often of a terrifying nature, may also be present. Delirium is supposed to be caused by the severe toxæmia affecting the higher cerebral centres. As delirium is thus evidence of a very severe toxic state, it tends to occur only in the most severe infections, particularly typhoid fever, smallpox, septicæmia and meningitis.

Delirium accompanying a fever is usually spoken of as a *febrile* delirium to distinguish it from delirium due to other causes (non-febrile). Delirium not associated with fever is a feature of such conditions as mental diseases, brain tumours, uræmia (renal failure), chronic alcoholism, etc. Poisoning with such drugs as belladonna and hyoscine also causes a marked delirium.

Lastly, delirium, either febrile or non-febrile, is usually more frequent and pronounced in elderly people.

15. **The Typhoid State.**—The typhoid state is a condition of extreme prostration, often with semi-consciousness and delirium, which may arise in any toxæmia of sufficient gravity. The typhoid state was first characteristically described in typhoid fever and so given its name, but it is seen in severe toxæmia apart from that due to typhoid fever.

Features.

    (*a*) Severe prostration.
    (*b*) Sordes (dry sores) around the mouth.
    (*c*) Semi-consciousness ; in some cases coma.
    (*d*) Coma vigil (a peculiar type of coma where the eyes remain open).
    (*e*) Delirium, often described as being of a low muttering type.
    (*f*) Incontinence of both urine and fæces.
    (*g*) Carphologia (ceaseless plucking at the bed-clothes).
    (*h*) Subsultus tendinum or jerking of the tendons on the back of the hands (often a fatal sign).

GENERAL NURSING CARE OF AN ACUTE FEVER

The general nursing details outlined below apply to any acute feverish illness, except that the isolation procedure is necessary only in infectious diseases. These general nursing details will be repeatedly referred to in other chapters when discussing acute diseases associated with fever.

The general management and nursing care of an acute feverish illness can conveniently be described under the following main headings :—

1. Isolation Procedure (necessary only in infectious diseases).
2. Rest.
3. Sleep.
4. Diet.
5. Skin and Pressure Areas.
6. Attention to the Mouth.
7. Incontinence.
8. Constipation.
9. Prevention of Venous Thrombosis.
10. Rigors.
11. Delirium.

1. Isolation Procedure.

The fundamental aim in isolation nursing is to prevent the spread of infection to other individuals, including the nurse herself.

(a) The patient is nursed in a separate isolation cubicle. Alternatively, in some cases of infectious disease in which adequate isolation precautions to prevent spread of the disease can be taken in the general ward, the patient may be *barrier nursed* in a general ward. When *barrier nursing* a patient a corner bed, near a window and as close as possible to the sanitary annex, should be chosen. The whole area inside the screen must be regarded as infected and all records and charts kept outside the isolation area.

Cleaning should be done by means of a vacuum cleaner whenever possible, but when this is not possible *damp* dusting only should be carried out. Damp tea leaves should be spread on the floor and the duster should be moistened with a disinfectant such as lysol. Dry dusting must never be done as it only helps to spread infection.

(b) When attending to the patient the nurse, or any person coming in contact with the patient, must at all times protect her clothes by the use of a gown, which should be placed immediately inside the cubicle doorway. The outside of the gown, which becomes infected, should be clearly distinguishable from the inside, which is not infected. Sufficient gowns should be available for the doctors and nurses.

(c) The nurse must pay particular attention to disinfecting her hands and nails, and scrubbing with a good nailbrush is essential.

Rinsing the hands in a suitable antiseptic is also advisable. The importance of thorough washing of the hands and nails after handling all infectious patients cannot be over-emphasised.

(*d*) Face masks should be worn in certain cases, especially when dealing with infants and puerperal women and when nursing surgical wounds. It is most important that the face mask should be close-fitting and made of fine material, with at least several layers if the masking is to be of any value.

Masks must never be worn around the neck or carried in the pocket.

(*e*) Which secretions and excreta are infectious depends on the individual infectious disease. In all cases where the respiratory system is affected, the saliva and sputum are particularly infectious. Here, therefore, infection is spread by coughing, sneezing and close proximity to the patient in conversation.

Where the infecting organism has affected the intestinal tract (as in enteric fevers and dysenteries) the fæces (urine also in enteric fever) are particularly infectious. The excreta in these cases must be mixed with an equal volume of 1 in 10 lysol for two hours before disposal. Soiled linen should be soaked in 1 in 80 lysol solution for twelve hours before it is sent to the laundry.

(*f*) Separate marked utensils (both feeding and sanitary) must be supplied for the patient's own use. A separate thermometer is also necessary.

(*g*) Suitable swabs of paper or gauze, which can be burnt after use, should be available for any nasal discharge. For infants the napkins should be destructible.

(*h*) For all cases of infectious disease, all utensils and bedding must be thoroughly disinfected before being used for other patients.

(*i*) A suitable notice should be posted outside the isolation cubicle to show that the patient is infectious and so prevent anyone entering unnecessarily.

2. Rest.

(*a*) In all cases except the very mildest the patient must be nursed in bed. Even in the very mildest cases, if isolation is necessary, bed may be the only possible way of ensuring it. A well-ventilated room or cubicle without draughts is essential. Adequate ventilation is important both in reducing the risk of spread of infection and in the comfort of the patient. The temperature of the room is best kept between 60° and 65° F.

(b) The clothes, especially around the neck and sleeves, must not be tight as this makes them difficult to remove, which distresses the patient.

(c) The position the patient is best nursed in depends on the nature of the illness. In any case where the lungs are likely to be affected, then the upright position is advisable. If there is any danger of acute heart damage, then the patient must be nursed at complete rest in the semi-recumbent position. Absolute rest, to ease the strain on the heart, is particularly essential for acute rheumatic fever and diphtheria patients.

Where there is no special reason for the adoption of any specific position, then the wishes and comfort of the patient should be considered. Usually a semi-upright position is most suitable. Elderly patients have a great tendency to slip down in bed and so cause a predisposition to the development of congestion of the lungs. This must be guarded against.

(d) Rest, both physical and mental, is essential for all ill cases; therefore quietness, with as little disturbance to the patient as possible, is necessary. No doubt many treatments in the shape of drugs, injections, aperients, etc., will be ordered by the doctor, but if these entail disturbing the patient every hour or so, then they defeat their own purpose. A complaint voiced by many patients is that they never get any rest owing to the continual washings, swallowing of " thousands " of tablets, and being pin-pricked like a pin-cushion. Although there is obvious exaggeration in these complaints there is no doubt that there is often some justification for them. Treatments, as far as possible, should be dovetailed to allow the maximum amount of rest and quietude to the patient, especially during sleeping hours.

3. Sleep.

Sleeplessness, or insomnia, is frequently present in any acute illness and prevents the patient from getting the rest essential for fighting his illness. The *causes of insomnia* fall under two main heads :—

> (a) Anxiety—or Psychical Causes.
> (b) Physical Causes.

(a) ANXIETY.—Anxiety or worry is a very frequent cause of sleeplessness during illness, and indeed it is only natural that the patient should be worried about himself when he is ill. In addition, a patient who is ill, especially if nursed in hospital in strange and somewhat frightening surroundings, is very inclined to weigh every word from the doctor and the nurse. An anxious look or shake of the head may therefore unwittingly convey to the patient the impression that his " last hours " have arrived. Equally, however, the nurse can, by a cheerful countenance, sympathy and reassurance allay the patient's anxiety and thus ensure mental rest and sleep.

(b) PHYSICAL CAUSES.—In many patients some trivial condition is often sufficient to cause insomnia. A stuffy atmosphere or, on the other hand, a draught may prevent sleep. The patient's bed-clothes may be creased or the position of the pillows uncomfortable. Noise or an unshaded light may also keep the patient awake. It must therefore be ensured that none of these conditions is present to interfere with the patient's sleep.

A raised temperature, which makes the patient hot and clammy, often keeps the patient awake, and tepid sponging and a change of night-clothes are often invaluable in these cases. Alternatively, the patient may feel cold, whereupon an extra blanket or a hot-water bottle will produce the desired effect. A hot drink (milk, Horlicks, Ovaltine, or Benger's) is very soothing and often induces sleep.

If insomnia is still present after all the above measures have been tried, then hypnotic drugs may have to be given under the doctor's instructions. Hypnotics are drugs which produce sleep, but it should be noted that if insomnia is present owing to pain, then analgesic or narcotic drugs may be necessary as the hypnotic drugs do not relieve pain. If a hypnotic is ordered it should be given reasonably early and not after the patient is worn out and tired from lack of sleep.

Pain is a very frequent cause of insomnia, and the general measures for the relief of pain are fully dealt with elsewhere (p. 535). In certain cases such simple measures as local heat (hot-water bottles or poultices) or light massage may be all that is necessary.

If the pain is not relieved by these measures, then an analgesic drug (aspirin, phenacetin, or codeine) may be ordered. In cases of very severe and acute pain narcotic drugs, which produce a deep sleep accompanied by the relief of pain, are necessary. Morphine is a most useful and widely used narcotic.

Many patients have a great fear of taking sleeping drugs in case they become addicted to their use. This anxiety may affect any good the drug may do ; therefore a brief word to the patient—that the use of sleeping drugs is only temporary and that as soon as his illness is over he will not require them—is desirable to relieve his anxiety on this score.

The most useful hypnotics are the barbiturates (medinal, soneryl, amytal), chloral hydrate and bromides, and paraldehyde. For children aspirin and chloral are most useful.

It is most important that hypnotics and especially narcotics (morphine) should be discontinued at the earliest opportunity to prevent drug addiction.

It must be stressed that in most cases of insomnia the general measures outlined above, without the use of drugs, are all that is necessary to promote sleep, and therefore all these general measures must be tried before drugs are given.

In addition to the above physical causes of insomnia, such symptoms as a cough and dyspnœa in diseases of the respiratory and circulatory systems, indigestion and hunger pains in gastro-intestinal diseases and pruritus (itching) in jaundice or skin diseases, may all interfere with sleep. These symptoms must be relieved by the various specific measures given under the individual diseases.

4. Diet.

A suitable diet in acute feverish illnesses is most important. The patients, especially if seriously ill, have little or no appetite, and yet adequate nourishment must be given to supply the bodily needs and replace wear and tear of tissues. In addition, owing to the excessive loss of fluid through sweating, usual in fever, it is also important that sufficient fluid be taken.

In the first few days in a case of severe fever the diet will of necessity consist mainly of fluids and semi-solids. At least 4 to 5 pints of fluid a day should be given. Fruit juices, weak tea and cocoa are all very useful in varying the fluid given. Milk is a most valuable food and easily assimilated. Some patients, however, develop a distaste for milk and it is therefore important to vary pure milk with milk jellies, custards, Bournvita, Horlicks, Ovaltine, or Benger's. Ice cream is usually well tolerated. If curds appear in the stools, or if the patient finds pure milk difficult to digest, citrating the milk (1 grain of sodium citrate to each ounce of milk) is useful.

In addition to fluids and milk, carbohydrate is given in liberal amounts to supply energy for the body. Carbohydrate, moreover, is easily digested and therefore of particular value in any acute illness. The carbohydrate can be given as glucose, ordinary cane sugar, syrup, honey, boiled sweets or chocolate.

Eggs are most useful as they are usually well tolerated and supply protein and fat.

As soon as possible, further additions must be made to the diet so as to maintain adequate nutrition. White fish, puréed vegetables and fruits, and white meat are usually fairly well tolerated after the initial acute stage. Particularly in a long illness, proteins must not be withheld for too long as they are essential for replacing the wear and tear of tissues.

It will be seen from the above that the type of food given is very important. So also are two other considerations. Firstly, too large an amount, even of a suitable type of food, is harmful as it overloads a digestion which cannot cope with it. Too large meals can therefore cause flatulence, epigastric pain and abdominal distension, which may give rise to respiratory and cardiac embarrassment. Frequent small feeds are the solution to this problem, as long as it is remembered that too frequent disturbance of the patient interferes with his rest and sleep. Within limits the patient's own appetite is a good guide to the amount of food required.

Secondly, it is essential that the food should be served in an attractive manner. Frequently good food is wasted because it is unappetisingly served. Care should therefore be taken to ensure that the food is attractive to the eye and palate as this will help the patient to take and digest sufficient nourishment.

Finally, in certain illnesses specific diets are laid down as a special item of treatment. Where these special items are necessary they will be discussed under the individual diseases.

5. Skin and Pressure Areas.

(a) In cases of high fever there is usually severe sweating which necessitates frequent changes of clothes. Again, sweating is very distressing to a patient, leading to restlessness and insomnia. As already stated, in these circumstances a tepid sponging with water at 70° to 80° F. is extremely comforting and conducive to sleep. Tepid sponging to reduce the temperature is essential in all cases of hyperpyrexia (temperatures over 105° F.).

(b) Pressure areas will require particular attention in all patients needing prolonged confinement in bed, and especially with elderly people, who are very prone to develop pressure sores. Frequent changes of position are most important. The importance of frequent changes of position to avoid pressure sores cannot be over-emphasised. Avoiding creases in the sheets and the provision of a comfortable mattress (rubber mattresses are very useful) are essential details. The presence of any paralysis or incontinence calls for extra care and attention if pressure sores are to be prevented.

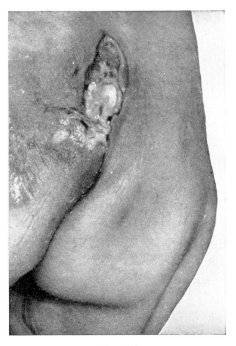

FIG. 14
Pressure sore.

6. Attention to the Mouth.

With fever of any degree the mouth is usually dry and very liable to become infected, with the result that inflammation may occur (stomatitis). Careful routine cleansing of the mouth should therefore be done at specific times during the day. Swabbing with some suitable solution is best, but this must be done gently as too vigorous swabbing will only do more damage. Suitable solutions for cleansing the mouth are soda bicarbonate (1 drachm to 1 pint of water), dilute lemon juice or glycothymoline.

Making sure that the patient is drinking an adequate amount of fluid is one essential way of ensuring a clean mouth.

7. Incontinence.

Incontinence of urine and fæces is often present in a severely ill patient, particularly if the patient is elderly. Incontinence as already stressed calls for special care in treating the skin, as pressure sores are very likely to develop. Again, incontinence of urine may also be caused by an overflow resulting from retention of urine, so a careful watch must be kept on the bladder to see that it is not distended. A distended bladder can be felt as a tender round swelling above the pubes. In these cases catheterisation with full aseptic technique will be necessary.

8. Constipation.

Constipation is a feature of most acute feverish illnesses with a few notable exceptions. As constipation may cause abdominal distension, with resultant discomfort to the patient, it must be treated and prevented if possible. Purgatives are drugs which cause bowel evacuation, and are ordered at the discretion of the doctor. Senokot and cascara are useful mild purgatives, whilst in some cases an enema may be ordered to relieve the constipation. It should be realised, however, that if a patient is on a fluid diet only it is not essential for the bowels to be opened every day. Excessive purgation in these cases can only be distressing to the patient.

Some patients are very prone to constipation and a few inquiries put to the patient at the onset of the illness may save a good deal of trouble later on. In these cases the nurse should find out from the patient what, if any, purgative he is in the habit of taking and should give this purgative, subject to the doctor's agreement.

9. Prevention of Venous Thrombosis.

In all cases of severe illness which necessitate prolonged confinement to bed, thrombosis in the deep veins, especially of the legs and pelvis, is always a danger. The important factors which predispose to deep venous thrombosis are sluggish circulation and trauma. (Severely ill patients, particularly elderly patients, tend to remain " fixed " in one position, which tends to lead to sluggishness of the circulation.) Deep venous thrombosis is also particularly liable to arise after operations.

The great danger of deep venous thrombosis is that the clot may break off, travel to the lungs, and thus cause pulmonary embolism which may prove fatal.

To prevent thrombosis, particular care must be taken that the patient's limbs are often moved, both passive and active movements of the limbs being necessary at intervals. Furthermore, the frequent movements of the limbs help to prevent the joints becoming fixed, a development which is very prone to occur with prolonged recumbency, especially with elderly patients.

10. Rigors.

The patient must be kept warm and adequately covered. Hot-water bottles may be required, especially at the onset before sweating

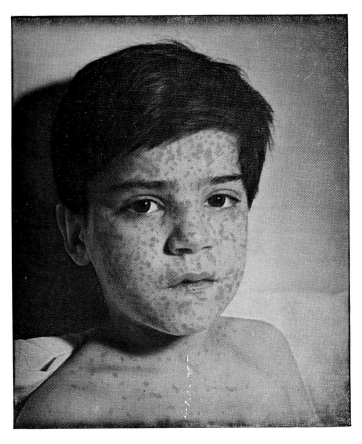

FIG. 15
Measles.

[*To face page* 47

starts. Great care must be taken, however, in the use of hot-water bottles especially with seriously ill and restless patients as they can easily burn themselves. When the patient is perspiring, tepid sponging will be necessary. A rigor in the course of an illness is most frightening to the patient, who should be told that there is nothing to be alarmed about and that the attack will soon pass.

Sedatives, such as chloral and bromides, may be ordered by the doctor.

11. Delirium.

Constant and skilled attention is necessary in all delirious cases. These patients are usually extremely restless and often try to get out of bed, which in their sick state may have serious effects. The nurse must try to restrain the patient from injuring himself, using the minimum of force, and relying as much as possible on persuasion and tact. In febrile delirium, cold compresses to the head are often useful and soothing. Bed-boards suitably padded to prevent injury may be necessary. In most cases sedatives will be required, and chloral, bromides or paraldehyde are often prescribed. In severe cases it may be necessary to give hyoscine or morphine by injection.

In all cases of delirium all the nurse's skill will be required to ensure that adequate fluids are taken. Elderly patients, who are particularly liable to become delirious when seriously ill, require special care over this question of fluid intake.

MEASLES

Cause.—Virus infection.

Spread.—Spread is by direct contact through droplet infection from sneezing or coughing. It is very contagious, especially in the catarrhal stage before the rash appears.

Incubation Period.—Ten to fourteen days.

Incidence.—The maximum incidence of the disease is between the ages of 8 months and 5 years. Attacks are commonest in winter and spring when widespread epidemics may occur.

Symptoms and Signs.

1. The onset is usually abrupt with the following catarrhal symptoms predominant :—

(*a*) Coryza.
(*b*) Conjunctivitis.
(*c*) Photophobia.
(*d*) Bronchitis.

With these symptoms the child gives a picture of running eyes and nose, coughing and sneezing. In some cases a laryngitis with hoarseness is present.

2. At this stage, before the rash appears, many cases will show the typical *Koplik's spots*. These are small white spots on the mucous membrane of the mouth beside the molar teeth. They often disappear when the rash comes out. Koplik's spots are seen only in measles.

3. The temperature rises on the first day, often to 100° to 103° F. It usually falls slightly on the third day, to rise again on the fourth day with the onset of the rash.

4. The rash appears first on the forehead and behind the ears, and soon spreads all over the face and body. The rash is a dusky red macular eruption which gives a bloated, swollen appearance to the face.

5. The rash gradually fades and is gone in a week whilst the temperature falls slowly. The infection varies in severity from mild to seriously ill cases.

Complications.

1. Broncho-pneumonia is the most important complication of measles and is responsible for most of the deaths. It is especially frequent in young children.

2. Acute gastro-enteritis. This is particularly liable to arise in infants and children under 2 years of age.

3. Conjunctivitis, blepharitis and corneal ulceration.

4. Otitis media and mastoiditis.

5. Stomatitis.

6. Inflammation of the brain and spinal cord (encephalomyelitis) is a rare complication of measles, as it is of many of the other infectious fevers.

Treatment.—The patient is nursed in strict isolation in a well-ventilated room. The usual nursing care as outlined in the general treatment of any fever case with regard to diet, bowels, sleep, etc., is given.

In view of the danger of conjunctivitis, corneal ulceration and stomatitis, particular attention should be paid to the eyes and mouth. If the eyes are discharging they should be bathed in warm water. Direct sunlight on the eyes should be avoided.

A careful watch must be kept on the respiration as any undue rise probably means the onset of the serious complication of broncho-pneumonia. Sulphonamides, penicillin or other antibiotics will be given if there is any suspicion of pneumonia or other bacterial complication.

Pain in the ear, discharge from the ear or swelling behind the ear will denote an otitis media or mastoiditis, and one of the antibiotic drugs will be given to clear up the inflammation. In those cases which do not rapidly clear up, incising the drum of the ear (*myringotomy*) to provide proper drainage may be necessary.

The patient is kept in bed until the temperature has been normal for several days at least and until all signs in the chest have gone. This may take several weeks in moderately severe cases.

All the clothes, linen, utensils, etc., are disinfected at the end of the illness as with any infectious case.

Preventive Treatment—Immunisation.

1. ACTIVE.—There is at present no way of conferring an active immunity to measles by artificial means.

2. PASSIVE.—A passive immunity to measles can be given by the injection of gamma globulin. Gamma globulin forms part of the proteins in serum and it has been found that the globulin fraction of the serum protein contains most of the antibodies against the measles virus.

If gamma globulin serum is given to contacts within five days of exposure to infection, an attack of measles can be completely prevented. If the gamma globulin is given between six and nine days after exposure, a modified mild attack of measles develops. In practice, full protection is usually given to infants under 2 years, where the danger of broncho-pneumonia and gastro-enteritis is greatest. Above the age of 2, unless the child is already ill with another disease, full immunisation is not usually carried out.

RUBELLA (German Measles)

Cause.—Virus infection.

Spread.—By direct contact and droplet infection on coughing, sneezing, etc.

Incubation Period.—Fourteen to nineteen days.

Incidence.—Adults as well as children are affected. The disease is most prevalent in spring and early summer.

Symptoms and Signs.

1. The onset is less acute than in measles and the patient is far

less ill. There are the general symptoms of a mild infection, namely, malaise, headache, nasal catarrh and a slight temperature.

2. The rash appears on the first day of the illness. It begins on the face and spreads to the trunk and limbs. It is a discrete, pink, papular eruption, not usually as confluent and widespread as in measles. Koplik's spots do not occur.

3. The occipital and cervical lymph glands are characteristically enlarged.

Course and Complications.—The whole illness is usually mild and complications are very rare. If, however, rubella occurs in the first three months of pregnancy, in a certain number of cases it causes congenital deformities in the fœtus, especially congenital heart disease.

Treatment.—Isolation is necessary (five to six days being sufficient) with the usual treatment for a mild fever case.

DIPHTHERIA

Cause.—Infection with the diphtheria bacillus, of which there are several strains, the gravis strain being the most severe.

Spread.—Mainly by droplet infection. Indirect spread (*e.g.,* from sucking infected pencils) also often occurs.

Incubation Period.—Short, two to four days.

Incidence.—Children are chiefly affected, although diphtheria may also be seen in adults, especially during epidemics. Winter is the most usual season for diphtheria.

Pathology.—The illness takes the form of a typical local lesion with a severe general toxæmia.

1. THE LOCAL LESION.—This is a membranous exudate which usually occurs in the throat, causing faucial diphtheria. Less often it is situated either in the nose (causing nasal diphtheria) or in the larynx (causing laryngeal diphtheria). Combined lesions may occur. In rarer cases, skin diphtheria may be present.

2. GENERAL TOXÆMIA.—The organisms remain in the membrane, but they produce a very powerful toxin which causes a general toxæmia.

The toxin particularly attacks (*a*) the heart muscle (myocardium), causing an acute myocarditis; (*b*) the nervous system, causing various forms of paralysis.

Common Types of Diphtheria :—

    (A) Faucial.   (B) Nasal.   (C) Laryngeal.

A. FAUCIAL DIPHTHERIA

As this is the commonest and severest type of diphtheria, it will be described first.

Symptoms and Signs.

1. The onset is insidious, the child looking pale and being off colour. The fever is usually only mild.

2. The patient generally complains of a sore throat, but in young children this symptom may be slight or even absent.

3. The pulse is rapid, much more so than one would expect from the mild degree of fever.

4. When the throat is examined a characteristic musty smell from the breath is noticed. The tonsils are covered with a greyish-white membrane which is hard to remove. In severe cases this membrane spreads on to the soft palate and pharynx. The extent and rapidity of spread of the membrane are a measure of the severity of the attack.

5. The tonsillar glands are nearly always enlarged and in severe cases the swelling in the neck may be so marked as to give rise to the " bull-neck " of diphtheria.

Diagnosis.—Culturing a throat swab in the laboratory will reveal the diphtheritic organism, but this takes time—at least twenty-four hours. Therefore, because delay in treatment is serious, the diagnosis is in every case made on the clinical signs. The slightest suspicion of the disease justifies treating the case as one of diphtheria.

Differential Diagnosis.—This is mainly to distinguish diphtheria from other causes of sore throat such as :—

1. ACUTE STREPTOCOCCAL TONSILLITIS.—Here the throat is much more painful and the temperature is higher. The exudate on the throat is usually patchy and does not take the form of an adherent membrane.

2. VINCENT'S ANGINA.—This causes a greyish ulceration of the throat, but the general signs of toxæmia are absent.

Complications of Diphtheria.

1. ACUTE MYOCARDITIS AND HEART FAILURE.—This is the commonest cause of death in diphtheria. Vomiting is one of the earliest signs of heart involvement and the onset of vomiting is therefore always a grave sign. The pulse usually becomes rapid, soft and often irregular. In some cases, however, the pulse may be slow and irregular owing to heart block.

With acute myocarditis the patient becomes restless, there is often a cyanotic tinge to the lips, and dyspnœa is also present. Examination of the urine is important and usually shows albuminuria and oliguria.

2. DIPHTHERITIC PARALYSES.—Various forms of paralysis occur in diphtheria as a result of the toxins damaging the nervous system.

(a) Paralysis of the soft palate. This usually develops in the second or third week and causes a " nasal " voice and regurgitation of food through the nose.

(b) Paralysis of the eye muscles. The patient cannot read as the eye does not focus on the print owing to paralysis of the accommodation muscles of the eye.

(c) Paralysis of the heart, pharynx and diaphragm. These forms of paralysis are very serious as they may cause death through heart or respiratory failure. The paralyses develop late in the disease—about the seventh week. Dyspnœa and difficulty in swallowing owing to the accumulation of mucus in the throat are the predominant signs.

(d) Peripheral neuritis. This type of paralysis is usually seen very late in the disease—after the seventh week.

Treatment of Faucial Diphtheria.

1. NURSING.

(a) The nursing of a diphtheria patient is most important and may mean the difference between recovery and death. The patient is nursed in strict isolation with all the usual precautions, as previously outlined.

(b) The patient is nursed at complete rest. Everything must be done for the patient, who must be fed, washed and carefully lifted on and off the bed-pan. The nursing measures for a patient with diphtheria are similar to those in acute rheumatic fever because in both illnesses an acute myocarditis is liable to develop.

(c) A careful watch on the pulse is necessary. Particular note must be taken of any undue rise or fall in the rate, or of any irregularity in the rhythm. Such findings must be immediately reported to the doctor, as these findings (especially if accompanied by vomiting) denote acute heart damage.

(d) In addition to paying particular attention to the pulse, similar close attention must be given to the respirations, and any difficulty in respiratory movement, especially if cyanosis is present, must be immediately notified to the doctor.

(e) A careful watch is kept on the output of urine as a fall in output may denote heart failure. A heavy deposit of albuminuria is also important.

(f) The diet should be soft and bland, and glucose is given in liberal amounts. If constipation develops, enemas are given instead of purgatives as they cause less strain.

2. MEDICAL TREATMENT.

(a) A throat swab is taken at the outset and sent to the laboratory for isolation of the organism. Anti-diphtheritic serum is, however, given as soon as the diagnosis is made on *clinical grounds* without waiting for the result of the swab. Any delay in giving serum may affect the prospects of recovery.

(b) Serum is given intramuscularly or, in very severe cases, intravenously. The dose depends on the severity of the illness, the average dose being about 24,000 units. In very severe toxic cases doses as large as 50,000 to 100,000 units, given intravenously, are needed. A small dose given early is more effective than a very big dose later.

(c) Paralysis of the pharyngeal muscles, as revealed by difficulty in swallowing, is treated by raising the foot of the bed in order to allow the excessive mucus, which quickly collects in the throat, to drain away. The excessive secretions will need to be continually cleared by a suction machine or by swabbing. The difficulty of feeding these patients has to be met by a nasal tube.

(d) Respiratory paralysis requires the use of a special respirator.

Course.—The course of the disease varies according to the severity and also according to whether or not cardiac damage or paralysis is present. Strict bed rest is usually continued for several weeks even in moderate attacks. After three to four weeks the patient is usually allowed to sit up in bed and feed himself. A continuing watch must, however, be kept on the pulse to see that there is no rise in the rate or any irregularity of rhythm. Convalescence must be prolonged especially in severe attacks.

B. NASAL DIPHTHERIA

This is the mildest form of diphtheria and there are usually few signs of toxæmia.

Symptoms and Signs.—The principal sign in nasal diphtheria is a nasal discharge which is serous and often bloodstained. Excoriation of the nose and upper lip may occur. The membrane may be visible when the nose is examined and a nasal swab will reveal the organism.

Treatment.—Nasal diphtheria rapidly responds to a small dose of diphtheria antitoxin, 8,000 to 16,000 units being sufficient, as the condition is mild with little toxæmia. The patient is usually allowed up after a few weeks.

C. LARYNGEAL DIPHTHERIA

This type of diphtheria is not so common as the faucial type but may occur with it or, less often, by itself. It is much less toxic than faucial diphtheria. The real danger of this variety is its liability to cause laryngeal obstruction. The membrane forms on the vocal cords and, if it grows sufficiently large, can block the laryngeal airway. Laryngeal diphtheria is seen most commonly in children up to the age of 5 years.

Symptoms and Signs.

1. Hoarseness with a croupy cough.

2. If the membrane causes obstruction, the breathing becomes laboured and *stridor* develops. At first the dyspnœa occurs in spasms, with relatively quiet breathing between the attacks.

3. In many cases, however, the stridor and laboured breathing become continuous. This is associated with cyanosis and restlessness, and the child gasps for breath. Recession, or a falling in of the lower ribs, develops. At this stage, if the obstruction is not relieved, the child dies of heart failure and exhaustion.

4. If faucial diphtheria is also present the child is extremely toxic and the whole outlook is very grave indeed.

Diagnosis.—The primary object is to distinguish laryngeal diphtheria from other causes of acute laryngitis or laryngeal obstruction occurring in children.

(*a*) ACUTE LARYNGITIS IN MEASLES.—Here the hoarseness is associated with the typical catarrhal signs of running eyes and nose, whilst, in addition, Koplik's spots may be present. When the rash appears the condition is obvious.

(*b*) ACUTE LARYNGO-TRACHEO-BRONCHITIS (CROUP).—This condition is becoming increasingly common and is probably caused by a virus, although superadded bacterial infection soon arises. The hoarse, croupy cough is accompanied by severe toxæmia. Tracheotomy may be necessary to maintain a clear airway. If diphtheria is suspected, antitoxin is given immediately.

(c) FOREIGN BODY.—An inhaled foreign body may cause laryngeal obstruction. In that case it is usually known that the child has inhaled something.

Treatment.—In any case of acute laryngitis with or without obstruction (*i.e.*, stridor and gasping respirations), where there is the slightest suspicion of diphtheria, anti-diphtheritic serum is at once given. The case is treated as one of diphtheria till the subsequent course and the result of the swab prove it is not.

The child is nursed as outlined under faucial diphtheria but, in addition, special watch must be kept to see that any laryngeal obstruction present does not distress the child too much through interfering with air entry. If this interference does arise (as shown by increasing stridor, cyanosis and sucking in of the chest wall), then operative measures to relieve the obstruction must be taken as an acute emergency.

Relief of Laryngeal Obstruction.

1. ASPIRATION of membrane is probably the best method when the membrane is the chief cause of the obstruction. Aspiration is effected by passing a special instrument, called a laryngoscope, into the mouth so that by suitable illumination the larynx can be seen. Then by using a suction pump the membrane can in many cases be removed.

2. TRACHEOTOMY.—A tracheotomy is an operation in which an opening is made in the midline of the neck into the trachea. Tracheotomy is indicated when aspiration of the membrane has been tried and has failed to relieve the obstruction. In addition, tracheotomy is usually required when the main cause of the laryngeal obstruction is inflammatory œdema and not membrane.

For the performance of a tracheotomy the child is rolled in a blanket (to keep it steady) and an assistant holds the head absolutely still with the neck extended. An incision is made into the trachea below the cricoid cartilage and special tracheal dilators are inserted to hold open the trachea. A tracheotomy tube is then inserted into the opening and tied in position by tapes around the neck. Next, a second inner tube is inserted which can be easily removed for cleansing.

The nursing of a tracheotomy patient calls for skilled and constant attention as the tracheotomy tubes are inclined to become blocked from the secretions and, if the airway is not immediately cleared, death from asphyxia will result. Blocking of the tube causes restlessness, stridor, cyanosis and laboured respirations, and at the first sign of any of these symptoms the inner tube must be removed and washed in bicarbonate solution. In addition to any emergency cleansing of the tube, periodic routine removal of the inner tube for cleansing should, of course, also be carried out.

Any discharge from the tube must be immediately removed by moistened gauze swabs and dissecting forceps. These swabs are infectious and must be burnt. It is important to realise the necessity for prompt and skilled attention to keep the airway clear at all times and all the necessary instruments, swabs and solutions must always be available at the bedside. It is usually advisable to have spare tracheotomy tubes and tracheotomy dilators also ready.

3. INTUBATION.—Intubation is sometimes used instead of a tracheotomy. Here a tube is inserted through the mouth and between the vocal cords into the larynx and left in position. The drawback with intubation, however, is that it is a very skilled procedure; furthermore, the tube is often coughed out and therefore frequently needs replacement.

PREVENTIVE TREATMENT OF DIPHTHERIA

1. **Passive Immunisation.**—This can be done effectively by injection of anti-diphtheritic serum but, as with all types of passive immunisation, the effect lasts only for a few weeks. Passive immunisation is therefore undertaken only to prevent diphtheria in a contact who is already ill and in whom the added strain of diphtheria might be a serious matter.

2. **Active Immunisation.**—Active immunisation against diphtheria is now carried out on a wide scale in most countries, with wonderful results in reducing the incidence of the disease. In Canada, for example, where nearly all the school children have been immunised, diphtheria is now a rare disease. In England, increasing immunisation is reducing yearly the number of cases. Immunisation against diphtheria and vaccination against smallpox have in fact been the two most successful procedures in preventive immunisation.

Before carrying out active immunisation, a *Schick* test is performed to see whether or not the person is already immune to diphtheria. In doing a Schick test a small dose of diphtheria toxin is injected into the skin of the forearm, and if the person is immune no reaction occurs at the site of the injection—which shows that the person's antibodies have destroyed the toxin. On the other hand, if the person is susceptible, a red area develops which may last up to a week. (Preliminary Schick testing is not, however, usually performed as a routine before active immunisation of children is carried out, as most young children are not immune to diphtheria.) Two or three injections of diphtheria toxoid are then given at monthly intervals and the antibodies developed produce a lasting immunity to diphtheria. (Toxoid is altered toxin, which will not cause an actual attack of diphtheria but nevertheless can stimulate the body's defences to produce lasting antibodies.) With children a boosting dose of toxoid is usually given when the child starts school to strengthen the immunity.

Diphtheria Carriers.—Diphtheria carriers are people who persistently harbour the diphtheria organism in their bodies and may thus spread the infection to others. The carrier state may develop in a person who has himself recovered from an attack of the disease or, alternatively, a person may carry the organism without ever having had diphtheria himself. Diphtheria bacilli usually persist in infected tonsils and sinuses or, less commonly, in discharges from the ear. Penicillin has been found to be of considerable value in clearing up the carrier state. Infected tonsils or sinuses should be surgically treated as necessary. Carriers should be isolated to prevent spread of infection.

WHOOPING-COUGH (Pertussis)

Cause.—An organism called the pertussis bacillus.

Spread.—Usually by droplet infection in coughing; less commonly the disease is spread by contact with infected clothes or other articles (fomites).

Incubation Period.—Seven to fourteen days.

Incidence.—The disease is most prevalent in spring and autumn. Children under the age of 5 are the usual sufferers, but adults may also be affected. Since the decline in the severity of scarlet fever and the reduction in the number of diphtheria cases through active immunisation, whooping-cough is nowadays the most serious acute specific fever in children.

Symptoms and Signs.

1. CATARRHAL OR PRE-PAROXYSMAL STAGE.—This stage usually lasts about a week, during which time the child appears to be

afflicted with a bad cold. Fever is often present, whilst the cough tends to be very persistent and may be associated with vomiting.

2. PAROXYSMAL STAGE.

(*a*) When this stage is reached there is no mistaking the nature of the illness. Paroxysmal attacks of severe coughing occur, the child going blue in the face and holding his breath. When it seems that the child must suffocate, a long, deep inspiration with a loud " whoop " takes place.

(*b*) Vomiting with the cough is very often present.

(*c*) Thick sticky mucus is expectorated.

(*d*) There may be as many as twenty or more of these bouts (which are especially frequent at night) in a severe attack.

Course.—The paroxysmal stage usually lasts for three or more weeks, the bouts gradually becoming less severe. The younger the child the more severe the disease, so that most of the deaths occur in children under 1 year of age.

Diagnosis.—This is obvious in the paroxysmal stage. Before this stage, whooping-cough should be suspected in any child with a severe cold and cough associated with vomiting. A swab suitably curved for insertion into the post-nasal region is taken and then cultured on a special medium in the laboratory, when it will reveal the whooping-cough bacillus in a large percentage of cases.

Complications.

1. BRONCHO-PNEUMONIA.—This is the outstanding complication of whooping-cough and is responsible for most of the deaths amongst infants.

2. BRONCHIECTASIS.—Collapse of a part of the lung may occur in the acute stage owing to the thick mucus obstructing a bronchus. If the lung does not re-expand, the permanent collapse may give rise to bronchiectasis.

3. GASTRO-ENTERITIS.—In children under 2 whooping-cough often leads to gastro-enteritis, particularly in the summer months when enteritis is prevalent.

4. CONVULSIONS.—Repeated convulsions are serious and may prove fatal.

Treatment.

1. In mild cases, where the paroxysms are few and the child's general health is good, the patient should be kept in the fresh air as much as possible.

2. In the more severe cases, with frequent paroxysms and fever, the child is put to bed. A well-ventilated room is particularly important in the treatment of whooping-cough.

3. Diet is of special importance because of the frequent vomiting. The child is best fed with small, frequent, light meals immediately after each bout of coughing. Skilled attention will be necessary to induce the child to take sufficient nourishment. This is especially so with infants. Routine bottle feeds may have to be abandoned and the infant fed whenever it will take its feeds.

4. To reduce the paroxysms of coughing, various drugs have been tried. Phenobarbitone, $\frac{1}{2}$ gr. twice a day ($\frac{1}{4}$ gr. b.d. for infants), may be effective.

5. Convulsions are best treated with oxygen and by giving phenobarbitone, 1 gr. immediately, followed by smaller doses afterwards. It is important that the sedatives should not be given in such quantities as to make the child too drowsy, as the cough reflex then becomes depressed with resultant retention of the thick bronchial mucus.

6. Penicillin is given at the first suspicion of pneumonia.

7. The tetracycline antibiotics are sometimes given in severe attacks as it is believed by some that these drugs reduce the number and severity of the paroxysms.

Preventive Treatment.—An effective vaccine is available for active immunisation. The vaccine is usually combined with that of diphtheria and three injections at monthly intervals are given. Immunisation is best started at about the age of 2 to 3 months, as whooping-cough has its highest fatality rate in the first year of life.

SCARLET FEVER

Cause.—Hæmolytic streptococcus.

Spread.—Mainly by droplet infection. Less often, fomites (infected articles such as toys, books, etc.) may be responsible. Milk infected by a carrier may cause a widespread outbreak of the disease.

The organism generally enters the body through the throat and a streptococcal sore throat is an initial symptom of the disease. In puerperal women the infection may occur via the genital tract— *puerperal scarlet fever.*

Incubation Period.—Two to four days.

Incidence.—Primarily in children, especially during the winter.

Symptoms and Signs.

1. The onset is nearly always sudden, with fever, severe headache, vomiting and sore throat.

2. The pulse rate is very fast, more so than one would expect from the degree of fever.

3. The throat is very red, and exudate is usually present on both tonsils, often giving the appearance of a membrane.

4. The tongue is heavily furred and the red papillæ seen through the fur gives the appearance referred to as the *strawberry* tongue. After a few days the tongue peels, becoming red and raw—*red strawberry* tongue.

5. RASH.—The rash appears on the second day and has the following characteristics :—

(*a*) It avoids the face, which is, however, flushed, except around the mouth. (This condition is the well - recognised *circumoral pallor.*)

(*b*) It appears first around the neck and chest and soon spreads rapidly all over the body.

(*c*) It is a bright red erythema which blanches on pressure.

(*d*) It fades in about a week, to be followed by the typical desquamation. Here the skin peels off, either in large scales or in a small form which produces " pin holes " in the skin.

Types.

1. SIMPLE.—This is the ordinary, relatively mild type with symptoms and signs as just described.

2. TOXIC.—Here severe toxæmia is present and many patients die. This form is now very rare in Great Britain but is still commonly seen in Eastern Europe.

3. SEPTIC.—In this type the septic complications are a predominant feature.

Diagnosis.—The diagnosis is usually made on the streptococcal sore throat accompanied by the erythematous rash. If the rash is so slight that it is missed, the occurrence of desquamation later on in the illness is suggestive of scarlet fever.

DICK TEST.—This is a similar test to the Schick test used in diphtheria. Scarlatinal toxin is injected into the skin, and if the person is susceptible to scarlet fever a bright erythema develops in twelve hours and is gone in twenty-four hours. The test can be used up to the third day or so of the disease if the toxin is inserted into an area of skin where no rash is present.

Complications of Scarlet Fever.—The complications of scarlet fever can be divided into two groups :—

      1. Septic.   2. Toxic and Allergic.

1. SEPTIC.—The septic complications are caused by the infection spreading to the surrounding tissues. They usually develop in the early stage of the disease, unlike the toxic complications which tend to arise in the second and third weeks. The main septic complications are :—

      (*a*) Septic cervical adenitis.
      (*b*) Otitis media, which may spread to cause mastoiditis.
      (*c*) Quinsy (peritonsillar abscess).

2. TOXIC AND ALLERGIC.—

      (*a*) Acute myocarditis and endocarditis. The heart involvement in scarlet fever is closely related to that in acute rheumatic fever and is treated in the same way.
      (*b*) Acute nephritis. This is identical with the ordinary form of acute nephritis described on page 411.
      (*c*) Arthritis.

Treatment.

1. The patient is nursed in bed with the isolation procedure and nursing care usual in a fever case. In view of the mild form of the present day scarlet fever, patients are not usually nursed in hospital where there is an added risk of cross-infection from other strains of hæmolytic streptococci.

2. Penicillin is most valuable in the treatment of scarlet fever and considerably reduces the risk of complications.

3. Isolation for two weeks is usually sufficient except where there are any septic discharges which may contain the organisms.

ERYSIPELAS

Cause.—Hæmolytic streptococcus.

Spread.—By direct contact, entry into the body usually being through a skin abrasion or wound.

Incidence.—Erysipelas was formerly a very common infection in hospitals and institutions, especially in surgical wards where infected wounds and abscesses spread the disease. Nowadays, however, with proper aseptic technique, and particularly with the introduction of the sulphonamides and the various antibiotics, the disease is much less common and can be quickly controlled.

Symptoms and Signs.

1. Erysipelas is most frequently seen in middle-aged and elderly people, and the presence of some debilitating disease or chronic alcoholism is particularly likely to give rise to the infection.

2. The onset is usually sudden, with fever, general constitutional upset and rigors.

3. The characteristic lesion is a bright red erythema of the skin which is swollen and tense with a clear-cut border. The most frequent site of this local lesion is the face, and it often spreads in a butterfly distribution over the nose and cheeks. Another common site is around the margin of a surgical wound.

Course and Treatment.—Before the use of sulphonamides and penicillin, erysipelas was a prevalent disease and often serious. Sulphonamides and penicillin, however, usually clear up the infection in a few days and thereby also reduce the risk of the infection spreading. The general treatment consists of bed rest and the routine care for an acute fever case.

TYPHOID FEVER

Cause.—Bacillus typhosus (*Salmonella typhosus*).

Spread and Incidence.—Typhoid fever is spread mainly through the contamination of water, milk, or food with sewage. Human carriers excrete the organisms in the fæces or urine, and if proper hygiene and sanitation are lacking, contamination of water or food results. For this reason typhoid fever is particularly likely to arise in armies during times of war and also in areas where adequate sanitation is lacking.

Incubation Period.—Usually ten to fourteen days.

Pathology.—There is a well-recognised pathology in typhoid fever.

1. It begins as a general septicæmia, with the organism growing in the blood.

2. Typical localised lesions then develop in the small intestine, the lymphoid tissue known as *Peyer's patches* showing the following changes :—

   (*a*) Inflammatory swelling in the first week.
   (*b*) Sloughing of the patches in the second week.
   (*c*) Separation of the sloughs in the third week.
   (*d*) Repair of the ulcers in the fourth week.

The above changes account for many of the customary complications seen in typhoid fever.

3. The other main pathological changes are :—

(a) Enlargement of the spleen.
(b) Inflammation of the gall-bladder.
(c) Acute myocarditis.
(d) Inflammation and abscesses of the bones.

Symptoms and Signs.

1. The onset is gradual, with slowly rising fever reaching a maximum by the end of the week of 102° to 104° F.

2. There are the usual signs of a severe fever, especially severe frontal headache, epistaxis, and marked weakness and fatigue.

3. The pulse is slow in relation to the height of the temperature.

4. Abdominal discomfort is usually present and the abdomen is distended and tender. Constipation is the rule at this stage although diarrhœa may occur.

5. By the end of the first week the patient appears severely ill and is in a state of physical and mental fatigue. He has a dry mouth and hot skin, and on the seventh day the characteristic rash occurs. This rash—the *rose spots*—appears at the end of the first week or the beginning of the second week, usually on the seventh day. The rash consists of small, round, papular rose areas which first occur on the chest and abdomen. The spots are scanty and successive crops appear.

6. In the second and third weeks the patient usually continues severely ill, and the temperature remains steadily high, often between 103° and 104° F.

7. Instead of constipation, diarrhœa is commonly present with the typical " pea soup " stools. These are watery and contain undigested food and often shreds of mucous membrane. In some cases, streaking with blood or a more obvious hæmorrhage may occur. It should be noted, however, that many patients with typhoid fever do not have diarrhœa but may be constipated throughout the illness.

8. The abdomen is usually more distended and tender. Abdominal pain may be complained of and, if this is at all severe, the possibility of a complicating perforation of the bowel must be considered.

9. In very severe infections the patient may relapse into the *typhoid state*, with a " low muttering " delirium, extreme prostration

and toxæmia. (The typhoid state has been fully described under the general symptoms of Acute Infectious Fevers.)

10. By the end of the third week or the beginning of the fourth there is usually a gradual but steady improvement in the patient's condition, and the temperature slowly falls to normal (by lysis). Convalescence is prolonged, and relapses, when the temperature rises and symptoms reappear, occur in approximately 10 per cent. of cases. Relapses are usually milder than the initial attack.

It should be remembered that the severity of typhoid fever varies markedly from a mild illness lasting a week or two to a fulminating infection.

COMPLICATIONS OF TYPHOID FEVER

Complications are very common in typhoid fever. As the main lesion is in the intestine it is natural that the main complications should arise here, but as there is also a general septicæmia, complications can and do occur in any system of the body.

1. **Intestinal Hæmorrhage.**—This complication usually arises towards the end of the second or during the third week. It is caused by the erosion of a blood vessel as a result of the sloughing and ulceration in the Peyer's patches.

The hæmorrhage varies in degree from a mere streaking of the stools with blood to more severe hæmorrhage where the stools become black and tarry. In very severe cases there may be a sudden flooding of bright red blood from the intestines.

In cases of severe hæmorrhage there is a sudden deterioration in the patient's general condition, with marked pallor, rise in the pulse and fall in the temperature.

2. **Intestinal Perforation.**—Perforation is a well-recognised but fortunately rarer complication, due to the ulceration of the bowels. It usually occurs at the end of the third week. There is sudden acute abdominal pain with signs of collapse and shock, including a rise in the pulse rate and a fall in the temperature. Vomiting may also occur. The abdomen is acutely tender and rigid.

3. **Meteorism (Tympanites).**—Meteorism is severe distension of the abdomen caused by the accumulation of flatus in the bowel. The abdominal distension may cause pressure on the already weakened heart.

4. **Acute Myocarditis.**—The toxæmia of typhoid fever is very prone to cause an acute myocarditis, and heart failure is in fact one

of the common causes of death in typhoid fever. A rapid soft pulse, often also irregular, is a warning of heart damage.

5. **Other Complications.**—Very many other complications are seen in typhoid fever of which the following are the most important :—

> (*a*) Broncho-pneumonia.
> (*b*) Acute Cholecystitis
> (*c*) Parotitis.
> (*d*) Thrombophlebitis.
> (*e*) Arthritis.

Diagnosis of Typhoid Fever.

In a well-developed typical attack by the second or third week the condition is fairly obvious, but it is important to realise that the degree of severity can vary enormously from really serious cases to the type where the person merely feels "off colour," with a mild fever.

It is important to confirm the diagnosis of typhoid fever at an early stage, both for the purpose of treatment and to prevent spread of the disease. Laboratory tests may help considerably in early diagnosis.

LABORATORY AIDS TO DIAGNOSIS.

1. A blood culture is often positive early in the disease. Several daily blood cultures should be taken, as when these are examined in the laboratory it may be possible to isolate the typhoid organisms. In the early stages of typhoid, blood culture is the best means of isolating the organism.

2. *Fæces.*—Routine specimens of fæces are sent to the laboratory for isolation of the organisms. A rectal swab may be used instead of a specimen of fæces.

3. *Widal reaction.*—This is a special test which is used not only in typhoid but also in several other infectious diseases as an aid to diagnosis.

As a result of the infection the body develops antibodies against the invading organisms. These antibodies take time to develop but can usually be found in appreciable amounts in the blood after the first week.

For purposes of this test the blood (serum) from the patient is mixed with actual known typhoid bacilli, and if typhoid antibodies are present in the serum an agglutination reaction occurs. This agglutination reaction arises only when organisms and their *specific* antibodies are brought together.

3

The Widal reaction has to be carefully interpreted, as if a person has in the past been inoculated (vaccinated) against typhoid fever, he will as a result have developed antibodies and will give a positive agglutination reaction.

4. *Urine.*—Typhoid bacilli may in some cases be excreted in the urine, which is therefore usually examined for the presence of the organisms. As, however, the organisms are not usually present in the urine till the third week, this examination is not of very much use in diagnosis.

5. *Blood Count.*—A decrease in the number of white blood cells (leucopenia) often occurs in typhoid, in contrast to the usual increase in white cells (leucocytosis) seen in most infections.

TREATMENT OF TYPHOID FEVER

1. **Isolation Procedures.**—The patient is nursed in strict isolation, all the usual measures to prevent spread of the infection being taken. Particular attention must be paid to the disposal of the stools and urine as the bacilli are excreted in these. All excreta must be allowed to stand in 1 in 10 lysol (or other suitable disinfectant) for two hours before disposal. The nurse must wear gloves when attending to the patient, and scrupulous washing of the hands and nails after every contact with the patient is essential.

All linen and bedding before being laundered must be soaked in a suitable disinfectant. Separate marked utensils must be provided and boiled after use.

2. **General Nursing.**—Typhoid fever is a prolonged and serious illness, and therefore special nursing care is needed to sustain the patient and prevent as far as possible the development of complications. Strict attention must be paid to all the details given under the general nursing care of a fever case (p. 38); the following points are the most important :—

(*a*) Everything must be done for the patient, who must be fed, washed and carefully lifted on and off the bed-pan, in order to avoid a strain on the heart, which may be affected in typhoid fever.

(*b*) A rubber mattress should be provided for all patients. Pressure sores must be prevented by detailed attention to all pressure areas.

(*c*) Stomatitis is a common complication and frequent attention to the mouth is necessary.

(d) If the diarrhœa is very severe, the use of tow to receive the excreta is less disturbing to a severely ill patient than frequent bed-pans.

(e) The stools must be examined daily for the presence of curds (see later) and blood. The presence of blood must be reported to the doctor at once. The importance of daily examination of the stools must be stressed.

(f) The pulse rate and temperature must be carefully watched, as any sudden change is a warning of a serious complication such as hæmorrhage, perforation, or heart failure.

(g) The abdomen should be examined daily for any undue distension (meteorism).

(h) Severe abdominal pain and vomiting should be at once reported as these symptoms suggest an intestinal perforation.

3. **Diet.**—Typhoid fever causes severe lesions in the intestinal tract with the consequential danger of hæmorrhage and perforation. As a result diet plays a most important role in the treatment of the disease. As far as possible a non-residue diet should be given but, at the same time, the patient must get sufficient nourishment to maintain his resistance.

(a) Milk (approximately 2 pints a day) is the foundation of the diet, though it must be remembered that whole milk may be difficult to digest. Abdominal distension or the presence of curds in the fæces call both for a reduction in the total amount of milk and also for citration (1 gr. to the ounce) of the milk. Also, as milk is monotonous it should be varied with custard, milk jellies and junket.

(b) Eggs, beaten up in milk or lightly boiled, rusks and butter, milk chocolate and a small amount of pounded white fish are all useful articles of diet that may be given.

(c) Sufficient fluid must be taken and plenty of glucose given in the feeds. Strained fruit juices which supply vitamin C are important.

(d) If severe abdominal distension or diarrhœa occurs, the solid foods may have to be left out of the diet for a short period.

(e) After the third week, when the danger of hæmorrhage and perforation is much less, more solid food should be added to the diet.

4. **Specific Treatment.**—Chloramphenicol (chloromycetin) is the only specific drug available. It reduces the general toxæmia and usually causes the temperature to fall to normal in three to four days. The danger of hæmorrhage and perforation, however, appears to remain nearly as great and, in addition, relapses do occur with

chloramphenicol therapy. Therefore all the general nursing care and dietary measures still form a most important part of the treatment.

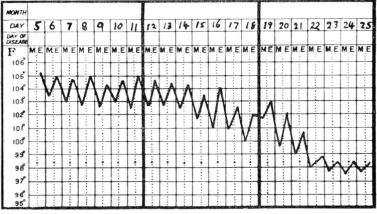

FIG. 16

Temperature chart from a case of uncomplicated typhoid fever, not treated with chloramphenicol. The temperature became normal on the twenty-third day.

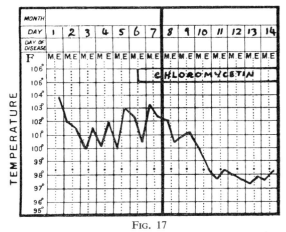

FIG. 17

Temperature chart from a case of typhoid fever showing the response to chloramphenicol.

Chloramphenicol is given in capsule form by mouth, the initial dose being about 1 gm., followed by 0·5 gm. (two capsules) every six hours for seven to fourteen days.

If a relapse develops, a further course of chloramphenicol (chloromycetin) is given for one week.

5. Treatment of the Complications.

(*a*) *Hæmorrhage.*—All solid food must be stopped and only fluids given. Sedatives, such as morphine, ⅛ to ¼ gr., may be necessary. If the hæmorrhage is severe a blood transfusion will be given.

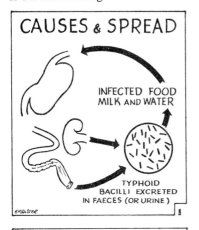

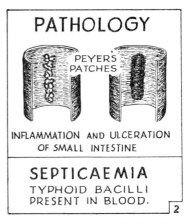

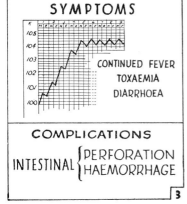

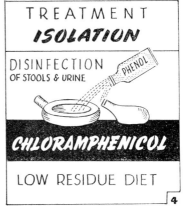

Fig. 18
Typhoid fever.

(*b*) *Perforation.*—Formerly all patients were immediately operated on to close the perforation. The mortality rate following operation is, however, so high that many patients with perforation are instead now initially treated medically with blood transfusions and antibiotics (streptomycin, terramycin, etc.) to combat peritonitis.

(c) *Tympanites.*—The presence of abdominal distension with pain usually means that the diet has been too irritating, and the milk and glucose should therefore be reduced. Turpentine stupes to the abdomen often give relief. Excessive diarrhœa may be present with tympanites and, if the above measures do not bring relief, a starch and opium enema is often given.

(d) *Hyperpyrexia and Delirium.*—These complications usually respond to tepid sponging; in addition, a hypnotic (such as one of the barbiturate drugs) is useful.

6. **Convalescence.**—Convalescence must be lengthy after such a prolonged illness as typhoid. The patient is not free from infection until the fæces and urine are free from the typhoid bacilli.

7. **Preventive Treatment.**—An active immunity to typhoid fever can be created by means of the highly effective vaccine available. It is necessary, however, to revaccinate once a year if an effective immunity is to be maintained. Vaccination against typhoid is usually practised in any circumstances wherein the sanitation and hygiene are such that they cannot be relied upon to prevent the disease arising. For troops during war and for people who, because of travel, may be exposed to contaminated food or water, typhoid vaccination is essential.

PARATYPHOID FEVERS

Paratyphoid fevers are caused by infection with the paratyphoid bacilli, referred to as A, B and C. These bacilli are very like the typhoid bacillus in their action. Paratyphoid fevers and typhoid fever are often grouped together under the heading of **enteric fever.** Typhoid fever, which formerly was much the commonest type of enteric fever seen in Great Britain, is now less common; on the other hand, paratyphoid B infection is now more prevalent.

Paratyphoid infection tends, on the whole, to be much less severe and toxic than typhoid, but the general symptoms and the treatment are all very similar. For this reason all that has been said about typhoid applies to paratyphoid fever. The exact diagnosis of the specific organism causing the enteric fever is made on bacteriological examination.

BACILLARY DYSENTERY

Cause.—Dysentery bacilli, of which there are several types including Sonne, Flexner and Shiga.

Spread.—The method of spread of the disease is similar to that of enteric fever. The bacilli are excreted in the fæces, and through defective sanitation and bad hygiene, food and water can then become contaminated. Flies, too, frequently cause contamination of food and are a prevalent mode of spread of the disease.

Incidence. — Although dysentery is commonest in tropical countries it is becoming more frequent in Great Britain, especially in camps, nurseries and large institutions subject to overcrowding. Sonne infections in children are commonly seen in this country. Flexner dysentery, which usually occurs in adults, is less common in Great Britain but is more severe. The most virulent infections are caused by the Shiga bacilli but these are rarely seen outside the tropics.

Pathology.—There is an acute inflammation of the large intestine with ulceration in severe cases.

Symptoms and Signs.

1. In Sonne dysentery in children the disease is usually mild, with few constitutional symptoms and only slight fever. The predominating signs are diarrhœa, with the passage of blood and mucus in the stools. The number of stools passed in the day rarely exceeds five or six. Slight abdominal colic is usually present.

2. In Flexner infections, toxæmia is more marked, with headache, loss of appetite, thirst and lassitude all present. Severe abdominal colic with the rapid onset of urgent diarrhœa are the main symptoms. As many as fifteen to twenty stools a day may be passed. The typical dysenteric stool is small and consists entirely of blood and mucus or muco-pus, with no fæcal matter present. In severe cases shreds of mucous membrane are present.

3. Shiga infections are usually accompanied by profound prostration and dehydration.

Diagnosis.—Laboratory examination of the stools or of a rectal swab is carried out in all cases and usually reveals the causative organism.

Treatment.

1. The usual nursing care and isolation precautions outlined under typhoid fever are necessary. The form of dysentery usually seen in Great Britain (Sonne) is highly infectious, and when dealing with the disease in children it is most important that different nurses should attend to the feeding and to the changing. Destructible napkins should be used.

2. In the acute stage a fluid diet is given, but as soon as the stools become more solid, additions to the diet are quickly made in the form of soft, bland, low-residue foods. For severe cases, where dehydration is present, intravenous fluids may be necessary.

3. The specific treatment is the administration of one of the tetracycline antibiotics which usually have a rapid curative effect. Alternatively, the sulphonamides may be given; formerly the low absorption group of sulphonamides (see p. 574) were used but nowadays equally good or better results are obtained using the absorbable sulphonamides.

4. The patient is considered infectious until successive bacteriological examinations of the stools are negative.

FOOD POISONING

Cause.—Food poisoning is caused by the contamination of food with bacteria, or with the toxins of bacteria. The most common causes of food poisoning are the Salmonella group of bacilli and the toxins produced by the Staphylococcus.

The rare form of food poisoning, known as *botulism*, is caused by the improper canning of foods.

Spread.—Food poisoning may arise through contamination of food due to lack of proper hygiene on the part of people who, whilst harbouring the organisms in their fæces, are engaged in handling food. Animals such as rats and mice may also infect food. Such foods as reheated pies, cooked meats and duck eggs are especially liable to contamination by Salmonella organisms, whilst cakes, custards and ham are most frequently infected by staphylococcal toxin.

Symptoms and Signs.

1. Food poisoning due to staphylococcal toxin causes a severe acute gastro-enteritis with vomiting, abdominal colic and diarrhœa. These symptoms usually start within a few hours of the eating of the offending food. Usually all the people who eat the food are similarly affected.

2. Food poisoning caused by the Salmonella bacilli produces a similar picture of an acute gastro-enteritis. The onset, however, is not so rapid as in staphylococcal poisoning, as it takes six to twenty-four hours to develop, and the symptoms may persist for a longer period—over several days.

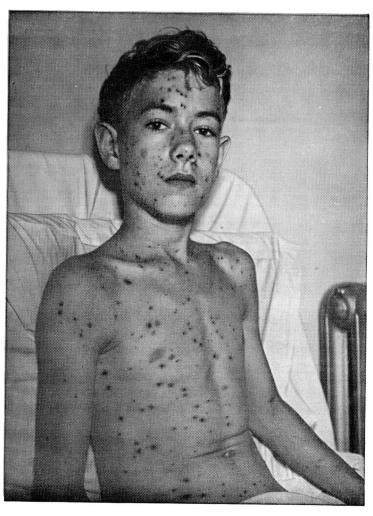

FIG. 19
Chickenpox showing polymorphic eruption.

[*To face page* 73

3. In botulism the symptoms usually develop about twenty-four hours after the poisoned canned food was eaten. The predominating symptoms are various forms of paralysis; in most cases the outcome is fatal.

Diagnosis.—The diagnosis of food poisoning is usually easily made when vomiting, abdominal pain and diarrhœa occur in several people after they have eaten the same food. Dysentery, which also causes abdominal colic and diarrhœa, is differentiated from food poisoning by the absence of vomiting and also by the presence of blood in the stools, which is rarely seen in food poisoning.

Treatment.—Most patients with food poisoning recover fairly rapidly with rest in bed and a fluid diet. If abdominal colic and diarrhœa are severe, a kaolin and opium mixture may be given.

In staphylococcal cases which do not quickly clear up, the antibiotics, erythromycin or terramycin, may be used with some effect. In Salmonella food poisoning there is no specific therapy, but chloramphenicol or the tetracycline antibiotics may be of value in some cases.

Preventive treatment is most important and entails the proper handling and storage of all foods. Full hygienic measures must be employed in all kitchens, and care taken to see that flies, rats and mice cannot get at the food. In addition, all people handling food must be free from any infection.

CHICKENPOX (Varicella)

Cause.—Virus infection.

Spread.—By droplet infection or by the hands and clothing of attendants.

Incubation Period.—Twelve to twenty-one days, usually fourteen.

Incidence.—The disease is very common, attacking all age groups, but especially children under 10. Chickenpox is most prevalent in autumn and winter.

Symptoms and Signs.

1. The onset is usually mild, the patient merely feeling " off colour," with a slight pyrexia. In children, quite often the first sign of the disease is the appearance of the rash.

2. The *rash* of chickenpox has the following characteristics :—

    (*a*) It appears first on the trunk, particularly the back, and then spreads to the face and limbs. The eruption is densest on the trunk and the upper parts of the limbs.

3 A

(b) Red papules appear first, which rapidly change to vesicles and pustules. Within a few days the pustules dry up and form scabs which quickly fall off.

(c) The rash appears in crops so that all types of lesion, papules, vesicles, pustules and crusts are seen together.

Complications.—Chickenpox is nearly always a mild disease, severe toxic types being very rare. The most frequent complication is infection of the rash through scratching.

Diagnosis.—The most important part in diagnosis is to distinguish a severe case of chickenpox from a mild case of smallpox. This differentiation usually rests on the order of appearance, the distribution and, in smallpox, the protracted development of the rash. The main points of difference are given under Smallpox.

Chickenpox may also be mistaken for various skin diseases like impetigo, urticaria and scabies.

Treatment.—Treatment of chickenpox is mainly concerned with the prevention of secondary infection of the lesions. In children the finger nails should be cut short and, if itching is severe, gloves or splints should be applied. The itching may be alleviated by using a soothing lotion such as calamine with 1 per cent. phenol. If the lesions are profuse, penicillin may be given to prevent secondary infection.

Isolation is necessary till all the crusts have separated.

SMALLPOX

Cause.—Virus infection.

Spread.—By direct contact and droplet infection through the respiratory tract. Contaminated clothing or other articles may also spread the disease. Smallpox is the most infectious of all known infectious fevers.

Incubation Period.—Twelve to fourteen days.

Incidence.—Smallpox occurs throughout the world, but is rare in countries where active measures (vaccination) are taken to prevent it. It is very rife, often causing widespread epidemics, in certain tropical countries. Outbreaks in Great Britain are usually the result of the arrival in this country of an unsuspected case from abroad. Smallpox affects all age groups.

Symptoms and Signs.—All grades of severity of the disease are seen. A typical attack of a moderately severe type will be described.

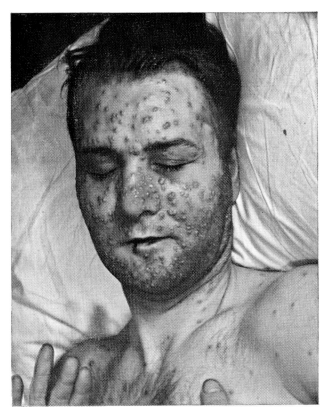

FIG. 20
Smallpox.

[*To face page* 74

1. STAGE OF INVASION.—The onset is sudden with all the symptoms and signs of a severe fever, including high pyrexia (103° to 104° F.), rigors, severe headaches and vomiting. The patient is usually seriously ill, with marked prostration.

2. STAGE OF ERUPTION.—The characteristic rash of smallpox has the following features :—

(a) It first appears on the face, then spreads to the arms, trunk and legs. The eruption is heaviest on the face, forearms and hands, and below the knees. On the trunk and upper portion of the limbs the rash is scanty.

(b) The eruption goes through well-defined stages. It starts, usually on the third day of the illness, as small red macules which quickly change to papules (flat, raised areas). These, after about two days, turn into vesicles (i.e., raised areas containing a clear fluid, like little water blisters). By the eighth day the vesicles become pustules, which, by the fifteenth day, dry up to form dark scabs. The scabs, when they fall off, leave deep pitted scars.

(c) All the lesions in smallpox develop approximately at the same time and not in separate crops, with the result that all reach each stage simultaneously.

During the pustular stage in particular the general constitutional symptoms become worse and the patient is extremely ill. Mental lethargy, prostration, dry mouth often with sordes, and extreme restlessness are features of this stage. In very severe cases all the symptoms of the " typhoid state " (p. 38) may develop.

3. STAGE OF CONVALESCENCE.—Owing to the serious nature of the disease, convalescence in smallpox must be prolonged. The crusts may be very persistent in the scalp and take weeks to separate.

Types.—The severity of smallpox varies considerably according to the virulence of the virus and whether or not the patient has been vaccinated in the past. The following types are usually described :—

1. VARIOLA MAJOR (UNMODIFIED SMALLPOX).—This is the classical severe form of the disease as described above. The most severe types of variola major are the confluent and hæmorrhagic.

2. MODIFIED SMALLPOX (VARIOLOID).—This type of smallpox occurs in people with a partial immunity derived from past vaccination. The disease is usually in a mild form ; the rash may be scanty and the severe constitutional symptoms seen during the pustular stage in unmodified smallpox do not occur.

3. VARIOLA MINOR (ALASTRIM).—This is a mild form of smallpox which is almost identical with modified smallpox. In variola minor, however, the mild nature of the disease is not due to a previous vaccination but to the fact that the smallpox virus is of a less virulent strain.

Complications of Smallpox.

1. BRONCHO-PNEUMONIA.—This is a very common complication of severe attacks of smallpox.

2. ACUTE MYOCARDITIS.

3. SEPTIC SKIN LESIONS.—Boils, abscesses and pressure sores are particularly liable to develop with a widespread pustular rash.

4. CORNEAL ULCERATION.

Diagnosis.—This is often very difficult, especially in the early stages. Confusion is particularly likely to arise between mild attacks of smallpox and severe attacks of chickenpox. In chickenpox, however, the rash appears first, and is heaviest on the trunk and scanty on the face, hands and feet. This is in marked contrast to the rash in smallpox. Also, the rash in chickenpox appears in *crops* with papules, vesicles, pustules and scabs all present at the same time.

In recent years it has become possible to isolate the virus in scrapings from the vesicles and pustules.

Treatment of Smallpox.

1. ISOLATION.—As mentioned earlier, smallpox is the most infectious of all diseases, and as a rule all cases are nursed in special hospitals. The strictest precautions are necessary to prevent the attendants from coming in contact with other people and so possibly spreading the disease. For this reason, special living quarters are necessary for all staff coming in contact with the patients. All such staff must themselves be rendered immune by vaccination.

The virus is present in the respiratory tract and skin lesions, so that gowns, masks and special hoods to cover the hair are necessary. Patients are isolated till all the scabs have separated and all the scars healed.

2. GENERAL NURSING.—The nursing of a patient with smallpox is most important, partly because of the severity of the disease and partly because there is no specific treatment available. All the routine nursing care of a severe acute feverish illness is necessary. Special points are :—

    (*a*) Complete rest is essential, particularly in view of the danger of heart involvement.

(b) Pressure sores and skin abscesses are especially liable to occur, so that extra care in the treatment of the skin and pressure areas is necessary. A rubber mattress should be provided.

(c) Oral hygiene and careful attention to the eyes must be carried out.

(d) Particular care must be exercised at all times to prevent the patient injuring himself, as delirium with extreme restlessness is a feature of severe attacks.

3. DIET AND DRUGS.—As the disease is protracted, as liberal a diet as the patient will take is given. Whilst there is no specific drug available, penicillin or one of the tetracycline antibiotics are helpful in reducing the risk of secondary infections and are therefore usually given as a routine.

Sedatives such as chloral or paraldehyde will be required for extreme restlessness or delirium.

4. PREVENTIVE TREATMENT OF SMALLPOX (VACCINATION).—It was in smallpox that the first brilliant instances of the prevention of disease by vaccination were obtained by Jenner. In vaccination against smallpox the vaccine used is a suspension of a virus which causes cowpox in cattle. The virus of cowpox (*vaccinia*) appears to be identical with the virus of smallpox except that its effect on human beings is much less virulent. Inoculating a person with a vaccine containing the virus of cowpox causes an attack of vaccinia. As a result the person becomes immune to the much more serious disease, smallpox.

The degree of immunity varies in different people. For this reason anyone who has been in contact with a case of smallpox, or is going to a country where the disease is prevalent, is revaccinated, unless successful vaccination has been carried out in the previous few months.

TECHNIQUE OF VACCINATION.—Calf lymph vaccine is used and it is essential that the lymph should be fresh. Various methods are employed, including a linear scratch and multiple-pressure pricks. The upper arm (or the thigh in women) is the site usually chosen, and the skin must first be cleansed with soap and water or acetone. Non-volatile antiseptics must not be used as they will destroy the virus. Strict asepsis is essential.

COURSE OF PRIMARY VACCINATION.—About the third to fifth day a red papule appears at the site of the vaccination. The papule becomes vesicular and later, by the eighth to the twelfth day, pustular, with an area of surrounding inflammation. The pustule soon dries up, forming a scab which separates in two or three weeks, leaving a scar. At the height of the reaction there may be slight general symptoms such as fever, malaise and irritability. The younger the person the fewer the reactions as a rule.

COURSE OF REVACCINATION.—The effects of revaccination are a considerable acceleration of the development of the local lesion which reaches its height by the fourth to eighth day. In addition the degree of the reaction is much smaller.

COMPLICATIONS OF VACCINATION.—The complications of vaccination are much less in young children, so that vaccination is usually advised in the first year, with revaccination at school age.

(a) *Generalised Vaccinia.*—Here generalised lesions occur on the body. Constitutional symptoms may be severe. Generalised vaccinia is seen only after primary vaccination.

(b) *Local Sepsis.*—This usually results from the child's scratching the site of the vaccination.

(c) *Post-vaccinal Encephalitis.*—This rare complication hardly ever arises in infants ; instead it generally follows primary vaccination in older children and adults. Severe headaches, high fever, vomiting and convulsions develop. Residual paralyses are infrequent in patients who recover.

MUMPS (Epidemic Parotitis)

Cause.—Virus infection.

Spread.—By droplet infection through the respiratory tract.

Incubation Period.—Twelve to twenty-eight days, usually seventeen days.

Incidence.—Mumps is chiefly seen in children between the ages of 5 and 15 years and also in young adults. Epidemics occur mainly in schools and institutions.

Symptoms and Signs.

1. In some cases the first sign of the disease may be the swollen face. Usually, however, the initial symptoms of pyrexia, headache and sore throat arise a few days before the characteristic swelling of the parotid glands.

2. The enlarged parotid glands produce a swelling below the angle of the jaw and the skin over the glands becomes tense and shiny. One gland is usually enlarged for a short time before the

other. There is often a complaint of pain on eating and it may be difficult to open the mouth.

3. The enlargement of the glands usually subsides within seven to ten days. The temperature falls when the glands begin to subside, which is generally within a few days.

Complications.

1. Orchitis, or inflammation of the testis, is a well-recognised complication which is most frequently seen in older children and adults. With the onset of orchitis, fever returns, with pain and swelling of the testis.

2. Rarer complications of mumps include mastitis (inflammation of the breast), oophoritis (inflammation of the ovary), pancreatitis and encephalitis.

Treatment.—There is no specific treatment for mumps. Children are nursed in bed till the temperature has subsided and are kept away from school until all the swelling has gone. Adults, however, in view of the likelihood of complications, are usually kept in bed for a longer period until all the parotid swelling has subsided. Aspirin or codeine may be needed to relieve pain. If chewing is difficult, a soft diet is given.

If orchitis develops cortisone or allied steroid often brings about rapid relief of the swelling and pain and is therefore usually prescribed.

INFLUENZA

Cause.—Virus infection of which there are several different strains.

Spread.—By droplet infection. Influenza is a highly infectious disease.

Incubation Period.—Short, one to three days.

Incidence.—Influenza occurs throughout the world in widespread epidemics, which vary considerably both in their clinical picture and fatality rates. Pandemics (world-wide epidemics), with a very high mortality rate, also occasionally occur—the last in 1918 when millions died of the disease. In more localised outbreaks influenza is fairly mild.

Symptoms and Signs.

1. The onset is usually sudden, with symptoms similar to those of the common cold or an acute bronchitis. The symptoms tend to vary, however, with different epidemics.

2. The general constitutional upset is more severe than one would expect with an ordinary cold. Headache, chills and lethargy are common.

3. A cough, sneezing, running eyes and nose, and laryngitis are usual symptoms.

4. Nausea, vomiting and abdominal pains are a feature of some outbreaks.

Complications.—Broncho-pneumonia is the most important complication and is responsible for most of the deaths. The pneumonia is usually caused by secondary infection with such organisms as the influenzal bacilli, streptococci and staphylococci. Elderly people are more prone to develop pneumonia.

Treatment.—All patients are best nursed in bed with the usual nursing care for a fever case. Isolation is not often possible owing to the rapidity of development of the disease and the difficulty of early diagnosis.

There is no specific treatment for influenza. Aspirin or codeine are useful for the headache. Penicillin or other antibiotics are usually given for the treatment of the secondary infections.

As the immunity to influenza lasts for a short period only, recurrent attacks are usual.

MENINGOCOCCAL FEVER

Meningococcal fever is also known as cerebrospinal fever and cerebrospinal meningitis. It is an acute infectious disease caused by the meningococcus. The infectivity of the disease varies a good deal and usually the cases occur sporadically. Under certain conditions, however, especially in overcrowded camps in times of war, epidemics do occur. The disease is spread by droplet infection, as the organisms are present in the upper respiratory tract.

In most cases of meningococcal fever the meninges bear the brunt of the infection, and an acute pyogenic meningitis develops with the characteristic signs as described in the chapter on Diseases of the Nervous System (p. 305). In some cases a characteristic hæmorrhagic rash may appear.

The diagnosis of meningococcal meningitis, as distinct from other forms of acute meningitis, is made by isolating the organism, which is found in the cerebrospinal fluid. The treatment is outlined under Meningitis, sulphonamides being the specific treatment in most cases.

OTHER INFECTIOUS DISEASES

So far we have discussed the most important infectious fevers seen in Great Britain. Other important infectious diseases are, as already stated, discussed later under the individual systems. It remains to mention briefly some of the more important infectious diseases which are rarely seen in Great Britain. Most of these occur in tropical or subtropical countries.

MALARIA

Malaria is still the commonest disease seen in tropical countries and, in the last century, was widespread throughout the world. Malaria is due to infection with a parasite called the plasmodium, of which there are several types causing respectively tertian, quartan and subtertian malaria. Subtertian malaria is the most severe and accounts for most of the deaths. The chief symptoms of malaria are recurrent high fever accompanied by severe rigors, profuse sweating, severe headaches and vomiting: in serious cases delirium and coma are also usually present. The spleen is characteristically enlarged. The diagnosis is usually made on the high recurrent fever with severe rigors and the finding of the parasite in the blood (a blood film suitably stained usually reveals the parasite).

The malarial parasite is conveyed to man by a certain species of mosquito (anopheles) which introduces the parasite into the blood when it bites. The eradication of malaria from most European countries has been effected by extermination of the breeding grounds of the anopheline mosquito, *i.e.*, by proper drainage of all stagnant waters. The measures for the prevention of malaria in tropical countries to-day consist of the proper drainage and, when this is not possible, of oiling the water to kill the young mosquitoes. In addition, precautions against being bitten by the mosquito (such as the use of nets and screens) are usually taken.

In areas where malaria is rife, suppressive therapy to protect against an attack of malaria may be given. Pyrimethamine (daraprim), amodiaquine (camoquin), proguanil (paludrine), or chloroquine (nivaquine, aralen) are all commonly used. For the treatment of an acute attack of malaria amodiaquine or chloroquine is given. With malaria due to *Plasmodium vivax* (benign tertian malaria) relapses are very likely, and in this type of infection amodiaquine therapy is followed by a course of primaquine.

UNDULANT FEVER (Brucellosis)

Undulant fever (also called Mediterranean fever and Malta fever from its prevalence in these areas) is occasionally seen in Great Britain. It is caused by infection with the brucella organisms, of which there are several types. The organisms are present in infected cows, pigs and goats, and the infection is carried to man through handling or ingestion of contaminated milk, cheese, meat, or pork. Farm workers and packing house employees are frequently affected.

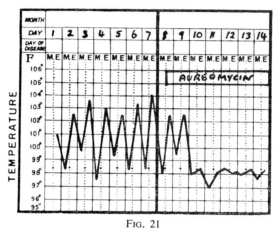

Fig. 21

Temperature chart from a case of undulant fever
showing a dramatic response to aureomycin.

The chief symptoms are a prolonged fever, often with few constitutional signs. Severe sweating and joint pains are a feature of many cases. The spleen is usually enlarged. The diagnosis is confirmed by finding the organisms in the blood (by means of a blood culture) or, more often, by an agglutination reaction similar to the Widal reaction of typhoid.

The specific treatment is the administration of one of the tetra-cycline antibiotics. In severe cases, streptomycin may also be given at the same time. Relapses are, however, commonly seen.

AMŒBIC DYSENTERY

In tropical and subtropical countries, in addition to the wide-spread bacillary forms of dysentery there is another common type caused, not by bacteria but by a parasite called the *Entamœba histolytica*. This amœbic parasite produces inflammation and ulceration of the colon, with severe diarrhœa and the passage of blood and mucus in the stools. A possible complication (which does not arise in bacillary dysentery) is that the amœbæ may travel to the liver to cause a hepatitis and often a liver abscess.

The diagnosis of amœbic dysentery is made by finding the amœbæ in the stools, and for this a fresh specimen of stool must be examined microscopically. It is often difficult to eradicate amœbæ from the body and various drugs are used in combination. In the acute stage, emetine injections (1 gr.) for three to five days are usually given, followed by a course of emetine bismuth iodide (E.B.I.), 3 gr. daily for twelve days. Other drugs, such as carbarsone (an arsenical preparation) and diodoquin, are often given as well as emetine. For amœbic hepatitis, chloroquine (nivaquine) is given in addition to emetine injections. Emetine injections are very toxic and the patient must be nursed at complete rest and a careful watch kept on the pulse rate and blood pressure.

Infection is usually spread through contaminated fruit, vegetables and water. The proper disposal of sewage and ensuring that the water supply is not contaminated are most important in prevention.

CHOLERA

Cholera is an extremely severe and often fatal disease seen in the tropics. It is caused by a bacillus called the *Vibrio comma*. Infection is spread through contamination of water in particular, and also of food. The disease occurs in large epidemics and the main features are an intense diarrhœa with watery stools containing shreds of mucous membrane from the intestinal wall—the typical " rice-water " stools of cholera. In addition, a rapid and severe dehydration sets in as a result of the loss of fluid from the body. The eyes become sunken, the skin pinched and dry, whilst severe cramps arise in the muscles owing to the dehydration and loss of salt.

The treatment of cholera lies in the urgent relief of the usual intense dehydration by the use of intravenous fluids. Streptomycin has been used with effect in the treatment of cholera.

TYPHUS FEVER

Included in the term *typhus fever* are many different forms, all of which are caused by a group of organisms called *Rickettsiæ*. These organisms are found in rats and other rodents, and are conveyed to man through the bites of lice, fleas, ticks and mites. The various forms of typhus are seen in different parts of the world under the names of tropical scrub typhus, Rocky Mountain spotted fever (America and Canada), Q fever (Australia, America) and epidemic typhus (Eastern Europe, Asia). The severity of the different forms varies in different outbreaks from a mild to a highly fatal disease.

The characteristics of most forms consist of a sudden abrupt high fever, severe toxæmia and a purpuric rash. The fever usually runs a course of two to three weeks. The forms of typhus which are spread by lice and rat fleas are especially prone to occur in overcrowded camps and institutions where there is a lack of proper hygiene.

In typhus fever general nursing care is most important in order to maintain the patient's resistance. The strictest measures are necessary to prevent the nurse herself and the other patients being bitten by any lice or fleas. Thorough delousing of all patients is necessary. The specific treatment of typhus consists of the administration of one of the tetracycline antibiotics or chloramphenicol, which have a rapid effect in most cases.

PLAGUE

Plague is a highly infectious and often fatal disease seen in tropical areas. It often occurs in widespread epidemics. It is caused by a bacillus which is found in rats and the infection can be conveyed to man by the bite of the rat flea. Two main forms are seen, the *bubonic* where the lymph glands become enlarged, and the *pneumonic* where the principal feature is a severe bronchopneumonia. In both types severe prostration and toxæmia are present and the death rate is high.

In preventing the spread of infection the suppression of rats and their eradication from ships (which can carry infected rats from one area to another) is most important. The treatment of an individual attack consists of the routine nursing care of a severe infectious fever and the administration of streptomycin, which is effective in plague.

LEPROSY

Leprosy which in former years was world-wide in distribution is nowadays mainly confined to Asia and certain parts of the Americas. The causative agent is a bacillus which is generally found in the nasal secretions. It is a chronic disease of which the main effects are on the skin and nerves. The face especially becomes thickened and nodular. In advanced cases destruction of the bones of the nose and face develops and blindness is also common. Affection of the nerves causes loss of sensation leading to trophic ulcers.

Most cases are segregated in special leper colonies so as to prevent spread of the disease. Active therapy consists of the administration of one of the sulfone drugs such as dapsone or the more recently introduced drug, thiambutosine.

RABIES (Hydrophobia)

Rabies is a virus infection which occurs in dogs and is transmitted to man by the bite of an infected dog. It is not seen in Great Britain owing to the strict quarantine enforced on dogs brought into the country. Dogs infected with the virus go mad and die. In man the chief symptoms are severe spasms of the muscles, especially of the throat, and swallowing or even the sight of food or water sets up these spasms: hence the name hydrophobia—fear of water. Death occurs through exhaustion and dehydration.

Preventive action consisting of vaccine treatment for people bitten by a mad rabid dog usually affords complete protection.

TETANUS (Lockjaw)

Tetanus is caused by bacteria which usually gain entrance to the body through wounds, especially deep penetrating stab wounds, e.g., from nails. The bacillus is most commonly present in soil and manure, and wounds so infected are particularly dangerous. The main symptoms are severe muscular spasms which usually start in the jaw muscles, causing difficulty in opening the mouth—lockjaw. The spasms then rapidly spread to other muscles so that the severe muscle spasms become generalised. Death results from exhaustion.

The widespread use of preventive inoculation with tetanus toxoid or antitoxin in all wound cases has reduced the incidence of the disease enormously. In treatment, sedation and curare to control the severe spasms are used, combined with large doses of tetanus antitoxin. In severe cases a tracheotomy may be necessary to ensure a clear airway.

CHAPTER III

TUBERCULOSIS

TUBERCULOSIS is caused by infection with an organism called the *tubercle bacillus*. There are two main types of this bacillus, the human and the bovine, which can be distinguished from each other in the laboratory by their different characteristics. Both are called *acid-fast bacilli*, as they resist the decolorising action of acid on the specimens stained so as to show up the tubercle bacillus under the microscope. Very few other bacteria are acid-fast, so this property is used to identify the organism.

In many cases of infection the tubercle bacilli may, however, be very difficult to find in the material taken for examination, and the diagnosis of tuberculosis is therefore often made on other grounds, such as X-ray examination.

Pathological Lesions caused by the Tubercle Bacillus.—Tuberculosis can affect most organs and tissues in the body, producing a wide variety of lesions of both acute and chronic types. In many ways it is like syphilis in this respect.

Essentially the pathological lesion (or change in the tissues) due to tuberculosis is an inflammatory one of rather a specialised type. The following stages are usually recognisable in a tuberculous lesion, but they may be modified according to the tissue involved. For example, the effects of a lesion in the lung are slightly different from those of a lesion in the bones.

1. **Tubercle Formation.**—The tubercle is a collection of small *endothelial cells* and *lymphocytes* around the bacilli. " Giant " cells typical of tuberculosis occur. These tubercles can gather together so that a wide area of tissue may be affected.

2. Two things may now occur :—

> (A) Caseation.
> (B) Fibrosis.

(A) CASEATION.—This is a breaking down, or necrosis, of the tubercles into a soft cheesy mass which may liquefy to form tuberculous pus. What happens next depends on where the lesion is : *e.g.*, if it is in the lungs, it can rupture into a bronchus and leave behind a cavity; if in a lymph gland, it can produce ulceration with discharge of tuberculous pus, forming a sinus.

(B) FIBROSIS.—Active fibrous-tissue formation can occur around the tubercles. The fibrous tissue constitutes an attempt by the body to wall off the infection and heal the lesion by scar-tissue formation.

In most cases caseation and fibrosis are present together. Marked caseation and slight fibrosis are evidence of severe infection and little effort on the part of the body to heal. Alternatively, when fibrosis is marked, then the disease is usually arrested or limited.

Another way of healing a tuberculous lesion is to lay down calcium in the caseated mass, whereupon the lesion calcifies.

Spread of Tuberculous Lesions within the Body.—Tuberculosis spreads in the body in the following ways :—

1. By direct spread within the tissues or organs, so that wide areas of tissue may be involved.
2. Tubercle bacilli are frequently carried by the lymphatics to the neighbouring lymph glands, and from there they can invade the blood-stream through the thoracic duct.

Mode of Entry of Tubercle Bacilli into the Body—Spread of Tuberculosis.

1. INHALATION THROUGH THE RESPIRATORY TRACT.—This is the commonest route of infection and accounts for nearly all cases of pulmonary tuberculosis. Human tubercle bacilli are expectorated in the sputum in many cases of pulmonary tuberculosis (open cases). Direct contact with such a case can and frequently does set up respiratory disease.

Another way in which pulmonary tuberculosis is frequently contracted is through inhaling dust which contains the tubercle bacilli. The bacilli can live for many months in dust so that they are a constant source of danger.

2. INGESTION.—Tuberculosis commonly affects cows and so the milk may become infected. Drinking such infected milk is a common cause of tuberculosis of the glands, bones and intestines. It is mainly because of the danger of drinking milk infected with the bovine type of tubercle bacilli that such great precautions are taken to provide a sterile milk by pasteurisation. This destroys any tubercle bacilli or other organisms that may be present—in addition to tuberculosis, enteric fever, scarlet fever and diphtheria

may all be spread through contaminated milk. Controlling the spread of tuberculosis in cows by destroying infected animals has also reduced the incidence of bovine tuberculous infections in man.

3. THROUGH THE SKIN.—This type of infection is not common, occurring mostly in butchers, veterinary surgeons, or others who handle infected material. It causes various types of skin lesions.

These then are the usual ways in which man is infected by tuberculosis: by direct contact with a case or inhaling infected dust which cause pulmonary tuberculosis, or by drinking infected milk which causes mainly gland and bone tuberculosis.

CLINICAL TYPES OF TUBERCULOSIS

PULMONARY TUBERCULOSIS

This is to-day by far the commonest type of tuberculosis. It occurs in various forms, according to the virulence of the organism and the powers of resistance of the individual. The following are in brief the main types of pulmonary tuberculosis (see also p. 189 et seq.).

1. Chronic Adult Type (Fibro-caseous Form).

Here caseation and fibrosis occur and it depends on the resistance of the individual which is the more marked. If fibrosis, the infection can be overcome without any really serious damage resulting, the only evidence of disease being a small " spot " seen in an X-ray of the chest, which, without causing much in the way of symptoms, can heal up, usually by calcifying.

On the other hand, when caseation is more in evidence than fibrosis, the disease may spread and the tuberculous pus formed may be coughed up, leaving a cavity in the lungs. In chronic cases the cavity is usually walled off by fibrous tissue. How much of the lung will be damaged before the patient recovers from the disease or dies of it will depend on the resistance of the individual and the treatment given.

2. Acute Pulmonary Tuberculosis.

(a) TUBERCULOUS PNEUMONIA.—This is rare to-day and is seen only in cases where the resistance of the individual is very low. Rapid spread of caseation occurs in the lungs with little or no evidence of healing fibrosis. It is very often fatal.

(*b*) MILIARY TUBERCULOSIS.—This is not, in fact, confined to the lungs but the main lesions may occur here, so that it is usually considered under the heading of pulmonary types. In miliary tuberculosis, tubercle bacilli invade the blood stream and the infection is thus widely disseminated through the body. Lesions resulting from blood-stream infection are usually seen in two places, the lungs and the meninges, causing miliary tuberculosis of the lungs and tuberculous meningitis. Both these diseases may be found together.

(*c*) TUBERCULOUS PLEURISY.—Tuberculous pleurisy, either dry or with fluid present, is a common form of infection. In young people most of the cases of pleurisy where there is no evidence of an underlying lung disease, like pneumonia, are caused by tuberculosis.

EXTRA-PULMONARY TUBERCULOSIS

As mentioned earlier, the tubercle bacilli can invade most organs and tissues and set up disease; therefore very many different forms of extra-pulmonary tuberculosis can occur. It is proposed here to mention only the more common forms.

1. **Tuberculous Glands.**—Tuberculous glands are usually caused by the ingestion of bovine bacilli in milk. This form of tuberculosis is becoming less frequent to-day owing to pasteurisation of milk and the present control of the disease in cows.

(*a*) TUBERCULOUS GLANDS IN THE NECK (Commonest Site).—The cervical glands enlarge and often caseate to form an abscess (*cold abscess*) which ruptures through the skin to become a chronic sinus.

(*b*) TUBERCULOUS INTESTINAL GLANDS.—Formerly very common, these are now becoming rare. They cause the disease tabes mesenterica wherein the mesenteric glands enlarge and cause abdominal pain and wasting.

2. **Tuberculous Disease of the Bones.**—Tuberculous disease of the bones is usually due to the bovine type of bacillus. It causes a chronic inflammation (osteitis) with abscess formation. This abscess can spread from the bone to invade the soft tissues. For instance, when the lumbar spine is involved, pus can track down the psoas muscle and a fluctuating swelling will appear in the groin (*psoas abscess*). Tuberculous disease of the spine is often known as *Pott's disease* of the spine.

3. **Tuberculous Disease of the Joints.**—This is not so common to-day as in former years. Any joint may be affected, with resultant chronic arthritis of the joint.

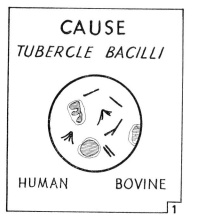

CAUSE
TUBERCLE BACILLI

HUMAN   BOVINE

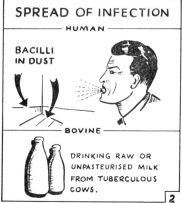

SPREAD OF INFECTION
HUMAN

BACILLI IN DUST

BOVINE

DRINKING RAW OR UNPASTEURISED MILK FROM TUBERCULOUS COWS.

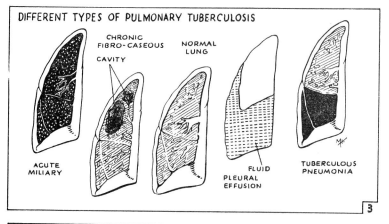

DIFFERENT TYPES OF PULMONARY TUBERCULOSIS

CHRONIC FIBRO-CASEOUS

NORMAL LUNG

CAVITY

ACUTE MILIARY

FLUID
PLEURAL EFFUSION

TUBERCULOUS PNEUMONIA

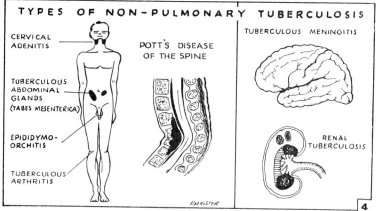

TYPES OF NON-PULMONARY TUBERCULOSIS

CERVICAL ADENITIS

TUBERCULOUS ABDOMINAL GLANDS (TABES MESENTERICA)

EPIDIDYMO-ORCHITIS

TUBERCULOUS ARTHRITIS

POTT'S DISEASE OF THE SPINE

TUBERCULOUS MENINGITIS

RENAL TUBERCULOSIS

HMALSTER

FIG. 22
Tuberculosis.

4. **Tuberculous Peritonitis.**—Tuberculous peritonitis is usually due to spread from the intestinal glands. The chronic inflammation of the peritoneum causes a large outpouring of serous fluid which produces an ascites (fluid in the peritoneal cavity).

5. **Tuberculous Meningitis.**—Tuberculous meningitis is a common form of tuberculous infection which produces a subacute type of meningitis.

6. **Renal Tuberculosis.**—In renal tuberculosis the pelvis of the kidney is affected. Typical symptoms are renal pain and hæmaturia. The disease commonly spreads by direct extension to the ureters and bladder.

7. **Tuberculous Disease of the Genital Organs.**—In males, the prostate, epididymis and testes are mainly involved, causing prostatitis and epididymo-orchitis. In females, the Fallopian tubes are usually affected, causing a tuberculous salpingitis.

8. **Miscellaneous Forms.**

(*a*) Tuberculous laryngitis, due to direct spread from a pulmonary lesion.

(*b*) Tuberculous skin disease. Lupus vulgaris and skin tuberculides are the common forms.

(*c*) Tuberculous ulceration of the tongue and tonsils.

(*d*) Tuberculous ulceration of the rectum (ischio-rectal abscess and fistula).

DIAGNOSIS OF TUBERCULOSIS

At this stage it is important to stress one very vital factor. Tuberculosis is a very common disease in many countries throughout the world and has been for a great many years. As a result, we are all being continually exposed to infection, and it is not hard to appreciate that most of us must, at one time or another, have actually been infected with the bacilli. But why, one may ask, did we not know of it if tuberculosis causes such widespread and serious disease ?

The answer is bound up in that difficult subject—the resistance of the individual and the development of an immunity to a disease. The majority of people by the time they reach adult life have been infected with the tubercle bacillus, but their resistance has been so high that no disease developed. The initial **primary infection,** as it is called, usually occurs in childhood or early adult life and causes serious disease in the body only in severely debilitated and undernourished people or when the infection is extremely heavy and persistent. That this primary infection has occurred can be proved by the presence of old, healed, calcified, tuberculous areas in the lungs, as revealed by X-ray examination.

We can also tell which people have been infected with the tubercle bacilli by means of a test known as the **Mantoux test.** Here 0·1 ml. of tuberculin (*i.e.*, the toxin produced by the bacilli) is injected into the skin, usually on the forearm, whereupon a red raised area develops in those people who have been infected with the tubercle bacilli. This is a positive Mantoux reaction. If no tuberculous infection is or has in the past been present, then a negative reaction will occur. This test is of value in the diagnosis of active tuberculosis in children, but less so with adults because so many people have been infected with the tubercle bacilli by the time they reach adult age that even a positive reaction may reveal merely a past and not a present infection.

In diagnosing tuberculosis, therefore, one must be careful to distinguish between active tuberculous disease and signs of old healed infection.

Steps in Diagnosis.

1. The most important step in diagnosis is to **isolate the actual bacilli,** but as mentioned previously, in many cases the bacilli are present in such small numbers that it may be difficult to do so.

The following materials are often examined for the presence of the tubercle bacilli.

(*a*) SPUTUM—in all cases of suspected pulmonary tuberculosis. Repeated examinations (perhaps as many as six to twelve) may have to be made to ensure not missing a positive test. In patients with suspected pulmonary tuberculosis who have no sputum, repeated gastric lavage first thing in the morning is often performed. The stomach washings are cultured for the tubercle bacilli, with success in many cases.

(*b*) PUS from a suspected abscess.

(*c*) FLUID from the pleural cavity in pleural effusions and from the peritoneal cavity in ascites.

(*d*) CEREBROSPINAL FLUID in a case of suspected tuberculous meningitis.

(*e*) URINE in renal tuberculosis. The whole of the first morning specimen of urine passed is necessary.

2. **X-ray Examination.**—This is of the greatest value, especially in pulmonary forms, as the earliest sign of tuberculous infection is

seen on the X-ray. It is for this reason that all over the country mass-radiography units have been set up, where people can be X-rayed in order to discover at the earliest possible moment any evidence of active tuberculosis even before it has caused symptoms.

X-rays of the bones, joints and renal tract also provide most valuable evidence of tuberculous disease.

TREATMENT OF TUBERCULOSIS

This depends on the form of the tuberculous disease and is discussed in detail under the appropriate section. The following general principles are important.

1. Tuberculosis is a chronic disease and treatment has to be prolonged. One of the most important parts of the treatment in all forms of tuberculosis is rest. This in most cases is best carried out in special hospitals for tuberculosis (sanatoria). Whereas in severe or chronic cases this may mean many months in hospital, in early cases treated by modern methods only the initial treatment need be carried out in hospital and the patient can then be supervised as an out-patient.

2. In any consideration of rest as a therapeutic measure we must include *mental rest* as well as physical. In such a prolonged disease as tuberculosis resulting in a long and tedious stay in hospital with anxiety about loss of work, the mental state of the patient has to be catered for. Tuberculous patients are often very irritable and restless and it is here that the nurse can play a big part, through sympathy and understanding, in relieving the tediousness and anxiety of the disease. Occupational therapy of a suitable nature is also of the utmost importance.

3. All cases of active tuberculosis are nowadays treated by chemotherapy. There are three drugs in common use.

Streptomycin is given by intramuscular injection while *isoniazid* (I.N.A.H.) and *para-aminosalicylic* (P.A.S.) are given by mouth. The drugs must always be given in combination as the tubercle bacillus rapidly becomes resistant to any of these drugs given on its own. Usually, for the first three months of treatment, streptomycin is given daily by injection and a combination of P.A.S. and I.N.A.H. given by mouth two or three times a day. After the first three months, if the condition is quiescent, streptomycin can be discontinued and oral treatment with P.A.S. and I.N.A.H. is maintained for about eighteen months.

Chemotherapy has revolutionised the whole outlook in all forms of tuberculosis. The majority of the acute severe forms of the disease, such as miliary tuberculosis can now be cured: before, most of these patients died.

4. Where possible, surgical removal of the diseased tissue (e.g., resection of the diseased part of the lung or removal of a severely infected kidney) may be carried out in suitable patients.

5. Collapse therapy such as artificial pneumothorax and pneumoperitoneum is nowadays rarely if ever performed in the treatment of pulmonary tuberculosis because of the success of chemotherapy. Selective thoracoplasty, whereby a varying number of ribs are resected to produce permanent collapse and thereby rest the diseased part of the lung, is still however used but to a much lesser extent.

Prevention of Tuberculosis.

It is in preventive measures that the ultimate hope of a real advance in reducing the incidence of the disease lies. Already, by providing a " clean " milk free from infection with tubercle bacilli, the incidence of certain types of bovine tuberculosis has been greatly reduced. It is, however, pulmonary tuberculosis that is so difficult to control at present owing to the expectoration of the bacilli from infected cases and the ability of the bacilli to survive for a long time outside the body.

The ideal measure to prevent spread of pulmonary tuberculosis would be to isolate all " open cases " (patients with tubercle bacilli in the sputum). In view, however, of the large number of such patients and the prolonged course of the disease, it is not practicable to carry out such isolation. This being so, to minimise the spread of infection all patients with pulmonary tuberculosis must be carefully instructed on how dangerous coughing and expectorating can be in spreading the disease. All patients must realise the importance of proper disposal of their sputum and handkerchiefs.

Avoidance of overcrowding, bad housing and undernutrition is of the utmost importance. Routine chest X-rays of all people who are exposed to the risk of tuberculosis (e.g., nurses, doctors and contacts with cases of tuberculosis) are also essential.

Immunisation.

At present the production of an active immunity from tuberculosis by means of a B.C.G. (*Bacille Calmette-Guèrin*) vaccine is being tried on a wide scale. This is particularly so in certain occupations, such as nursing and medicine. Only those people who have a negative Mantoux reaction, showing that they have not already been infected with the tubercle bacilli, are vaccinated. After vaccination a repeat Mantoux test usually shows that the reaction has become positive.

In addition to its use for those nurses and medical students who are Mantoux negative, B.C.G. vaccination of children is also being encouraged. In some countries vaccination shortly after birth is now compulsory and the results appear to be very good. B.C.G. vaccination seems to be of definite value in the prevention of tuberculosis.

CHAPTER IV

VENEREAL DISEASE

SOME diseases occur mainly through sexual intercourse and to these the generic term *venereal disease* is applied. There are about six of these diseases but only two are prevalent in the western countries—syphilis and gonorrhœa—the remainder are more rife in tropical areas.

SYPHILIS

Cause.—Syphilis is caused by a spirochæte called the *Treponema pallidum.*

Spread.—In most cases infection occurs during sexual intercourse, but in a small minority of cases infection is the result of handling infected material (non-venereal infection). An important point with regard to the spread of infection is that the spirochæte, which enters the body through the skin or mucous membrane, can do so only through an abrasion or crack in these areas.

Incidence.—Syphilis is widespread throughout the world, affecting all age groups, but especially adults. A congenital form occurs when the fœtus is infected by a syphilitic mother.

Pathology.—Syphilis affects most organs and tissues and can cause widespread damage. The main lesion is a chronic inflammation which, in healing, causes scarring and weakening in many vital areas.

The arteries are commonly affected, with a consequential danger of thrombosis in these vessels.

Syphilitic lesions tend not to heal completely of their own accord, with the result that the disease is both chronic and progressive if untreated.

Symptoms and Signs.—Syphilitic disease can be divided into three stages :—

1. Primary Stage.

Here the outstanding sign is the initial syphilitic sore or **chancre.** This is most common on the penis in males and on the labia in females. The sore is hard, indurated, and bleeds easily. It causes enlargement of the neighbouring lymph glands.

Other less common sites for the primary sore are the lips and fingers. The sore usually heals in a few weeks.

2. Secondary Stage.

The secondary stage begins a few weeks after the appearance of the primary sore and lasts up to two years. In this stage generalised blood infection occurs, producing several different types of lesion :—

(a) Syphilitic rashes—usually papular or maculopapular. They are symmetrically placed on both sides of the body, are ham-coloured and never itch.

(b) Generalised enlargement of the lymph glands.

(c) Mouth lesions—thin, narrow, white linear ulcers which give rise to the typical " snail-track " ulcers. The tongue may be red, inflamed and fissured (glossitis).

(d) The hair may fall out—syphilitic alopecia.

(e) Anæmia.

(f) General constitutional symptoms of fever, headache and malaise may occur.

(g) Syphilitic meningitis and cerebral thrombosis—meningo-vascular syphilis.

3. Tertiary Stage.

This stage may start as early as two years or as late as fifteen years after the primary sore. In the tertiary stage the disease becomes localised in one or more systems.

The main effects are :—

(a) SKIN LESIONS.—Deep ulcers (gummata) develop, especially on the legs.

(b) BONE LESIONS.—A chronic inflammation of the bones (osteitis) may arise causing a boring pain over the affected bone which is often worse at night. The long bones are most commonly affected.

(c) HEART LESIONS.—These may take several forms :—

(i) Stretching and weakening of the aortic valve ring which causes an aortic incompetence.

(ii) The chronic inflammation and resulting fibrosis of the aortic valve ring may involve the mouths of the coronary arteries. This leads to diminished blood supply to the heart muscle and so may be one cause of the syndrome angina pectoris.

4

(iii) Stretching and weakening of the aorta can progress to produce a wide dilatation known as aneurysm of the aorta. The aneurysm can occur in any part of the aorta.

(*d*) NEURO-SYPHILIS.—In the tertiary stage the central nervous system is commonly invaded so that either of two diseases may develop :—

> (i) Tabes dorsalis.
> (ii) General paralysis of the insane.

(*e*) GUMMA OF THE MOUTH, THROAT AND TONGUE.—Gummatous ulceration causes widespread destruction of the bones of the face and nose. Perforation of the soft palate also occurs. The tongue shows a diffuse glossitis which causes a white hard induration of the surface, called *leucoplakia*.

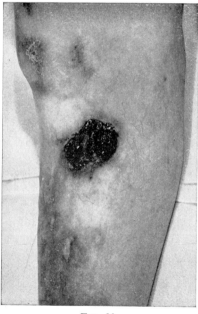

FIG. 23

Typical punched-out gummatous ulcer in the tertiary stage of syphilis. The site of the ulcer in the upper part of the leg contrasts sharply with the common varicose ulcer which usually occurs in the lower part of the leg.

Diagnosis of Syphilis.

1. The primary sore or chancre on the genitals is typical and is rarely mistaken. The spirochæte can be found in the serum taken from the sore.

The specific blood tests for syphilis, of which there are very many, become positive a few weeks after the appearance of the primary sore. The commonest blood tests for syphilis are the **Wassermann** and **Kahn** tests.

2. In the secondary stage, with its symmetrical, ham-coloured, non-itching rashes, enlarged lymph glands and ulcers in the mouth, the blood tests are always positive. In cases of cerebral thrombosis in a young adult, syphilis should always be suspected as a cause.

3. In the tertiary stage the blood tests are often negative. Aneurysm of the aorta is nearly always due to syphilis and may be accompanied by syphilitic aortic incompetence.

Neuro-syphilis is described in a later section.

In any deep chronic ulcer the possibility of syphilis should be investigated.

Treatment of Syphilis.

1. In the primary and secondary stages the nurse must take full precautions to prevent spread of infection, particularly to herself. As mentioned under spread of the disease, handling either infected dressings or the syphilitic lesions themselves can spread the disease. The smallest scratch on the skin is sufficient to allow the spirochæte to enter the body. Rubber gloves and gowns must always be used in dealing with cases in the primary or secondary stages. All dressings must be burned and the patient's feeding and washing utensils must be kept separate. In the tertiary stage there is no danger of spread of infection.

2. The specific treatment for syphilis is the administration of penicillin. Many different schemes of dosage are at present in use, but in the main large total doses of six million units are given over a period of about ten days. Procaine or benzathine penicillin are most commonly used. Nearly all patients respond to penicillin therapy alone.

CONGENITAL SYPHILIS

Syphilis may be transmitted to the fœtus by an infected mother. If this happens in the early months of pregnancy, then a miscarriage often takes place. Alternatively the infant may be born dead ; thus syphilis may be a cause of stillbirth.

Symptoms and Signs.—1. The infant may be born with signs of disease, and if so the infant usually dies. These infants are often wasted and premature.

2. Snuffles due to syphilitic rhinitis (inflammation of the nose) is a very common early sign, usually occurring in infants of about 3 to 6 weeks old.

3. Rashes are also common at 3 to 8 weeks, especially around the napkin area and genitals. Very typical also is a rash on the

palms and soles.   Cracks and fissures round the mouth also often appear at this stage.

4. Bone lesions may cause inflammation of the epiphyseal ends of the bone.

5. Hair may be abundant with bald patches—" syphilitic wig."

6. Later signs often appear at about 6 years of age :—

(a) Hutchinson's notched teeth (notches are present on the permanent upper central incisors).

(b) Periostitis, causing sabre-shaped tibiæ.

(c) Eye changes—interstitial keratitis, leading to blindness.

(d) Mental deficiency.

(e) Neuro-syphilis.   Tabes dorsalis and general paralysis of the insane can occur in young people owing to congenital infection.

The appearance of the child is one of stunted growth and mental development.   Deformity of the nose and mouth due to ulceration may be present.

Treatment.—1. Penicillin is the specific drug to be used as in acquired syphilis, and is given by intramuscular injection.

2. Isolation of the child is necessary to prevent infection of others. The nursing details are as outlined under acquired syphilis.

3. Careful feeding and nursing of the infant are necessary as the child is usually undernourished and wasted.

4. For interstitial keratitis, hydrocortisone eye drops or ointment are instilled at frequent intervals, usually four-hourly, for several weeks in addition to the use of penicillin therapy.   The pupil must also be kept dilated by the use of atropine during the treatment.

GONORRHŒA

Cause.—Gonorrhœa is due to infection by the gonococcus, which is an organism causing an acute, purulent inflammation.

Incidence.—It is a widespread disease, especially common in time of war, as is all venereal disease.

Spread.—Gonorrhœal infection usually occurs in one of two forms :—

(A) Gonorrhœa in the adult through sexual intercourse.

(B) Gonorrhœal infection in the eyes of newborn infants whose mothers have active acute gonorrhœa.

(A) **Gonorrhœa in the Adult.** This may be :—

    1. Acute.
    2. Chronic.

1. ACUTE.—The main lesions in acute gonorrhœa are as follows :

   (a) Acute inflammation of the urethra (acute urethritis) in the male and of the cervix of the uterus in the female. This inflammation causes a thick, purulent, yellow discharge often combined with painful micturition, and is the predominating sign of gonorrhœa.

   (b) The inflammation often spreads to neighbouring organs, causing prostatitis and epididymo-orchitis in the male, and salpingitis and oophoritis in the female. The latter leads to pelvic peritonitis.

   (c) Blood-stream infection develops in some cases, resulting in :—

      (i) Septicæmia, with the organisms growing in the blood. This may be associated with an infective bacterial endocarditis and also a meningitis.

      (ii) Acute arthritis (" gonococcal rheumatism ").

      (iii) Inflammation of the eyes. Iritis and conjunctivitis are common.

2. CHRONIC.—In the late stages the common results of gonorrhœa are a urethral stricture and chronic prostatitis with prostatic abscess in the male, and in the female, chronic salpingitis with sterility.

(B) **Gonococcal Ophthalmia of Infants.**

The gonococcus may set up an acute inflammation of the eyes in an infant as a result of contamination during its birth in cases where the mother suffers from acute gonorrhœa.

Severe conjunctivitis, iritis and corneal ulceration can result and lead to blindness. The presenting sign is a discharge from the eyes of a newborn infant. This may, however, be caused by organisms other than the gonococcus, but in all cases swabs from the eyes are taken to establish the causative organism.

Treatment of Gonorrhœa.

1. PROPHYLACTIC. — Formerly penicillin or sulphacetamide (albucid) drops were usually instilled into the eyes of the newborn infant to prevent ophthalmia. Nowadays, however, antenatal care,

by detecting cases of active gonorrhœa, is the most important item in the prevention of gonococcal ophthalmia of infants.

2. CURATIVE.

(*a*) Practically all acute cases of gonorrhœa will respond to one or two injections of procaine penicillin. In the chronic stages of gonorrhœa, penicillin, in larger doses for a longer period, is also very effective.

(*b*) In the chronic stages, if a urethral stricture is present, dilatation with bougies is performed.

(*c*) For infants with ophthalmia, penicillin is also the best treatment. If only one eye is affected the good eye must be protected by a shield (Buller's shield) and the infant should lie on the affected side.

(*d*) The importance of proper isolation in all cases of active acute gonorrhœa must be stressed. Any discharge present contains the gonococci, therefore the greatest care must be taken in handling all dressings or soiled linen.

All cases of discharge from the eyes in newborn infants must be treated with the strictest isolation procedure. Infection can spread with the utmost rapidity to other infants unless the greatest care is taken. It should be remembered that eye discharges are seen in infants which are caused by other organisms than the gonococcus, *e.g.*, by streptococci or staphylococci. These cases are also extremely infectious and must be treated with strict isolation technique to prevent spread of infection.

CHAPTER V

DISEASES OF THE CIRCULATORY SYSTEM

INTRODUCTION.—The heart acts as a pump to propel the blood throughout the body. The arteries and veins form the pipe-lines by means of which the blood is carried to all organs and tissues and returned to the lungs and heart. The blood in the arteries is the fresh oxygenated blood which supplies the necessary oxygen to all the tissues. The blood in the veins, which contains the waste product from the tissues, carbon dioxide, is carried back to the right side of the heart and is pumped into the lungs by the right ventricle via the pulmonary artery. In the lungs the blood gives up the carbon dioxide, which is expelled into the air, and takes up oxygen. The revitalised blood is now carried to the left side of the heart to be once more pumped into the arteries by the left ventricle.

The heart cycle is divided into two periods—systole and diastole. The systolic period is when the heart is contracting to propel the blood into the lungs and out into the arterial circulation. The right and left ventricles contract at the same time. As can be readily understood, the pulmonary and aortic valves are open during systole to allow the blood to pass through. The atrio-ventricular (auriculo-ventricular) valves (mitral and tricuspid), however, are closed. This is to prevent blood being forced back into the atria (auricles) when the ventricles are contracting. When the ventricles cease to contract the period of rest or diastole begins. At this stage the pulmonary and aortic valves close to prevent wasteful regurgitation of blood back into the ventricles. On the other hand the atrio-ventricular valves, which were closed during systole, now open to refill the empty ventricles in time for the next systole of the heart. The function of the valves is therefore to prevent a wasteful backward flow of blood.

THE PULSE

When the heart beats an impulse is transmitted to the aorta which travels in a wave-like fashion into all the arteries. This impulse can be easily felt when an artery lying near the surface is palpated. In practice the most convenient place to feel this impulse is over the radial artery at the wrist. Feeling the arterial beat is known as " taking the pulse," and is, like taking the temperature, one of the most important routine examinations made. In fact, taking the pulse is so important that it is carried out at frequent intervals with all patients. Why is taking the pulse so important ? Because by taking the pulse we can learn a great deal about the heart's action, and so about the patient's condition. Of course this information can be obtained by listening over the heart with special earphones, known as a stethoscope. This is indeed a routine procedure carried out by doctors in the examination of all patients, but as it is a more complicated technique, it does not fall into the province of the nurse except in certain special circumstances.

In taking the pulse three separate points are to be noted :—

      1. Rate.

      2. Rhythm.

      3. Force.

1. Rate.

The pulse rate tells one the rate of the heart except in those cases where there is an abnormal irregular heart action (see p. 146). The normal pulse rate in adults at rest is about 60 to 80 beats a minute, usually averaging 70. An increase in the heart rate above the normal is known as a **tachycardia** and means that, for some reason, the heart is beating faster than is normal. There are very many causes of a tachycardia but we may conveniently divide them into three groups.

(a) INCREASED METABOLISM CALLING FOR INCREASED OXYGEN REQUIREMENTS.—Any increase in bodily function calls for an increase in oxygen, the essential fuel of the body, and to supply this the heart beats faster to increase its output. This explains the tachycardia of all physical and emotional (fear, excitement, anger) effort. Fever, which is present in all infections and many other types of disease, is associated in nearly all instances with an increased metabolism, and so with a tachycardia. Severe pain likewise causes a tachycardia. In the disease thyrotoxicosis, which creates a marked increase in bodily metabolism, a rapid tachycardia is a feature.

(b) REDUCTION IN THE OXYGEN-CARRYING POWER OF THE BLOOD.—If, for any reason, the capacity of the blood to carry the necessary oxygen to the tissues is much reduced, the heart beats faster. This increases the circulation rate and so makes the reduced number of red cells and hæmoglobin present do more work. This accounts for the tachycardia in anæmias. In cases of shock and hæmorrhage, where the blood volume is reduced and consequently the oxygen-carrying power of the blood, a constant tachycardia is present. The increase in the pulse rate is a most valuable guide to the severity and progress of the shock or hæmorrhage, and it is a routine procedure to take hourly or half-hourly pulse readings. If the rate increases or remains high it is an indication that the hæmorrhage or shock is continuing. Alternatively, a slowing in the pulse rate means that the shock or hæmorrhage is stopping.

(c) HEART DISEASE.—The third main cause of a tachycardia is disease in the heart. In all cases of heart failure the heart is weakened and is unable to pump out into the circulation the normal amount of blood at each beat. To compensate for this and thus supply sufficient oxygen to the tissues, the heart beats faster. Apart from the tachycardia due to heart failure there are also several common types of abnormal irregular heart action associated with a tachycardia (see p. 146). These may or may not be accompanied by actual failure of the heart.

Bradycardia means slowing of the heart rate. Most cases of slowing of the pulse to below 60 beats a minute are due to the irregular heart action known as heart block. Overdosage of some drugs, such as digitalis (which produces a heart block) or morphine, also causes a bradycardia. Lastly, certain diseases of the central nervous system associated with an increased intracranial pressure cause a slowing pulse rate. These diseases include meningitis, cerebral tumour and head injuries.

2. Rhythm.

When taking the pulse the nurse should note whether it beats with a regular rhythm as the normal pulse should. When the pulse is irregular the term *irregular heart action* is used. There are many causes of this, but as the whole subject is one of importance it is dealt with at length later on (p. 146). It is sufficient to state here that when the heart's action is very irregular, the pulse rate may be a fallacious guide to the heart rate. In such circumstances, to obtain the true heart rate it is necessary to listen directly over the heart with a stethoscope. *Auricular fibrillation* is the commonest and most important irregular heart action in which it is often necessary for the nurse to count the heart rate by this means.

4 A

3. Force.

Much is often made of the degree of fullness or volume of the pulse and also of the compressibility or tension. So many factors are, however, involved here that it is inadvisable for the nurse to read too much into these characteristics of the pulse. With practice the nurse will gradually learn what the normal force of the pulse should be. Note should be made, however, if the pulse is very soft and thready, because if so, it is a good indication that the blood pressure is low and may point to such conditions as shock, hæmorrhage, or heart failure.

The Normal Blood Pressure.

In adults the normal *systolic* blood pressure at rest varies on an average from 110 to 150 mm. of mercury. The *diastolic* blood pressure, which measures the blood pressure when the heart is resting, varies from 70 to 90 mm. of mercury.

The blood pressure is taken by a special instrument called a sphygmomanometer.

INDIVIDUAL DISEASES OF THE HEART

Causes of Heart Disease.—There are numerous causes of heart disease but there are seven common causes :—

1. Congenital heart disease.   5. Coronary artery disease.
2. Rheumatic heart disease.   6. Pulmonary heart disease.
3. Syphilitic heart disease.   7. Hypertension.
4. Thyrotoxic heart disease.

CONGENITAL HEART DISEASE

By this is meant an imperfect development of the heart during fœtal life leading to various deformities. There are many types of these and some are so severe that they are incompatible with life, the child either being born dead or dying soon after birth. Less severe deformity of the heart may be compatible with a short period of life : in milder cases still, the normal span of life may be only slightly reduced. The common types of defect which are met with are :—

1. Abnormal opening in the septum separating the auricles or ventricles—called **patent interauricular** and **interventricular septum.**

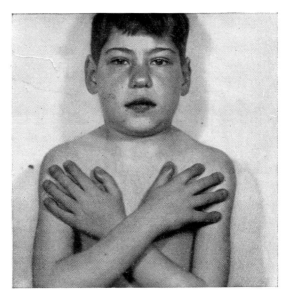

Fig. 24
Congenital heart disease.

[*To face page* 107

2. **Patent Ductus Arteriosus.**—The ductus arteriosus is a normal communication present between the pulmonary artery and aorta which, during foetal life, " shunts " the blood so that it by-passes the lungs which are not expanded. Soon after birth this opening normally closes to allow all the venous blood to go through the lungs, but in some cases it remains open, so causing signs of congenital heart disease.

3. **Pulmonary Stenosis.**—The pulmonary valve may be blocked so that it obstructs the blood going to the lungs from the right ventricle. This is commonly associated with other defects such as a patent septum between the ventricles, and is in these cases given the name of **Fallot's Tetralogy.**

4. **Coarctation of the Aorta.**—In this form of congenital lesion there is a marked narrowing of the arch of the aorta so that the flow of blood into the lower parts of the body through the normal channels is inadequate. The intercostal and other arteries become much bigger and join up with arteries in the lower part of the body so as to carry sufficient blood into the lower limbs. The dilated intercostal arteries may be seen on the chest. Coarctation of the aorta causes a severe hypertension in the upper limbs but not the lower.

Symptoms and Signs common to many Congenital Heart Lesions.— There are several symptoms and signs which lead one to suspect the presence of a congenital heart lesion.

1. AGE OF PATIENT.—In infancy or early childhood a heart lesion is probably congenital because other causes of heart disease do not occur or are very rare. Stunted growth and evidence of mental deficiency are often associated with severe congenital heart disease.

2. CYANOSIS.—This is especially marked around the lips, ears and fingers. Cyanosis may be due to the mixing of the arterial and venous blood as the result of an abnormal connection between the right and left sides of the heart. If the venous blood flows into the left side, there will be an abnormal amount of unoxygenated blood in the arterial system, which causes cyanosis. Cyanosis may also be caused by a poor circulation in the lungs so that there is insufficient oxygen uptake from the lungs. Cyanosis is so marked a feature of many types of congenital heart disease that the term *blue baby* is often used to describe these patients.

3. CLUBBING OF THE FINGERS.—The ends of the fingers and even the toes are often enlarged and may look like " drum-sticks." The

cause of this clubbing is unknown. It is also seen in some chronic respiratory diseases.

Diagnosis.—The diagnosis of congenital heart disease is made on the presence of severe cyanosis, clubbing of the fingers, dyspnœa and characteristic heart murmurs in an infant or young child. To diagnose the exact *type* of congenital lesion present is, however, except with the commoner types, more difficult. The marked advance in recent years of surgical treatment of congenital heart disease has, however, made such exact diagnosis of increasing importance in order to establish whether or not the lesion is of a type amenable to surgical treatment (not all types are).

To help in the diagnosis, specialised X-ray examinations are often carried out after injecting an opaque dye into a vein. The dye outlines the heart and its various chambers, and any abnormality may thus be visualised. This form of X-ray examination is called *angiocardiography.*

Complications.—In many types of congenital heart disease one of the commonest complications is bacterial endocarditis. This is very common in patent ductus arteriosus where infection occurs in the connection between the pulmonary artery and the aorta. It is also likely to complicate coarctation of the aorta.

Treatment of Congenital Heart Disease.—Until recent years very little could be done for congenital heart disease, but now, owing to important advances in surgery, many patients can be improved and some cured.

1. Surgery has produced the most dramatic results in cases of patent ductus arteriosus. The duct is ligatured, thus removing any abnormal strain and also preventing the development of bacterial endocarditis. Bacterial endocarditis which has already supervened on congenital heart disease is treated with penicillin or other antibiotics (p. 117).

2. In patients with Fallot's tetralogy an anastomosis between the pulmonary artery above the level of the stenosis and one of the main arteries, like the subclavian, is made. This allows a more adequate flow of blood into the lungs and dramatically relieves the cyanosis.

In severe cases of pulmonary stenosis with no septal defects a *valvotomy* may be performed to widen the stenosed pulmonary valve and thus allow a free flow of blood into the lungs.

3. In cases of coarctation of the aorta, successful removal of the obstructed part of the aorta has been carried out.

4. More recently, successful repair of auricular septal defects has been carried out.

RHEUMATIC HEART DISEASE

Rheumatic heart disease is the most important cause of heart disease in young and middle-aged people. Rheumatic heart disease occurs in two main forms:—

(A) Acute.   (B) Chronic.

A. ACUTE RHEUMATIC HEART DISEASE

Acute rheumatic heart disease usually occurs in the course of **acute rheumatic fever**, but, in addition, the disease *chorea*, which is dealt with under Diseases of the Nervous System, is allied to rheumatic fever in that rheumatic heart disease often follows an attack of chorea.

Cause.—The cause of acute rheumatic fever is not definitely known but it is associated in some way with streptococcal infection. It usually follows a streptococcal sore throat after a lapse of seven to twenty-one days. One attack gives no immunity; in fact there is a definite susceptibility to recurrences. Most cases occur in young children and the disease is unusual after the age of 25. The younger the patient and the more frequent the attacks, the greater the liability that permanent heart damage will result.

Pathology.—Rheumatic fever is a general infection but it particularly affects:—

1. The heart, causing (*a*) acute rheumatic endocarditis and (*b*) myocarditis and often pericarditis.
2. The joints, causing a non-suppurative arthritis.

(*a*) RHEUMATIC ENDOCARDITIS.—Endocarditis is an inflammation of the endocardium of the heart, affecting particularly the valves of the heart. Endocarditis (valvular disease of the heart), as we shall see later, has many causes, but rheumatic endocarditis is the commonest form in young and middle-aged people.

Characteristic lesions called vegetations occur on the valves as a result of the endocarditis. Vegetations are small clots (thrombi) which look like a row of beads on the valves. These vegetations are composed of fibrin, red cells and platelets, and in contrast to the vegetations which form in bacterial endocarditis, comparatively rarely break off to travel in the circulation and cause embolism,

The valves themselves become swollen and distorted owing to the inflammation.

Acute rheumatic endocarditis produces few signs of its own apart from a blowing murmur in the heart. The presence of an endocarditis in the course of acute rheumatic fever is inferred

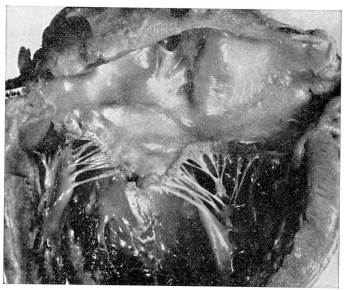

Fig. 25
Acute rheumatic endocarditis of the mitral valve showing the typical row of bead-like vegetations.

from the associated acute myocarditis which causes a rapid and occasionally irregular pulse.

(b) RHEUMATIC MYOCARDITIS AND PERICARDITIS.—In the acute stage of rheumatic heart disease the heart muscle (myocardium) is affected and acute myocarditis is present. Acute myocarditis is of particular importance because death in the acute stage of rheumatic heart disease is usually due to failure of the heart muscle. The unduly rapid and occasionally irregular pulse seen in rheumatic fever is a most important sign of an underlying acute myocarditis.

Inflammation of the pericardium (pericarditis) occurs generally in the more severe cases of acute rheumatic fever. The pericarditis may be dry or wet (pericardial effusion). A large pericardial effusion may press on the heart causing severe embarrassment to an already damaged heart (see p. 144).

Symptoms and Signs of Acute Rheumatic Fever.

1. The onset is often preceded, as mentioned earlier, by a sore throat seven to twenty-one days beforehand.

2. There is general malaise with a high temperature and heavy sweating. The profuse perspiration may cause a sweat rash.

3. The involvement of the joints is very characteristic and the diagnosis of acute rheumatic fever is often made on the joint lesions alone. Pains occur over the affected joints, the typical feature being their *flitting* nature so that different joints are affected at different times. There is swelling and tenderness of the affected joints but seldom to any severe degree. The joints never suppurate as in cases of septic arthritis.

4. The main signs of heart involvement are the very rapid pulse rate and the presence of heart murmurs. The pulse rate is faster than one would expect from the degree of fever, and the rhythm may be irregular. Any irregularity of the pulse must be carefully noted by the nurse as it may be one of the few signs of heart damage.

5. RHEUMATIC NODULES.—These are small fibrous nodules which occur around the joints and tendons, usually behind the elbows, on the back of the scalp, or ankles. They are tender and painful and their presence usually denotes a severe attack affecting the heart.

Treatment of Acute Rheumatic Fever.

1. NURSING.—In the acute stage the patient is kept at complete rest in bed. Everything is done for the patient in the way of feeding, washing and all other necessities. Any sudden exertion may throw a strain on the heart, which, as already stressed, is very liable to be affected in most patients with acute rheumatic fever. As may be realised the nursing of these cases is often very difficult when the patient is a child and has recovered from the acute joint pains. Children find lying still in bed very tedious. It requires a good deal of skill and attention to see that these patients continue to lie quiet and do not sit up in bed and so throw a strain on the heart. The importance of keeping rheumatic fever patients lying still and quiet must be stressed.

If the joints are unduly swollen and painful, wrapping in warm cotton-wool is often most useful to relieve the pains. The affected joints should be protected from the weight of the bed-clothes by bed-cradles.

During the acute stage of the fever light diet only will be needed which will be increased as the acute symptoms subside.

2. DRUGS.—There is no specific cure as yet for acute rheumatic fever although *sodium salicylate* dramatically relieves the joint pains and lowers the temperature. Salicylates have little or no effect on the heart lesions. The drug is usually given in 15 to 30 gr. doses four-hourly. Toxic symptoms may occur from the large doses of salicylates used, but no real harm results as these toxic symptoms rapidly subside when the drug is reduced. Buzzing in the ears (tinnitus), deafness, nausea and vomiting are the usual toxic symptoms noticed.

It is now usual to prescribe a prolonged course of penicillin for many years after an attack of rheumatic fever as there is some evidence that giving penicillin may prevent recurrences. Cortisone or allied steroids are sometimes given in very severe attacks of rheumatic fever accompanied by carditis as it is believed that in some cases the heart lesions may resolve more quickly with steroid therapy.

Convalescence.—Complete rest in bed is enforced until the active stage of the disease is over. This is usually revealed by the return of the pulse rate to normal and by means of a special test known as the **blood sedimentation rate.** When the pulse rate and the blood sedimentation rate have been normal for several weeks, the patient is allowed to feed himself, later to wash himself, and then to sit out of bed for short periods. In severe attacks it may be many months before the patient is allowed to sit out of bed.

SUBACUTE RHEUMATISM OF CHILDREN

In addition to the acute type of rheumatic fever described above there is another common form known as subacute rheumatism of children. Here there is little constitutional upset, the child usually being described as " off colour." There is mild aching in the joints with little or no swelling. This subacute form of rheumatic fever is, however, just as important as the acute, as both give rise to the same liability to chronic heart disease. The treatment of subacute rheumatism of children is the same as for acute rheumatic fever except that convalescence may not have to be so prolonged.

It should be understood that whenever the term *acute rheumatic fever* is used in relation to heart disease, the subacute form is included.

B. CHRONIC RHEUMATIC HEART DISEASE
(Chronic Rheumatic Valvular Disease or Chronic Rheumatic Endocarditis)

Chronic rheumatic heart disease follows the acute stage but many years may elapse before the effects are noticed. Most cases of chronic rheumatic heart disease therefore have a history of acute or subacute rheumatic fever, or chorea, in childhood. In some cases, however, there is no history of the acute stage of the disease, and in these patients it is presumed that the symptoms in the acute stage were so mild that they escaped notice.

Pathology.—In chronic rheumatic heart disease it is the valves that are particularly damaged, chronic inflammation causing thickening, distortion and loss of the normal elasticity. As a result the valves cannot function properly.

Two main effects follow this chronic inflammatory change :—

1. The valves may adhere together, causing a narrowing of the valve opening and obstruction to the flow of blood. This is usually known as stenosis of the valve.

2. Because of the loss of elasticity and distortion of the valve the latter may not close properly, so that a leakage or regurgitation of blood results. This is known as incompetence of the valve.

Chronic rheumatic valvular disease may affect all the valves of the heart but those most commonly damaged are the mitral and aortic valves. A **mitral stenosis** and **aortic incompetence** are the conditions which most commonly arise, although mitral incompetence and aortic stenosis also occur. Quite often mitral stenosis and aortic incompetence develop in the same patient.

Symptoms, Course and Treatment.—Until heart failure results from the added strain on the heart, chronic rheumatic valvular disease may cause few symptoms. Valvular lesions are easily diagnosed, however, if the heart is listened to with a stethoscope, whereupon the characteristic murmurs are heard. Indeed, the first indication of a valvular heart lesion may appear during the course of some routine examination, *e.g.*, for military service or insurance purposes, the patient having previously been unaware of any disease. Enlargement of the heart may also be found owing to the compensatory muscular hypertrophy which takes place to overcome the strain on the heart. In mild cases the patient may suffer little disability and live to an advanced age, but with severe lesions heart failure develops, with death following a few years later.

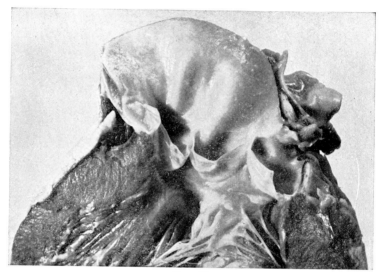

FIG. 26

Normal aortic valve showing the thin elastic cusps. (Compare with Fig. 27.)

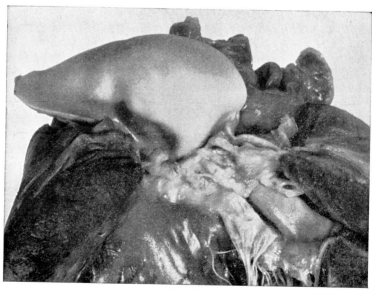

FIG. 27

Chronic rheumatic endocarditis of the aortic valve causing marked distortion and deformity of the valve.

During the prolonged period when there are no symptoms (the condition having perhaps been discovered only through some routine examination), the patient is advised to avoid any undue exertion which might tax the heart too much and so precipitate heart failure.

The operation of *mitral valvotomy* is often carried out in the treatment of mitral stenosis. The stenosed valve is dilated, thus relieving the obstruction. Young patients with progressive and severe dyspnœa and no gross enlargement of the heart are particularly suitable for operative treatment. The initial results of valvotomy have been most encouraging. Valvotomy has also been performed with good immediate results in patients with aortic stenosis.

Complications of Chronic Rheumatic Valvular Disease.

1. HEART FAILURE.—Heart failure, as just mentioned, is the usual outcome of most cases of rheumatic valvular disease. Heart failure is fully discussed later (see p. 133). In those cases where there is a mitral stenosis, irregular heart action in the form of auricular fibrillation is usually present. Auricular fibrillation and its treatment with digitalis are discussed later (see p. 148).

2. EMBOLISM.—In cases of mitral stenosis, particularly if they are accompanied by auricular fibrillation, a clot (thrombus) may form in the enlarged left auricle of the heart. This clot often becomes dislodged with the result that it travels in the circulation, finally most frequently lodging in a cerebral artery, so causing cerebral embolism (one form of apoplexy); the embolus also frequently lodges in a peripheral artery of a leg, giving rise to peripheral embolism and its resultant gangrene of the leg.

Pulmonary embolism may also arise in rheumatic valvular heart disease when heart failure develops. Here the embolus usually comes from thrombosed veins in the legs or pelvis as a result of the sluggish venous circulation which is a feature of heart failure.

3. **Subacute Bacterial Endocarditis.**—This important complication of rheumatic valvular heart disease will be discussed at length.

Subacute bacterial endocarditis is nearly always caused by one organism, the non-hæmolytic streptococcus called the *Streptococcus viridans*. It is important to note that this organism never attacks perfectly normal valves—only those already diseased, usually from rheumatic endocarditis or some congenital lesions. The organisms settle on the valves and cause large vegetations much bigger than those seen in acute rheumatic endocarditis. The vegetations are very easily dislodged into the blood stream to cause the emboli typical of this form of endocarditis.

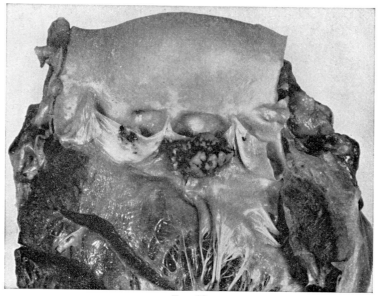

FIG. 28

Subacute bacterial endocarditis showing the typical large, loosely adherent vegetations on the aortic valve. This photograph should be compared with Fig. 25 showing the smaller, more firmly adherent vegetations of rheumatic endocarditis.

Symptoms and Signs.

1. The case most often starts as one of prolonged pyrexia of obscure origin until other signs develop to make the diagnosis clear. The fever is usually high and accompanied by rigors and sweating. These signs are in fact those of a septicæmia, caused by the *Streptococcus viridans* being actually present in the blood stream.

2. The disease is a serious one and the patient is ill and anæmic from the toxæmia.

3. At some period, signs of embolism from the dislodged vegetations appear in most cases. The exact signs depend, of course, on the organs affected by the emboli. The following are the sites most commonly involved :—

BRAIN.—Paralysis in the form of a hemiplegia (paralysis of one side of the body) usually occurs, the patient lapsing into coma for a temporary period.

KIDNEYS.—Emboli lodging in the kidneys cause pain in the loins with blood in the urine (hæmaturia).

SKIN.—Multiple small emboli are common in the skin, producing petechial spots or larger purpuric hæmorrhages. These petechial hæmorrhages are especially common in the nails.

4. In addition to the above there are always murmurs to be heard when the heart is examined by the doctor with a stethoscope. These murmurs are due to the changes in the valves.

Diagnosis.—The diagnosis is often difficult in the early stages when the only sign may be a continuing fever. Aids to diagnosis are :—

1. The presence of a heart murmur.

2. A positive blood culture. To obtain this a small amount of blood (2 ml.) is withdrawn from a vein under strict asepsis to prevent contamination. The blood is put into a blood culture bottle, which contains a special medium (usually glucose broth) to aid the growth of bacteria. The organisms may thus be isolated as the organism is present in the dislodged vegetations which are present in the blood stream. Several blood cultures are often necessary before the bacteria are isolated.

Treatment of Subacute Bacterial Endocarditis.—The discovery of penicillin and other antibiotics has completely changed the outlook in subacute bacterial endocarditis. Before their introduction most of these patients died, but now very many of them recover. Penicillin is to-day the drug of choice; large doses are needed—at least one million units a day in divided doses—and if there is no response (as seen by failure of the temperature to return to normal), then much larger amounts—such as five million units a day—are often given. In resistant cases other antibiotics may be given along with penicillin, for instance, streptomycin. Whatever drug or combination of drugs is used, treatment has to be continued for a prolonged period—at least six weeks.

The usual nursing care of a seriously ill patient is of course necessary. As the illness is a long one, every care and attention to pressure areas is necessary. The high fever, often with rigors, may require tepid sponging.

SUMMARY OF THE COURSE OF RHEUMATIC HEART DISEASE

The usual history is the onset in childhood of acute rheumatic fever, or chorea, which is allied to rheumatic fever. During the attack of acute rheumatic fever or chorea the heart is often damaged.

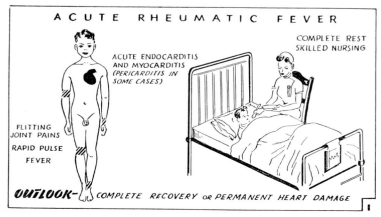

ACUTE RHEUMATIC FEVER

ACUTE ENDOCARDITIS
AND MYOCARDITIS
(PERICARDITIS IN
SOME CASES)

COMPLETE REST
SKILLED NURSING

FLITTING
JOINT PAINS

RAPID PULSE

FEVER

OUTLOOK— COMPLETE RECOVERY OR PERMANENT HEART DAMAGE

1

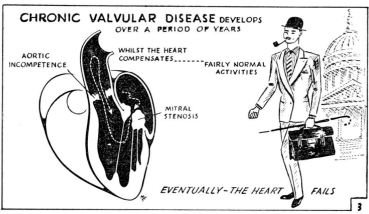

CHRONIC VALVULAR DISEASE DEVELOPS
OVER A PERIOD OF YEARS

WHILST THE HEART
COMPENSATES------

AORTIC
INCOMPETENCE

FAIRLY NORMAL
ACTIVITIES

MITRAL
STENOSIS

EVENTUALLY—THE HEART   FAILS

3

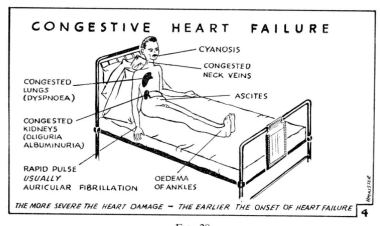

CONGESTIVE HEART FAILURE

CYANOSIS

CONGESTED
NECK VEINS

CONGESTED
LUNGS
(DYSPNOEA)

ASCITES

CONGESTED
KIDNEYS
(OLIGURIA
ALBUMINURIA)

RAPID PULSE
USUALLY
AURICULAR FIBRILLATION

OEDEMA
OF ANKLES

THE MORE SEVERE THE HEART DAMAGE — THE EARLIER THE ONSET OF HEART FAILURE

4

FIG. 29
The course of rheumatic heart disease.

The acute heart lesions may completely clear up when the acute rheumatic fever is over. In many cases, however, after the acute rheumatic fever is over and when to all intents and purposes the child appears to be quite fit, the acute rheumatic endocarditis continues to smoulder, and after a lapse of many years becomes chronic. This chronic endocarditis gives rise to valvular heart disease (usually mitral stenosis or aortic incompetence, or both) in early adult life. At first little disability occurs, the heart compensating for the added strain by myocardial hypertrophy. Gradually, however, signs of failure of the heart develop, causing in the early stages shortness of breath on moderate or severe exertion only. Later, however, marked dyspnœa, cyanosis and œdema occur. Whether or not heart failure will develop early, *i.e.*, within a few years of the initial attack of rheumatic fever, depends on the severity of the damage to the heart. In milder cases heart failure may not occur till middle age or even later still.

In addition to heart failure, embolism (either arterial or pulmonary) and subacute bacterial endocarditis may complicate chronic rheumatic valvular heart disease.

SYPHILITIC HEART DISEASE

Syphilis causes a chronic inflammation of the tissues and organs which results in fibrosis or scarring. The ascending aorta is commonly affected and this produces a marked weakening of the arterial wall. The high pressure on the aorta causes the weakened wall to stretch and eventually gross dilatation results. These changes in the ascending aorta may affect the heart in the following ways :—

1. The marked dilatation of the aorta, which is known as *aneurysm* of the aorta, usually stretches the aortic valve opening and thus produces an aortic incompetence.

2. The syphilitic fibrosis commonly affects the mouths of the coronary arteries (which originate in the first part of the aorta) and so obstructs the flow of blood through these arteries. This, as will be seen when angina pectoris is discussed, may have a serious effect on the heart. Sudden death is a well-recognised feature of syphilitic angina.

Diagnosis.—The presence of aortic incompetence in a middle-aged or elderly person with no evidence of rheumatic heart disease should be suspected as being due to syphilis. The presence of aneurysm is detected by X-ray examination, when the dilated aorta is seen.

In many cases of syphilitic heart disease the specific blood tests (Wassermann and Kahn) are positive.

Treatment.—In the early stages, before the onset of heart failure, antisyphilitic treatment with penicillin is usually given. When failure occurs this is treated in the usual way. The treatment of syphilitic heart disease is, on the whole, very unsatisfactory.

THYROTOXIC HEART DISEASE

Thyrotoxicosis, which is due to overactivity of the thyroid gland, is very liable to damage the heart by causing a degeneration of the myocardium. There is usually a persistent tachycardia and very often an irregular heart action of the type known as *auricular fibrillation.* The pronounced tachycardia is caused by a marked increase in the general metabolism produced by the overactivity of the thyroid gland. Increased metabolism means increased work for the body, and this calls for more oxygen. To supply this the output of the heart has to be increased, and this is brought about by the heart beating faster, *i.e.,* tachycardia. If the thyrotoxicosis is allowed to go untreated, permanent damage with congestive heart failure very often develops.

Diagnosis and Treatment.—This will be more fully discussed under Diseases of the Ductless Glands. The patient may be given one of the antithyroid drugs such as carbimazole (neo-mercazole), or else operation to remove part of the thyroid is undertaken. Radioactive iodine is also used. Any congestive heart failure or auricular fibrillation present is treated on the usual lines.

CORONARY ARTERY DISEASE

Arteriosclerosis (atherosclerosis) is a degenerative disease of the arteries which is seen most commonly in the second half of life. It frequently affects the coronary arteries; the vessels become thickened and narrowed, thus reducing the blood supply to the myocardium. In the early stages the reduced blood supply may be sufficient for normal activity, but extra exertion produces symptoms of heart disease, usually in the syndrome known as angina pectoris. Again, the thickened degenerated vessels are very liable to become the site of thrombosis, and the condition of coronary thrombosis then arises. The two clinical effects of coronary arteriosclerosis are, therefore, angina pectoris and coronary thrombosis.

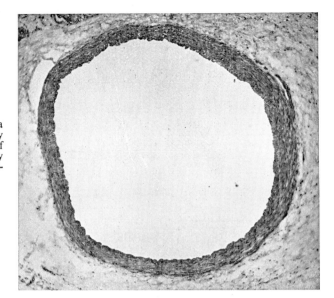

FIG. 30

Photomicrograph of a normal coronary artery showing the width of the lumen of the artery in relation to the thickness of the walls.

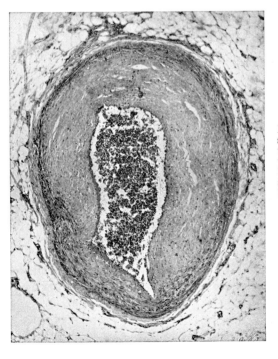

FIG. 31

Photomicrograph of an arteriosclerotic coronary artery showing the marked thickening of the wall which results in diminished blood supply to the heart. In addition, in this case, a thrombus has formed in the coronary artery blocking the circulation.

ANGINA PECTORIS

This is a clinical syndrome produced by a reduction in the blood supply to the muscle of the heart. When a muscle has to work with a deficient oxygen supply a severe cramping pain occurs. This pain, due to oxygen deficiency, is common to all muscles : an example can readily be provided by applying a blood-pressure cuff to the arm and opening and shutting the hand several times. This, after a time, brings on severe pain in the hand which is due to the lack of oxygen caused by cutting off the blood supply by the blood-pressure cuff.

In angina the pain is characteristically felt across the upper part of the chest and it most frequently radiates down the left arm. It may also radiate into the right arm, into the neck, or, more rarely, into the upper abdomen. It is of a dull, gripping nature. It results from exertion, the patient usually stating that he notices it when he goes up an incline or climbs stairs. The pain is relieved by rest. The patient usually stops and after a minute or so the pain passes off. It is only in very advanced cases that the pain comes on at rest.

Causes of Angina.—The majority of cases are due to arteriosclerosis of the coronary arteries. Another common cause is syphilitic narrowing of the mouths of the coronary arteries, causing obstruction to the blood flow. As the pain is produced by a lack of oxygen supply to the muscle, angina is also seen in some cases of severe anæmia where there is an oxygen deficiency.

Treatment of Angina.—There is no specific treatment which cures angina and all measures merely relieve the pain and try to prevent extra strain on the damaged heart. The patient is warned to make no exertion which will bring on the pain. This, in many cases, means altering his mode of living. Apart from physical exertion, the patient must also be advised of the danger of overexcitement or emotional upset, both of which increase the work of the heart considerably. Patients suffering from angina are often of a highly strung nature and inclined to worry. This anxiety factor must be overcome and, in addition to the usual advice to the patient to " take things more easily," sedative drugs such as small doses of phenobarbitone are useful. Diet is also of importance in angina. Obesity, if present, throws an added strain on the heart, and therefore a low calorie diet is given to reduce the patient's weight to normal or slightly below normal. Individual meals must always be light, because a heavy meal increases the work of the heart to an appreciable extent ; indeed, anginal pain may be noticed after a heavy meal, the patients imagining they suffer from " indigestion."

Several drugs, apart from the sedatives already mentioned, are used in the treatment of angina, all of which act by producing a dilatation of the coronary arteries and thus improving the blood supply to the heart. Amyl nitrite is in the form of a capsule, which the patient crushes, then inhaling the drug. Glyceryl trinitrate (trinitrin) ($\frac{1}{130}$ gr.) is in the form of a tablet, which is allowed to dissolve under the tongue. Longer-acting nitrites may be used in conjunction with trinitrin, *e.g.*, pentaerythritol tetranitrate (Peritrate, Mycardol), which is given in doses of 10 to 20 mgm. three times a day.

CORONARY THROMBOSIS

Coronary thrombosis is a complication of coronary arteriosclerosis in that a clot is very likely to occur in the roughened and narrowed arteries. The clot cuts off the blood supply to the area of the myocardium supplied by the affected artery. The heart muscle undergoes the changes described under infarction (p. 6). The severity of the condition depends on how large a part of the myocardium is involved and may vary from sudden death to a moderately serious illness.

Symptoms and Signs.—The onset is often very sudden but there may be a previous history of angina pectoris, as the cause of both conditions is in most cases the same. The patient experiences a very severe pain in the upper part of the chest which, though similar to the pain of angina pectoris, differs in the following respects :—

(*a*) It lasts much longer, hours or days instead of minutes.

(*b*) It comes on usually at rest and not on exertion.

(*c*) The pain is often accompanied by vomiting.

(*d*) It is often associated with the signs of shock, the patient being cold and clammy, and the pulse fast and feeble.

(*e*) The blood pressure falls and difficulty in breathing and cyanosis may be present.

Diagnosis.—Severe attacks of angina may be difficult to distinguish from the milder attacks of coronary thrombosis. In most cases, however, the diagnosis of coronary thrombosis may be confirmed by an electrocardiogram. This is a tracing of the heart's action taken by means of a special instrument which records the electrical impulses from the heart beats. If the heart is normal, a typical tracing is produced; in coronary thrombosis the normal electrocardiogram is altered in a specific manner.

In coronary thrombosis there is usually a marked rise in the level of transaminase in the blood and estimations of the serum transaminase (S.G.O.T.) are usually carried out for the first three or four days to confirm the diagnosis.

Course and Complications.—Some patients may die in their first attack and the nurse should realise that coronary thrombosis is a frequent cause of sudden death. In other cases repeated attacks occur and chronic heart failure develops. The causes of death and the chief complications in coronary thrombosis are :—

(*a*) HEART FAILURE.

(*b*) RUPTURE OF THE HEART.—This may arise owing to the pressure of the blood in the heart forcing a way through the severely damaged muscle out into the pericardial sac.

(*c*) EMBOLISM.—In some cases of coronary thrombosis the endocardium overlying the infarcted muscle becomes inflamed and roughened (endocarditis). A further clot is then very liable to occur over the damaged endocardium and to form what is called a mural (wall) thrombus in the heart cavity. This mural thrombus may become detached, travel in the arterial circulation and lodge in some artery, thus causing embolism. The cerebral arteries are frequently affected, so giving rise to one cause of apoplexy (stroke), with its usual residual paralysis. Another common site for embolism is a peripheral artery of the lower limbs, resulting in gangrene of that part of the limb deprived of its blood supply.

Pulmonary embolism also frequently occurs in coronary thrombosis. In these cases the clot usually comes from the veins in the legs.

Treatment of Coronary Thrombosis.

1. From the description of the disease and the grave possibilities that may arise it will readily be understood with what great care the patients have to be nursed. Absolute rest is required, which means that everything possible must be done for the patient. In severe attacks even so slight a strain as turning in bed or reaching out for a drink from an awkwardly situated bedside locker may prove too much for a badly damaged heart. The patients must be told that they must ask for all their requirements and not try to do things for themselves. This is important as some patients, not knowing the seriousness of their illness, may try to be helpful and " not bother the nurse."

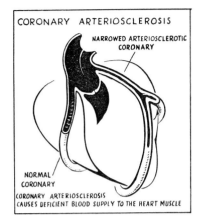

CORONARY ARTERIOSCLEROSIS

NARROWED ARTERIOSCLEROTIC CORONARY

NORMAL CORONARY

CORONARY ARTERIOSCLEROSIS CAUSES DEFICIENT BLOOD SUPPLY TO THE HEART MUSCLE

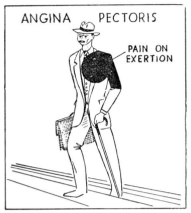

ANGINA PECTORIS

PAIN ON EXERTION

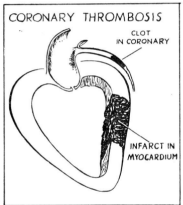

CORONARY THROMBOSIS

CLOT IN CORONARY

INFARCT IN MYOCARDIUM

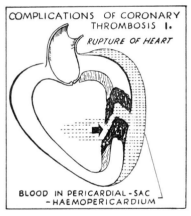

COMPLICATIONS OF CORONARY THROMBOSIS I.

RUPTURE OF HEART

BLOOD IN PERICARDIAL-SAC -HAEMOPERICARDIUM

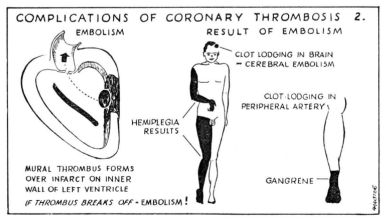

COMPLICATIONS OF CORONARY THROMBOSIS 2.

EMBOLISM

RESULT OF EMBOLISM

CLOT LODGING IN BRAIN - CEREBRAL EMBOLISM

CLOT·LODGING IN PERIPHERAL ARTERY

HEMIPLEGIA RESULTS

MURAL THROMBUS FORMS OVER INFARCT ON INNER WALL OF LEFT VENTRICLE

IF THROMBUS BREAKS OFF - EMBOLISM!

GANGRENE

FIG. 32
Coronary artery disease.

The diet must be light, as a heavy meal throws too great a strain on the heart. Similarly constipation, which may cause abdominal distension and also straining at stool, produces a very considerable

TABLE IV

	HEPARIN.	PHENINDIONE, WARFARIN, DICOUMAROL.
Administration	By intravenous injection every 4 to 6 hours, or intramuscularly every 8 to 12 hours.	By mouth in single or divided doses.
Rapidity of action	Immediate.	18 to 48 hours for full effect. Phenindione and warfarin take effect in 24 to 36 hours and dicoumarol in 36 to 48 hours.
Danger . .	Hæmorrhage.	Hæmorrhage, especially hæmaturia.
Antidote .	Immediately neutralised by intravenous injection of 5 ml. of protamine sulphate.	Vitamin K_1, 5 to 20 mgm. orally or intravenously, repeated if necessary. Takes 2 to 6 hours to act. Blood transfusions essential with severe hæmorrhage.
Clinical use .	Best given at onset of attack of thrombosis till phenindione or other drugs take effect.	Better than heparin for long-term treatment, as they can be given by mouth.
Control . .	...	Prothrombin estimations (a form of clotting time) essential.
Average dose .	Depends on the clotting time. Usually 5,000 units every 4 to 6 hours intravenously, or 12,500 units every 12 hours intramuscularly.	Depends on the preparation used and on the prothrombin time. Phenindione: 200 mgm. on first day, 100 mgm. on second day. Maintenance doses are usually 50 to 200 mgm. daily. Warfarin: 35 to 50 mgm. as initial dose. Maintenance doses are usually 3 to 15 mgm. daily. Dicoumarol: 300 mgm. on first day, 200 mgm. on second day, followed by daily maintenance doses of 50 to 100 mgm.

strain on the heart and must be avoided at all costs. A regular aperient such as senokot is very useful. It should be remembered, however, that the bowel habits of different people vary a good deal, some people requiring frequent aperients whilst others seldom need drugs in order to have a bowel action. Again, many people have found from experience that a particular aperient is always effective whilst others are not. The nurse should therefore anticipate any possible difficulties with regard to the bowels and ask the patient what, if any, aperient he has been accustomed to take and, if the doctor approves, should use that aperient.

2. In severe cases, with breathlessness and cyanosis, oxygen will be given. Morphine ($\frac{1}{4}$ gr.) will be needed for the severe pain and shock, and repeated injections are often necessary in the first day or so. In addition to relieving the pain and shock, morphine provides much needed rest and allays anxiety.

In profoundly shocked patients, attempts must be made to raise the blood pressure. Intramuscular injections of metaraminol (aramine) or mephentermine (mephine) are often successful, but sometimes noradrenalin (levophed) has to be given by intravenous drip. If possible, the systolic blood pressure should be maintained above 100 mm. of mercury.

3. ANTICOAGULANT DRUGS.—These drugs are very useful in that they may prevent the extension of the clot in the coronary artery and, also, even more important, may lessen the risk of embolism, either arterial or pulmonary. Anticoagulant drugs act by increasing the clotting time of the blood and so reduce the likelihood of further clot formation. There are many different anticoagulant drugs available, but those in most frequent use at present are probably heparin, phenindione (Dindevan), marcoumar, dicoumarol and warfarin sodium (marevan). Heparin has an immediate action and is, therefore, often given at the onset of an attack of thrombosis and then followed by any of the other drugs. Phenindione, warfarin, and dicoumarol, provided that there is skilled laboratory control, produce a more constant and satisfactory action than heparin. Moreover, heparin has the disadvantage of having to be given by injection at frequent intervals. The properties and use of heparin and the other anticoagulants are summed up in Table IV (p. 126). Certain drugs, such as aspirin, must be avoided, whilst oral antibiotics should be given only with great care while the patient is taking anticoagulant drugs as they increase the danger of hæmorrhage.

The patient is kept in bed for at least four weeks, and in severe cases for much longer. The return to normal activity must be very gradual. In view of the permanent underlying coronary arterio-sclerosis, the instructions outlined under angina must be carried out.

The use of long term anticoagulant therapy over an indefinite period to try and prevent further attacks of coronary thrombosis is at present being tried, so far with promising results.

As there is some evidence that a diet containing a high proportion of saturated fats (dairy fats such as butter, eggs, meat fat and cheese) increases the cholesterol in the blood and predisposes to atherosclerosis, the patient may be prescribed a diet which restricts the amounts of these fats. Certain unsaturated fats (vegetable oils such as corn (maize) oil), which are thought not to be harmful, may replace the saturated (dairy) fats in the diet.

Nicotinic acid or triparanol can also be given as tablets to reduce the blood cholesterol where this is too high.

PULMONARY HEART DISEASE

Chronic diseases of the lungs, most commonly chronic bronchitis and emphysema, may in severe cases cause heart failure. This is due to the added strain on the heart of pumping the blood through the diseased lungs. When heart failure develops as a result of chronic bronchitis and emphysema it is treated in the usual manner as described later. Unfortunately the treatment of the lung condition itself is not very effective.

HYPERTENSION (High Blood Pressure)

Hypertension is one of the commonest and most important diseases in medicine. To illustrate its importance it is enough to say that almost a quarter of all deaths in elderly people are due to hypertension or its complications. A raised blood pressure may be caused by many different diseases, e.g., chronic nephritis, toxæmias of pregnancy and tumours of the adrenal gland. In the vast majority of cases of hypertension, however, no definite cause can be found. This type of hypertension is given the name **essential hypertension.**

Many different theories have been put forward to try and explain the cause of essential hypertension, and at present the main focus of attention is the kidneys. When there is a diminished blood supply to the kidneys (renal ischæmia), these organs excrete a substance into the blood called *renin*. Renin interacts with other substances in the blood to cause a widespread constriction of the arteries, which in turn causes a raising of the blood pressure. This sequence of events has been proved in experimental work on animals, when clamping the renal arteries brings about a renal ischæmia and renin is excreted. The blood pressure of the animal then rises. The difficulty in accepting this theory as the explanation of essential hypertension in man is that it does not explain what causes the initial renal ischæmia, *i.e.*, it does not explain why the blood supply to the kidneys was deficient in the first place.

However, whatever may be the exact cause of the raised blood pressure there is no doubt that certain factors are involved: there

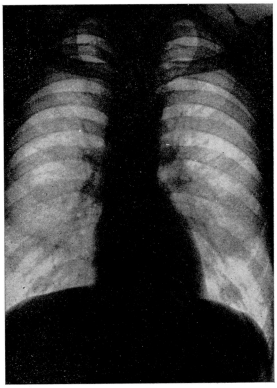

FIG. 33

X-ray showing the shape and size of the normal heart and also the X-ray appearance of the normal lungs.

is a strong familial tendency in most cases, and excessive strain, especially mental strain, also plays a part.

Pathology.—The effects of the increased pressure in the arteries are numerous and in most cases serious.

1. The left ventricle of the heart enlarges and hypertrophies to counteract the extra pressure in the arteries. Eventually, if the strain becomes too severe the heart cannot cope and heart failure sets in.

2. The renal arteries, owing to increased pressure, become

5

thickened and narrowed, which leads to a diminished blood supply to the kidneys. This causes in turn a loss of function and may lead to chronic renal failure (uræmia).

3. The raised pressure commonly causes rupture of certain arteries, especially the cerebral arteries. This results in cerebral hæmorrhage (apoplexy or stroke).

4. The continuous raised pressure often aggravates or predisposes

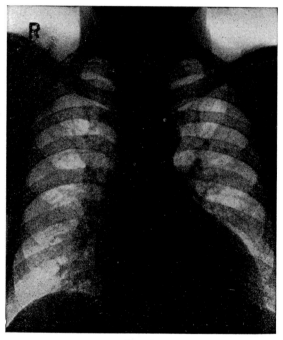

FIG. 34

X-ray showing a markedly enlarged heart due to hypertension.

to sclerotic changes in the arteries with the result that angina pectoris, coronary thrombosis and cerebral thrombosis are all frequently seen in association with hypertension.

Symptoms.—Hypertension is often present for many years— perhaps ten or fifteen—during which it causes few symptoms. Headache, giddiness, ringing in the ears and epistaxis are the commonest early symptoms. Eventually, however, owing to the

CAUSE

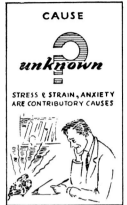

unknown

STRESS & STRAIN, ANXIETY ARE CONTRIBUTORY CAUSES

SYMPTOMS

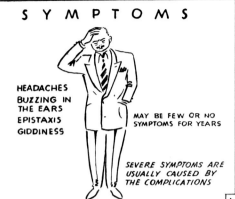

HEADACHES
BUZZING IN THE EARS
EPISTAXIS
GIDDINESS

MAY BE FEW OR NO SYMPTOMS FOR YEARS

SEVERE SYMPTOMS ARE USUALLY CAUSED BY THE COMPLICATIONS

COMPLICATIONS

SPHYGMOMANOMETER

HIGH B·P
200

NORMAL B·P
140

THE ADDED STRAIN ON THE HEART FROM THE EXCESSIVE ARTERIAL PRESSURE CAUSES —

ENLARGEMENT OF THE HEART

EVENTUALLY THE HEART FAILS —
CONGESTIVE HEART FAILURE

HYPERTENSION
AGGRAVATES OR PREDISPOSES TO
CORONARY ARTERIOSCLEROSIS

NARROWED ARTERIOSCLEROTIC ARTERIES CAUSE DEFICIENT BLOOD SUPPLY.

results ANGINA PECTORIS
CORONARY THROMBOSIS

CEREBRAL HAEMORRHAGE (STROKE)

EXCESSIVE ARTERIAL PRESSURE RUPTURES A CEREBRAL ARTERY

HYPERTENSIVE KIDNEY DISEASE

A FEW CASES OF HYPERTENSION DIE OF RENAL FAILURE (URAEMIA)

FIG. 35
Hypertension.

persistently increased pressure against which the heart has to work, heart failure develops.   In addition, the patients may complain of anginal pain resulting from coronary arteriosclerosis, since hypertension predisposes to the occurrence of coronary arteriosclerosis.   For the same reason, coronary thrombosis is common in hypertensive people, whilst another frequent result of hypertension is apoplexy caused by a cerebral hæmorrhage.

In severe cases of hypertension attacks known as *hypertensive encephalopathy* may arise.   Severe headaches, vomiting, convulsions and paralysis are usually present.   These attacks are also particularly frequent in the form of hypertension called **malignant hypertension.** Here, in contrast to the prolonged course of the more usual type of essential hypertension (often called benign essential hypertension to contrast it with the malignant form), the whole tempo of the disease is much more rapid and death takes place within a few years of the onset.   The kidneys are especially affected in malignant hypertension and renal failure (uræmia) is a frequent feature.   Malignant hypertension also tends to affect much younger people than the benign form.

Treatment.—There is no specific cure for hypertension.   As mental strain is an important factor, patients are advised to avoid as far as possible all worry and emotional upsets and to lead a relatively quiet life.   Sedatives such as phenobarbitone are very useful to relieve strain.   If obesity is present, a reduction in weight is advisable and a low calorie diet should be prescribed.   Venesection of a pint of blood at periodic intervals is often useful in reducing a high blood pressure for a short time.

Patients with the more severe grades of hypertension are treated with hypotensive drugs.   Unfortunately most of the hypotensive drugs at present available are very liable to cause severe side-effects when given in doses large enough to be effective.   New drugs are continually being introduced in an effort to provide effective hypotensive therapy with a minimum of side-effects.

The hypotensive drugs most frequently used at present include :—

(*a*) Guanethidine (ismelin) 10 to 20 mgm. once a day as an initial dose, gradually increased until the blood pressure is controlled.   It acts by relieving sympathetic nerve constriction of blood vessels and can lead to a dangerous fall in blood pressure after exercise.   Another drug of this type is darenthin (bretylium).

(b) Mecamylamine (inversine) and pentolinium (ansolysen) are occasionally used where ismelin is ineffective. They are efficient in lowering the blood pressure but give rise to severe constipation, dryness of the mouth and blurred vision.

(c) Rauwolfia and its alkaloid reserpine (serpasil) are milder hypotensive agents with a sedative effect. If given for too long a time, severe mental depression and trembling of the hands may result.

The action of these hypotensive drugs is greatly enhanced when the oral diuretic chlorothiazide (saluric), or one of its derivatives, is given at the same time.

During the initial period of stabilisation on hypotensive drugs, care must be taken to increase the dose only gradually, since the blood pressure may fall suddenly. If the patient is in the ward, the blood pressure must be recorded daily.

CHRONIC HEART FAILURE

We have so far discussed the common causes of chronic heart disease and we have seen that many heart diseases cause symptoms only when failure of the heart develops. Before this stage the diagnosis of many forms of heart disease depends on the presence of signs which definitely indicate that the heart is not normal. Such signs include heart murmurs, irregular heart action and an enlarged heart. X-ray examination usually confirms or establishes the presence of an enlarged heart which, in nearly all cases, means that the heart is permanently damaged. Lastly, an electrocardiogram may show evidence of a diseased myocardium, particularly if it has been caused by coronary artery disease.

Chronic heart failure is usually the result of long-standing chronic heart disease which eventually affects the heart by severe strain over a long period. The heart usually enlarges and the muscle hypertrophies to overcome the added strain. This allows the heart for a time to act more efficiently. The stage is reached, however, when the enlargement and hypertrophy of the heart result in a severe weakening of the myocardium, and at this time heart failure develops.

If the strain on the heart is on the left side only, as commonly occurs in some heart diseases, then the left side of the heart may fail while the right side may continue to function normally. This stage is called left heart failure. Ultimately, however, failure of the left side of the heart throws a burden on the right side and this in turn fails, whereupon right heart failure, or as it is more often termed, *congestive heart failure*, arises.

LEFT HEART FAILURE

Here, as noted above, the strain is on the left ventricle. This commonly occurs in :—

(a) Hypertension.

(b) Aortic valvular disease.

(c) Coronary artery disease.

Symptoms and Signs.—These are caused by failure of the left ventricle to pump the blood from the left side of the heart into the arterial system, with the result that as the right side of the heart continues to function properly, blood accumulates in the lungs causing severe congestion. We have then a condition wherein the right side of the heart continues to pump blood into overloaded and congested lungs.

The cardinal symptom is dyspnœa, which occurs on any moderate exertion. It may also come on, however, at night, waking the patient up from sleep gasping for breath, so that he has to sit up in bed, and often goes to an open window for more air. Gradually the attack passes off. These attacks are called paroxysmal nocturnal dyspnœa or **cardiac asthma.** The signs present depend on the cause of the left heart failure and may include a raised blood pressure, or signs of aortic valvular disease, such as murmurs. In addition, the pulse is usually rapid and may be irregular in rhythm. In all cases of left heart failure the left ventricle of the heart is enlarged. It should be noted that the signs of gross congestion in the venous system and the œdema, which are both so prominent in congestive (right-sided) heart failure, are absent at this stage.

Treatment.—For the attacks of cardiac asthma, morphine ($\frac{1}{4}$ gr.) combined with atropine ($\frac{1}{100}$ gr.) is of great value and usually relieves the attack fairly quickly. In addition to morphine, oxygen must be given. Another drug of value is aminophylline (0·25 gm. given intravenously or 0·5 gm. intramuscularly).

Between the attacks the patient should be advised not to over-exert to any extent that would cause undue dyspnœa and so increase the strain on the already overladen heart. A low salt diet and diuretics as in congestive failure may be ordered to reduce the congestion in the lungs.

CONGESTIVE HEART FAILURE

Congestive heart failure is the stage when the right side of the heart has ceased to function efficiently in pumping the blood from

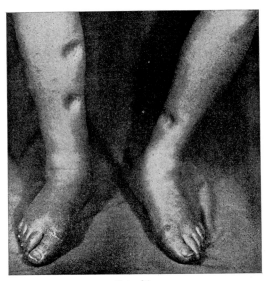

FIG. 36
Pitting œdema of the legs in a case of
congestive heart failure.

the right side of the heart and venous system, forward, into the lungs. Therefore the blood becomes dammed back in the venous system so that severe congestion arises. Hence the descriptive term *congestive failure.*

Causes.—The seven common causes of chronic heart disease, which may all eventually give rise to congestive failure, have already been given (p. 106). Some of these diseases may first cause left heart failure, whilst in others the right side of the heart is affected from the start. For instance, in chronic chest diseases, especially chronic bronchitis and emphysema, congestive (right-sided) failure develops without going first through the stages of left heart failure.

Symptoms and Signs.

1. DYSPNŒA.—This is the cardinal symptom of congestive heart failure as it is of left heart failure. In congestive failure, however, the degree of dyspnœa is much more severe and usually occurs even on mild exertion, such as walking up an incline, climbing a flight of stairs, or walking fast on the flat. In very severe cases the patient may even be breathless lying in bed. Here the peculiar type of breathing known as Cheyne-Stokes respirations may be present; the respirations wax and wane so that there are periods of deep, gasping respirations followed by periods of very quiet breathing. Cheyne-Stokes breathing denotes an advanced degree of failure.

2. CYANOSIS.—This is due to the stagnation of the blood in the venous system, and also to the severe congestion in the lungs causing imperfect oxygenation of the blood.

3. THE PULSE.—In congestive failure the pulse is usually rapid and may be regular or irregular. The commonest type of irregularity of the pulse met with is auricular fibrillation.

4. The veins in the neck are distended and stand out owing to the venous congestion.

5. The congested lungs, in addition to producing the cardinal symptom of dyspnœa, also cause a cough and often hæmoptysis. The latter is, however, never very severe.

6. The kidneys are also congested and this leads to a diminished output of urine (*oliguria*). The urine is usually highly concentrated, dark in colour, and contains albumin.

7. Congestion of the stomach and the intestines produces symptoms of dyspepsia, such as nausea, heartburn and vomiting.

8. ŒDEMA.—Œdema means the presence of fluid in the tissues. In congestive heart failure the fluid accumulates owing to the increased pressure in the venous circulation which forces fluid from the veins into the tissues. As the pressure in the venous circulation is greatest in the lower part of the body, œdema is usually first noticed around the ankles when the patient is up and about. In the later stages the fluid increases so that the legs become grossly swollen.

If the patient is in bed the œdema is usually most marked around the sacrum, producing the well-known sacral cushion or pad. This is because while the patient is in bed the sacral area becomes the lowest part of the body and the fluid sinks into this area.

The fluid may also accumulate in the different cavities of the body, such as the pleural cavity, producing what is known as a hydrothorax, and in the peritoneal cavity causing *ascites*.

In contrast to the œdema which is present in kidney disease—renal œdema—the face is never affected. This is because, as mentioned above, cardiac œdema is due to the increased pressure in the veins which causes the fluid by the force of gravity to settle in the lowest parts of the body.

Increased venous pressure is thus an important factor in the causation of cardiac œdema. In addition, there is the question of salt retention. In cardiac failure the kidneys fail to excrete salt properly and this retention of salt in turn causes retention of water.

TREATMENT OF CONGESTIVE HEART FAILURE

1. **Nursing.**—The patient is nursed at complete rest sitting up in bed. Patients with heart failure are unable to lie flat as this increases the congestion of the lungs and so increases the dyspnœa. A bed-table on which the patient can lean is very useful. In many cases, however, the patient prefers to sit up in a chair so as to avoid the slipping down which may occur in bed. In addition, special beds known as cardiac beds, to keep the patient well propped up in a sitting position, are available.

2. **Diet.**—This is of great importance in the treatment of congestive failure. Firstly, the diet must be light and easily digestible so as to avoid overloading the already congested gastro-intestinal system. Obesity, which throws an extra strain on the heart, will call for a further reduction in the diet. Secondly, the restriction of salt is essential. In congestive failure the kidneys fail to excrete salt properly, which is therefore retained in the body. Retention of salt causes a retention of water; therefore restricting salt is most valuable in relieving and preventing œdema. Usually a moderate restriction of salt will suffice to get rid of the œdema. No salt must be used in cooking or added at table, and very salty foods such as bacon, pickled meats, sausages, kippers, haddock, and gravies must be avoided. For a few patients, however, an even more restricted salt diet is needed and here all the foods containing more than a minimum of salt must be omitted from the diet (see Fig. 38). A very low salt diet usually contains about 500 mgm. of sodium a day, whilst a moderate low salt regime contains

5 A

approximately 1,000 mgm. of sodium daily. A list of the sodium content of the more common foods is given on pages 642 and 643. Special low sodium foods are usually available for patients on a restricted sodium intake. An intake and output chart should be kept and the patient weighed regularly, so as to observe how quickly he is eliminating fluid from his body.

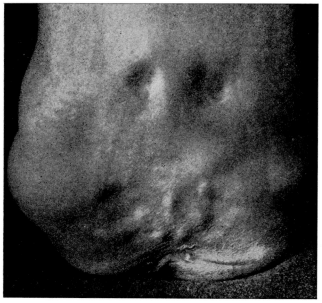

Fig. 37

Characteristic sacral pad of œdema in a case of congestive heart failure.

3. **Bowels.**—An aperient should be given to keep the bowels open and so prevent constipation and abdominal distension, with their added strain on the heart. The use of a commode at the bedside often causes less strain to patients than a bed-pan. Whenever a patient finds difficulty in using a bed-pan the commode should be substituted, the doctor's permission having, of course, first been obtained. Much more use should be made of the commode as opposed to the bed-pan than is customary in hospital practice to-day. To see patients perched precariously on a bed-pan which they obviously find impossible to use is a most unhappy sight, particularly with patients who are seriously ill. A most valuable

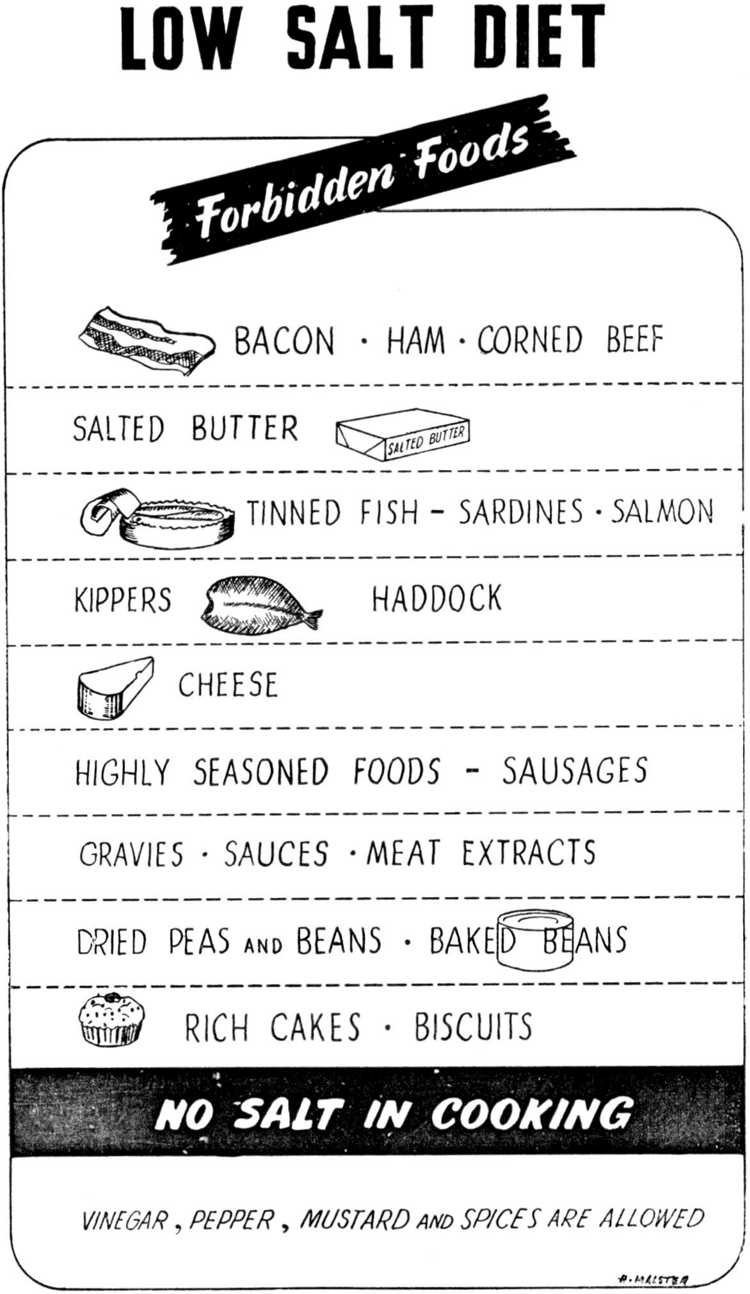

LOW SALT DIET

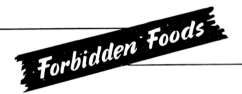

Forbidden Foods

 BACON · HAM · CORNED BEEF

SALTED BUTTER

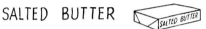 TINNED FISH – SARDINES · SALMON

KIPPERS   HADDOCK

 CHEESE

HIGHLY SEASONED FOODS – SAUSAGES

GRAVIES · SAUCES · MEAT EXTRACTS

DRIED PEAS and BEANS · BAKED BEANS

 RICH CAKES · BISCUITS

NO SALT IN COOKING

VINEGAR , PEPPER , MUSTARD and SPICES ARE ALLOWED

A. MALSTER

FIG. 38

aid in the difficult problem of the bed-pan is the Bohmansson chair in which the patient can be wheeled to the lavatory and the chair (which has a hole in the seat) fits over the pan. The patient, therefore, does not have to be lifted off the chair.

4. **Oxygen.**—Oxygen is needed to improve the oxygen content of the blood and thereby relieve the cyanosis. It also, for the same reason, relieves the dyspnœa. To be of any value it must be given properly in adequate concentration. Oxygen is best given by means of an oxygen tent or in an emergency by a B.L.B. mask. It is most important that no open flame should come in contact with the oxygen owing to the risk of fire. For this reason smoking must be stopped and the patient warned about this danger.

5. **Drugs.**—Several drugs are used in the treatment of heart failure but there are three drugs of special value :—

> (*a*) Morphine.
> (*b*) Diuretics.
> (*c*) Digitalis.

(*a*) MORPHINE.—Morphine is given to ensure a good night's sleep and thus much needed rest. Most patients with heart failure before coming under treatment have probably lacked sleep for some time. Morphine in $\frac{1}{4}$ gr. doses is usually necessary for the first few nights, after which milder hypnotics such as the barbiturates (medinal or amytal) will probably be sufficient. It is essential to see that the patient does fall asleep. In congestive failure due to chronic bronchitis and emphysema, morphine is best avoided owing to its depressant action on the cough reflex.

(*b*) DIURETICS.—These are used to reduce the œdema and so relieve the congestion. At present the following diuretics are most frequently used.

(i) Mercurial diuretics. Mersalyl is given intramuscularly approximately every three days in doses of 1 to 2 ml. and later on, as the œdema subsides, weekly. Mercaptomerin sodium (thiomerin) and meralluride are mercurial diuretics which can be given subcutaneously. The advantage of subcutaneous therapy is that, where necessary, the patients can be taught to give their own injections. Oral mercurial diuretics, such as chlormerodrin, tend to have too many side-effects, such as nausea, vomiting and diarrhœa. The diuretic action of mersalyl can often be increased if ammonium chloride, another diuretic drug is given beforehand (2 gm. orally).

Toxic Effects.—Mercurial diuretics are toxic drugs and may

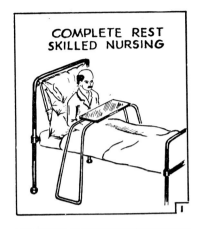

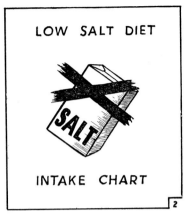

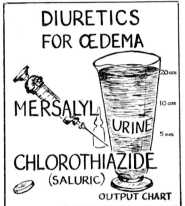

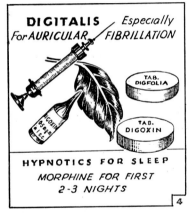

FIG. 39

Treatment of congestive heart failure.

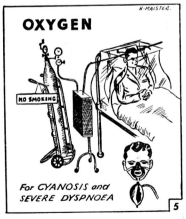

cause stomatitis, gastro-intestinal upset and skin eruptions. The most important toxic effect is, however, on the kidneys, which may give rise to dehydration, uræmia and severe albuminuria. For this reason, mercurial diuretics are never used in the treatment of œdema due to acute nephritis.

Another serious side-effect from the use of mercurial diuretics combined with rigid salt restriction is the *salt depletion syndrome*, in which there is a severe fall in the body salt with serious results. It is therefore most important to recognise as early as possible the symptoms of salt depletion so that it can be treated by giving salt. (The salt depletion syndrome is discussed fully on page 461.)

In addition to salt depletion, rigid salt restriction and intensive mercurial therapy can lead to potassium and chloride deficiency with symptoms of severe muscle weakness, lethargy and mental confusion. (Potassium depletion is discussed on page 462.)

(ii) Chlorothiazide and its derivatives. The greatest advance in the treatment of œdema has been the introduction of the very potent diuretic chlorothiazide, which has the advantage over mersalyl of being fully effective when given by mouth, thus obviating the need for injection therapy with most patients. Also, unlike the mercurial diuretics, chlorothiazide does not cause renal damage and can therefore also be given to patients with œdema caused by kidney disease.

Chlorothiazide (Saluric) is given in doses of 0·5 gm. to 1 gm. twice daily for three to five days a week according to the severity of the œdema. Hydrochlorothiazide (hydrosaluric, esidrex) and hydroflumethiazide (naclex, hydrenox) are similar but much more potent preparations so that the usual dose of these drugs is 25 mgm. to 50 mgm. twice daily for three to five days a week.

Particular care must be taken to watch for signs of salt (sodium) and potassium deficiency when large doses and prolonged therapy with these drugs are given. Potassium supplements such as potassium chloride, orange juice or salt-free marmite may be given as a routine when prolonged therapy with chlorothiazide is given.

Chlorothiazide and its derivatives are also very liable to increase the danger of digitalis overdosage when chlorothiazide and digitalis are given together. It is essential therefore to keep a careful watch for signs of digitalis poisoning in all patients on both chlorothiazide and digitalis and the dose of digitalis must be reduced if necessary. The importance of watching for signs of digitalis overdosage in these circumstances must be stressed.

(iii) Spironolactone (aldactone) antagonises the hormone aldosterone and so causes loss of sodium and fluid from the kidneys. It is expensive and hence is reserved for cases not responding to chlorothiazide or mersalyl.

The best means of telling when the patient is responding to diuretic therapy or, on the other hand, beginning to develop œdema is regular weighing. As soon as they are fit, patients with heart failure should be weighed once or twice weekly.

(c) DIGITALIS.—This drug is of great benefit in the treatment of congestive failure. As will be seen later, digitalis is the specific drug used in controlling auricular fibrillation, and the most dramatic results are obtained in those cases of congestive failure accompanied by auricular fibrillation. Digitalis is, however, also of value in those cases of failure not associated with auricular fibrillation. The use of digitalis is fully described later (p. 148).

6. **Mechanical Measures for the Removal of Œdema.**—In most cases the measures outlined above will remove the œdema even when there is fluid in the pleural or peritoneal cavities. In a few cases, however, œdema fluid may persist and it then becomes necessary to aspirate the fluid. For removal of a hydrothorax, a needle is inserted between the ribs into the pleural cavity and suction applied by means of a syringe and two-way adaptor, or by one of the many forms of suction apparatus available. Paracentesis abdominis (aspiration of an ascites) is performed by inserting a small trocar and cannula through the abdominal wall, under the strict aseptic technique used for any operation. The site for the insertion of the trocar is either midway between the symphysis pubis and umbilicus, or in either flank. The trocar is withdrawn and a rubber tube attached to the cannula to allow the fluid to drain into a suitable receptacle at the side of the bed. As the fluid subsides an abdominal binder is progressively tightened. It is essential that the bladder should be emptied before carrying out a paracentesis abdominis to avoid damage to that organ. All patients, therefore, must be catheterised as a preliminary measure. For the removal of fluid from the tissues in some intractable cases, Southey's tubes are available. These are small metal tubes which are inserted into the œdematous legs and allow the œdema to drain. The danger of this procedure is the risk of sepsis. Southey's tubes, which were in frequent use before the discovery of the mercurial diuretics, are only very occasionally required nowadays.

7. **Venesection.**—This measure is very useful in some cases to relieve the congestion in the venous circulation. A pint of blood is rapidly withdrawn by using a large-bore intravenous needle. It is essential for the blood to be taken off quickly if venesection is to be effective.

8. **Convalescence.**—When the œdema has subsided and the congestion in the lungs improved, a very gradual return to a limited activity is started. With the treatment outlined above, the patient may be able to get about again and even do light work. However it is very likely that the patient will relapse, as in most cases the heart disease causing the failure cannot be cured.

DISEASES OF THE PERICARDIUM

PERICARDITIS

Diseases of the pericardium are uncommon and the most frequent is an inflammation—pericarditis. Pericarditis may be dry or wet (pericardial effusion). The diagnostic sign of pericarditis is the coarse to and fro rub heard over the heart.

1. **Rheumatic Pericarditis.**—Rheumatic fever is the commonest cause of pericarditis and there are always present, in addition, an acute endocarditis and myocarditis. The presence of pericarditis denotes a severe infection. Rheumatic pericarditis may be dry or wet, but any effusion is always serous.

The treatment of rheumatic pericarditis is as outlined under acute rheumatic fever. If a large effusion is present, the patient is often most comfortable when sitting up in bed, leaning forward on a bed-table. A rheumatic pericardial effusion seldom causes so much pressure on the heart that it has to be aspirated.

The patient with a rheumatic pericarditis is always very ill and toxic and therefore requires the utmost care and attention from the nurse for all his needs.

2. **Purulent Pericarditis.**—Pericarditis with a purulent effusion is usually due to spread from a pneumonia in the left lung. A high swinging temperature and rigors in a patient with pneumonia not responding to treatment are suggestive of this rare complication. If the pericarditis does not respond to penicillin or other such drugs, operation to drain the pericardium may be necessary.

3. **Chronic Constrictive Pericarditis.**—Chronic constrictive pericarditis is rare and it differs from all other types of pericarditis in being chronic. Dense adhesions form around the heart,

constricting it and so preventing it from functioning properly. The cause of the adhesions is unknown. Many cases have been successfully operated on, the adhesions being cut and the embarrassment to the heart thus relieved.

4. **Acute Non-specific (Benign) Pericarditis.** — This type of pericarditis has become increasingly common in recent years. The exact cause is unknown, but it is believed to be a virus infection. Symptoms of respiratory infection (cough, pain in the chest on breathing) are often present. The condition usually clears up quickly and leaves no permanent cardiac damage. Antibiotics, such as the tetracyclines, have yielded good results in some cases.

5. **Tuberculous Pericarditis.**—This is comparatively rare and may be associated with pulmonary tuberculosis. A large pericardial effusion, often bloodstained, is usually present. The patient is treated with streptomycin and allied drugs.

6. Pericarditis often occurs in coronary thrombosis, when it requires no special treatment. Nor is special treatment needed for the terminal pericarditis seen in the late stages of uræmia (renal failure).

VALVULAR HEART DISEASE

When discussing the individual causes of heart disease it was seen that the valves of the heart are frequently damaged and that many different types of valvular lesion can arise. It is convenient here to summarise the main types and features of valvular heart disease.

1. **Rheumatic Valvular Heart Disease.**—All the valves of the heart may be affected, but usually it is the mitral and aortic valves that are particularly involved. Stenosis (obstruction) or incompetence (leakage) of the valves may result. Mitral stenosis and aortic incompetence are the commonest lesions met with. Mitral incompetence and aortic stenosis also occur.

Rheumatic valvular heart lesions are the most important cause of heart disease in young and middle-aged people.

2. **Syphilis.**—Syphilis causes the condition known as aneurysm of the aorta in which there is a marked dilatation of the aorta. When the first part of the ascending aorta is affected, the aortic valve becomes stretched and regurgitation of blood through the valve occurs, *i.e.*, aortic incompetence. Syphilis never affects the mitral valve.

3. **Arteriosclerosis** (Atherosclerosis).—Arteriosclerosis is a degenerative disease of the arteries which is frequently seen in later life. When it affects the aorta it also tends to spread to the aortic valves to produce thickening and distortion. The result of arteriosclerotic changes on the aortic valve is either an aortic incompetence or a stenosis.

4. **Congenital Heart Disease.**—Various valvular lesions are the result of congenital disease in fœtal life. The valve may be abnormal owing to improper development, or deformities of the valves may occur from fœtal endocarditis. A stenosis of the pulmonary valve, either alone or combined with other lesions, is a common congenital valvular lesion.

IRREGULAR HEART ACTION

Physiology of the Heart Action.—The heart normally beats at a regular rate, usually between 70 and 80 times a minute. There is a specialised conducting mechanism in the heart which is responsible for the proper initiation and conduction of the heart impulse. The cardiac impulse normally starts in the upper part of the right auricle, in what is called the *sino-auricular node* or pacemaker of the heart. The impulse quickly fans out over both auricles causing them to contract. The impulse now passes to a second area of specialised tissue known as the *auriculo-ventricular node*, which lies close to the septum between the auricles. From here the impulse passes to the ventricles by a special pathway in the intraventricular septum called the *bundle of His.* The latter divides up into two branches, right and left, to carry the impulse to both ventricles. The contraction of the ventricles is therefore normally controlled by an impulse which arises in the auricles, thus causing the auricles and ventricles to beat at the same rate and in a regular fashion. When the conducting pathway is diseased, so that the passage of the impulse is interfered with, the auricles and ventricles may, however, cease to beat at the same rate. In extreme cases, where disease in the conducting pathway may completely block the passage of all impulses from the auricles to the ventricles, the latter start to beat on their own accord and at their own rate. It should be noted that this ventricular rate is not around 70 to 80 beats a minute but is approximately 30 beats a minute.

The pacemaker of the heart, the sino-auricular node, is under the influence of two nerves—the vagus, which slows, and the sympathetic, which quickens the heart rate.

Types of Irregular Heart Action.—The following are the more common forms of irregular heart action :—

1. Sinus Arrhythmia.	4. Heart Block.
2. Extrasystoles.	5. Paroxysmal Tachycardia.
3. Auricular Fibrillation.	6. Auricular Flutter.

SINUS ARRHYTHMIA

Sinus arrhythmia is a very common condition wherein there is an increase in the rate of the heart on inspiration, with a corresponding slowing of the heart rate on expiration. It is most frequently seen in young children. It is of no significance and is not a sign of heart disease.

EXTRASYSTOLES

Extrasystoles are one or more extra or premature beats which occur before the next normal beat is due. After the premature beat there is usually a long pause in the heart action. This premature or extra beat may be so weak that the impulse does not travel to the pulse at the wrist so that there is a missed beat. If the extrasystoles are very numerous the patient may complain of palpitations due to the irregular heart action.

Causes.—The causes of extrasystoles may be conveniently divided into two groups, important and unimportant.

1. IMPORTANT.—Here the extrasystoles are of significance and there is usually heart disease present.

(*a*) In acute myocarditis due to acute rheumatic fever and diphtheria, the presence of extrasystoles is a most important sign of heart involvement and is a warning of the extreme care and attention necessary in nursing these patients. The other irregular heart action seen under these circumstances is heart block, which has the same significance (p. 150).

(*b*) Thyrotoxicosis, by its effect on the heart, commonly causes numerous extrasystoles as well as auricular fibrillation.

(*c*) Digitalis poisoning. Overdosage with digitalis often produces an extrasystole after every other heart beat so that a characteristic coupling of the pulse rhythm occurs—pulsus bigeminus. The presence of this irregularity calls for a reduction in the dose of the drug.

2. UNIMPORTANT.—Extrasystoles are often present without any evidence of heart damage and no significance need then be attached to them. In dyspepsia, excessive smoking, or anxiety states, extrasystoles are common.

AURICULAR FIBRILLATION

Auricular fibrillation is the most important type of irregular heart action and after extrasystoles it is also the most common. Auricular fibrillation is usually associated with heart disease.

Instead of the normal orderly contraction of the auricles which follows when the cardiac impulse starts in the sino-auricular node, the auricles undergo a very rapid twitching called fibrillation. There is no proper contraction of the auricles. The ventricles are continuously stimulated by these rapid twitchings but respond only to the stronger impulses. The result is that the ventricles contract in a most irregular fashion both as regards the rate and force.

Causes.

1. Rheumatic heart disease, usually associated with mitral stenosis, is the commonest cause before the age of 50.

2. Thyrotoxicosis, when the auricular fibrillation may recur in paroxysmal attacks or may be permanent.

3. Coronary arteriosclerosis and hypertension in later life.

Auricular fibrillation may be caused by any form of heart disease, but the above are the most frequent causes.

Symptoms and Signs.—The diagnostic clinical sign is the complete irregularity of the heart's action in both the rate and the force. The rate in untreated cases is often 120 to 160 beats a minute. There is in most cases a difference between the rate as counted by the pulse at the wrist and that counted directly over the heart with a stethoscope, which is known as a " pulse deficit." The pulse deficit may be as much as 20 beats a minute. The pulse deficit is caused by some heart beats being too weak to be transmitted to the pulse at the wrist.

As most cases of auricular fibrillation are associated with heart disease, signs of the latter are usually present. Very often the onset of auricular fibrillation precipitates congestive heart failure.

Treatment.—The specific drug in the treatment of auricular fibrillation is **digitalis.** The two most commonly used preparations of digitalis are the powdered digitalis leaf and digoxin. Digitalis leaf is available in tablet form in two strengths of ½ and 1 gr. Digoxin is available in tablets of 0·25 mgm. each and also in ampoules of 0·5 mgm. for intravenous use.

ACTION OF DIGITALIS.—Digitalis delays the conduction of the cardiac impulses in the heart thus reducing the number of impulses reaching the ventricles, so that slowing of the heart rate results. In effect digitalis produces a form of heart block. Slowing the ventricles makes their action stronger and more efficient.

DOSAGE.—The dose of digitalis depends on the urgency of the case. The faster the heart rate and the more severely ill the patient, the larger the initial dose of digitalis must be so as to hasten the action of the drug.

1. *Urgent Cases* with heart rate of 140 or over and severe heart failure present. In these cases speed of action is essential, so an initial dose of 0·5 to 1 mgm. of digoxin is given intravenously.

The intravenous dose of digoxin begins to have effect within an hour. Oral therapy with 0·5 mgm. is continued at six-hourly intervals until the apex rate is slowed to 85 to 80 beats a minute. The dose is then reduced to a maintenance level of 0·25 to 0·5 mgm. daily.

2. *Severe Cases (but less urgent than above):* heart rate under 140 but over 100 a minute. Here, too, a rapid action is also required, and so comparatively large doses of digitalis are needed. Intravenous therapy is, however, not necessary. An initial dose of 1 mgm. of digoxin by mouth is given, followed by 0·5 mgm. at six-hourly intervals till the apex rate is 85 to 80 beats a minute. Then the daily maintenance dose is prescribed.

3. *Non-urgent Cases:* heart rate of 100 beats or less a minute. In these cases there is no urgency and large doses of digitalis are not necessary. It is sufficient to give 0·25 mgm. of digoxin three times a day till the heart rate is 85 to 80 and then to give the maintenance dose.

Instead of digoxin the powdered digitalis leaf may be given, 1½ gr. of the leaf being substituted for each 0·25 mgm. of digoxin.

SIGNS OF DIGITALIS POISONING.—Digitalis is a toxic drug and overdosage causes poisoning. As digitalis is used so frequently it is important that the nurse should be fully aware of the signs of digitalis overdosage :—

1. Loss of appetite, nausea and vomiting.
2. Very slow pulse rate, usually under 60.
3. Coupled beats—pulsus bigeminus (due to the presence of extrasystoles).

Notes on Digitalis Therapy.

1. If the pulse rate drops to 60 or under in a patient on digitalis the drug must be discontinued. The doctor will advise when the digitalis may be recommenced (usually when the pulse rises to normal) and in what dosage.

2. The dose of digitalis varies not only according to the urgency of the case but also according to the age and weight of the patient. Younger and heavier people require larger doses, but large doses of digitalis should be given only with great care to elderly and debilitated people.

3. Vomiting occurring at the start of digitalis therapy is usually caused by the associated heart failure and not by the drug. However, vomiting, especially if accompanied by a slow pulse, after the patient has been on digitalis for several days, is most probably due to digitalis overdosage.

4. When large doses of digitalis are given the patient must be closely watched so that the drug may be reduced as soon as the heart rate has slowed to 85 to 80 beats a minute. The pulse rate is not, however, an accurate guide to the heart rate in rapid auricular fibrillation, as so many beats do not get through to the pulse at the wrist owing to the pulse deficit. It is essential, therefore, to count the rate directly over the apex of the heart with a stethoscope as well as counting the pulse. In urgent cases on large doses of digitalis, simultaneous two-hourly readings at the apex of the heart and at the pulse are necessary.

5. Digitalis overdosage is especially liable to develop in patients having also the potent oral diuretic chlorothiazide or its derivatives as these drugs enhance the effect of digitalis. Therefore extra care must be taken to watch for signs of digitalis overdosage in all patients having both digitalis and chlorothiazide. *This is very important.* Most patients having both drugs will require much smaller doses of digitalis.

QUINIDINE IN AURICULAR FIBRILLATION.—Quinidine differs from digitalis in that it can convert the irregular heart rhythm to a normal one. Quinidine, however, is a very toxic drug and extreme care is therefore necessary in selecting the type of case for quinidine therapy. Any evidence of congestive heart failure or marked enlargement of the heart is a definite contraindication to the drug. The danger with this drug is the likelihood of embolism and sudden death. The type of case most suitable for quinidine therapy is thyrotoxic auricular fibrillation persisting after thyroidectomy.

HEART BLOCK

Disease affecting the conducting mechanism of the heart may interfere with the proper conduction of the cardiac impulse, so that blocking of the beats may occur. There are very many different types of heart block but it is sufficient for the nurse to know the main types. In *incomplete* heart block, isolated impulses fail to reach the ventricles from the auricles; consequently the ventricles fail to contract, with the result that a beat is missed or dropped. The rhythm of the heart rate in incomplete heart block is usually irregular. In *complete* heart block no impulses reach the ventricles from the auricles and the ventricles beat at their own independent rate, usually about 30 beats a minute. The rhythm of the heart in complete block is regular.

Causes.

1. Coronary arteriosclerosis.
2. Digitalis poisoning.
3. Acute myocarditis in acute rheumatic fever and diphtheria.

The nurse should be aware of the possibility of heart block due to digitalis overdosage, and a pulse rate under 60 in a patient on digitalis calls for omission of the drug. The nurse, while taking the pulse as a routine measure, will perhaps be the first to detect the early signs of heart block caused by digitalis poisoning. Again, while taking the pulse in cases of acute rheumatic fever and diphtheria, dropped beats producing an irregular pulse may first be noticed by the nurse. As this irregularity of the pulse may be one of the few signs of heart damage in acute rheumatic fever or diphtheria its great importance should be noted.

Treatment.—In severe heart block due to digitalis poisoning, *i.e.*, pulse rate under 60, the drug should be stopped till the pulse begins to rise again and a reduced maintenance dose given thereafter. Atropine, $\frac{1}{100}$ gr. subcutaneously, is often useful in severe digitalis poisoning.

In the other causes of heart block no specific treatment is needed apart from the treatment of the underlying condition.

STOKES-ADAMS SYNDROME

In Stokes-Adams syndrome the ventricles fail to contract for a period as the result of a severe degree of heart block. In most of these patients coronary arteriosclerosis is the cause of the heart block. In severe cases the patient falls unconscious and a convulsion or fit may occur, usually with cyanosis. If the heart fails to beat within two minutes the patient dies; less severe attacks usually cause a feeling of faintness and giddiness with a transient " blackout."

Treatment.—In many cases ephedrine, $\frac{1}{2}$ to 1 gr. three times a day, is useful as it tends to quicken the heart rate. Aminophylline tablets, 0·1 gm. three times a day, are also useful and cortisone can be tried. In severe attacks, if the patient is unconscious, adrenaline (1 ml.) may have to be injected direct into the heart.

PAROXYSMAL TACHYCARDIA

Paroxysmal tachycardia is a common irregularity of the heart but is not often seen by the nurse, as most of these patients do not require in-patient hospital treatment. Paroxysmal tachycardia is not usually associated with any other evidence of heart disease.

Symptoms and Signs.

1. Sudden onset of extreme tachycardia so that the heart beats about 180 to 200 times a minute and never less than 160.

2. Rhythm of the heart is absolutely regular.

3. The attack may last from several minutes to several hours, or even in severe cases for days. During the attack the patient may complain of palpitations and/or dyspnœa.

4. The attack passes off as suddenly as it occurs.

Treatment.—Pressing on the vagus nerve in an effort to slow the heart rate may occasionally stop an attack. Pressure on the vagus may be exerted either directly over the nerve in the side of the neck or indirectly by painful pressure over the eyeballs. If these methods do not succeed digitalis is usually given, which frequently stops an attack. If digitalis fails to have effect, quinidine is then usually tried. To prevent attacks which would otherwise frequently recur, digitalis or quinidine may be given for an indefinite period.

AURICULAR FLUTTER

Auricular flutter is rare. It is due to the same causes as auricular fibrillation and has a similar type of action except that the heart is often regular instead of irregular. The treatment is the same as for auricular fibrillation, *i.e.*, digitalis.

DISEASES OF THE BLOOD VESSELS

(A) THE ARTERIES

There are three common diseases of the arteries met with in medicine :—

    1. Arteriosclerosis (Atherosclerosis).

    2. Syphilitic Arterial Disease.

    3. Thrombosis and Embolism.

ARTERIOSCLEROSIS (ATHEROSCLEROSIS)

Cause.—Arteriosclerosis is a very common condition most frequently found in middle-aged and elderly people. The exact cause of arteriosclerosis is unknown, but certain factors do appear to play an important role in the causation of the disease.

1. There is a strong hereditary basis.

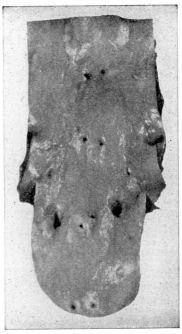

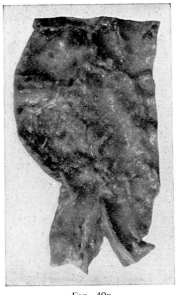

FIG. 40B
Arteriosclerosis of the aorta showing the thickened, roughened and ulcerated wall. It is easy to see how clots can form on such damaged arterial surfaces.

FIG. 40A
Photograph showing part of the normal smooth wall of the aorta.

2. Certain diseases predispose to this lesion, *e.g.*, diabetes is very often associated with arteriosclerosis.

3. High blood pressure (hypertension). This very common disease is distinct from arteriosclerosis, but there is some evidence that its presence aggravates or predisposes to the development of arteriosclerosis. Both conditions, however, may occur independently of each other.

4. The possible part played by the fat content of the diet in the causation of arteriosclerosis is now being investigated. It is believed that an excessive consumption of animal (saturated) fats

(bacon, butter, cream, fat of meat) and a low intake of vegetable (unsaturated) fats may predispose to arteriosclerosis.

Pathology.—Arteriosclerosis is known as a degenerative disease and causes thickening and narrowing of the arteries owing to changes in the inner wall of the vessels. Localised deposits of fatty material appear on the inner surface of the arteries, forming large patches known as atheromatous plaques. These plaques narrow the smaller arteries and so they cause deficient blood supply to organs and tissues. Atheromatous plaques are also very liable to break down and form ulcers. Thrombosis may then develop as a result of the roughening and ulceration of the inner coat of the arteries. Lastly, arteriosclerotic changes which commonly affect the aorta may spread down to the aortic valve to cause an incompetence or stenosis of the valve.

Symptoms and Signs.—The symptoms and signs caused by arteriosclerosis are due to :—

1. The effect of the disease on the blood supply to the organs or tissues supplied by the arteries.

2. The thrombosis which is liable to occur in the diseased arteries.

In many arteries arteriosclerosis may have little effect, but in the following sites arteriosclerosis produces well-recognised diseases :—

(*a*) In the *coronary* arteries where it causes :—

      (i) Angina pectoris.

      (ii) Coronary thrombosis.

(*b*) In the *cerebral* arteries where it causes cerebral thrombosis (one form of apoplexy or " stroke ").

(*c*) In the *leg* arteries where it causes :—

      (i) Intermittent claudication, *i.e.*, severe pain in the legs on exertion owing to the diminished blood flow through narrowed arteries.

      (ii) Peripheral thrombosis with gangrene of the limb.

(*d*) In the *aortic valve* where it causes aortic incompetence or stenosis.

Treatment.—There is no specific treatment for arteriosclerosis. Any factors such as stress or strain which aggravate the condition should be avoided. The early recognition and treatment of diabetes is of importance in reducing the danger of arteriosclerosis. Any condition such as angina due to arteriosclerosis is treated on the usual lines. For intermittent claudication, vasodilator drugs, such as phenoxybenzamine (dibenyline), are useful.

The efficacy of a diet low in fats, especially animal fats, in minimising the effects of arteriosclerosis is being tried.

SYPHILITIC ARTERIAL DISEASE

Syphilis may set up a chronic inflammation in any artery. In most cases the result of syphilitic inflammation in the arteries is scarring and weakening of the vessel wall. The pressure in the

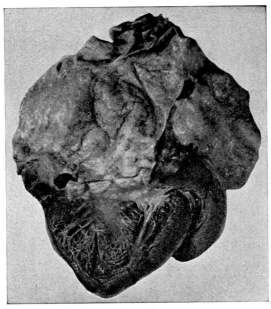

FIG. 41

Advanced syphilitic aneurysm of the first part of the aorta with the characteristic gross dilatation of the aorta. The aortic valve cusps are thickened and separated from each other, causing aortic incompetence.

arteries acting on the weakened walls eventually produces a marked dilatation of the artery known as an aneurysm. Syphilis is a common cause of aneurysm, the only other common causes being the congenital type seen in the cerebral arteries, traumatic aneurysm, and aneurysm due to arteriosclerosis.

The most frequent sites for syphilitic aneurysm are the ascending aorta and the arch of the aorta.

1. Aneurysm of the Ascending Aorta.

An aneurysm in this part of the aorta is commonly associated with an aortic incompetence, as the widened aorta stretches the aortic valve opening. Angina pectoris is also frequent as syphilitic scarring narrows the openings of the coronary arteries which branch off from this part of the aorta. A boring pain from erosion of the ribs and sternum may be present too.

2. Aneurysm of the Arch of the Aorta.

Severe dilatation of this part of the aorta often presses on the various structures in the mediastinum, producing typical symptoms. It may press on :—

(a) The trachea, causing a stridor and cough which is often brassy.

(b) The great veins, producing cyanosis and œdema of the head, neck and arms.

(c) The nerves, producing hoarseness due to the paralysis of the laryngeal nerve, or severe girdle pains from pressure on the intercostal nerves.

(d) The œsophagus, causing difficulty in swallowing (dysphagia).

Diagnosis.—In most cases of aneurysm the diagnosis can be confirmed by X-ray examination in which the dilated artery may be seen. In addition, the specific blood tests for syphilis (Wassermann and Kahn tests) may be positive.

Treatment.—In advanced cases of aneurysm only palliative treatment is possible. In those cases which have been diagnosed early, antisyphilitic treatment (penicillin) is given.

THROMBOSIS AND EMBOLISM

1. Arterial Thrombosis.

Thrombosis is clotting in a blood vessel. Apart from certain special arterial cases thrombosis is usually seen in the veins. The circulation in the arteries is normally too rapid for a clot to occur, but in the veins a sluggish circulation is not uncommon. However, when there is severe disease of an artery, particularly arteriosclerosis (atherosclerosis), thrombosis does occur; it is also found as a result of injury to an artery.

The main types of arterial thrombosis are :—

(a) Coronary thrombosis in arteriosclerotic coronary arteries.

(b) Cerebral thrombosis in arteriosclerotic or, less often, syphilitic cerebral arteries.

(c) Thrombosis in arteriosclerotic arteries of the lower limbs.

Coronary and cerebral thrombosis have already been fully described elsewhere; there remains for discussion thrombosis in peripheral limb arteries. In advanced cases of arteriosclerosis with gross narrowing of the arteries due to atheromatous plaques and also roughening of the inner wall, thrombosis may supervene and

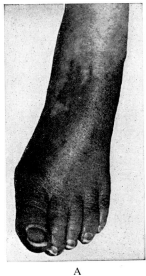 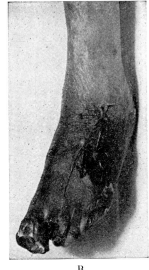

A   Fig. 42   B

A, Peripheral embolism. Early changes in the foot due to an embolus lodging in the popliteal artery. The foot is mottled blue and dead cold, and the patient is unable to move it. The onset is marked by extreme pain. In this case the arterial embolus was dislodged from the heart, the patient having had a coronary thrombosis twelve days before.
B, A later stage of arterial embolism of the leg showing advanced gangrene. The foot is black and necrotic.

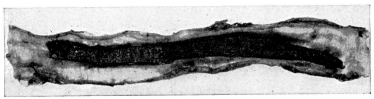

Fig. 43

Excised portion of the femoral artery showing a part of an embolus which completely blocked the circulation to the leg.

completely obstruct the already partially blocked vessel. Complete obstruction of the arterial blood supply results in gangrene or death of the tissues supplied by the affected vessels. This form of gangrene is often called *senile* gangrene, as it usually occurs in elderly people

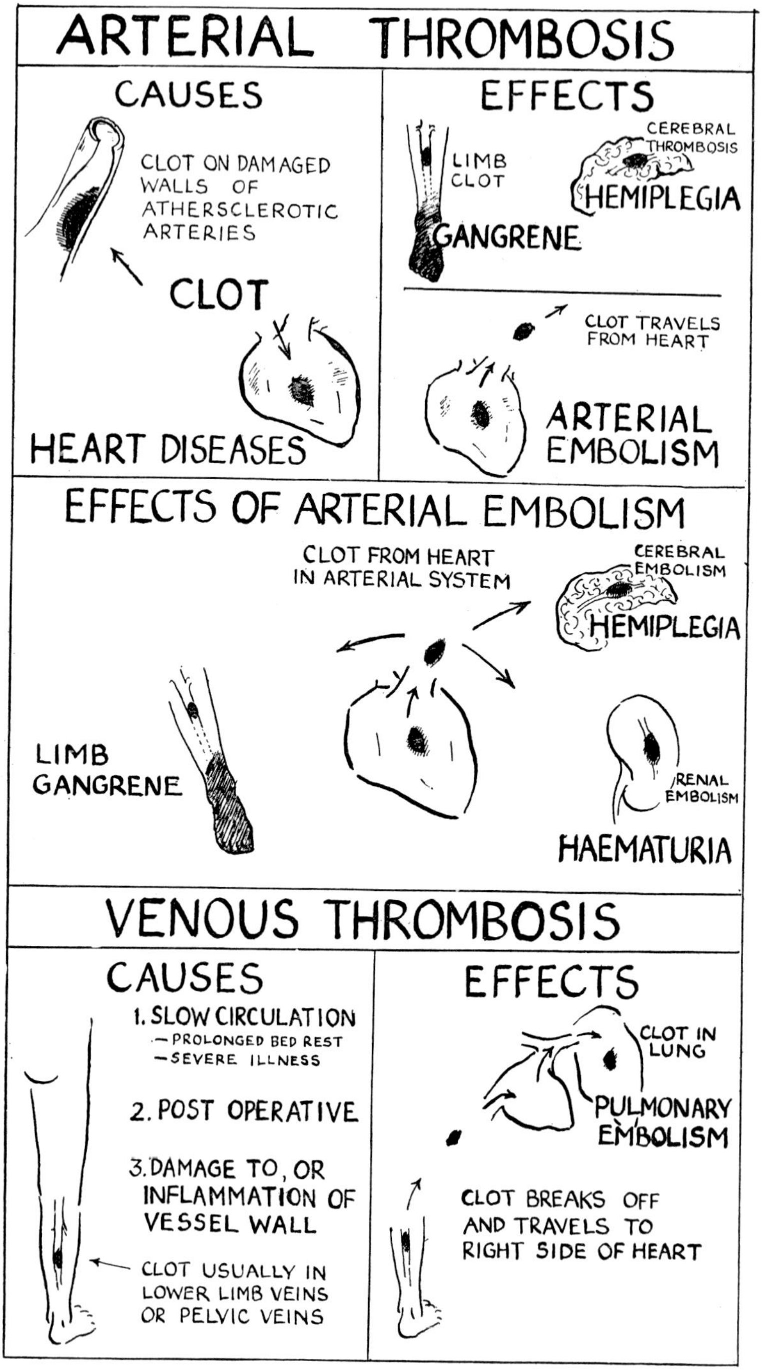

FIG. 44
Thrombosis and Embolism.

158

with advanced arteriosclerosis. The disease diabetes mellitus is a potent predisposing cause to arteriosclerosis and gangrene.

2. Arterial Embolism.

Embolism in the arterial circulation is usually due to a clot becoming detached from the left side of the heart and travelling in the circulation, finally to lodge in an artery. There are three conditions which frequently give rise to a clot in the left side of the heart and so may cause arterial embolism :—

(a) *In mitral stenosis* with auricular fibrillation a clot (thrombus) may form in the left auricle.

(b) In *coronary thrombosis* a clot may form on the endocardium of the heart over the damaged muscle (mural or wall thrombus, see p. 124).

(c) In *subacute bacterial endocarditis* the large vegetations on the valves are easily and repeatedly dislodged to travel in the circulation. These small emboli may then lodge in the skin, kidneys, brain, etc. (p. 116).

In the cases of (a) and (b) the embolus most frequently lodges in an artery in the brain, leg, kidney, or mesentery. In the brain it causes cerebral embolism with its consequential paralysis, usually in the form of a hemiplegia. In a peripheral artery of the leg it completely cuts off the blood supply causing severe pain in the leg, which becomes white, cold, paralysed and later gangrenous. The changes brought about by arterial thrombosis and embolism are essentially the same except that in embolism the changes are much more dramatic and usually more complete owing to the sudden onset.

THROMBO-ANGIITIS OBLITERANS (BUERGER'S DISEASE)

Thrombo-angiitis obliterans, although not as common as the arterial diseases already described, is not rare. For some unknown reason it rarely affects women. The exact cause is unknown and the only factor of established importance is that smoking appears to play a part. The underlying cause of the symptoms is the deficient blood supply to the affected limbs which is the result of the marked narrowing of the diseased arteries. The lower limbs are most commonly affected, the patient experiencing pain in the calves on exertion (intermittent claudication) which disappears with rest. (This pain is similar in type to that of angina pectoris, which is also due to deficient blood supply—ischæmia.) In the later stages gangrene sets in, usually starting in the toes. Gangrene is often precipitated by exposure to cold or to injury.

The treatment of thrombo-angiitis obliterans is unsatisfactory as there is no specific cure. The patient must take great care to avoid both the slightest injury to the feet and exposure to cold. Scrupulous attention to keeping the feet dry, warm and clean is essential. The nails must be trimmed with extreme care to avoid the slightest cut. If the patient is confined to bed special care must be taken to avoid pressure sores.

The operation of lumbar sympathectomy to cut the constricting sympathetic nerves is of value in early cases. When gangrene occurs a high amputation is usually necessary.

For the relief of pain sedatives such as codeine or aspirin are needed. Morphine or other habit-forming drugs must not be given. The patient must give up smoking.

RAYNAUD'S DISEASE

In contrast to thrombo-angiitis obliterans, Raynaud's disease is usually seen in women and very rarely in men. Furthermore, it usually affects the fingers and seldom the feet, whereas the effect of thrombo-angiitis obliterans is precisely the opposite. Raynaud's disease is due to spasm of the arteries of the fingers and hands, causing deficient circulation. The hands first go blue and then dead white and feel numb. Exposure to cold is the usual cause of these symptoms. In severe cases gangrene may develop, but it is not as common a complication as in thrombo-angiitis obliterans.

In the treatment of Raynaud's disease protection from cold is most important. In severe cases sympathectomy may result in marked improvement. The vasodilator drugs, phenoxybenzamine (dibenyline), tolazoline (priscol), ronicol and hydergine, may be of value in relieving the symptoms.

(B) THE VEINS

PHLEBITIS

Phlebitis, or inflammation of a vein, is a very common condition, especially in the lower limbs. Apart from the cases in which it occurs of its own accord for no obvious reason, phlebitis also frequently arises during prolonged serious infections such as typhoid fever, as a result of injury to a vein (such as may occur during an operation), and during the puerperium.

If a superficial vein is affected it produces localised swelling, redness and pain. In the case of a deep-seated vein, marked œdema or swelling of the affected area and pain are the most prominent features. The chief danger in a deep venous phlebitis is the likelihood of a clot forming in the inflamed vein, whereupon the condition of *thrombophlebitis* arises. If this happens, *i.e.*, if a thrombus forms in cases of phlebitis, there is a risk that the clot may become dislodged, travel through the venous system, and lodge in the lungs, so causing pulmonary embolism.

VENOUS THROMBOSIS

Thrombosis frequently complicates a phlebitis but it may also arise of its own accord. Any condition that produces a slowing of the venous circulation creates a predisposition to the formation of a clot in the veins. Such slowing of the venous circulation is frequently seen in patients who are confined to bed for a long time, particularly if they do not move about in bed. It is for this reason that venous thrombosis often develops in patients after *major operations*, especially in elderly people who are more reluctant to alter their position in bed.

Congestive heart failure, because of the resultant slowing of the venous circulation, also predisposes to venous thrombosis.

In many cases of venous thrombosis, especially where there is no evidence of phlebitis, the symptoms and signs may be so slight that the first indication of the condition may be the occurrence of pulmonary embolism, the clot having become detached and travelled to the lungs. In the post-operative cases the thrombus most commonly forms in the deep calf or pelvic veins. As a result the patient may notice a sense of heaviness or slight pain in the calf, whilst slight swelling may be present. It is important to realise that the pain and swelling may be minimal even though a potentially dangerous thrombosis is present. Due weight should therefore be given to these slight signs. In these patients a low-grade fever is also often present; after operation the presence of a slightly raised temperature for no obvious reason should arouse suspicion of a deep venous thrombosis.

Treatment of Phlebitis and Thrombosis.—In the case of a superficial phlebitis the danger of pulmonary embolism is so very rare that it is unnecessary to put all patients to bed. In mild cases a supportive elastic dressing may be all that is required. In the cases of deep venous thrombosis where there is a very definite danger of

6

embolism, complete rest to the affected limb is essential; a splint or sandbags are the most useful means of immobilising the limb, and a bed-cradle to take the weight of the clothes off the affected limb is also advisable. In post-operative patients, where the risk of embolism is great, anticoagulant drugs may be given to lessen the clotting power of the blood, thus, by preventing the further spread of the thrombosis, reducing the risk of embolism. Heparin, phenindione, warfarin and dicoumarol are the most useful anti-coagulant drugs for this purpose.

Preventive treatment in those conditions likely to cause a venous thrombosis is most important. Early movement of the lower limbs combined with massage, to prevent undue slowing of the circulation, is most important. Elderly patients, who are especially reluctant to move about in bed, must be urged to undertake active movements. After major operations the patients must be encouraged to move their legs and not lie fixed in one position. Early ambulation after operation also reduces the risk of thrombosis and embolism.

SUMMARY

1. Many of the diseases which affect the heart produce permanent changes which may in time interfere with efficient cardiac function. Most of the changes arising in the heart as a result of these diseases throw a strain on the heart which increases the amount of work it has to do. The heart compensates for this added strain and work by hypertrophy of its muscle (myocardial hypertrophy). Eventually, however, after perhaps many years, the strain may become too great whereupon the heart ceases to act efficiently and heart failure results. This heart failure may affect the left side of the heart only, provided that the strain is only on the left side. In left-sided heart failure the main symptoms are breathlessness on exertion and the characteristic attacks of nocturnal dyspnœa—cardiac asthma. Most cases of left heart failure ultimately, however, cause failure of the right side of the heart too, when the term " congestive heart failure " is used. Congestive heart failure may also result from an initial and direct strain on the right side of the heart. The main results of congestive heart failure are severe congestion of the venous system and lungs, both due to the heart's inability to pump the blood efficiently throughout the body. Congestion in the lungs causes severe breathlessness and cyanosis. Another characteristic sign in these cases is the œdema, which is most marked in the legs when the patient is up, and over the sacrum when the patient is in bed. The œdema is caused by the increased venous pressure forcing fluid into the tissues and also by the retention of salt in the body.

2. There are several diseases which commonly affect the heart, causing permanent heart disease and eventually heart failure.

(a) Hypertension, or high blood pressure, is perhaps the most common and important disease which affects the heart. The high pressure in the arteries overloads the heart so that after many years heart failure results—at first left heart failure and ultimately congestive failure.

(b) Arteriosclerosis (atherosclerosis) is a very frequent degenerative disease which may affect all the arteries. It causes a thickening and narrowing of the arteries. Arteriosclerosis very often occurs in the coronary arteries with two possible main effects :—

(i) Owing to the narrowing of the arteries the blood supply to the heart is diminished, thus interfering with efficient cardiac function. The clinical picture in these cases is one of severe pain over the heart on exertion— angina pectoris.

(ii) Owing to the narrowed and roughened artery wall, thrombosis in the coronary arteries is a frequent occurrence. Important changes (infarction) develop in the myocardium because of the loss of blood supply, and in severe cases sudden death or heart failure may result. Coronary thrombosis and angina pectoris very often occur in the same patient, as the cause of both, in most cases, is the same. When arteriosclerosis affects the aorta it often involves the aortic valves to cause thickening and distortion, and aortic stenosis and incompetence therefore often result from arteriosclerosis.

(c) Chronic respiratory diseases, especially the very common diseases, chronic bronchitis and emphysema, throw a strain on the right side of the heart and frequently cause congestive heart failure.

Hypertension, coronary arteriosclerosis and chronic bronchitis and emphysema are the most important and frequent causes of heart disease in later life. In younger people, however, the most important causes of chronic heart disease are acute rheumatic fever and its allied disease chorea. Acute rheumatic fever, for some unknown reason, particularly attacks the heart, causing both acute and chronic disease. In the acute stage acute myocarditis and endocarditis occur and sometimes acute pericarditis. The acute endocarditis is liable to become chronic and then permanent changes take place in the valves. Two main effects are seen : (i) a narrowing of the valve opening (stenosis) and (ii) an incompetence of the valve because the valve leaflets have lost their elasticity and cannot close properly. The valve lesions most commonly resulting from chronic rheumatic endocarditis are mitral stenosis and aortic incompetence. These valvular lesions cause heart failure, though often only after a considerable interval, perhaps as long as twenty or thirty years.

(d) In addition to the above main causes of chronic heart disease there are three other well recognised causes :—

(i) Syphilis affects the heart mainly through its effect on the ascending aorta. Syphilis causes a chronic inflammation with scarring of the aorta (and indeed it may have the same effect on many arteries in the body). The wall of the aorta becomes stretched from the pressure in the aorta acting on the weakened walls, and gross dilatation or aneurysm results. The aortic valve opening also becomes stretched and the result is an aortic incompetence. The second main effect of syphilis on the heart is to cause narrowing of the mouths of the coronary arteries (which arise from the first part of the aorta) by the syphilitic scarring. This results in a deficient blood supply to the heart and so is another important cause of angina pectoris.

(ii) Thyrotoxicosis, where the metabolism or work of the body is greatly increased owing to oversecretion of the thyroid hormone, may cause heart disease, as the heart, which has to work much harder, may fail.

(iii) Because of improper development of the heart in fœtal life various abnormal-
ities are met with which give rise to heart disease. Abnormal openings
between the auricles and ventricles, stenosis of the pulmonary valve,
and a persistence of the ductus arteriosus after birth are some of the
more common lesions. These congenital heart lesions tend to produce
a typical clinical picture in the child of marked cyanosis (blue baby),
clubbing of the fingers and breathlessness.

3. (a) In addition to chronic heart disease discussed above, acute heart
disease also occurs. It has already been stated that acute rheumatic fever (and
chorea) particularly affect the heart, causing acute myocarditis, endocarditis and
often pericarditis.

(b) Diphtheria is also especially liable to cause an acute myocarditis. Unlike
acute rheumatic heart disease, however, it does not cause permanent heart damage.
In acute heart disease due to either rheumatic fever or diphtheria, the main sign of
heart changes is a very rapid and often irregular pulse. The irregularity of the
pulse may be due to such disorders of the heart's action as extrasystoles (extra
beats) or heart block (missed or dropped beats).

(c) Finally, acute heart disease is commonly caused when bacteria gain
entrance to the blood stream and settle on the valves (usually already damaged)
to give rise to a bacterial endocarditis. In most cases one type of bacteria is
present, the Streptococcus viridans, causing the clinical picture of subacute bacterial
endocarditis. Rheumatic endocarditis and congenital heart lesions are the
conditions most often complicated by bacterial endocarditis.

4. Diseases which affect the heart in the several ways mentioned above may
also alter the regular heart rhythm and so cause various types of irregular heart
action. The most important and common irregularity is that called auricular
fibrillation, when the heart rate is usually fast and wholly irregular in both time
and force (strong beats and weak beats). Any of the diseases which affect the
heart may be associated with auricular fibrillation, but particularly rheumatic heart
disease and thyrotoxicosis.

Extrasystoles, when extra beats occur causing irregular rhythm, are very
common and may be of little significance. On the other hand, when they occur
in the course of acute rheumatic fever and diphtheria, extrasystoles are of great
significance as they indicate underlying heart damage. In patients on digitalis,
extrasystoles (especially after every second beat when they produce a coupling of
the pulse—pulsus bigeminus) are a definite sign of digitalis overdosage.

Digitalis overdosage may also cause a second type of irregular rhythm known
as heart block. Here impulses from the auricles fail to get through to the ventricles
and the result is dropped beats. There may be occasional dropped beats (incomplete
heart block) or, in some cases, all the impulses from the auricles may be blocked
so that the auricles and ventricles beat independently (complete heart block).
Heart block causes a slow pulse and any pulse rate under 50 is usually due to one
form or other of heart block. Heart block, like extrasystoles, may also be the
only sign of underlying heart damage in acute rheumatic fever and diphtheria.
Heart block is also a common result of coronary artery disease.

5. Thrombosis in the arteries is most commonly seen in arteriosclerosis.
Coronary thrombosis has already been mentioned. Thrombosis also frequently
occurs in the cerebral arteries, causing one form of apoplexy, whilst gangrene in the

lower limbs is often seen in elderly people owing to thrombosis in arteriosclerotic leg arteries. Arteriosclerotic gangrene is particularly prevalent in diabetes.

Arterial embolism occurs in cases of coronary thrombosis from a thrombus detached from the heart. It is also seen in bacterial endocarditis, where the characteristic vegetations on the valves are easily dislodged, and in mitral stenosis with auricular fibrillation. Embolism may occur in any artery but is particularly frequent in the cerebral arteries and peripheral limb arteries. The result of embolism is to cut off the blood supply to the affected tissues which leads to rapid loss of function—gangrene. The changes in embolism are the same as in thrombosis except for the rapidity of onset.

6. Thrombosis in the veins is a very common condition, occurring especially in cases where the venous circulation is sluggish or as a result of injury or inflammation of a vein. In all serious diseases requiring prolonged bed rest, especially in elderly people, and after major operations, a deep venous thrombosis may form in the leg or pelvic veins. The danger is that this thrombus may become detached and travel to the lungs, so causing pulmonary embolism.

Treatment of Heart Disease.

1. Chronic heart disease in most cases gives rise to congestive heart failure. The treatment of congestive failure is, therefore, most important and the fundamental bases of treatment are : rest, the avoidance of strain on the heart, and relief from the congestion and the œdema. Digitalis, in controlling the auricular fibrillation which often precipitates heart failure, frequently delays the occurrence of failure for many years. Digitalis is a toxic drug and recognition of the signs of overdosage is most important. A slow pulse rate under 60 (often accompanied by coupled beats), nausea and vomiting are particularly important signs. Two-hourly readings of the heart rate are essential in all cases on large doses of digitalis.

Diuretics and salt restriction to relieve the œdema, sedatives (especially morphine in the early stages), and oxygen for the cyanosis and extremes of dyspnœa are all of the utmost importance.

2. Before gross heart damage and failure develop much can be done in some diseases to minimise or prevent such damage.

(a) Prolonged and absolute rest and skilled nursing are most important in rheumatic fever to prevent both death from acute heart failure and the development of chronic rheumatic valvular disease.

(b) Frequent movements, both passive and active, of the lower limbs in all cases of prolonged bed rest considerably reduce the risk of venous thrombosis and so of pulmonary embolism. After operations, early movements of the limbs and getting the patient out of bed as soon as possible likewise lessen the danger of post-operative embolism.

Recognition of the early signs of a deep venous thrombosis (especially common in the calf veins) is also of great value. After operations slight pain and tenderness in the legs, often with a slight irregular fever, are important warning signs of a deep venous thrombosis. Anticoagulant treatment, given early, may prevent embolism.

(c) Treating thyrotoxicosis by removal of the thyroid gland, antithyroid drugs, or radioactive iodine may often restore the heart to normal.

(d) The recognition and treatment of syphilis in the early stages will prevent syphilitic heart disease in later years. Penicillin is the most valuable drug in the treatment of syphilis. Prolonged observation after treatment is necessary to make sure that all signs of the disease have been eradicated.

(e) Absolute rest and skilled nursing care in coronary thrombosis will often prove the decisive factor in recovery from the acute attack. Many of these patients where the underlying coronary disease is not advanced may live useful and active lives for very many years following the attack. Anticoagulant drugs to prevent spread of the thrombosis and also to lessen the risk of embolism are important.

3. Subacute bacterial endocarditis, which complicates rheumatic endocarditis and congenital heart lesions, is frequently cured by penicillin and other antibiotics such as streptomycin.

4. Surgery has produced dramatic results in some cases of congenital heart lesions. Ligating a patent ductus arteriosus results in a permanent cure. In cases of pulmonary stenosis, surgery also often produces remarkable relief from the extreme cyanosis and breathlessness, so that these children can lead much more active lives. In mitral and aortic stenosis surgery (dilating the stenosed valve) has also proved of benefit in relieving progressive dyspnœa.

SUMMARY OF SOME ROUTINE PROCEDURES UNDERTAKEN IN DISEASES OF THE CIRCULATORY SYSTEM

1. Intake and Output Fluid Chart.

In all cases of congestive heart failure and in all cases on diuretics or restricted fluid intake.

2. Cardiac Apex and Pulse Chart.

Simultaneous recordings of the rate of the heart by stethoscope and pulse readings, in cases of very rapid auricular fibrillation on large doses of digitalis.

3. Blood Pressure Recording.

(a) For diagnosis in all cases of heart or indeed most diseases.

(b) In the control of hypotensive treatment for hypertension when frequent recordings are made with the patient standing.

4. X-ray Examination.

(a) To determine the size of the heart and any alteration in its shape.

(b) To confirm the presence of a pericardial effusion.

(c) To confirm and estimate the amount of fluid in the chest (hydrothorax) in cases of congestive heart failure.

5. Electrocardiography.

(*a*) To confirm the diagnosis of coronary thrombosis.

(*b*) To differentiate the various forms of irregular heart action.

(*c*) To confirm the presence of heart involvement in acute rheumatic fever and severe cases of diphtheria.

(*d*) To aid in the diagnosis of such heart diseases as congenital heart lesions and myxœdema.

6. Estimation of Serum Transaminase (S.G.O.T.).

To confirm the diagnosis of coronary thrombosis, which causes a raised transaminase level in the blood.

7. Aspiration of Hydrothorax and Ascites.

To relieve pressure from a hydrothorax or an ascites in cases of congestive heart failure not resolving on mercurial diuretics.

8. Venesection.

(*a*) To relieve congestion of the lungs in heart failure, especially where caused by hypertension.

(*b*) To lower a very high blood pressure in cases of hypertension.

9. Circulation Time.

In the diagnosis of heart disease, estimation of the circulation time is valuable. Circulation time is always increased above the normal in all cases of heart failure.

10. Aspiration of Pericardial Effusion.

(*a*) To relieve pressure on the heart in cases of large pericardial effusions.

(*b*) To drain a purulent pericardial effusion.

SUMMARY OF IMPORTANT DRUGS USED IN DISEASES OF THE CIRCULATORY SYSTEM

1. **Anticoagulants** (heparin, phenindione, warfarin, sinthrome, tromexan, dicoumarol, marcoumar).
Coronary thrombosis.
Venous thrombosis.
Pulmonary and arterial embolism.

2. **Antithyroid Drugs** (carbimazole, thiouracil).
Thyrotoxic heart disease.

3. **Cortisone and Allied Drugs** (prednisone, prednisolone, dexamethasone).

   Acute rheumatic fever.

4. **Digitalis and Digoxin.**

   Auricular fibrillation.
   Congestive heart failure.
   Paroxysmal tachycardia.

5. **Diuretics** (mersalyl, chlorothiazide, hydrochlorothiazide, hydroflumethiazide).

   Congestive heart failure.   Left heart failure.

6. **Hypotensive Drugs** (reserpine, darenthin, ismelin, inversine).

   Hypertension.

7. **Drugs to raise Blood Pressure** (aramine, mephine and noradrenaline).

   Coronary thrombosis, for severe shock.

8. **Morphine.**

   Congestive heart failure.   Coronary thrombosis.

9. **Penicillin.**

   Subacute bacterial endocarditis.   Syphilitic heart disease.

10. **Quinidine.**

    Auricular fibrillation not accompanied by heart failure; especially useful in thyrotoxic auricular fibrillation.
    Paroxysmal tachycardia.

11. **Salicylates.**

    Acute rheumatic fever.

12. **Streptomycin.**

    Subacute bacterial endocarditis (combined with penicillin).

13. **Vasodilator Drugs** (amyl nitrite, trinitrin, peritrate, mycardol, dibenyline, priscol, ronicol).

    Angina pectoris.   Raynaud's disease.

14. **Drugs to lower Blood Cholesterol** (nicotinic acid, triparanol).

    Atherosclerosis.

CHAPTER VI

DISEASES OF THE RESPIRATORY SYSTEM

ANATOMY AND PHYSIOLOGY.—The respiratory system includes the nose, air sinuses, pharynx, larynx, trachea, bronchi and the lungs. The whole purpose of this system is to allow the intake of pure fresh air into the lungs and to discharge the used-up air after it has performed its function. By this means the blood in the lungs is brought into as close contact as possible with the inspired air and can take up the oxygen which is vital for the proper maintenance and function of practically every organ and tissue in the body.

We have seen, in discussing diseases of the heart, that the function of the heart is to pump the blood and that of the blood vessels is to carry it throughout the body so that every organ obtains a liberal supply of oxygen. This oxygen is carried in the red cells of the blood. In using up oxygen each organ and tissue gives off in exchange carbon dioxide as a waste product, which is passed into the venous blood, carried in the veins and eventually collected in the right side of the heart. From there it is pumped into the lung capillaries. Here this waste product, carbon dioxide, can be given off into the air in the minute air spaces in the lungs. These minute air spaces are called alveoli.

THE MECHANISM OF RESPIRATION.—Air is drawn into the lungs by the act of inspiration. During inspiration the chest cavity is inflated by contractions of the respiratory muscles attached to the bony cage of the chest, which pull out the ribs. The diaphragm descends during the act of inspiration, and this further helps to enlarge the chest cavity and so inflate the lungs. The lungs in expanding suck in air through the respiratory passages into each and every alveolus, and so allow the oxygen to be taken up and the waste product, carbon dioxide, to be given off. At the end of the inspiration the intercostal muscles and the diaphragm relax and allow the chest wall to fall back, thereby deflating the lungs. In addition, the elasticity of the lungs themselves, by exerting a pull on the chest wall, also plays an important role in expelling the air. This expulsion of air from the lungs is known as expiration.

CONTROL OF RESPIRATION.—Respiration is controlled through

the respiratory centre in the medulla of the spinal cord, which, through its influence on the nerves supplying the respiratory muscles and the diaphragm, can increase or decrease the act of respiration. Diseases which involve the respiratory centre may thus affect the act of respiration. Furthermore, for the normal control of respiration the amount of carbon dioxide in the blood is most important. Even a slight increase in the amount of carbon dioxide stimulates the respiratory centre to increase the rate and depth of the respirations. A marked reduction in the oxygen content of the blood also stimulates the respirations.

COMMON SYMPTOMS OF DISEASES OF THE RESPIRATORY SYSTEM

Many of the diseases affecting the respiratory system produce common symptoms and signs. In view of their importance it is convenient at the outset to mention these.

1. **Cough.**—This is a very common symptom seen in most diseases of the respiratory tract and usually due to some form of irritation. There are various types of cough, such as moist or dry, depending on whether the cough is accompanied by sputum or not. The short suppressed cough associated with pleurisy is characteristic. Here the act of coughing causes pain owing to the movement of the inflamed pleura, and so the cough is cut short by the pain.

2. **Sputum or Phlegm.**—Sputum is an excretion from the lining mucous membrane of the respiratory passages. According to the nature and extent of the disease the sputum varies in amount and character. In the early stages of disease sputum may be absent, appearing later when the lesion in the respiratory tract has progressed. The sputum may be a clear white colour, when it is called *mucoid*. In such cases the sputum is usually the result of minor irritation of the respiratory passage. In more severe lesions, especially inflammatory diseases, the sputum is frankly purulent. Where actual destruction of tissue is present the sputum may be bloodstained owing to erosion of a blood vessel.

Some diseases of the lungs are associated with chronic widespread damage to the lung tissue, and in these cases abundant purulent sputum, often offensive and bloodstained, is present. Such diseases are bronchiectasis, lung abscess, lung cancer and advanced tuberculosis.

3. **Dyspnœa.**—Dyspnœa means difficulty in breathing or as it

is most usually called, breathlessness. The underlying cause in most cases is a deficiency of oxygen. Any disease which interferes with the proper uptake of oxygen stimulates the respiratory centre, so that an increase in the respirations occurs to try and overcome this oxygen deficiency. Apart from diseases primarily involving the lungs, other diseases, especially heart failure, can cause dyspnœa. In heart failure, owing to the impaired action of the heart, the circulation through the lungs becomes slower so that congestion of the lungs results and seriously interferes with the proper uptake of oxygen. In addition, any disease which makes the respiratory act painful may cause dyspnœa.

4. **Cyanosis.**—This was discussed in connection with heart failure, when it was seen to be caused by a deficiency of oxygen in the blood giving rise to the bluish colour known as cyanosis. In many chest diseases there is a deficient intake of oxygen which causes cyanosis. Cyanosis usually means a fairly severe degree of involvement of the respiratory system.

5. **Pain.**—This is usually due to the pleurisy (inflammation of the pleura) which accompanies many forms of chest disease. The inflamed layers of the pleura when rubbed together during respiration cause pain.

6. **Hæmoptysis.**—Coughing up blood is called *hæmoptysis* and may vary from mere staining of the sputum, as mentioned above, to frank blood. The coughing up of blood is a most important sign, and in most cases denotes a serious chest disease, especially pulmonary tuberculosis and carcinoma of the lung.

DISEASES OF THE UPPER RESPIRATORY TRACT

The upper respiratory tract is usually taken to include the nose, sinuses, pharynx and trachea. Diseases affecting this part of the respiratory tract are extremely common, and many of them are described in textbooks on surgery. For instance, chronic enlargement of the tonsils and adenoids, sinusitis, etc., are not discussed here.

The common medical diseases which affect the upper respiratory tract include the following :—

1. Acute Coryza.
2. Acute Tonsillitis.
3. Acute Tracheitis.
4. Laryngitis.
5. Hay Fever.

ACUTE CORYZA (The Common Cold)

This, as will be known, is an extremely common condition. The cause is a virus which is very infectious and spreads rapidly from person to person. One attack produces no immunity or resistance in the body, so that further attacks can and, of course, do occur.

Symptoms and Signs.—These will already be familiar and need little description. The essential feature is an inflammation of the nasal passages, known as *rhinitis*, which produces a running nose and sneezing. Running eyes are also common and, perhaps, a mild conjunctivitis. The inflammation often spreads to involve the pharynx and trachea and so set up a pharyngitis and tracheitis with resulting huskiness, sore throat and cough.

Course and Prognosis.—Most cases clear up within a few days and the only danger is that infection may spread down to affect the lungs and thus cause a pneumonia. This is likely to occur only in patients in debilitated states, especially elderly people and young infants.

Treatment.—Most people " walk off " a cold and have their own particular remedy. All treatment is purely symptomatic, *i.e.*, to relieve the symptoms, because as yet there is no specific cure. Inhalants such as menthol or benzedrine often give relief to the congestion in the nose. Hot sweet drinks are suitable and aspirin or Dover's powders at night, 5 to 15 gr., are often helpful. It is only in severe attacks or for people who are likely to develop complications that bed rest is needed.

ACUTE TONSILLITIS (Acute Streptococcal Throat)

This is a very common infection, especially in any institution where large numbers of people are closeted together. The cause is most often the hæmolytic streptococcus, but other organisms can cause an acute tonsillitis.

Symptoms and Signs.

1. The onset is usually sudden, with a general feeling of malaise, fever and headache.

2. The patient complains of a sore throat and difficulty in swallowing. The throat is often described as feeling very dry.

3. When the throat is examined it will be found to be inflamed and red and usually white spots (*exudate*) are present on both tonsils.

4. In some cases a *peritonsillar abscess* forms which produces a large and very painful swelling in the mouth. *Quinsy* is a frequently used name for a peritonsillar abscess.

Diagnosis.—This is fairly obvious in most cases on account of the presenting complaint of a sore throat. Difficulties, however, often arise in the case of infants and young children. Here, even with children old enough to give an account of their symptoms, a soreness of the throat is seldom complained of. The presenting symptoms in young children are usually fever, malaise and abdominal colic; the latter may give rise to a mistaken diagnosis of acute appendicitis.

Examination of the throat in sick children is therefore most important as a routine, whether or not a sore throat is complained of. The nurse should have readily available a spatula and suitable illumination (torch) for the doctor when he is examining all sick children. It is convenient here to add that, as well as the throat, the ears are always examined as a routine in all sick children. An auriscope of suitable size should therefore also be to hand.

There are two other diseases that give rise to sore throats and symptoms like those in acute streptococcal sore throat and it is important to differentiate between them :—

1. DIPHTHERIA.—Here the symptoms are very similar except that the patient is usually more ill and toxic, and the pulse more rapid. There is also the characteristic membrane in the throat, which does not occur in most cases of acute tonsillitis. A throat swab will reveal the diphtheritic organisms.

2. VINCENT'S ANGINA.—This produces a sore throat with greyish ulceration on the tonsils. Signs of fever or toxæmia are absent or mild, except in severe cases. The organisms responsible can be isolated by taking a throat swab.

Treatment.

1. The patient is put to bed and a throat swab is taken in all cases to confirm the presence of the hæmolytic streptococcus or other organism; also to exclude the diphtheria bacillus as a cause. If there is any suspicion of diphtheria the case must be isolated and treated as such.

2. Diet has to be light, with plenty of hot drinks, which are soothing to the throat. If the latter is very painful, especially in cases of peritonsillar abscess, kaolin poultices to the neck are very comforting.

3. In all except the mildest cases either sulphonamides or penicillin will probably be given. In any case where diphtheria is suspected as the cause of the acute sore throat, the specific diphtheria antitoxin must be given without waiting for the result of the throat swab. Any delay in giving antitoxin in a suspected case of diphtheria may have disastrous consequences.

4. If a peritonsillar abscess is present and does not subside rapidly on the above treatment it will need to be opened. This is done by means of sharp-pointed sinus forceps or a short-bladed knife.

ACUTE TRACHEITIS

Inflammation of the trachea may occur :—

1. In association with certain of the infectious fevers, such as measles or influenza.
2. With the common cold.
3. As a primary infection in itself.

Symptoms and Signs.—The general signs of infection, including fever, malaise and headache, are present. In addition, the patient complains of a typical sore feeling behind the sternum. A dry or slightly moist cough is also common.

Treatment.—This is similar to that for acute tonsillitis.

LARYNGITIS

(A) Acute Laryngitis.

Causes.

1. Acute infectious fevers, particularly measles, diphtheria and influenza.

2. The common cold, acute tracheitis, or acute bronchitis may all cause an acute laryngitis.

Symptoms and Signs.—In addition to the general signs of infection, including malaise, fever and headache, there is the characteristic huskiness of voice and hoarseness. In some cases there may be almost complete loss of voice. The throat is sore and there is an accompanying dry cough.

Diagnosis.—The diagnosis of laryngitis is usually obvious, but it is important to distinguish those cases which are due to measles and diphtheria. The examination of the mouth will show any Koplik's spots, thus identifying the case as one of measles, as also would, of course, the presence of a morbilliform rash. In diphtheria there is in most cases the characteristic membrane present in the throat, but in a few patients this may be absent. If there is any suspicion that the laryngitis might be due to diphtheria the case is treated as such till a definite diagnosis is made.

Treatment of Acute Laryngitis.—The patient is nursed in bed in a well-ventilated atmosphere, but avoiding draughts. If it is thought that the laryngitis may be due to measles, diphtheria, or any other infectious fever, then proper isolation precautions are taken and, in addition, any specific treatment, *e.g.*, antitoxin, given.

The diet should be light, with plenty of soothing hot drinks. Some patients with laryngitis find a steamy atmosphere soothing, and inhalations from an inhaler or a steam tent may be used. Friar's balsam, 1 drachm to the pint of water, is the most commonly used inhalant.

If the case is a severe one, with high temperature and signs of toxicity, penicillin or another antibiotic may be given. It is very rarely, except in cases of diphtheritic laryngitis, that obstruction to the breathing occurs requiring tracheotomy.

(B) Chronic Laryngitis.

Causes.

1. Prolonged over-use of voice as in singers.
2. Tuberculous laryngitis.
3. Syphilitic laryngitis.
4. Malignant disease of the larynx.

Symptoms and Treatment.—The predominating complaint is one of chronic progressive hoarseness, eventually leading to loss of voice. In all cases of chronic hoarseness an examination of the throat and vocal cords will be made by means of a laryngoscope. By this means the exact nature and cause of the laryngitis can usually be identified.

The treatment will naturally vary according to the cause. In those cases due to over-use of the voice, prolonged rest is usually sufficient to restore normal conditions. In tuberculous patients there is usually an advanced pulmonary tuberculous lesion as well, which requires the appropriate treatment as outlined on page 192. Sedative lozenges containing opium are useful for the pain.

In syphilitic laryngitis, penicillin is given. In malignant disease of the larynx, operation or radium therapy is carried out unless the disease has spread too far, in which case only palliative sedatives can be given.

HAY FEVER

Hay fever is one of the allergic diseases, like many cases of asthma and urticaria. In hay fever the patients are sensitive to the grass pollens and when they come in contact with them the typical symptoms of hay fever develop.

Symptoms and Signs.

1. The onset is always at a specific time of the year—in England in the month of May, when the new grasses grow.

2. Paroxysmal attacks of sneezing, associated with a running nose and running eyes, occur. The bouts of sneezing may last in some cases for hours on end. There is usually severe congestion of the nasal passages and eyes.

Treatment.—Local treatment to relieve the nasal congestion, such as inhalation of menthol or benzedrine, is very useful. Antihistamine drugs have proved of great benefit. Numerous preparations are available and newer ones are continually being introduced (see p. 591). At present antistin, anthisan, benadryl, dibistin, histantin, phenergan and sandosten are all in common use. Some are more powerful than others, whilst some patients find one drug more effective than others. Usually 1 to 4 tablets a day are given. As all these drugs have a hypnotic action as well, sleeping drugs, such as barbiturates, should not be given at the same time.

More recently hydrocortisone in the form of a nasal spray or snuff has given very good results in the treatment of hay fever.

To prevent attacks, desensitisation may be effected by means of gradually increasing doses of the offending pollens injected subcutaneously. The injections have to be started several months before the hay fever starts in May and stopped when the new grass pollens grow. The effect, unfortunately, only lasts for one to two years.

DISEASES OF THE LOWER RESPIRATORY TRACT

BRONCHITIS

A) **Acute Bronchitis.**

This is a very common condition indeed, in which inflammation of the bronchi occurs. A variety of organisms may cause the attack, especially streptococci, pneumococci, influenzal organisms, etc. There are several factors which predispose to acute bronchitis, particularly a damp climate and stuffy and dust-laden atmospheres. It is very common in infants and elderly people and more frequent in winter.

Bronchitis fairly constantly occurs in several infectious fevers, especially measles, influenza and whooping cough.

Symptoms and Signs.

1. There are the symptoms of a mild fever such as malaise, headache and loss of appetite.

2. A cough is an early symptom and is associated with a moderate amount of mucoid or purulent sputum.

3. There may be soreness or pain beneath the sternum caused by an accompanying inflammation of the trachea.

4. The respirations are usually a little fast and somewhat laboured, but except in serious cases there is no severe dyspnœa or cyanosis.

5. When the chest is examined, alterations in the normal breath sounds are heard which enable the doctor to diagnose the condition.

Course.—The disease usually subsides fairly rapidly in a few days with proper treatment, and is serious only in young children and elderly people where the inflammation may spread and cause a broncho-pneumonia. Repeated attacks of acute bronchitis may, however, give rise to chronic bronchitis with much more serious consequences.

Treatment of Acute Bronchitis.—The patient is put to bed and kept warm in a well-ventilated atmosphere. Light fever diet is given with plenty of drinks. Aspirin and Dover's powders will probably be found useful, and on this treatment most cases will subside rapidly.

Expectorants, *i.e.*, drugs to increase expectoration of sputum, may be ordered, especially if the sputum is thick and difficult to bring up. If, however, there is a dry persistent cough without sputum (which may occur when the condition is subsiding) then a sedative linctus will prove of most value. The severe cases with a high temperature which do not respond rapidly to the above treatment will require treatment with penicillin (or other antibiotic) or sulphonamides.

(B) Chronic Bronchitis.

The chronic stage of bronchitis is extremely common in the British Isles, especially in men. It is difficult to say what exactly causes the condition but probably many factors play a part. Repeated attacks of acute bronchitis, a damp climate, working in a moist and dust-laden atmosphere are all important contributory causes.

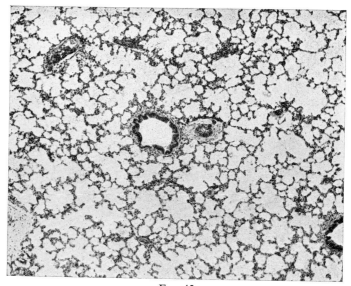

Fig. 45
Section through a normal lung showing the clear empty
air sacs (alveoli).

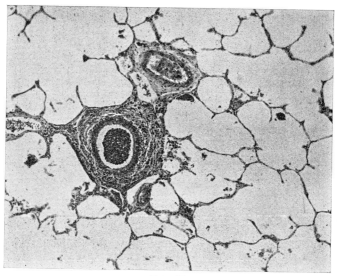

Fig. 46
Emphysema of the lung showing the characteristic thin-walled and
distended alveoli.   Bronchitis is also present, as shown by the
inflammatory exudate inside the bronchus.

In practically all cases of chronic bronchitis there is also present a change in the lungs known as **emphysema**. Chronic inflammation of the bronchi, such as is present in chronic bronchitis, produces a chronic cough which eventually after many years causes a severe strain on the lung tissue resulting in distension and thinning of the fine alveoli (air spaces) of the lungs. To this distension and thinning of the lung tissue the term *emphysema* is given, and it is important as it in turn can cause heart failure.

It is appropriate here to distinguish the condition often seen in surgical diseases known as *surgical emphysema*. Here, air is present in the subcutaneous tissues, causing swelling and typical crackling sounds when the skin is touched. It is most often seen as a complication of fractured ribs and seldom requires any special treatment.

Symptoms and Signs.

1. The patient is usually a middle-aged or elderly man who has had a " weak chest " for some time and has had to go to bed nearly every winter for several weeks with an attack of acute bronchitis. The attacks recur until eventually throughout most of the winter and occasionally in summer he suffers from chest trouble.

2. He complains of a persistent cough and sputum, the latter being either mucoid or muco-purulent.

3. Dyspnœa, except in the very early stages, is always present and is mainly due to the commonly associated emphysema.

4. With the passage of the years the disease becomes progressively worse ; the dyspnœa increases and eventually congestive heart failure may develop owing to the added strain thrown on the heart by the diseased lungs.

Treatment of Chronic Bronchitis.

1. FOR THE ACUTE EXACERBATION.—During the attacks when acute bronchitis is added to the more chronic condition the patient is put to bed and treatment as outlined under Acute Bronchitis is given. The danger in these attacks is the development of broncho-pneumonia. After a few weeks the acute episode subsides and the patient is left with the chronic residual symptoms.

2. FOR THE CHRONIC STAGE.—There is no definite cure for chronic bronchitis and emphysema, and the measures taken are for the relief of the symptoms and to prevent, as far as possible, the acute exacerbations. The patient's occupation should be one, if possible, that enables him to avoid damp smoky atmospheres and also any undue exposure in wet weather. As this is very difficult

to achieve in a damp climate, the patient is often advised to go to a dry climate, where the disease frequently improves. In practice this very useful advice can be carried out only in exceptional cases. Smoking is best avoided if possible, as it aggravates the disease.

If the cough is dry and irritating a sedative linctus is given, while if it is moist expectorants may be used to ease the production of the sputum. If heart failure develops this is treated on the usual lines. With severe and frequently recurring attacks of bronchitis prolonged treatment over months with sulphonamides or antibiotics may be given to try and prevent further recurrences.

PNEUMONIA

In this very common condition there is an inflammation of the alveoli of the lungs caused by various micro-organisms. These include the different types of pneumococci and also streptococci, staphylococci, the influenzal bacilli and certain viruses. In addition the tubercle bacillus causes a specific type of pneumonia.

Pneumonia may be conveniently classified into the following main types :—

BACTERIAL PNEUMONIAS

1. Lobar Pneumonia.
2. Broncho-pneumonia.
3. Tuberculous Pneumonia.

VIRUS PNEUMONIA

1. Primary Atypical Pneumonia.

LOBAR PNEUMONIA

Pathology.—In this form of pneumonia one whole lobe of a lung is affected. There are very characteristic and typical changes in the diseased lobe, which becomes solid and airless owing to the inflammation. The term *consolidation* is used to denote these pathological changes. In addition the pleura lining the affected lobe is often inflamed, giving rise to one form of pleurisy.

Symptoms and Signs.

1. The *onset* is sudden, with a high fever (often 102° to 104° F.), and is in many cases accompanied by shivering attacks (rigors). A severe *pain* in the chest over the affected lobe of the lung is present owing to the frequently accompanying pleurisy. This pain characteristically catches the breathing so that the patient is nervous of

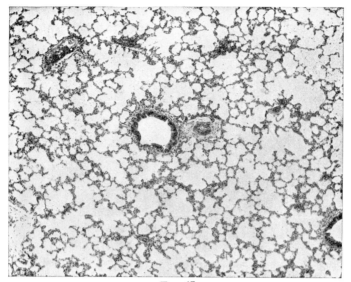

FIG. 47

Section through a normal lung showing the clear empty
air sacs (alveoli).

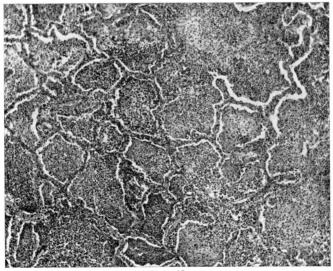

FIG. 48

Lobar pneumonia. The alveoli are completely filled with inflammatory
exudate (white blood cells, fibrin and some red cells). The alveolar
walls are thickened owing to congestion and œdema. The solid airless
state of the lung in pneumonia is known as consolidation.

taking a deep breath. For this reason also the *cough*, which is always present, is short and suppressed.

2. The face is flushed and *herpes febrilis* is very commonly present on the lips or cheek. This is a small group of vesicles clustered together which after a few days crust and resolve. Herpes febrilis is most commonly associated with lobar pneumonia or the common cold.

The *respirations* are rapid and the *alæ nasæ* (nostrils) may be seen to move with respiration. This sign is important as it denotes a fairly serious disease of the respiratory system. The pulse rate rises, but not to the same extent as the respirations.

3. After a day or so the cough becomes moist with the typical *rusty* sputum, the colour being due to altered blood. The sputum is very thick and tenacious and often adheres to the side of the sputum mug.

4. In severe cases the breathing may be very distressed and cyanosis is present. In these severe attacks delirium may also occur.

5. When the doctor examines the chest with a stethoscope, typical alterations in the breath sounds over the consolidated lobe are heard which in conjunction with the above symptoms allow a ready diagnosis to be made. X-ray examination of the chest may be carried out to confirm the diagnosis and also to watch the resolution of the pneumonia. The solid lobe shows up on X-ray as a dense shadow.

Course.—In the days before the discovery of sulphonamides and penicillin the illness usually ran a course lasting from seven to nine days. Suddenly about the seventh day or so there occurred an abrupt change in the patient's condition when after being very ill his temperature dropped, the respirations became calm and the signs of toxæmia vanished ; what is known as a crisis had taken place. To-day this course is not usually seen as specific treatment has altered the whole course of the disease.

Complications.—These are much less common to-day because of the specific treatment. If the patient is not responding to treatment as evidenced by the failure of the temperature to return to normal then one of the following complications should be suspected :—

1. Empyema. Here there is a purulent effusion in the pleural cavity, see page 188.

2. Lung abscess.

3. Rarely, purulent pericarditis or meningitis.

Treatment of Lobar Pneumonia.

1. NURSING : GENERAL MEASURES.—The patient is usually nursed propped up in bed, supported by pillows, as this position gives the maximum amount of ease to the respirations. A well-ventilated warm room is of particular value and adds greatly to the patient's comfort. The clothes should be light and loose, especially around the neck and sleeves, and must be easily removable. This point about clothing is of great importance, not only in pneumonia but in any severe illness in which the chest or heart may have to be examined from time to time during the course of the illness. To see the nurse struggling to remove tight clothes over the head and shoulders in an ill patient is a most distressing and unnecessary sight.

In severely ill patients, and especially with elderly people, constant attention will be needed to overcome their great tendency to slip down in the bed with the consequent likelihood of their developing congestion of the lungs. In these cases also, careful watch must be kept on their fluid balance as left to themselves they tend to sleep and take very little fluid. Fluid must be given in adequate amounts and glucose fruit drinks and milk will be found very useful. Depending on the severity of the case, diet will be light and nourishing as for any general infection and increased as necessary.

Careful attention to the mouth as in all cases of fever will be necessary. Gentle swabbing and adequate fluids are most important in keeping the mouth clean.

Elderly patients particularly will have to be carefully treated, with constant attention to all pressure areas to prevent the development of pressure sores. A mild purgative to open the bowels and prevent abdominal distension which might further aggravate the laboured respirations is given at the onset of the illness.

In all cases of severe dyspnœa and cyanosis, oxygen will be needed. For the pain, if this is severe and persistent, a kaolin poultice to the affected side (never on the front of the chest) is useful. If insomnia is present a hypnotic such as medinal, soneryl, or chloral hydrate is given.

2. SPECIFIC TREATMENT.—As mentioned earlier specific treatment has now almost completely changed the whole course and outlook of cases of pneumonia, not only in this particular form of pneumonia but also in the other forms as will be seen later. From being a severe illness with fatal results in many cases it has now become a relatively minor illness with the severe symptoms lasting perhaps a couple of days only. There are, however, exceptions to this,

especially with infants and elderly people when the condition may well be serious in spite of specific therapy.

The specific treatments for lobar pneumonia are penicillin, sulphonamides, or the tetracycline antibiotics. The bacteria in the sputum are cultured and their sensitivity to the various agents is determined. At present penicillin or one of the sulphonamides is most extensively used since most bacteria are sensitive to them. Penicillin is given by mouth (phenoxymethyl penicillin—penicillin V) 60 to 125 mgm. four-hourly to six-hourly or by intramuscular injection,

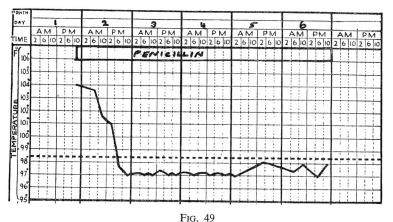

Fig. 49

Temperature chart from a case of lobar pneumonia showing the dramatic response to penicillin.

100,000 units six-hourly. Occasionally it has no effect and one of the other antibiotics or sulphonamides has to be given.

Sulphonamides are widely used in the treatment of pneumonia and are fully effective when given by mouth. The main drawback with sulphonamides is the liability to toxic reactions. The importance of an adequate fluid intake, stressed earlier under the general nursing of pneumonia, becomes greater still when sulphonamides are used. Crystallisation of these drugs in the kidneys, with the danger of anuria and renal failure, is prevented by an adequate fluid intake.

The preparations of sulphonamides most commonly used at present are sulphadimidine (sulphamezathine), sulphafurazole (gantrisin), sulphadiazine and the sulphonamide mixtures (sulphatriad). The doses and administration of these drugs are as outlined on page 575.

The tetracycline antibiotics are also very effective in pneumonia and are given in capsule form by mouth.

Penicillin, sulphonamides, or whatever drug has been used is continued till the temperature has been normal for two to three days.

BRONCHO-PNEUMONIA (ASPIRATION PNEUMONIA)

In this form of pneumonia it is believed that scattered areas of collapse (atelectasis) usually develop, which then become infected, with resultant inflammation of the lungs.

Broncho-pneumonia or aspiration pneumonia shows the following features :—

1. In broncho-pneumonia instead of one whole lobe of a lung being involved, there are patchy areas of pneumonic consolidation scattered throughout both lungs.

2. Broncho-pneumonia is more common in infants and elderly people, often as a complication of some other illness, especially chronic bronchitis. It is the form of pneumonia which usually complicates the acute infectious fevers (measles, whooping cough) and operations.

3. The onset is usually not so sudden and pain in the chest from an associated pleurisy is often absent.

4. Empyema is a much less common complication than in lobar pneumonia. However, the pneumonic changes may persist longer and the condition of delayed resolution or unresolved pneumonia may arise. In these cases permanent damage may result, such as fibrosis of the lungs.

Treatment.—This is exactly the same as for lobar pneumonia. The patients are likely to be more severely ill because infants and elderly people are more commonly affected, and because broncho-pneumonia is very often a complication of some other illness.

TUBERCULOUS PNEUMONIA

This is an uncommon form of acute pulmonary tuberculosis, very rapid in onset and carrying a high mortality rate. As it is a variety of Pulmonary Tuberculosis it is more conveniently discussed under that heading (p. 88).

VIRUS PNEUMONIA

This form of pneumonia is due not to bacteria but to a virus. In this way it differs from the types of pneumonia previously described. It causes symptoms very like those described under lobar pneumonia, but the signs in the chest are very few and unlike those found in the other types of pneumonia.

Virus pneumonia is suspected if, in addition to the absence of typical signs in the chest, there is no response to penicillin or sulphonamides, as these drugs have no effect on virus infections. The tetracycline antibiotics or chloramphenicol are sometimes prescribed for virus pneumonia although their use is of doubtful value. The tetracycline antibiotics are given by mouth, 150 to 250 mgm. six-hourly. The dose of chloramphenicol is 500 mgm. six-hourly by mouth. The antibiotics are continued until the temperature has been normal for two to three days.

The tetracycline antibiotics may cause nausea and diarrhœa and, less often, a serious ileo-colitis may develop (see p. 582). Chloramphenicol may, on rare occasions, cause aplastic anæmia.

PLEURISY

Pleurisy or inflammation of the pleura is a very common disease occurring in many different forms and due to many causes.

Causes.
1. Tuberculosis.
2. Pneumonia.
3. Carcinoma of the bronchus.

Types.
1. Dry pleurisy.
2. Pleural effusion (wet pleurisy).
3. Empyema.

TUBERCULOUS PLEURISY

This form of pleurisy caused by the tubercle bacilli may be either wet or dry, and it accounts for nearly all the cases of pleurisy occurring in young adults without any other sign of disease in the lungs. For this reason tuberculous pleurisy is often known as primary pleurisy.

Symptoms and Signs.

1. The onset is usually sudden, with pain in the chest accompanied by the general signs of fever, including headache and malaise. The pain in the chest characteristically catches the breathing and may be quite severe.

2. A dry cough often cut short by pain is very common.

3. When the chest is examined the diagnostic pleural *friction rub* is heard. This is a coarse grating sound occurring with the breath sounds and is due to the inflamed layers of the pleura rubbing together. (This rub is analogous to the pericardial rub diagnostic of pericarditis.)

4. In many cases the dry stage may develop into a pleural effusion, when a large amount of fluid due to the inflammatory changes accumulates in the pleural cavity. The fluid may cause no symptoms additional to those just mentioned, and its presence is then diagnosed by the signs in the chest, by X-ray examination, or by putting a needle into the pleural cavity and withdrawing fluid.

In some patients, however, the quantity of fluid present may be so large that it causes embarrassment to the breathing, and then severe dyspnœa and cyanosis occur.

5. The fluid, if present, in tuberculous pleurisy is nearly always clear and straw coloured. It is serous and never purulent, except in those rare cases associated with severe, advanced, underlying pulmonary tuberculosis. In a few cases the fluid may be bloodstained.

Course.—Tuberculous pleurisy usually resolves in a matter of weeks, and in most cases there is little or no evidence of obvious underlying disease in the lungs. The general condition of these patients is good, but in some cases, perhaps after a lapse of months or years, evidence of pulmonary tuberculosis develops.

Treatment.—As mentioned above, the pleurisy usually soon resolves, whilst the fluid present usually disappears without the need for aspiration, which is necessary in tuberculous patients only if signs of embarrassment to the breathing occur. As, however, the great danger is the development of pulmonary tuberculosis, treatment must be prolonged. The keynote of treatment is rest in bed with full diet. Nearly all patients are treated by a prolonged course of chemotherapy with streptomycin, para-aminosalicylic acid or isoniazid as for patients with pulmonary tuberculosis (see p. 193). After all the signs in the chest have cleared up and the temperature has been normal for many weeks, graduated exercise is allowed.

These patients are kept under observation for several years, with periodic chest X-rays to diagnose any pulmonary tuberculosis at the earliest moment.

PNEUMONIC PLEURISY

In discussing lobar pneumonia it was stated that in nearly all cases there is an inflammation of the pleura overlying the affected lobe of the lung. This pleurisy accounts for the pain in the chest common in pneumonia. Apart from this pain the symptoms and signs of the pneumonia overshadow those due to the pleurisy. No special comment is necessary in most cases of pneumonic pleurisy, the treatment being that of the underlying pneumonia.

In a small percentage of cases, however, a pleural effusion occurs as a complication of the pneumonia and in these cases the fluid is usually purulent. The term **empyema** is used to denote purulent effusions, and by far the commonest cause of empyema is pneumonia. Less commonly, as stated under Tuberculous Pleurisy, advanced pulmonary tuberculosis can cause a tuberculous empyema.

When empyema occurs as a complication of pneumonia the condition is recognised by failure of the temperature to fall with specific treatment and also by the signs of fluid in the chest (the latter being usually confirmed by X-ray examination). Aspiration of the fluid by inserting a large needle between the ribs under a local anæsthetic reveals that the fluid is purulent. Culturing the fluid in the laboratory will isolate the causative organism, generally the pneumococcus, streptococcus, or staphylococcus.

Treatment.—Only the treatment of empyema calls for special comment, as the usual dry form of pleurisy associated with pneumonia rapidly responds to the general treatment of the pneumonia. Once it has been established that a purulent effusion is present, as much as possible of the fluid is removed by aspiration with a large-bore needle. After the aspiration a large dose of penicillin, such as 500,000 units in 10 to 20 ml. of sterile saline, is inserted into the pleural cavity.

Repeated aspirations with the instillation of intrapleural penicillin are usually necessary. Penicillin, as outlined in the treatment of pneumonia, is of course continued. With this treatment most of the cases will clear up completely. In the remainder, mainly where the fluid is too thick to be adequately aspirated with a needle, drainage of the pleural cavity by resecting a small portion of rib and inserting a large special tube (Tudor Edwards') is necessary. The tube has to be left in for many weeks, gradually shortened, and finally removed when no more pus remains in the chest.

It may be stated that penicillin and the other antibiotics have changed both the frequency and treatment of empyema. It is now becoming much less common, and when it does occur many of the cases respond to aspiration alone. Before penicillin, nearly all cases of empyema had to have rib resection and prolonged drainage.

PLEURISY DUE TO CARCINOMA

Carcinoma of a bronchus often spreads to involve the pleura and usually causes a pleurisy with effusion. The characteristics of the pleural effusion are that it accumulates rapidly and often needs aspiration to relieve the embarrassment to the respirations. It is generally a clear, serous, or a hæmorrhagic, fluid. More rarely, carcinoma can cause a purulent effusion.

The treatment of pleurisy with effusion due to carcinoma is generally purely palliative, as at this stage the carcinoma has probably spread too far to allow any radical form of therapy. Repeated aspirations of the chest are often necessary and sedatives for any pain present are given.

HYDROTHORAX

Hydrothorax is the name given to fluid which is present in the pleural cavity but not as a result of inflammation of the pleura. The fluid is therefore not an exudate and is known as a transudate. By far the commonest cause of a hydrothorax is congestive heart failure, and then the effusion may need removal if the general treatment does not clear it up. Rarer causes of a hydrothorax are—as part of a general renal œdema in cases of nephritis, and from pressure on the veins in the chest as with mediastinal tumours.

PULMONARY TUBERCULOSIS (Phthisis)

Pulmonary tuberculosis is caused by infection of the lungs with the tubercle bacillus. As was seen in the general discussion on tuberculosis (Chap. III), pulmonary lesions are due almost entirely to the human form of the tubercle bacillus, as distinct from the bovine type which is mainly responsible for glandular and bone tuberculosis. It was also seen that the usual route of infection in pulmonary tuberculosis is either by direct contact with a case of pulmonary tuberculosis or by inhalation of dust containing the organism.

Pathology.—The tubercle bacilli lodge in the lungs and set up a chronic inflammation of a specific type. The bacilli produce areas of infiltration which have a characteristic tubercle formation ; hence the name for the organism. These areas of disease are very likely to break down into cheesy pus which is known as *caseation,* and a small chronic abscess is then formed. This may burst into one of the bronchi with the result that a hole or cavity may occur in the lung tissue. As the condition is of a chronic inflammatory nature, the lungs react by forming fibrous tissue in an effort to heal the disease. This fibrous tissue may produce a dense and widespread fibrosis in the lung. Usually in the chronic form of the disease both fibrosis and caseation are present.

The infection in the lungs usually starts, for some unknown reason, in the upper parts or apices of the lungs. It may start on one side and spread to other parts of the same lung, or cross to the other side to involve the opposite lung.

Clinical Forms of Pulmonary Tuberculosis.

(A) Chronic Fibro-caseous Tuberculosis.
(B) Tuberculous Pneumonia.
(C) Miliary Tuberculosis.

(A) CHRONIC FIBRO-CASEOUS TUBERCULOSIS

This is the most common form seen in clinical practice. The disease sets up the specific lesions in the lungs, and there are also signs of general toxicity. These two factors combine to give rise to the various symptoms and signs.

Symptoms and Signs.

1. THE ONSET.—This is in most cases an insidious development over weeks or months, and the earliest symptom is a *cough*, at first dry but later moist with varying amounts of sputum. In some cases there is a previous history of either wet or dry pleurisy, as tuberculous pleurisy often foreshadows a pulmonary lesion.

2. There is usually a steady and progressive *loss of weight* and this is associated with general malaise and fatigue.

3. A persistent *pyrexia* is present, characteristically raised in the evening and lower in the morning. The evening pyrexia is accompanied by heavy night sweats. The pulse rate is also fast.

4. HÆMOPTYSIS.—In some patients one of the first signs may be a cough associated with a bloodstained sputum or perhaps a more copious hæmoptysis. The blood is typically bright red and frothy and afterwards the sputum is tinged with blood for several days.

Diagnosis.—Any person, especially a young adult, who has a chronic cough associated with a persistent loss of weight, and particularly if there is any history of spitting up blood, should immediately be suspected of suffering from pulmonary tuberculosis. In these patients an X-ray examination of the chest should be made. This will in all cases show whether or not tuberculosis is present. It should be noted that changes are revealed by X-ray examination which are diagnostic of tuberculosis even before the patient complains of any symptoms ; therefore the earliest diagnosis of tuberculosis is made on X-ray examination.   If there is a history of any of the

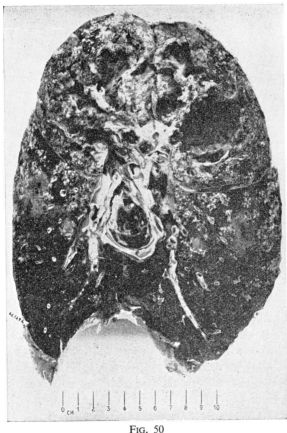

FIG. 50

Advanced fibro-caseous tuberculosis of the lung showing large ragged cavities in the apex of the lung.

symptoms mentioned above and the patient has been known to be in contact with a case of tuberculosis, then the probability of tuberculosis is very high.

Treatment.

1. PREVENTIVE.—This is the most important step in the long-term policy of trying to reduce the incidence of pulmonary

tuberculosis. Good hygienic measures and prevention of over-crowding, which decrease the risk of infection, are of the utmost importance. Any person known to have been in contact with a case of tuberculosis is usually X-rayed to make sure that he has not contracted the disease. In many districts large scale X-ray measures are now being adopted to diagnose the early cases of tuberculosis who have no symptoms and who are unaware that they are sufferers from this disease. This is done by what is known as *Mass Miniature Radiography*, whereby large numbers of people can be X-rayed in a minimum of time ; any suspected cases so found are then fully examined by more detailed measures. By this means many previously unsuspected cases of pulmonary tuberculosis have been found in their early stages, with a consequentially improved outlook for the patient and quicker return to full health.

Vaccination with a vaccine prepared from a modified form of the tubercle bacilli, often known as the B.C.G. vaccine, has also been used. It is done only with those patients whose Mantoux reaction is negative. (For further details, see section on General Tuberculosis.)

Lastly, all known patients with pulmonary tuberculosis who have the organism present in their sputum (" open " cases) are as far as possible isolated until they become " closed " cases (*i.e.*, the sputum no longer contains tubercle bacilli) and therefore not infectious. It is not always possible, however, to carry out this ideal procedure in practice.

All patients with tubercle bacilli present in their sputum must be warned of the danger of spreading the infection to others by coughing and expectorating. Coughing in people's faces and indiscriminate spitting must at all costs be avoided.

2. CURATIVE.

(*a*) *General Nursing Measures.*—Except in the very chronic cases with very few symptoms of toxicity, all patients are given prolonged bed rest. This is particularly essential in the early stages. Treatment is, as far as possible and if conditions allow it, best carried out in special hospitals known as sanatoria. In certain cases, however, they may be nursed in general hospitals, but if so, full precautionary measures against spread of infection must be adopted. They should be nursed in a separate cubicle or a special ward, and their crockery must be marked, kept separate and adequately sterilised. Their sputum must be disposed of in a proper and safe manner, *i.e.*, by being burnt. Disposable containers for the sputum made from cardboard are better than the permanent enamel sputum mugs which need continued, repeated sterilisation.

The room should be well ventilated with plenty of fresh air, and the patient should be kept warm and away from draughts. The patient's general resistance has to be built up by good diet.

In view of the chronic prolonged nature of the illness, which requires a long stay in hospital, it is not surprising that these patients are at times irritable and depressed. Great patience, sympathy and kindness are required in nursing them and form an essential part of the treatment. An irritable impatient person is not getting the proper rest necessary to overcome his illness. Occupational therapy plays a large and valuable role in the treatment of chronic pulmonary tuberculosis.

(b) *Chemotherapy.*—There are at present three drugs in common use in the treatment of pulmonary tuberculosis. These are :—

> (i) Streptomycin.
> (ii) Isoniazid.
> (iii) Para-aminosalicylic acid (P.A.S.).

(i) **Streptomycin.**—Streptomycin is one of the most effective drugs so far discovered in its action against the tubercle bacillus. It has, however, two disadvantages : the tubercle bacillus becomes resistant to it (" drug-fast ") after a period (usually within a few months), and in addition it is a toxic drug. In large doses, streptomycin causes severe and lasting damage to the eighth cranial (auditory) nerve, resulting in deafness and giddiness (vertigo) which can be so severe that when up the patient may reel about like a drunken person. In the doses now used in the treatment of tuberculosis, however, these toxic effects are seldom seen. Streptomycin may also cause a dermatitis of the hands in nurses and doctors as a result of their contact with the drug when preparing the injections.

Owing to the resistance which the tubercle bacillus develops against streptomycin it must never be used alone in the treatment of pulmonary tuberculosis. However, if para-aminosalicylic acid (P.A.S.) or isoniazid is combined with streptomycin, drug resistance rarely occurs.

The usual dose of streptomycin is 1 gm. intramuscularly daily or on alternate days, continued for many months.

(ii) **Isoniazid.**—This is a very effective drug. Like streptomycin,

7

however, bacterial resistance to isoniazid soon develops so that it, too, is never used alone, but is always combined with streptomycin or P.A.S.

In the doses usually employed, isoniazid has so far shown few toxic effects, but constipation, muscular twitching and, more serious, peripheral neuritis (polyneuritis) have been known to occur.

Isoniazid is given by mouth in 50 mgm. tablets, the usual daily dose being 200 to 300 mgm.

(iii) **Para-aminosalicylic Acid (P.A.S.).**—This drug is much less

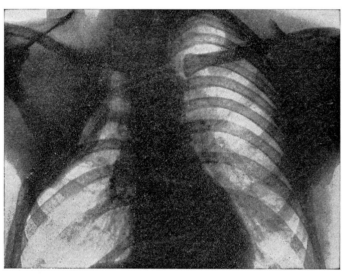

FIG. 51

X-ray after a partial thoracoplasty for pulmonary tuberculosis. This shows how cutting the right upper ribs produces a collapse of the upper part of the lung and so closes a tuberculous cavity.

effective in its action against the tubercle bacillus than streptomycin or isoniazid and its sole use is in conjunction with these drugs to prevent bacterial resistance. P.A.S. is given by mouth in large doses of up to 12 to 15 gm. daily.

CHOICE OF DRUGS.—In the initial stages, streptomycin by injection is given together with a combination of P.A.S. and isoniazid in tablet or granule form by mouth. After about three months, if there is real improvement, streptomycin can often be discontinued and treatment continued with combined P.A.S. and isoniazid for a further period of about eighteen months.

(*c*) *Surgical Treatment.*

(i) **Pulmonary Resection.**—In recent years resection of the diseased part of the lung in suitable patients has been increasingly performed with good results. Patients with localised lesions, especially cavities which do not heal rapidly on chemotherapy, are often so treated.

(ii) **Thoracoplasty.**—This is a major operation for which varying numbers of ribs are resected so that the chest wall caves in and collapses part of the underlying lung. This collapse of the underlying part of the lung is permanent. Nowadays, with the marked success of chemotherapy, thoracoplasty is much less often needed.

The other forms of collapse therapy such as artificial pneumothorax and artificial pneumoperitoneum are rarely if ever performed today as chemotherapy has obviated the need for such procedures.

(B) TUBERCULOUS PNEUMONIA

This form of pulmonary tuberculosis is much more acute and is very serious and frequently fatal. The patients may be suspected of having an ordinary pneumonia and the condition may be realised only when they fail to respond to the normal treatment for this disease. X-ray examination and the finding of tubercle bacilli in the sputum will establish the diagnosis. Prolonged chemotherapy as outlined earlier is given. The general measures for pneumonia with, in addition, isolation precautions are necessary. Tuberculous pneumonia is fortunately rare.

(C) MILIARY TUBERCULOSIS

Miliary tuberculosis is an acute generalised blood-stream infection and thus is not confined to the lungs. As, however, the lungs or the meninges bear the brunt of the infection, it is convenient to discuss this type of tuberculosis here.

Acute miliary tuberculosis occurs mainly in people with poor resistance or little immunity to the tubercle bacillus. Thus a person living in a country with little or no tuberculosis, who travels to another country where tuberculosis is common, may develop the acute florid types of tuberculous infection, such as miliary tuberculosis, tuberculous pneumonia, or tuberculous meningitis. An example of this is the common incidence of these acute forms of tuberculosis in Negroes who come from certain parts of Africa

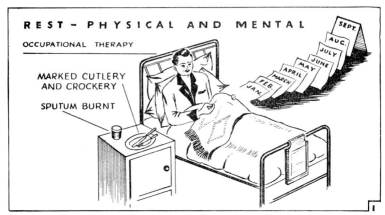

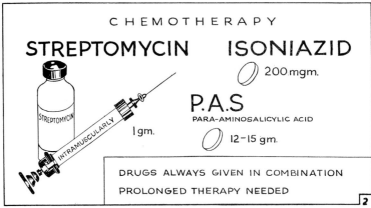

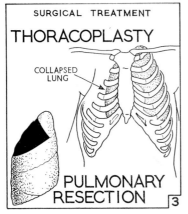

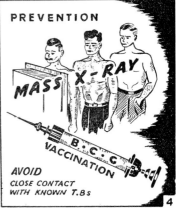

FIG. 52

The treatment of chronic pulmonary tuberculosis.

where tuberculosis is rare to live in Europe where the disease, and so the liability to infection, is common.

Symptoms and Signs.

1. The disease usually starts as a pyrexia of unexplained origin.

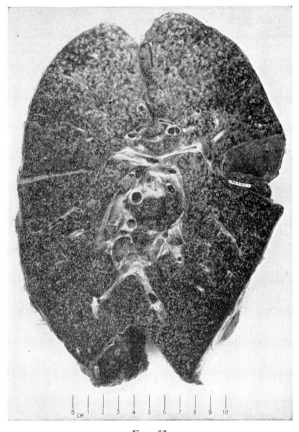

FIG. 53

Acute miliary tuberculosis of the lungs showing the tubercles, characteristically small and evenly disseminated throughout the lung.

The fever is prolonged and typically higher in the evening. The onset is gradual, lasting some weeks with the general signs of fever increasing. Headache, malaise, night sweats and loss of appetite are very common.

2. With the full development of the disease the patient becomes acutely ill, with extreme toxæmia, rapid feeble pulse, dry furred tongue and delirium. The "typhoid state" of a severe general infection is common in this disease.

3. The physical signs, until the later stages, are few or non-existent, and so diagnosis is difficult. Ultimately, signs of either

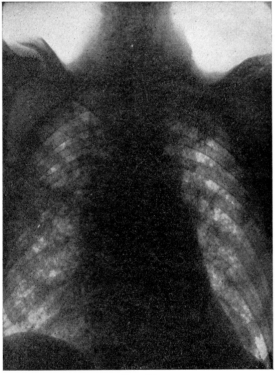

FIG. 54

X-ray of acute miliary tuberculosis of the lungs showing the typical fine mottling—"snowstorm" appearance.

pulmonary or meningeal infection develop. An X-ray examination of the chest at this stage shows the characteristic "snowstorm" appearance due to the widespread tuberculous infiltration of the lungs. In the stage of meningeal involvement all the signs of tuberculous meningitis are present (p. 305).

Treatment.—Before the use of chemotherapy nearly all patients died, except for a very few of a more subacute miliary type. Now many patients recover, as do some cases of tuberculous meningitis where formerly all died. Prolonged chemotherapy, such as streptomycin, isoniazid and para-aminosalicylic acid is given.

As these patients are acutely ill, often delirious, and prolonged in course, all the skill and patience of the nurse will be necessary in nursing the patients. All the detailed care described under the treatment of an acute fever is essential.

SUMMARY OF THE TREATMENT OF PULMONARY TUBERCULOSIS

The emphasis is on prevention, and so on the early diagnosis of the case and the limiting of the spread of the disease. For early diagnosis the value of mass miniature radiography, especially for people exposed to tuberculosis, is great. B.C.G. vaccine has proved of value and is being used on an increasing scale especially in children and those, such as nurses and medical students, exposed to infection.

The main treatment once the disease has developed is rest and a prolonged course of chemotherapy for many months at least, usually six to nine or longer. Streptomycin, isoniazid and para-aminosalicylic acid are given in various combinations. (Other drugs, such as viomycin, have as yet a limited and not clearly defined place in the treatment of pulmonary tuberculosis.)

Collapse therapy is far less often required to-day since the introduction of chemotherapy has revolutionised the whole outlook and progress of the disease. Artificial pneumothorax and artificial pneumoperitoneum are rarely if ever performed to-day. Thoracoplasty and pulmonary resection are the two surgical procedures most often used at present. Persistent cavitation is the usual indication for collapse therapy or pulmonary resection.

In a chronic and debilitating disease like tuberculosis, the value of such general measures as full diet, good surroundings, occupational therapy, sympathy, kindness and understanding in the small matters that become important during a prolonged illness cannot be too vigorously stressed.

ASTHMA

Asthma, or bronchial asthma to give it its full title to distinguish it from cardiac asthma, is a very common disease. It comes into the category of the allergic diseases, which are in the main due to hypersensitiveness to some foreign protein. This foreign protein may be present in a variety of substances, such as the pollen of flowers, dust, hair, feathers, certain foodstuffs, drugs, etc. The other common forms of allergic disease include urticaria, hay fever and some types of eczema. Why one person develops asthma as a form of sensitivity to a foreign protein in some article and another person develops urticaria or eczema is still a mystery.

There are two other important factors in the precipitation of an asthma attack. Infection, especially of the respiratory tract, will often lead to asthma; and an emotional upset, such as a family quarrel or a disappointment, can also be responsible.

Symptoms and Signs.—The symptoms of asthma are caused by the offending articles causing a spasm of the smooth muscle of the bronchioles. This spasm, as will be realised, causes difficulty in the maintaining of a proper airway and so the patient's breathing becomes distressed and laboured.

The disease usually begins typically with sudden attacks of dyspnœa, which become progressively more severe until the respirations are laboured and characteristically wheezy. The attacks vary in duration from a few minutes to hours, days, or even weeks, and they may be of all grades of severity. Any long-standing case may be complicated by chronic bronchitis, and ultimately by heart failure.

Diagnosis.—This is usually easy. Paroxysmal attacks of wheezing respiration recurring over many years, with good health in between the attacks, make the condition obvious.

Treatment.

1. OF AN ATTACK.—Various measures are adopted, depending on the severity of the case. It is usually found that many of these patients, in view of the chronic nature of their illness, will have their own pet remedies.

(*a*) In mild cases ephedrine by mouth ($\frac{1}{2}$ to 1 gr.) may be sufficient.

(*b*) Isoprenaline (neo-epinine, neodrenal), which is similar in action to adrenaline, may be given in the form of inhalations or in tablet form for putting under the tongue.

(*c*) If both these methods fail and also at the start of any severe attack, injections of adrenaline will be needed. Both the dose and the frequency will depend on the response, and in some severe cases repeated injections, perhaps every fifteen minutes or even more often, may have to be given. The usual amount given is approximately 3 to 8 minims subcutaneously.

Another most useful drug used in the treatment of asthma is aminophylline. In severe attacks 0·25 gm. is given intravenously. In less severe attacks an aminophylline suppository is usually sufficient.

In the few very severe and prolonged attacks of asthma (status asthmaticus) which do not respond to adrenaline and aminophylline injections, cortisone or allied drugs, such as prednisone, prednisolone, dexamethasone, may be used with very good results.

(d) Any evidence of cyanosis, such as may occur in severe long-standing cases associated with chronic bronchitis, calls for oxygen administration.

2. TO PREVENT ATTACKS.—This is difficult in practice. Some few patients by avoiding contact with a known substance or articles which cause asthma can so prevent attacks. In a small proportion of other cases detailed tests of sensitivity to numerous foreign proteins can elicit the offending substance. In such cases by avoiding this substance if possible or alternatively by giving gradually increasing injections of the offending substance (desensitisation) attacks of asthma can be prevented. However, the vast majority of patients do not come in either of the above categories and prevention of the attacks is very difficult or impossible.

The patient's resistance should be kept as high as possible and anything likely to bring on an attack of respiratory disease, such as a soaking, damp atmosphere, etc., should be avoided. Any signs of sepsis (especially of the nose or teeth), which may aggravate attacks, should be treated. On the whole the treatment of asthma is rather unsatisfactory, and though many of these patients go from one form of treatment to another in an effort to clear up the condition, as yet there are no great hopes of a complete cure.

CARCINOMA OF THE LUNG

The lung is becoming an increasingly common site for malignant disease. The carcinoma arises in the bronchus of the lung. There is now strong evidence that prolonged cigarette smoking predisposes to lung cancer.

Symptoms and Signs.

1. It is more common in middle-aged or elderly people and men

7 A

are affected much more frequently than women probably because in the past men smoked cigarettes more frequently than women.

2. The onset is usually gradual with a persistent cough. Later on this cough may be associated with sputum which may be blood-stained. When the disease is more extensive it may produce collapse of the lung or a pleural effusion, whereupon the respirations will become laboured and there will be severe dyspnœa.

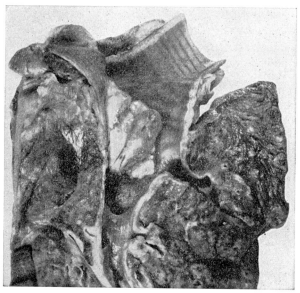

Fig. 55

Section of a lung showing a large carcinomatous growth in the bronchus of the lung just below the bifurcation of the trachea.

3. Associated with the chronic cough and sputum are usually progressive loss of weight, energy and appetite.

4. In the early stages very few signs will be found on examination of the chest.

Diagnosis.—This may be very difficult in the early stages when, as mentioned above, very few signs are present. Any case of persistent cough, especially in a middle-aged or elderly man, and particularly if accompanied by bloodstained sputum, should, however, be suspected as a possible case of carcinoma of the lung. Full investigations will then be carried out, and to start with an X-ray of the chest may reveal a shadow due to the tumour. If, however, the X-ray is normal or inconclusive, as happens particularly in early cases, a **bronchoscopy** will be performed.   Here, by passing a metal tube direct into the trachea and upper parts of the main bronchi it is possible in many cases to see the actual growth and also to take a piece of it away for examination in the laboratory.

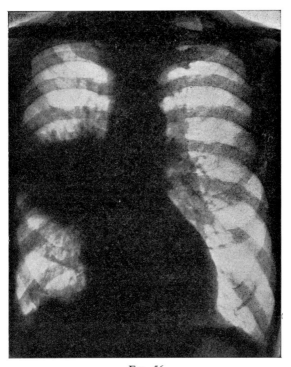

FIG. 56

X-ray showing a large shadow in the middle of the right
lung due to a carcinoma of the lung.

For more advanced cases the diagnosis is usually easy.   All cases of recurring pleural effusions, especially hæmorrhagic effusions, where there is no evidence of tuberculosis are very likely to be due to carcinoma ; so also is any unexplained collapse of the lung. X-ray examination in these advanced cases often shows a large shadow due to the growth.

Treatment.—The high death rate from carcinoma of the lung, as with carcinoma in many other parts of the body, is due to the difficulty in diagnosing the condition in the early stages.   In most patients by the time the growth has produced sufficient symptoms and signs to establish the diagnosis, the lesion has spread too far to be removed by operation. Early cases have been cured by removal of the affected lung (pneumonectomy).

In the later stages only palliative treatment is possible. Sedatives for relief of any pain are necessary. Repeated aspirations of the effusion which is often present are also frequently necessary.

BRONCHIECTASIS

When the bronchi become dilated and widened owing to disease the condition of bronchiectasis is present.

Causes.—Any chest condition which gives rise to a chronic inflammation or any chronic strain on the lungs can produce a dilatation of the bronchi. Therefore, bronchiectasis is usually a disease secondary to other chest conditions.

The chest diseases which usually create a predisposition to bronchiectasis are :—

1. Chronic bronchitis : here the chronic cough and inflammation cause a weakening of the bronchial walls.

2. Any continued inhalation of septic matter (as in cases of chronic sinusitis or severely septic teeth) or of certain types of dust (as in pneumoconiosis).

3. Any tumour, foreign body or other disease causing obstruction to the bronchi can lead to a dilatation of the bronchi.

4. Congenital weakening of the bronchial walls as seen in the type of bronchiectasis in young people, known as congenital cystic disease of the lungs.

Symptoms and Signs.—There are two main stages of this disease:—

1. The Dry Stage.
2. The Wet Stage.

1. THE DRY STAGE.—In this stage the only symptoms may be a chronic cough with scanty sputum and little else in the way of other symptoms and signs. There may be, however, in some patients, repeated slight attacks of hæmoptysis. The diagnosis is made with certainty only after a specialised form of X-ray examination of the lungs (see later).

2. THE WET STAGE.—Here more characteristic symptoms and signs develop with severe paroxysms of coughing and copious

foul sputum, especially in the morning. There are general signs of toxæmia with loss of energy, appetite and weight : there may be the dyspeptic symptoms of nausea and vomiting, and clubbing of the fingers may occur. (Here the terminal phalanges of the fingers

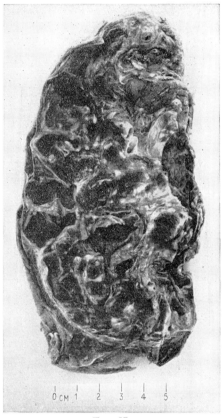

FIG. 57
Very advanced bronchiectasis showing large cavities throughout the lung.

may become enlarged and thickened, until in severe cases they look like drum-sticks. The reason for this change is unknown. We have seen that it also occurs frequently in cases of congenital heart disease.)

In later stages when the disease is advanced the patient is very toxic with marked dyspnœa and cyanosis.

Diagnosis.—In the early dry stage the diagnosis can be confirmed only by X-ray examination of the chest after inserting an opaque oil into the bronchi (*bronchogram*). The bronchi can then be outlined and if they are dilated and widened above the normal the diagnosis of bronchiectasis is confirmed. For the more advanced cases the diagnosis is usually fairly obvious, owing to the typical symptoms

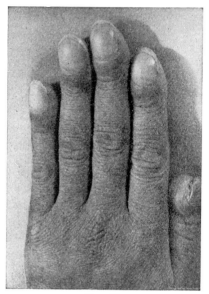

FIG. 58
Clubbing of the fingers in a case of
bronchiectasis.

and signs, especially the chronic cough, copious sputum and the clubbing of the fingers.

Complications.

1. Broncho-pneumonia.

This is the most common complication and is the usual termination of most cases.

2. Cerebral abscess.

Septic purulent emboli may travel from the lungs into the arteries and to the brain to cause a cerebral abscess.

Treatment of Bronchiectasis.—The treatment, except in early cases and in those which are confined to one lung, is unsatisfactory. In the early stages, by clearing up the cause if possible, prevention of any more serious spread of the disease may be avoided. In patients

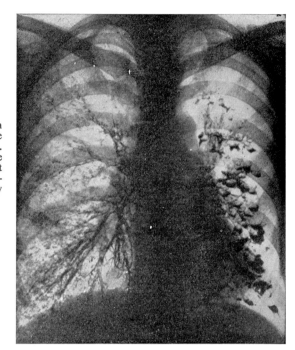

FIG. 59

X-ray after the instillation of opaque iodine into the bronchi (bronchogram). The outlined bronchi in the right lung are normal, but in the left lung bronchiectatic cavities are clearly visible.

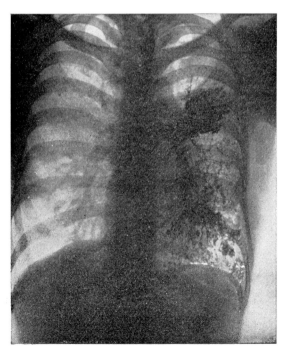

FIG. 60

Bronchogram from another case of bronchiectasis showing dilatation and cavitation of the bronchi in the upper lobe of the left lung.

where the disease is confined to one lobe or one lung, surgical treatment by way of removal of the affected area has resulted in a permanent cure. (This is usually possible only in children and young adults.)

In the later stages, and in those patients where the condition has spread to the second lung, no definite cure can be effected. General measures to build up the patient's resistance are adopted, such as good diet and living conditions. Any infection of the teeth, nose, or sinuses which may be aggravating the condition must be cleared up.

One important part of the treatment is to try and keep the affected areas of the lungs as dry as possible. This can be done by postural drainage. If, for instance, the lower parts of the lungs are affected, then the patient is " tipped up " so that the foul sputum is brought up more easily on coughing. The patient can be tipped up by elevating the foot of the bed with the patient lying flat on the bed, or else by the patient leaning forward over the edge. Special beds are available which allow easy posturing of the patient.

During the commonly seen acute exacerbations of the disease due to infection, antibiotics or sulphonamides are most valuable to clear up the secondary infection present.

COLLAPSE OF THE LUNG (Pulmonary Atelectasis)

Collapse of the lung is not a primary disease in itself, but is caused by any disease or condition which obstructs the bronchi or interferes with the respirations. Either blockage of a bronchus or interference with the expansion of the lungs in the respiratory movement causes the affected lung or parts of the lung to collapse into a solid airless condition. This interferes with the normal respirations and causes varying degrees of distress according to the extent of the collapsed lung area.

Causes.

1. Most commonly, pulmonary collapse calling for immediate treatment is seen post-operatively. Here, sedation due to the anæsthetic depresses the cough reflex and allows thick mucus to collect, which then obstructs the bronchi causing varying degrees of collapse. Infection of the bronchi which causes excessive mucus increases this likelihood of post-operative pulmonary atelectasis.

2. Pulmonary collapse is also always a constant danger in prolonged coma and, as in post-operative collapse, calls for energetic measures in prevention and treatment.

3. Carcinoma of the bronchus commonly causes atelectasis.

4. A foreign body lodging in a bronchus.

5. Paralysis of the respiratory muscles, as seen in poliomyelitis and diphtheritic paralysis, can cause pulmonary collapse, but this form calls for specialised treatment, usually in an artificial breathing apparatus, and is discussed under the individual diseases.

6. Again, it should be remembered that any fluid or air accumulating in the pleural cavity can cause collapse of the lung by pressure from outside.

Symptoms and Signs.—Most of the diseases causing pulmonary collapse are discussed under the individual headings, so only the very common form occurring post-operatively calls for special mention here.

After operation the patient is often described as being " chesty," with a cough, pain in the chest and difficulty in breathing. If the collapse is extensive, the dyspnœa is more severe ; it causes distress to the patient and is accompanied by cyanosis. In most cases a fever is present. Examination of the chest reveals the presence and extent of the atelectasis, and this is usually confirmed by an X-ray of the chest.

Treatment.

1. PREVENTION.—This is by far the most important part of the treatment. Any evidence of chest infection will naturally call for a postponement of the operation, if at all possible. Pre-operative breathing exercises in all patients subject to chest trouble are most valuable.

Routine encouragement of all post-operative patients to breathe deeply will reduce the incidence of atelectasis appreciably. In this connection also, early movement, frequent change of posture and getting the patient up as soon as possible are important.

Tight bandaging coming up over the lower ribs is a very common cause of post-operative pulmonary collapse, and the nurse should be particularly careful to see that any bandaging does not interfere with the respiratory movements. This is of especial importance in all upper abdominal operations.

2. TREATMENT OF ACTUAL COLLAPSE.—Deep breathing and coughing exercises every hour for a few minutes are very useful.

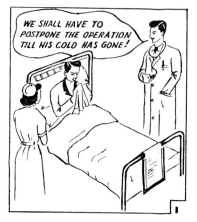

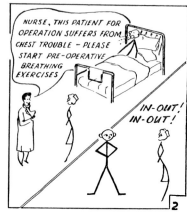

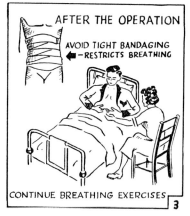

FIG. 61

The prevention and treatment of pulmonary collapse.

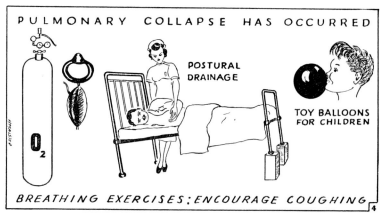

Inhalations of oxygen are useful especially if dyspnœa or cyanosis is present. Postural drainage, by tipping the patient so that the collapsed area (usually the base of the lung) is uppermost, often dislodges a thick plug of mucus and expands the lung. This procedure is possible only in some cases, depending on the severity of the operation and the general condition of the patient. It is, however, a very useful and most effective measure whenever it can be applied. Chest percussion (or clapping) by a skilled physiotherapist is often combined with postural drainage.

Blow-bottles, or blowing up toy balloons in the case of children, also help to expand the lung and are often used in conjunction with deep breathing exercises.

If all the above measures fail to re-expand the affected area, then one of the several methods of aspiration of the bronchial tree will be necessary. Passing a firm rubber catheter through the nose and into the trachea allows suction to be applied and so dislodges the thick mucus. Even if the tube cannot be passed into the bronchi, bouts of coughing occur which may be sufficient to bring up the plugs of mucus. If the above measures fail and the collapse is severe, causing acute distress and continued cyanosis, bronchoscopy will enable the obstructing mucus to be aspirated.

PULMONARY EMBOLISM (Pulmonary Infarction)

Pulmonary embolism is a most important condition, especially from a nurse's point of view, as preventive measures play a large part in minimising the frequency of the disease.

Pulmonary embolism is caused by a clot detaching itself in some part of the venous circulation, travelling in the veins, and lodging in the pulmonary artery or one of its branches. With the obstruction to the pulmonary circulation so produced, infarction of the lungs or part of the lungs, depending on the site of the lodgment of the embolus, occurs.

Causes.

1. Venous thrombosis, especially in the large deep veins of the lower limbs and pelvis. Thrombosis in a vein occurs in several circumstances, *e.g.,* in elderly people with slow circulation, particularly with heart failure. Prolonged rest in bed owing to a major illness or operation is also a very frequent cause.

2. Trauma to the large veins, especially in the lower abdomen during operations in this area, predispose to thrombus formation.

3. In the puerperium a venous thrombosis is often seen—" white leg of pregnancy."

4. In congestive heart failure a thrombus may form not only in one of the veins but also in the right side of the heart. This is particularly likely in heart failure associated with auricular fibrillation.

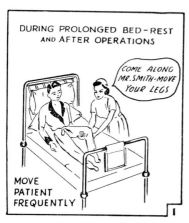

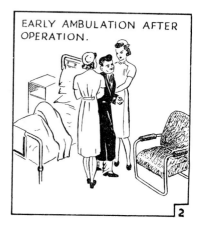

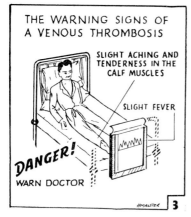

FIG. 62

The prevention of pulmonary embolism.

It is from thrombosis in the deep veins, particularly the calf and pelvic veins, that embolism is most likely to arise. Thrombophlebitis of the superficial veins is much less dangerous.

Symptoms and Signs.—The usual history and course of events is as follows : the patient may have recently undergone an operation and appear to be progressing satisfactorily, or may have had a severe illness and been confined to bed for some time. In these patients there may be evidence of a venous thrombosis in a lower

2. Severe ⎮
patient is put ⎮
for himself. ⎮
light diet is gi⎮

Most patie
as this is the ⎮

Very few ⎮
itself, so that
hæmorrhage t⎮

To allay tl
rest, sedatives
medinal (10 gr
the cough rel
lungs to beco
coughing is a
a mild sedativ
is useful.

PULN

Fibrosis o⎮
response to i
chronic inflam
inflammatory
type) and br⎮
where fibrosis
is called pneu
exposure to c⎮
from constant
dense diffuse ⎮

The people

1. Anthi
2. Stone
3. Steel
4. Asbes

In all these
dust disease o⎮
with chronic ⎮
reveals a typi
pulmonary tul
a danger to al

limb, with swelling, tenderness and slight pain in the affected leg. On the other hand there may be no such signs, or the signs may be so slight that they have escaped notice. A low-grade fever with no obvious cause is, however, often present in deep venous thrombosis and so should be viewed with great suspicion. Suddenly the patient may collapse with cyanosis and gasping respirations and die within a few minutes. Here a large embolus, sufficient to block the main pulmonary artery and so the whole pulmonary circulation, is present.

In other cases the embolus is somewhat smaller and produces severe dyspnœa, cyanosis and great distress. Pain in the chest is common, and later a cough with frank hæmoptysis develops. In milder cases still, the patient may complain of a slight pain, cough and bloodstained sputum.

Treatment of Pulmonary Embolism.

1. PROPHYLACTIC.—Any measures which will avoid or minimise the risk of a venous thrombosis are very valuable. Early movement of the legs in post-operative patients and early ambulation are most important. In any long-standing or severe illness, especially in elderly people, passive and active movements of the legs must be undertaken early. The nurse should look upon this as every bit as much a part of the routine as, say, washing the patient. Of course, if there is any contra-indication to movement of the limb, such as a fracture or a wound, this must be taken into consideration.

If there are signs of venous thrombosis, such as pain, tenderness, or swelling of the leg, then anticoagulant therapy with heparin, phenindione (dindevan), warfarin, marcoumar, or dicoumarol is usually given. This is to prevent further spread of the thrombosis and so lessen the risk and severity of pulmonary embolism. It is important to stress that the signs of a deep venous thrombosis may be very slight, and that particular notice must therefore be taken of slight pain or tenderness in the calf, where a thrombus is especially likely to occur. This slight pain or tenderness accompanied by a low-grade fever is of particular importance, as already noted.

2. WHEN EMBOLISM HAS OCCURRED.—In cases of a large embolus resulting in sudden death nothing can be done. In other cases, oxygen to relieve the cyanosis and dyspnœa is of great value. Sedatives are usually needed for the pain and also to allay the acute anxiety and shock present. Pethidine or morphine are usually given. Anticoagulant drugs, such as phenindione (Dindevan), are generally given to prevent further emboli.

Hæ
disease
occurr(
streake
are brc

Causes,

1.]
cause c
hæmop
and un
2. (
particu
3. (
cause c
4. I
5. (
and *pul*
Dia,
temesis
difficult
Table \

1. The t
    red,
2. There
    am(
    witl
    afte
3. Usual
    dise

If th
is not o
chest w
establisl

Treatme

1. A
other th

the pleural cavity present. X-ray examination will confirm the presence of air.

Treatment.—For most patients rest in bed is all that is required. The air is quickly absorbed and the lung underneath expands. In very severe cases with urgent dyspnœa associated with cyanosis, some of the air must be removed from the chest to relieve the tension. This can be done quickly by putting a needle between the ribs into the pleural cavity, attaching a long rubber tube to the end of the needle and inserting the end in water. Air can also be removed by means of an artificial pneumothorax apparatus, but reversing the usual procedure and sucking air out instead of putting it in.

In most cases the lung expands quickly without any special treatment. In a few cases the pneumothorax recurs, and surgical measures to prevent this may have to be undertaken.

A SUMMARY OF THE CAUSES AND TYPES OF COUGH AND SPUTUM

It has been seen in discussing the various chest diseases that a cough and sputum are practically constant symptoms in most cases. It may therefore be useful to the nurse if the main types of both cough and sputum, as seen in the more common and important chest conditions, are summarised (Table VI, p. 219).

SUMMARY OF SOME ROUTINE PROCEDURES UNDERTAKEN IN DISEASES OF THE RESPIRATORY SYSTEM

1. Sputum Examination.

(*a*) Estimation of the total twenty-four hour specimen.

    (i) Bronchiectasis.

    (ii) Lung abscess.

(*b*) Bacteriological examination.

    (i) All cases of suspected pulmonary tuberculosis for the tubercle bacillus. Repeated examinations necessary till positive result obtained.

    (ii) Pneumonia for the causative organism.

(*c*) Examination for carcinoma cells in suspected cases of carcinoma of the bronchus.

TABLE VI

DISEASE.	COUGH.	SPUTUM.
(A) Acute		
Acute bronchitis .	Dry and irritating in early stages, later moist.	Mucoid; in some cases muco-purulent.
Pneumonia . .	Dry and painful in early stages, owing to the associated pleurisy.	Typically rusty from altered blood, and extremely viscid and tenacious; later more purulent.
Pulmonary embolism	Usually associated with pain in the side of chest.	Usually frank hæmoptysis or heavily blood-stained sputum.
Pleurisy . . .	Dry and painful, catches the breathing.	*Nil.*
Laryngitis . .	Husky cough with hoarse-ness.	*Nil* or scanty mucoid.
Whooping cough .	Paroxysmal with long inspiratory whoop or stridor.	Thick, tenacious mucoid.
(B) Chronic		
Chronic bronchitis .	Persistent, moist; worse in winter.	Frothy, mucoid, or purulent, rarely blood-stained.
Pulmonary tubercu-losis.	Chronic, persistent; moist except in early stages.	Usually purulent and bloodstained, with frank hæmoptysis in many cases. Thick pus in the form of plugs, often called " num-mular " sputum.
Chronic lung abscess	Persistent, frequent, irri-tating.	Very purulent, usually frank pus, and may be bloodstained. Has typical foul smell and affects breath.
Bronchiectasis . .	Cough usually worse on first rising in the morn-ing. Moist, but may be dry in the early stages.	In early stages may be scanty; often frequent slight hæmoptysis. In late stages very copi-ous, purulent and foul as in lung abscess.
Carcinoma . .	Persistent and progres-sive.	Scanty; often repeated small hæmoptysis. Rarely more massive hæmorrhage.
Pressure on the trachea (aneurysm of the aorta, car-cinoma).	Loud, brassy, ringing.	Usually *nil.*
Paralysis of the vocal cords or paralysis of the respiratory muscles.	Soft, " cow-like," often described as " non-explosive."	*Nil* or mucoid.
Hysteria . . .	Loud, barking.	*Nil.*

2. Throat Swabs.

Bacteriological examination for causative organisms in all cases of sore throats, especially for diphtheria bacilli, hæmolytic streptococci and Vincent's organisms.

3. X-ray Examination.

To confirm the diagnosis and observe progress in most lung diseases, especially tuberculosis, pneumonia, pleurisy, carcinoma and all cases of hæmoptysis.

4. Aspiration of Pleural Fluid.

(a) For diagnosis.

(i) To determine the type of fluid present, especially whether purulent or serous.

(ii) To isolate any organism present.

(iii) For the presence of carcinoma cells in malignant pleural effusions.

(b) For treatment.

(i) To drain all cases of purulent effusions.

(ii) To relieve pressure on the heart and lungs in cases of large effusions, particularly in congestive heart failure, malignant effusions and, more rarely, in cases of tuberculous effusions.

5. Bronchography.

Filling the bronchi with an opaque oil which outlines the bronchial tree on X-ray examination.

(a) Bronchiectasis.

(b) Collapse of a bronchus usually due to carcinoma.

6. Bronchoscopy.

(a) For diagnosis.

In all cases of suspected carcinoma of the bronchus.

(b) For treatment.

(i) To remove a foreign body in the bronchi.

(ii) To aspirate a thick plug of mucus which may be causing a post-operative collapse of lung.

SUMMARY OF IMPORTANT DRUGS USED IN DISEASES OF THE RESPIRATORY SYSTEM

1. **Adrenaline.**

   Asthma.

2. **Aminophylline.**

   Asthma.

3. **Anticoagulant Drugs** (phenindione, marcoumar, dicoumarol, warfarin, sinthrome).

   Pulmonary embolism.

4. **Antihistamine Drugs** (antistin, anthisan, benadryl, dibistin, phenergan, etc.).

   Hay fever.

5. **Chloramphenicol.**

   As for penicillin.

6. **Demethylchlortetracycline** (ledermycin).

   As for penicillin.

7. **Cortisone and Allied Drugs** (prednisone, prednisolone, dexamethasone).

   Asthma.

8. **Ephedrine.**

   Asthma.

9. **Expectorant Drugs.**

   Bronchitis, pneumonia and bronchiectasis.

10. **Hydrocortisone.**

    As for cortisone and, in addition, hay fever.

11. **Isoniazid.**

    Pulmonary tuberculosis (combined with streptomycin or P.A.S.).

12. **Isoprenaline** (neo-epinine, neodrenal, aleudrin).

    Asthma.

13. Lincti.

All conditions associated with a non-productive irritating cough, especially in pleurisy, laryngitis and carcinoma of the bronchus.

14. Oxytetracycline (terramycin).

As for penicillin.

15. Para-aminosalicylic Acid (P.A.S.).

Pulmonary tuberculosis (combined with streptomycin or isoniazid).

16. Penicillin.

Bacterial infections of the respiratory tract, especially pneumonia, empyema, lung abscess, tonsillitis, etc.

17. Streptomycin.

Pulmonary tuberculosis (combined with isoniazid or P.A.S.).

18. Sulphonamides.

Bacterial infections, as for penicillin.

19. Tetracycline (achromycin, tetracyn).

As for penicillin.

CHAPTER VII

DISEASES OF THE ALIMENTARY SYSTEM

DISEASES OF THE MOUTH

STOMATITIS

STOMATITIS is an inflammation of the mucous membrane of the mouth and is a condition of particular importance to the nurse, because she can do so much to prevent it.

Causes.

1. Any prolonged fever or general illness, especially in infants and elderly people.

2. Thrush (infection with a fungus, *Oidium albicans*). This produces a form of stomatitis seen most frequently in infants.

3. A severe ulcerative stomatitis may accompany the gingivitis caused by Vincent's organisms.

4. Metallic poisoning. The continued use of mercury, bismuth or gold may give rise to a severe form of stomatitis.

Symptoms and Signs.—The mouth in stomatitis is red and swollen and the patient complains of soreness, especially on eating. In severe forms there may be actual ulceration, often with sloughs, and in these cases the patient is usually seriously ill and toxic. Excessive salivation and bleeding may also be present. The infection may also spread along the parotid ducts to cause inflammation of the parotid gland (*parotitis*).

In thrush white spots, very like milk clots, are seen on the mucous membrane of the mouth.

Treatment.

1. PREVENTIVE.—Most cases of stomatitis can be prevented and it is here that the nurse plays such an important role. In any fever (especially if prolonged) or in any severe general illness, dryness of the mouth frequently results from the reduced flow of saliva. This dryness combined with reduced mastication is very liable to cause

a stomatitis. For this reason every care and attention must be paid to proper mouth toilet (p. 45). Apart from the essential routine cleansing of the mouth and teeth (or dentures), another most important preventive measure is to ensure that the patient drinks enough. Fruit juices are most useful in stimulating the flow of saliva.

Some cases of stomatitis are caused by unclean feeding utensils, particularly the form of stomatitis seen in infants, which is known as *thrush*, and is due to dirty feeding bottles and teats. Meticulous care in the proper sterilisation of all bottles and teats is essential, especially where a number of infants are congregated together, *e.g.*, in hospitals or nurseries.

2. CURATIVE.—Local treatment for an established stomatitis consists of gentle swabbing with some mild solution like soda bicarbonate, thymol or hydrogen peroxide. Local treatment must be carried out with extreme gentleness otherwise more harm than good is done. Mouth washes (potassium chlorate, thymol or weak permanganate of potash) are also useful.

Penicillin helps to combat the infection and also to prevent spread to the parotid gland.

Any specific cause of the stomatitis such as mercurial or bismuth poisoning must be dealt with by stopping the drug and, in addition, dimercaprol (B.A.L.) is given in severe cases.

Finally, it must be stressed once more that for all cases of stomatitis, prevention is better than cure.

GINGIVITIS

Inflammation of the gums is known as gingivitis and may arise under the same conditions as cause stomatitis. The presence of decayed teeth predisposes to the development of gingivitis. A fairly common form is that caused by infection with Vincent's organisms, when the gingivitis may also be accompanied by tonsillitis (*Vincent's angina*) and stomatitis.

The treatment of gingivitis consists of proper care of the teeth and all the routine mouth toilet mentioned under stomatitis. Penicillin is most beneficial for Vincent's infections.

Bleeding from the gums is commonly present in certain blood diseases, especially leukæmia and purpura. Scurvy due to vitamin C deficiency is another cause of such bleeding.

DISEASES OF THE TONGUE

The appearance and condition of the tongue are very important in medicine. In many diseases, both local and general, the tongue is affected and proper examination of the tongue may therefore be very helpful in diagnosis and treatment. In health, the tongue is normally clean and is protruded in the midline when the patient is asked to put out the tongue. In most general illnesses, especially those associated with fever, the tongue is usually dry and coated with a thick fur. In nearly all cases of acute abdominal inflammation *e.g.*, acute appendicitis, the tongue is coated and the presence of a clean tongue is therefore very much against the diagnosis of acute appendicitis. In any condition where the patient has not been taking adequate fluids the tongue tends to become dry. A very dry tongue with a hard leathery appearance is commonly seen in cases of *uræmia*.

GLOSSITIS

Inflammation of the tongue (glossitis) occurs characteristically in several illnesses : (*a*) scarlet fever, (*b*) anæmias, especially pernicious anæmia, and (*c*) vitamin deficiency, particularly of the B complex.

The tongue in glossitis is red and looks rather glazed. The patient complains of soreness of the tongue.

The treatment of glossitis is that of the underlying cause.

ULCERATION OF THE TONGUE

The commonest cause of a severe persistent ulceration of the tongue is malignant disease. Here, the ulcer is very hard and quite often the neighbouring lymph glands are enlarged and hard. Syphilis and tuberculosis are other less common causes of ulceration of the tongue.

PARALYSIS OF THE TONGUE

Paralysis of the tongue is commonly seen with a hemiplegia, which is generally due to apoplexy (stroke).

DISEASES OF THE SALIVARY GLANDS

The salivary glands are the parotid, the submaxillary and sublingual. Their function is to aid digestion ; and their secretion, saliva, also acts as a lubricant in the mastication of food. The constant secretion of saliva has a very essential cleansing effect.

The salivary glands may be affected by various diseases. The commonest are :—

1. **Epidemic Parotitis (Mumps).**—This is an acute infectious disease caused by a virus. Both parotid glands become markedly swollen and the patient complains of difficulty in opening the mouth. There are, in addition, the general signs of a fever. Mumps is dealt with fully on page 78.

2. **Suppurative Parotitis.**—A suppurative inflammation of the parotid glands is usually the result of insufficient care of the mouth in the course of a severe and debilitating illness. Typhoid fever, measles and malignant cachexia are particularly prone to give rise to a septic parotitis.

3. **Stones.**—Stones may form in the various salivary glands causing pain and swelling in the glands, especially after eating. The stones can usually be seen on X-ray examination. Surgical removal is necessary.

DISEASES OF THE ŒSOPHAGUS
DYSPHAGIA

Most diseases which affect the œsophagus give rise to the symptom, difficulty in swallowing (dysphagia).

Causes of Dysphagia.

1. **Foreign Body in the Œsophagus.**—This is a common cause of dysphagia, and in these cases there is a typical history of something sticking in the throat after the patient has eaten. A fish bone is the commonest foreign body giving rise to dysphagia.

2. **Carcinoma of the Œsophagus.**—Carcinoma arising in the œsophagus is not uncommon, usually occurring in middle-aged or elderly people. The dysphagia is progressive, the patient complaining of increasing difficulty in swallowing foods, until finally only liquids can be taken. In the later stages the patient is wasted and anæmic from lack of nourishment.

3. **Pressure on the Œsophagus from without.**—The conditions which most commonly cause dysphagia through pressure on the œsophagus are :—

       (*a*) Malignant growths in the mediastinum.

       (*b*) Retrosternal goitres.

       (*c*) Aneurysms of the arch of the aorta.

4. **Stricture of the Œsophagus.**—This usually follows the swallowing of corrosive poisons (strong acids and caustic alkalis).

5. **Cardiospasm (Achalasia).**—As a result of disturbance of the nervous control of the sphincter of the œsophageal opening into the stomach, failure of the sphincter to relax and allow food to pass

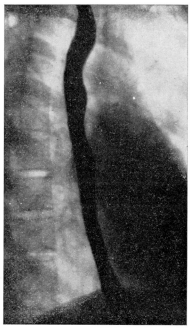

FIG. 64

X-ray showing the appearance of the normal œsophagus after a barium swallow.

into the stomach is sometimes seen. Cardiospasm occurs most commonly in women; dysphagia with recurrent vomiting are the main symptoms. The symptoms are, however, not as progressive as in carcinoma.

6. **Paralysis of the Œsophageal Muscles (Bulbar Paralysis).**— In polio-encephalitis and myasthenia gravis, difficulty in swallowing may arise as a result of a paralysis of the œsophageal muscles.

7. **Hysteria.**—In young girls particularly hysteria may cause a dysphagia with the characteristic symptom of a suffocating lump in the throat. Another typical finding in hysterical cases is that the

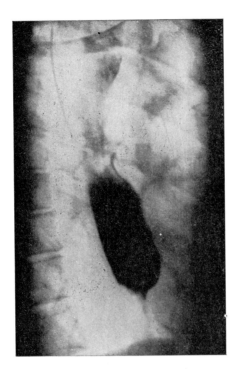

FIG. 65

X-ray (barium swallow) showing barium held up by a carcinomatous stricture in the lower part of the œsophagus.

FIG. 66

X-ray (barium swallow) showing the gross dilatation of the œsophagus in an advanced case of cardiospasm (achalasia).

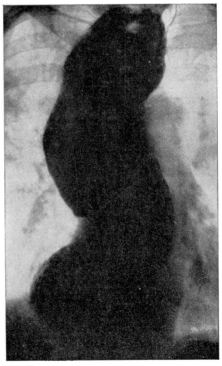

patient complains of equal difficulty in swallowing fluids and solids ; this is never the case in non-hysterical dysphagia.

Diagnosis.—When dysphagia arises after the swallowing of a fish bone or a corrosive poison, the cause is obvious. In the less acute cases an X-ray is usually taken while the patient is swallowing opaque barium (*barium swallow*). By this means the site and type of the obstruction is often seen. In cases where the X-ray is not conclusive it may be necessary to pass an instrument called an œsophagoscope directly into the œsophagus, whereupon a direct view of any lesion present can be obtained.

Treatment.—A foreign body is removed by operation. Cases of carcinoma were until recent years invariably fatal, but now early cases have been successfully operated on. In some cases of cardio-spasm, dilatation of the sphincter by bougies is undertaken, but in others an operation to divide the muscles around the cardiac sphincter may be performed. If there is a retrosternal goitre this is removed by operation.

In many cases of dysphagia, *e.g.*, advanced carcinoma, only symptomatic treatment can be given. In these the diet is important, as on the one hand foods cannot be swallowed, whilst on the other the patient must be given sufficient nourishment. The basis of the diet is therefore milk, which may be varied by the addition of Benger's, Ovaltine or Horlicks. Eggs beaten up in the milk, puréed vegetables and butter are also very useful.

In the late stages of incurable dysphagia when no food can be swallowed, the patient may have to be fed by means of a gastrostomy. Here, by operation, a tube is tied into the stomach, the patient being fed through this tube. The food given must of course be in liquid or semi-liquid form.

DISEASES OF THE STOMACH AND DUODENUM

DYSPEPSIA

The stomach is very readily upset both by diseases directly affecting the stomach and also by any general illness. In addition any nervous tension or anxiety frequently causes gastric upset ; most people have experienced loss of appetite, vague discomfort in the stomach, a feeling of biliousness, and similar symptoms when they are under some strain, *e.g.*, before an examination, interview or taking up a new job.

Many different terms, such as *dyspepsia* or *indigestion*, are used to describe the common symptoms met with in disorders of the stomach, and it may be best at this stage to describe these general symptoms of dyspepsia.

1. **Pain.**—Varying degrees of pain occur in most diseases of the upper gastro-intestinal tract and usually the pain is related to food, *i.e.*, it tends to occur at a specific time interval after meals. Indigestible foods, such as fried fats, rich carbohydrates and spices are especially likely to give rise to pain or discomfort. The pain is most frequently felt in the epigastrium.

2. **Nausea and Vomiting.**—These symptoms are of common occurrence in gastric diseases. Severe pain caused by gastric lesions is particularly liable to be followed by vomiting, which often, however, relieves the pain. Recurrent vomiting, especially of blood (**hæmatemesis**), is a most important symptom, denoting some serious gastro-intestinal disease.

Vomiting is also, however, a frequent symptom in non-gastro-intestinal diseases, and for this reason a general approach to the subject of vomiting is given on page 538.

3. **Loss of Appetite.**—This symptom, which occurs in both gastro-intestinal and other diseases, varies a good deal in frequency and severity. Persistent loss of appetite accompanied by progressive loss of weight usually denotes some severe disease such as cancer of the stomach.

Pain, vomiting and loss of appetite are the symptoms which are most often present in the more important diseases causing dyspepsia. In addition, however, the following symptoms are very frequent, particularly in the less important diseases which cause dyspepsia.

4. **Flatulence** is the distension of stomach or intestines with gas, which is then brought up or passed by rectum.

5. **Heartburn** is the well-known burning sensation which rises from the stomach to the throat. It is often accompanied by the regurgitation of a small amount of acid (sour) fluid into the mouth.

6. **Water-brash** is the term used to describe the clear fluid, like saliva, which suddenly wells up in the mouth. Water-brash is probably due to swallowed saliva which is formed in excessive amounts in some diseases of the stomach. The morning vomiting seen in cases of chronic gastritis, especially in chronic alcoholism. is a severe form of water-brash.

GASTRITIS

Gastritis means an inflammation of the lining mucous membrane of the stomach. It occurs in two main forms, acute and chronic.

1. **Acute.**—Acute gastritis is usually caused by some severe dietary indiscretion, such as overindulgence in alcohol or eating unsuitable food. Again, bacteria ingested in food or drink may cause an acute gastritis (food poisoning).

In most cases of acute gastritis there is also an accompanying inflammation of the intestines (enteritis) and therefore, for the sake of convenience, acute gastro-enteritis is discussed later under Diseases of the Intestines.

2. **Chronic.**—Prolonged dietary indiscretions, such as constantly irregular meal-times or, particularly, eating highly spiced and indigestible foods, are a frequent cause of chronic gastritis. In many of these cases the gastritis precedes a peptic ulcer. Strong tea and coffee may also give rise to gastritis, whilst another frequent cause is chronic alcoholism.

In addition to the above dietary causes, certain chronic infections can also lead to a chronic gastritis, e.g., chronic sinusitis and bronchiectasis, where the continued swallowing of purulent matter may irritate the gastric mucous membrane.

The symptoms of chronic gastritis are mainly those outlined under dyspepsia. Loss of appetite with early morning vomiting are features of most cases. Flatulence and heartburn may also occur.

The treatment is, first, to clear up the cause wherever possible, i.e., to clear up any infection or correct the dietary indiscretions. Then the treatment is similar to that outlined under peptic ulcer, except that the initial period of rest in bed with a strict diet may be replaced by the more liberal post-ulcer regime.

PEPTIC ULCER

Peptic ulcer is an extremely common disease and includes the following types :—

1. **Gastric Ulcer.** —Gastric ulcers are usually situated on the lesser curve of the stomach. Ulcers on the greater curvature of the stomach are much less common.

2. **Duodenal Ulcer.**—Duodenal ulcers occur only in the first stage of the duodenum.

3. **Anastomotic Ulcer.**—After the operations of gastro-enterostomy or partial gastrectomy, which are often performed in the treatment of gastric or duodenal ulcers, a recurrent ulcer may form at the site of the anastomosis. This type of ulcer is called an anastomotic ulcer.

Cause.—The exact cause or causes of peptic ulcer are unknown, but certain well-recognised factors are present in most cases.

1. AGE, OCCUPATION AND HEREDITY.—Peptic ulcer is primarily a disease of adult life and is rare in children. Ulcers are commonest in people who have very worrying occupations or who, for whatever reason, are subject to tension and anxiety. Heredity is also a factor as peptic ulcer tends to occur in families.

2. EXCESSIVE ACID IN THE STOMACH.—It is known that ulcers never occur where hydrochloric acid is not present : on the contrary, in the vast majority of cases of peptic ulcer there is an excessive acid secretion, *i.e.,* hyperchlorhydria. (*Hypochlorhydria* and *achlorhydria* are terms used for diminished and absent acid secretion respectively.) The exact relation of excess of acid to the causation of ulcers is, however, not definitely known because not all people with a hyperchlorhydria develop ulcers.

Symptoms.

1. PAIN.—This is the most important symptom. It is usually felt in the epigastrium and has definite characteristics.

(*a*) It is related to meals and especially heavy meals, coming on either after a meal or just before a meal. It tends to occur more quickly after a meal in cases of gastric ulcer than in those of duodenal ulcer.

(*b*) It is, however, temporarily relieved by food, especially with duodenal ulcer, and the patient therefore often complains that the pain is a *hunger pain.* The pain is often described as burning in character.

(*c*) The pain may occur at night, waking the patient from his sleep.

2. OTHER SYMPTOMS.—Vomiting often occurs, especially if the pain is severe. Other common symptoms are heartburn and flatulence. The appetite is usually good, except in some cases of gastric ulcer where the patient may be afraid to eat for fear of bringing on the pain. There is usually no loss of weight, unlike cases of carcinoma of the stomach.

One of the most remarkable features of peptic ulcer is that the symptoms come on in attacks which may last for several weeks and then clear up completely even without any treatment, only, however, to recur after an interval usually of two or three months. These recurring attacks may go on for years, becoming more severe and more frequent until eventually the patient goes to the doctor for treatment.

Physical examination of the patient usually reveals very little, except for localised tenderness to palpation in the epigastrium.

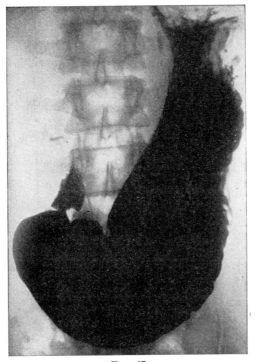

FIG. 67
X-ray (barium meal) showing the appearance of the
normal stomach.

Diagnosis of Peptic Ulcer.—The diagnosis can often be made on the basis of a typical history taken in conjunction with the finding of localised tenderness over the ulcer. The following investigations, however, are usually carried out to confirm the diagnosis :—

1. **X-ray Examination.**—A specialised X-ray examination, known as a *barium meal,* will show up the stomach and duodenum and

8 A

usually also any ulcer that may be present. After suitable preparation the patient is examined under an X-ray screen immediately
after drinking barium sulphate (the patient must have nothing
to eat or drink for six hours before the X-ray; in addition,
all medicines should have been stopped). Barium is opaque
to X-rays and it therefore outlines the whole stomach and

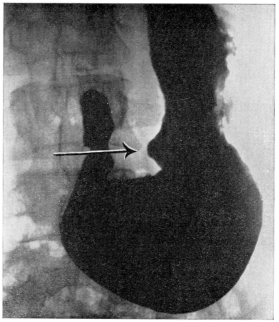

FIG. 68
X-ray (barium meal) showing an ulcer on the lesser
curvature of the stomach.

duodenum. In this way an ulcer crater may be seen. Occasionally,
however, even though an ulcer is present, the X-ray may not
reveal it.

2. **Test Meal.**—It was mentioned earlier that excessive acid in
the stomach was a very important factor in the causation of peptic
ulcer. Excessive acid in the gastric juice is therefore a confirmatory
finding in patients with symptoms suggestive of ulcer. Other
findings of importance in a test meal examination are an excessive
quantity of gastric juice in the fasting patient (resting juice) and the
presence of blood. An excess of resting juice is seen where there is

any delay in emptying of the stomach. This delay and the resultant large amount of resting juice may be caused by spasm of the pylorus due to a nearby ulcer, or pyloric stenosis from scarring in the healing of an ulcer.

Blood in the gastric juice is very suggestive of an ulcer or of malignant disease.

Before a test meal the patient fasts from the previous night, and in the morning a fine narrow tube called a *Ryle's tube* is passed into the stomach. The resting gastric juice is removed by aspirating with a syringe, and it is most important that all the resting juice should be removed. In this connection it should be noted that the tube often becomes blocked and if this is overlooked a large part of the resting juice may be left in the stomach. A blocked tube should be suspected in all cases where less than 10 ml. of resting juice are obtained. Washing out the tube with a few millilitres of distilled water or altering the position of the tube either up or down will, in most cases, allow the complete removal of the resting juice.

After removal of the resting juice a meal to stimulate the flow of gastric juice is given. There are three forms of test meal in common use—the *alcohol, gruel* and *histamine* meals. The alcohol meal, wherein 50 ml. of 7 per cent. alcohol are given, is that most often used. For the gruel meal, two tablespoonfuls of oatmeal are added to a quart of water and the mixture boiled till it is reduced to one pint. The mixture is then strained through muslin before use. For the histamine test meal 0·5 mgm. of histamine is injected subcutaneously. Histamine is the most powerful stimulant of the gastric juice and quite often the histamine test meal will show the presence of hydrochloric acid when the alcohol or gruel meal fails to do so. Frequently, the first two specimens of the alcohol test meal are tested for the presence of free hydrochloric acid by congo red paper which should turn from red to blue if hydrochloric acid is present. If no hydrochloric acid is present (*i.e.*, if the congo red paper remains red) histamine is injected.

The histamine test meal is also used in the diagnosis of certain anæmias such as pernicious anæmia and simple achlorhydric anæmia, which always show a complete absence of hydrochloric acid in the gastric juice (achlorhydria).

In all three forms of test meal 5 to 10 ml. of the gastric contents are withdrawn, usually every half hour for two and a half hours or until nothing further can be aspirated. All the specimens are then sent to the laboratory where the amount of acid is estimated and the presence of blood carefully looked for.

More recently it has been found possible to tell whether there is hydrochloric acid present in the gastric juice or not without the need to pass a tube into the stomach. This is called a " tubeless test meal." A dye, diagnex, is given by mouth and the urine subsequently passed collected over a two-hour period.

3. **Examination of the Fæces.**—In most cases of peptic ulcer, specimens of fæces are sent to the laboratory for examination for the presence of blood. The presence of blood in the motion is a most important sign, indicating bleeding from some source in the gastro-intestinal tract. With slight bleeding from the stomach or upper part of the intestinal tract the motion may appear normal in colour to the naked eye, because any blood present is intimately mixed with the motion. For this reason the blood is spoken of as hidden or **occult.** By chemical examination, however, the blood can be detected. When fæces are sent for examination for occult blood it may be necessary to keep the patient on a meat-free diet for three days beforehand, as meat may give a misleadingly positive result.

In cases of severe bleeding from the upper gastro-intestinal tract the motions become black and " tarry " from the large amount of altered blood present. Black tarry motions from upper gastro-intestinal hæmorrhage are known as **melæna.**

In contrast to the effect of hæmorrhage from the upper gastro-intestinal tract, blood in the motion in lower intestinal bleeding is bright red and is usually on the outside of the specimen, e.g., in carcinoma of the lower colon, hæmorrhoids and colitis.

In peptic ulcer the presence either of occult blood in the fæces or particularly of a melæna means that the ulcer is active (not healed) and therefore requires strict diet and rest. In treating a case of peptic ulcer, weekly occult blood examinations are usually made as a routine measure to follow the progress of healing.

4. **Gastroscopy.**—In cases where the diagnosis is still in doubt after the above investigations have been made, a gastroscopy may be performed. A gastroscope is a flexible tube with a system of lighting attached to it, by means of which a direct view of the interior of the stomach may be obtained when the instrument is passed down the œsophagus into the stomach. A gastric or anastomotic ulcer may thus be seen, and in some cases the differentiation between a non-malignant and a malignant ulcer made.

TREATMENT OF PEPTIC ULCER

The treatment of peptic ulcer can be divided into :—

(A) Medical.

(B) Surgical.

(A) Medical Treatment.

1. REST.—There appears to be little doubt but that rest is the most important factor in the healing of ulcers. At the beginning of treatment rest is essential and if possible the patient should be put to bed for at least several weeks. Rest in bed usually considerably hastens healing of the ulcers.

As many patients with peptic ulcer have some anxiety or worry, this must be treated if necessary with sedatives.

2. DIET.—The importance of diet in the treatment of ulcers is not at present agreed upon by all, as it is believed by some that diet does not have a very appreciable effect on the ultimate healing of ulcers. Nevertheless, there is little doubt but that the majority of patients obtain relief from their symptoms more quickly when a suitable diet is given.

The most important aspects of the diet are that it should contain bland non-irritating foods, and in particular that large meals should be avoided as they cause spasm and distension of the stomach with consequent pain. In planning a diet it also must be remembered that many patients find that food often relieves their pain and conversely, going long hours without food causes pain. Therefore the principal aim in the diet is to give small meals of a bland non-irritating type at frequent intervals.

The basis of an ulcer diet is milk, and about two pints a day are necessary. A glass of milk or milky drink such as Benger's, Ovaltine or Horlicks is given between the main meals and before going to sleep. The main meals should not contain fried, greasy foods, which usually upset the patient, or highly spiced foods, such as curries, stews and pickles. Suitable items of diet include all milky drinks, boiled or baked vegetables, boiled or grilled lean meat and fish, and cream cheese. Coarse vegetables are best avoided.

Carefully worked out detailed diets may fail in practice unless it is remembered that each patient must be treated individually. Patients with severe pain will tolerate the most rigid diet, whilst others with only slight pain will not. Again it must be emphasised that the patient as a whole and not just his ulcer must be treated. The anxiety factors, as pointed out earlier, are very prominent in ulcer patients, who therefore require kind and sympathetic nursing. The nurse can play a most important role in this respect. For example, in most patients the pain disappears after a few days' rest in bed on a bland diet. These patients imagine that because their symptoms have gone, the ulcer must have healed, with the result that they are anxious to get up and return to work. Continued assurances to the contrary are needed in dealing with these patients, and the nurse as well as the doctor can do a great deal in this respect.

3. DRUGS.—(a) **Alkalis** (often called antacids) play a valuable role in the treatment of peptic ulcer. They are given to neutralise the hydrochloric acid which, as mentioned before, is one of the main factors in causing the ulcer. Many different types of alkalis are used, those most commonly employed to-day being magnesium trisilicate, aluminium hydroxide gel, aluminium glycinate and various combinations of calcium and magnesium carbonate.

The dose of magnesium trisilicate is 5 to 30 gr. in a mixture or powder. Aluminium hydroxide is given in a cream (60 to 120 minims), and in tablet form in 5 to 10 gr. doses, whilst aluminium glycinate is usually given in tablet form in 0·9 gm. doses. Alkalis are usually given either after or between meals.

(b) *Antispasmodic and Antisecretory Drugs.*—Drugs which relieve the muscle spasm caused by the ulcer are often helpful in combating the pain. Belladonna and atropine are two very useful drugs in this respect. Belladonna is usually given in 10 to 15 minim doses and gradually increased till the patient begins to have relief from his pain. If signs of overdosage, such as dryness of the mouth or slight blurring of vision, occur the dosage must be reduced. Atropine is given in initial doses of $\frac{1}{20}$ to $\frac{1}{100}$ gr.

Anticholinergic drugs, such as propantheline (pro-banthine) can be used to depress the secretion of hydrochloric acid and relieve muscle spasm, and are usually prescribed in addition to diet and antacid therapy.

(c) *Sedatives* such as phenobarbitone ($\frac{1}{2}$ gr. twice a day). These are useful in overcoming the anxiety factor.

(d) *Vitamin C* in the form of ascorbic acid (100 to 200 mgm. daily). This is a useful addition to the diet, which may be low in this vitamin.

Course and After-treatment.—In most cases, after a week in bed, the patient's symptoms completely clear up. After three or four weeks, according to the initial severity of the attack, the patient is allowed up for most of the day.

The patient is instructed to eat regular meals; in particular not to over-eat and to rest after his main meals. He should keep to a bland non-irritating diet and take a milk drink in between the main meals.

FOODS TO AVOID AT ALL TIMES.

(*a*) Too highly spiced foods.

(*b*) All hard indigestible foods.

(*c*) All highly flavoured sauces and condiments.

(*d*) All fried, greasy and fatty foods.

(*e*) Pips and skins of fruit.

(*f*) Coarse vegetables.

(*g*) Strong drinks of any sort, including strong tea and coffee and alcohol.

Smoking is best avoided, or if this is impossible it should be allowed only after meals, never on an empty stomach.

(B) Surgical Treatment of Peptic Ulcer.

Surgical treatment is nearly always carried out in cases of :—

1. Perforated ulcer. This is usually a surgical emergency and an immediate operation is nearly always performed.
2. Pyloric stenosis. With an established stenosis medical treatment is of no avail.

Surgical treatment is usually *advised* in the following cases :—

1. Chronic ulcers which have failed to respond to medical treatment as outlined above.
2. Cases which have been complicated by hæmorrhage on more than one occasion, especially in elderly patients.
3. Cases of gastric ulcer where there is any suspicion of malignancy.

COMPLICATIONS OF PEPTIC ULCER

1. Hæmorrhage.
2. Perforation.
3. Pyloric Stenosis.
4. Malignant Change.

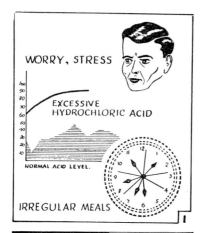

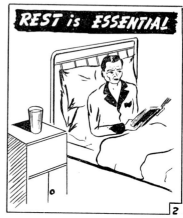

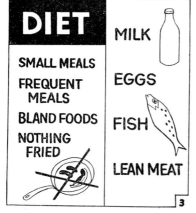

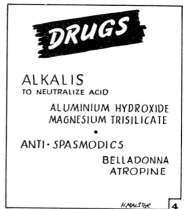

FIG. 69
Peptic ulcer

1. Hæmorrhage (Hæmatemesis and Melæna).

The ulcer may erode a blood vessel and thus give rise to hæmorrhage. In gastric ulcers the blood is usually vomited (hæmatemesis), but sometimes it is passed instead through the intestines, making the motions black and tarry (melæna). Hæmorrhage from duodenal ulcers usually takes the form of a melæna. As mentioned earlier (p. 236), a slight bleeding from peptic ulcer is often discovered only by chemical examination of the fæces for occult blood.

If the hæmorrhage is large it is accompanied by signs of collapse and shock :—

(a) The skin becomes cold and clammy.

(b) The pulse becomes very rapid.

(c) The patient is usually very restless.

(d) There is a severe drop in blood pressure.

In hæmatemesis the blood is dark red and may be mixed with food (compare with Hæmoptysis, p. 214). When the hæmorrhage is copious, blood can be clearly seen in the vomit, but if the hæmorrhage is not so large the blood may be intimately mixed with food and partially digested, whereupon the descriptive term *coffee ground vomit* is often used. (In carcinoma of the stomach the hæmorrhage is often in the form of " coffee grounds.")

Treatment of Hæmorrhage.

(a) GENERAL MEASURES.—If the hæmorrhage is large the patient is shocked and measures to overcome this must at once be taken. The patient is kept at absolute rest ; in severe hæmorrhage raising the foot of the bed is very useful. Adequate warmth is necessary, but care must be taken to avoid overheating, which only makes the condition worse. (For this reason a radiant heat cradle should be avoided.) To relieve the shock and any pain, and also to allay anxiety, a sedative such as morphine ($\frac{1}{4}$ gr.) should be given. A half or one-hourly pulse chart is kept. This is a guide to the patient's progress, as if the hæmorrhage goes on the pulse rate continues to rise. The blood pressure, too, is taken at fairly frequent intervals, a falling blood pressure, like a rising pulse, being an indication of continued hæmorrhage.

If the abdomen becomes distended, as may happen with a large hæmorrhage, a small enema may be ordered. To keep the stools soft and prevent straining, one or two ounces of liquid paraffin

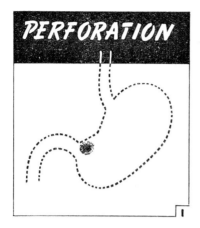

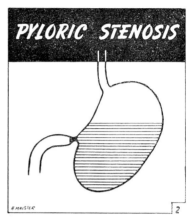

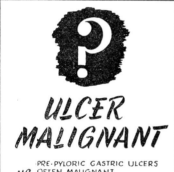

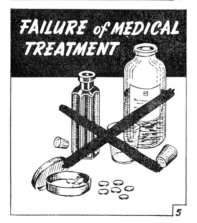

Fig. 70

The indications for surgical treatment of peptic ulcer.

daily are useful. The patient must be warned against straining at stool as this may restart bleeding.

(*b*) DIET.—Whether or not the patient is given food by mouth depends on the doctor in charge. In former days the patient was usually forbidden to take anything by mouth except sips of water or milk, but in recent years a more liberal diet has been allowed.

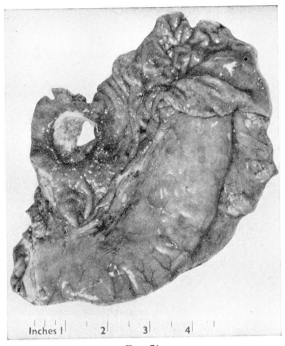

FIG. 71

A large chronic gastric ulcer which failed to heal under medical treatment and was removed by operation (partial gastrectomy).

The usual practice is to allow food by mouth as for patients with an acute ulcer—that is, small frequent feeds of a bland non-irritating variety. Some patients feel like eating more than others, and in the first few days it is wise to accede to the patient's wishes within the limits of the diet mentioned.

(*c*) TRANSFUSIONS.—In patients with copious hæmorrhage with severe shock, as revealed by a persistently rapid pulse of over 100, a systolic blood pressure below 100 mm. of mercury and restlessness, a blood transfusion is immediately given of at least two pints or more, according to the severity of the case. Of course, before the blood is given all the usual precautions must be taken—blood grouping, determination of the Rh factor and cross-matching. A strict watch must be kept for transfusion reactions.

With patients who do not immediately require a transfusion close observation of the pulse rate and blood pressure, as already mentioned, is essential, as if the hæmorrhage continues a blood transfusion may become necessary.

(*d*) SURGICAL INTERVENTION.—In most patients the hæmorrhage subsides with the above treatment, but it does persist in a minority of cases, usually in elderly patients with large chronic ulcers. The arteries in elderly people are more likely to be arteriosclerotic and therefore do not contract down so readily in order to control the bleeding. In these elderly patients with persistent hæmorrhage, surgery may be advised after the shock has been overcome with adequate transfusions of blood. Partial gastrectomy is the operation of choice.

Other Causes of Hæmatemesis and Melæna.—Before leaving the discussion of hæmorrhage as a complication of peptic ulcer it is convenient here to mention the other causes of hæmatemesis and melæna. It should be remembered, however, that in 90 per cent. of cases the cause is peptic ulcer.

(*a*) Cancer of the stomach.

(*b*) Cirrhosis of the liver.

(*c*) Banti's disease.

(*d*) Blood diseases (purpura, leukæmia, vitamin K deficiency).

(*e*) Swallowed blood, *e.g.*, from epistaxis or following operations on the nose and throat.

2. Perforation.

Here the ulcer ruptures through into the peritoneal cavity, perforation being one of the common causes of an " acute abdomen." There is shock with severe and agonising pain. When the patient is examined the abdomen is found to be held absolutely rigid. Peritonitis can quickly supervene if an immediate operation is not performed.

3. Pyloric Stenosis.

A chronic ulcer, when it heals, produces scar tissue. If the ulcer is situated near the pylorus the scar tissue may obstruct the pyloric opening, thus causing a pyloric stenosis. In severe cases very little food may pass through into the duodenum. Usually there are the following symptoms and signs :—

(a) Vomiting is frequent and copious, a history of vomiting of food eaten on a previous day being most characteristic of stenosis.

(b) The loss of weight varies with the degree of the stenosis, but it is very marked in the severe cases.

(c) Constipation is usually present.

(d) The resting juice withdrawn when a test meal is done is large in amount, perhaps as much as 20 to 30 oz.

(e) Barium meal examination will show that the stomach is very dilated and there is great delay in emptying.

The treatment for pyloric stenosis is operation, either a partial gastrectomy or gastro-jejunostomy being done.

4. Malignant Change.

Malignancy arises only with gastric ulcers, as duodenal ulcers never become malignant. When a gastric ulcer becomes malignant the symptoms become more constant and severe.

CARCINOMA OF THE STOMACH

The stomach is a common site for carcinoma, the disease arising most frequently in middle-aged or elderly people.

Symptoms and Signs.—The symptoms of carcinoma of the stomach are very like those of peptic ulcer, *i.e.*, epigastric pain, nausea and vomiting, but there are the following differences :—

1. The pain is usually much more persistent, instead of recurring in the periodical attacks typical of a non-malignant ulcer.

2. Loss of appetite is an early and fairly constant symptom.

3. There is progressive loss of weight. With uncomplicated peptic ulcer, loss of weight is absent or slight.

4. Anæmia is more constant.

5. Rest and diet which rapidly clear up the symptoms of a simple ulcer have little effect on carcinoma of the stomach.

6. In most cases of peptic ulcer any slight bleeding, as detected

by occult blood examination of the fæces, soon stops with rest and diet. This is not so with carcinoma; persistence of occult blood in the fæces when the patient is on rest and diet is a reason for strong suspicion of carcinoma. A hæmatemesis due to carcinoma usually takes the form of " coffee ground " vomit.

7. Jaundice may be present in the very late stages owing to the spread of the growth to the liver.

Diagnosis.—The diagnosis is usually made on the above

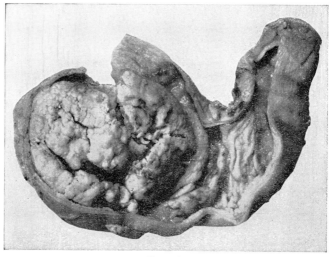

Fig. 72
Very advanced case of carcinoma of the stomach showing a large fungating tumour.

symptoms; the development, for the first time, of indigestion or gastric symptoms in middle-aged or elderly people is particularly significant. A barium meal examination in most cases confirms the diagnosis. A test meal usually shows an achlorhydria, whereas in the majority of cases of peptic ulcer there is an excess of acid *i.e.,* hyperchlorhydria. Blood may also be present in the test meal specimens.

Gastroscopy is useful in distinguishing a malignant from a non-malignant gastric ulcer. In many cases, however, the diagnosis can be confirmed only at operation, and when there is any suspicion that an ulcer is malignant, operation is performed. As mentioned earlier, duodenal ulcers never become malignant.

Treatment.—The only hope of a cure is in the complete removal of the cancer by operation.   Unfortunately, with the majority of patients, by the time they come to operation the cancer has spread too far to be wholly removed.   The prognosis, therefore, is usually bad except for the few patients who come to operation early.

PYLORIC STENOSIS

It has already been seen that one of the possible complications of peptic ulcer is pyloric stenosis.   Another well recognised form of stenosis is:—

CONGENITAL HYPERTROPHIC PYLORIC STENOSIS

This form of stenosis occurs in the first few weeks of life, and nearly always, for some unknown reason, in boys.   The pylorus becomes thickened and hypertrophied from muscle spasm, until eventually a severe degree of stenosis is present.

Symptoms and Signs.

1. The infant is usually perfectly normal for the first week or so of life, after which persistent vomiting after nearly every feed begins. The vomiting is typically described as being **projectile** in nature, the feed being forcibly expelled for some distance.

2. The baby is hungry and greedy for his feeds.

3. Constipation is always present and the stools are usually small and dark green in colour (" hunger " stools).

4. From the lack of nourishment the baby loses weight and becomes dehydrated, the skin becomes pinched and the eyes and fontanelle become sunken.

5. If the baby is examined under a good light and during a feed, *peristaltic waves* will be seen in the upper abdomen.   These waves are due to the contractions of the stomach forcing the food against the stenosed pylorus.

In most cases a firm, hard contracting tumour is felt in the pyloric region.   This tumour is the hypertrophied pylorus.

Diagnosis.—The diagnosis is usually easily made on the characteristic symptoms and the finding of visible peristalsis and a pyloric tumour.   It is essential to stress that the baby must be examined during or after a feed.   The only other condition likely to be confused with this is one where, instead of a definite stenosis being present, there is spasm of the pylorus, causing similar symptoms. In these cases the infant is usually a girl and the symptoms are not so severe, rapidly responding to medical treatment.

Treatment of Congenital Pyloric Stenosis.

1. MEDICAL.—In early cases medical treatment may suffice. This consists of :—

(*a*) Daily gastric lavage to empty the distended stomach.

(*b*) Antispasmodic drugs, given either as drops (eumydrin) or as lamellæ placed on the tongue (pylostropin). The drops and lamellæ, which are both atropine preparations, are given fifteen to twenty minutes before each feed. The dose of eumydrin is 1 to 3 drops of the alcoholic solution.

(*c*) If dehydration is present, extra fluid should be given subcutaneously.

2. SURGICAL.—In those cases where medical treatment has been tried and failed, and at once in all severe cases, an operation to relieve the stenosis is performed. *Ramstedt's* operation, which is usually done under a local anæsthetic, is a simple procedure. An incision down to the mucous membrane is made into the hypertrophied pylorus, thus relieving the stenosis.

Post-operative feeding is very important. Glucose saline is given several hours after the operation starting with drachm doses hourly, and after four such doses, increasing to 2 drachms. Milk feeds, preferably with breast milk, are given eight to ten hours after the operation, commencing with $\frac{1}{2}$ oz. every one and a half hours. Twenty-four hours after the operation the milk feeds are increased to 2 oz. three-hourly, and to 3 oz. three-hourly after forty-eight hours. After this the appropriate diet for the infant's age is given.

One of the greatest post-operative dangers is gastro-enteritis and therefore every care must be taken over cleanliness in feeding. An enteritis can also arise from too rapid an increase in the post-operative feeds.

DIAPHRAGMATIC HERNIA (Hiatus Hernia)

The commonest cause of diaphragmatic hernia is where a portion of the stomach protrudes through the œsophageal opening (hiatus) in the diaphragm into the thoracic cavity. Symptoms usually arise in middle or late life and include upper abdominal pain. The pain

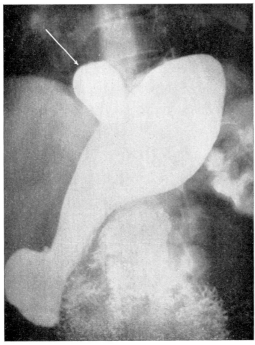

FIG. 73

Hiatus hernia. The herniated portion of the stomach can be clearly seen lying in the thoracic cavity above the diaphragm.

is especially likely to occur after meals and on lying down. Hæmorrhage, either hæmatemesis or melæna, and a resultant anæmia are also frequently seen.

The diagnosis of hiatus hernia may be confirmed by a barium meal examination, when part of the stomach will be seen protruding above the diaphragm. Medical treatment may be sufficient in some patients ; a bland diet similar to that used in peptic ulcer is given, and the patient is instructed to avoid lying down soon after a meal and, in addition, to sleep in a semi-upright position. An operation to repair the opening in the diaphragm is necessary in patients with severe symptoms who do not respond to medical measures.

DISEASES OF THE INTESTINES

Introduction.—There are three main symptoms which usually arise when the intestines are the seat of disease and it is necessary to deal in detail with two of them. The three main symptoms are :—

(A) Abdominal Colic.
(B) Constipation.
(C) Diarrhœa.

(A) ABDOMINAL COLIC

Pain is a constant feature of most intestinal diseases and is usually " colicky " in nature. By this is meant pain which gradually increases in intensity and then completely eases off. The pain comes and goes in frequent spasms. Pain in intestinal disease may, however, also be of a more persistent nature.

(B) CONSTIPATION

Constipation means delay in the evacuation of the bowels. It is important to remember, however, that the bowel habit varies considerably from person to person. Constipation may not be present even if the bowels are opened only once in two days or even longer. When definite constipation is present the motions passed are not only infrequent but also usually hard and dry.

Causes.—These are extremely numerous. The most usual are as follows :—

1. **Habit.**—Normally the desire to empty the bowel is experienced after a meal owing to the reflex bowel action called the gastro-colic reflex. In most people the gastro-colic reflex is most active after breakfast. If the desire to defæcate is ignored the reflex impulse soon loses its force, and as a result the fæces are retained. The retained fæces then become dry and hard from loss of water and so more difficult to pass. Thus a vicious circle develops.

Habit constipation is seen most often in people who rush off to work or to school without allowing sufficient time for a proper evacuation of the bowel. " Habit constipation " is by far the commonest type met with.

2. **Inadequate Diet.**—If the diet contains too little of the foods which resist complete digestion, the fæces become too small to

excite normal peristaltic action and so constipation results. Foods which do resist complete digestion and which form sufficient bulk to stimulate the intestinal peristalsis are often termed *roughage*, and include green vegetables, cereals and fruits.

In addition to lack of roughage, insufficient fluid intake by rendering the stools dry and hard will also cause constipation.

3. **Any acute general illness,** especially if accompanied by fever.

4. **Local causes in the intestines.**

(*a*) Any inflammation of the rectum, *e.g.*, hæmorrhoids or anal fissures, may result in constipation owing to the pain caused by evacuation.

(*b*) Tumours of the bowel may cause obstruction and thus lead to constipation. The constipation caused by tumours of the intestines often alternates with diarrhœa.

(*c*) Adhesions or bands, especially after operations, may cause obstruction.

Treatment.—Any organic cause, such as anal fissures, tumours, adhesions, etc., must be treated by the appropriate surgical measures. The treatment of constipation resulting from an acute general illness is dealt with on page 46. In the commonest types of constipation, due to faulty habits and bad diet, correction of these usually leads to rapid improvement.

In the initial stages of treatment, drugs to help evacuation of the bowel (purgatives, aperients) may be used but should be discontinued as soon as possible. The most commonly used drugs are given on page 611.

In more severe cases of constipation, especially in children or in the elderly, the lower bowel is filled with inspissated fæces and a suppository or an enema may be used to induce evacuation. A glycerin or bisacodyl (dulcolax) suppository can be inserted into the rectum but should be allowed time to dissolve before defæcation is attempted. Where this fails, an enema of warm water or warm normal saline can be used.

Very hard fæces may be softened by an olive oil enema, 3 to 8 oz. of warm oil being left in the rectum for several hours if possible. A soap and water enema afterwards is useful.

(C) DIARRHŒA

When unformed stools are passed, diarrhœa is said to be present. Diarrhœa is a common and important symptom of intestinal disease, its severity and nature varying according to the disease.

It is impossible here to give all the causes of diarrhœa, but a classification of the main causes is useful.

1. Causes of Acute Diarrhœa.

> (a) Acute gastro-enteritis.
>> Alcoholic.
>> Dietetic.
>> Food poisoning.
>> Chemical poisoning.
>> Infective gastro-enteritis of infants.
>
> (b) Enteric fevers.
>
> (c) Dysenteries.
>
> (d) Functional (simple nervous diarrhœa).

2. Causes of Chronic Diarrhœa.

> (a) Inflammatory diseases.
>> Ulcerative colitis.
>> Regional ileitis (Crohn's disease).
>> Diverticulitis.
>> Tuberculosis.
>
> (b) Carcinoma of the bowel.
>
> (c) Cœliac disease and Sprue.
>
> (d) Vitamin B deficiency (Pellagra).
>
> (e) Thyrotoxicosis.

For the purpose of diagnosing the cause of diarrhœa, and also of watching the effects of treatment, the character of the stools is of great importance and a summary of the main characteristics of the stools in the different diseases is given at the end of the chapter. First, however, in the following pages, some of the individual diseases causing changes in the stools are dealt with.

ACUTE GASTRO-ENTERITIS

Acute inflammation of the stomach (Gastritis, see p. 231) is often accompanied by inflammation of the small intestine (enteritis), so giving rise to the condition called gastro-enteritis. It is convenient to discuss the disease under two heads : (1) in adults and (2) in infants.

1. Gastro-enteritis in Adults.

The predominant symptoms in all cases are acute vomiting and diarrhœa, often accompanied by abdominal colic and perhaps fever. Acute alcoholism is a frequent cause of acute gastro-enteritis, as also is overindulgence in highly spiced or other unsuitable foods. Food infected with the Salmonella (food poisoning) organism is also responsible for many outbreaks of acute gastro-enteritis ; reheated pies and sausages and duck's eggs are common sources of infection. Food Poisoning is discussed on page 72. Rarer causes of acute gastro-enteritis are arsenical or mercurial poisoning. Severe enteritis may also occur during the administration of broad spectrum antibiotics, such as the tetracycline antibiotics. (See p. 582).

In most cases of gastro-enteritis the symptoms soon subside. All that is necessary is to keep the patient on a fluid diet till the vomiting and diarrhœa stop and then to give a bland non-irritating diet for a few days. In any case that does not settle within a day or so or whenever several cases occur together, the stools must be sent to the laboratory to find out whether any organisms of Salmonella food poisoning, dysentery or enteric fever are present. In all such cases strict isolation procedures must be carried out, especially with regard to disposal of stools.

2. Gastro-enteritis of Infants.

Gastro-enteritis presents a special problem when it arises (as it frequently does) in infants, because it may have a serious effect on the baby and also in many cases is extremely infectious.

The digestive system of an infant is very easily disturbed, not only by diseases of the gastro-intestinal tract itself but also by disease of any other part of the body. Gastro-enteritis of infants is therefore often divided into two groups : (a) Cases due to disease outside the gastro-intestinal tract—parenteral gastro-enteritis ; and (b) those due to diseases of the gastro-intestinal tract itself—enteral gastro-enteritis.

(a) PARENTERAL GASTRO-ENTERITIS.—Any general infection of an infant may be accompanied by vomiting and diarrhœa, e.g., measles, whooping cough, bronchitis, pneumonia, etc. In all these conditions the primary disease is obvious. There are, however, certain infections in which vomiting and diarrhœa are the predominating signs and, therefore, unless specifically looked for, the existence of the primary disease may in these cases not be realised. Thus infections of the ear (otitis media), the urine (pyelitis) and the throat (tonsillitis) may all appear to be cases of gastro-enteritis.

Parenteral gastro-enteritis usually responds to treatment of the primary disease, but where the vomiting and diarrhœa are severe it may be necessary to give weaker milk feeds. In the less common cases where the gastro-enteritis is very severe, with dehydration also present, the treatment is the same as for acute infectious gastroenteritis.

(*b*) ENTERAL GASTRO - ENTERITIS.—Gastro-enteritis in infants which is due to disease in the gastro-intestinal tract is often caused by improper feeding. Simple overfeeding may upset the infant's digestive system and so give rise to colic, vomiting and diarrhœa, whilst too strong a milk mixture or excessive use of sugar in the feeds are also common causes of gastro-enteritis. These dietetic forms of gastro-enteritis usually rapidly respond to correct feeding.

Much more serious are the acute forms of gastro-enteritis caused by intestinal infections, the commonest of which are acute bacillary dysentery (usually due in infants to the Sonne organism) and acute infective gastro-enteritis (summer or epidemic diarrhœa). Severe enteritis may develop during the administration of the tetracycline antibiotics (see p. 582). Acute Bacillary Dysentery is discussed on page 70.

ACUTE INFECTIVE GASTRO-ENTERITIS OF INFANTS
(Summer Diarrhœa)

Cause and Incidence.—The cause is unknown but is probably some as yet undiscovered organism (although in some cases coliform bacilli have been identified as the cause). Acute infective gastro-enteritis is most highly infectious to other infants, and if a case occurs in a ward or nursery it can spread with lightning rapidity to the other children. It is most prevalent in the summer months when the weather is hot, and for this reason is often known as summer diarrhœa. In an epidemic there may be many serious cases with fatal results. Again, it can complicate other diseases in infants, especially whooping cough and measles. Infection is probably spread through lack of cleanliness in preparing a feed, bad hygienic conditions, overcrowding and flies.

Symptoms and Signs.

1. The disease is usually seen in children under 2 and is particularly serious in infants under 1 year. It is a much less common and serious disease in breast fed as opposed to artificially fed infants.

2. The onset may be very abrupt, the infant being well one moment and in a matter of hours seriously ill. The severity of

the attack varies from a mild rapidly cured condition to a fulminating fatal disease.

3. The infant vomits his feeds and this vomiting is persistent. Diarrhœa sets in quickly and the stools are characteristically frequent, watery and green in colour. In severe cases the stools may be a bright orange colour and extremely frequent.

4. The infant is very lethargic and signs of dehydration rapidly appear in any severe case, *i.e.*, the eyes become sunken, the fontanelle depressed and the skin when pinched remains in a fold. The whole aspect of the child is one of severe toxicity and lethargy. Fever may also be present.

5. Broncho-pneumonia is a common complication.

Treatment.—Acute infective gastro-enteritis must be treated as a *medical emergency* for two reasons :—

1. To prevent spread to other children.
2. To prevent the disease becoming worse with the consequential great risk of a fatal outcome.

1. To Prevent the Spread of the Disease.—The strictest isolation precautions must be taken at once. The first sign of green watery stools in a child in any institution calls for immediate isolation. This point cannot be stressed too much and its importance must be fully understood. Full isolation technique as described on page 39 must be undertaken. Gowns, masks and gloves must be worn, and the nurse must pay particular attention to washing her hands after attending to the infant. A receptacle containing a disinfectant, in which to put all soiled napkins and linen, must be placed beside the cot. The nurse who attends to the child's toilet should not also handle bottles, teats or the feeding utensils either of the affected infant or other children.

2. Curative Measures.

(*a*) *Warmth.*—The infant must be nursed in a warm well-ventilated room. Adequate warmth is essential.

(*b*) *Initial Period of Starvation.*—This is necessary in all cases, and during this time only boiled water, glucose water or some such solution as Hartmann's is given by mouth. The total amount of fluid required in the twenty-four hours should be calculated on the basis of $2\frac{1}{2}$ oz. of fluid per pound body-weight plus an additional amount of 5 to 15 oz. to overcome any existing dehydration. Thus an infant of 10 lb. needs $10 \times 2\frac{1}{2} = 25$ oz. of fluid plus the amount necessary to overcome the dehydration.

These feeds must be given in small frequent amounts to prevent recurrence of the vomiting and also to avoid tiring the infant. To carry out these measures will call for all the skill and attention that the nurse can give. Usually the feeds are given at three or four hourly intervals.

(c) *Treatment of dehydration.*—To infants with severe dehydration, *i.e.*, with marked lethargy, sunken eyes, depressed fontanelle and pinched skin, fluid must be given by the intravenous route as soon as possible. Delay in giving intravenous fluid in these cases can be fatal. Intravenous therapy is also necessary in those cases where even boiled water is not tolerated by mouth. Half-strength saline, glucose-saline or Hartmann's solution are the usual types of fluid given intravenously.

(d) *Feeding.*—After the preliminary period of starvation, which usually varies from twelve to thirty-six hours according to the persistence of vomiting and the frequency of stools, milk feeds are started. At first one part of milk diluted in three or four parts of water is given, as the infant will not tolerate stronger feeds. If the infant keeps down the feeds, then the concentration of milk in each feed is gradually increased until finally the infant is taking full strength milk mixtures appropriate to its age. It usually takes approximately two to three days to re-establish normal feeds.

Breast milk is the ideal milk for an infant, but when an infant who is artificially fed is recovering from an attack of gastro-enteritis, it is best to keep it on a half-cream milk for a short period as too much fat is not well tolerated.

(e) *Drugs.*—Different antibiotics have been used with success in some cases of infective gastro-enteritis. Oral neomycin has proved of value in cases due to coliform organisms. Oral streptomycin, chloramphenicol and the tetracycline antibiotics may be useful in others.

ULCERATIVE COLITIS

In ulcerative colitis there is severe inflammation with ulceration of the mucous membrane. The cause is not known.

Symptoms and Signs.

1. The disease is most common in young and middle-aged people. It is a chronic condition which may temporarily clear up spontaneously or under treatment, only to recur.

2. Chronic diarrhœa, with watery stools containing blood and mucus, is the main complaint. In severe cases the stools may be as frequent as ten to twenty a day and may consist entirely of blood and pus with no fæcal matter.

3. Abdominal colic accompanies the diarrhœa and the abdomen is very tender to the touch.

4. The patient is toxic, wasted and anæmic.

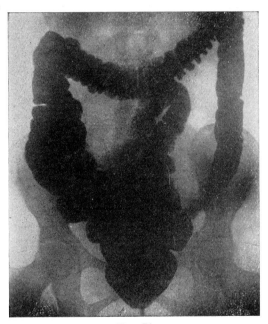

FIG. 74

X-ray (barium enema) showing the appearance of the normal colon.

Diagnosis.—The diagnosis is usually easily made on the characteristic symptoms and confirmed by **sigmoidoscopy**. A sigmoidoscope is a metal tube with a light attached, by means of which the lower colon can be seen. In cases of ulcerative colitis the mucous membrane will appear grossly inflamed and ulcerated. A sigmoidoscopy is also an important means of excluding other causes of chronic diarrhœa with the passage of blood in the stools, especially carcinoma of the lower colon.

9

Complications.

1. Strictures. In the course of healing, strictures may develop. In severe cases of colitis these strictures may be so extensive as to cause intestinal obstruction.

2. Multiple polyposis. Large numbers of polypi are seen in a small percentage of cases. The particular importance of multiple

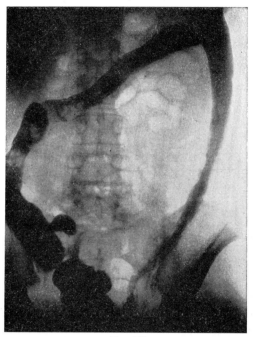

FIG. 75

X-ray (barium enema) from a severe case of chronic ulcerative colitis showing the narrowed tubular appearance of the colon and the absence of the normal haustral markings.

polyposis lies in the malignant change which may occur in the polypi.

3. Rectal abscesses and fistulæ.

4. Anæmia (as a result of the loss of blood in the stools).

5. Avitaminosis. A vitamin deficiency of particularly vitamins B and K may arise, because, owing to the severe inflammation, the vitamins may cease to be formed in the bowel or absorbed from it.

Treatment of Ulcerative Colitis.

Ulcerative colitis is a chronic disease which, in spite of all known treatment, may recur from time to time. In most cases of ulcerative colitis there is some underlying anxiety factor.

1. REST.—In all acute cases the patient is nursed in bed till any fever present has subsided. Nor is the patient usually allowed up till the number of stools passed in the twenty-four hours has decreased to four or five. The period of rest in bed may last for many weeks, or even months, in severe cases.

2. DIET.—Diet is most important in the treatment of ulcerative colitis, the main aim being to provide a low residue diet, *i.e.*, a diet which will be completely digested in the small intestines and leave no irritating residue in the colon. All raw fruits and vegetables and anything with pips and skins must be avoided. All tough, hard, stringy meats are also bad. In addition, fried greasy foods, highly spiced foods and sauces, which are all likely to upset the digestion, are not given.

It is most important, however, that the diet should be as nourishing as possible and any prolonged period on an inadequate diet must be avoided. Of course, in the initial stages with an acutely ill patient a light diet only is possible, and at this stage milk, boiled or poached eggs, mashed potatoes, custards, toast and butter are given. This diet must, however, be supplemented as soon as possible by steamed fish, lean tender meats and strained orange or tomato juice. Later when the stools are not so frequent or watery, well-cooked and strained cereals, stewed fruit and vegetables in the form of purées are added to the diet. Whole protein foods in the form of powdered proteins (casilan, hepovite) may be given with advantage as these patients lose abundant protein in the stools.

3. DRUGS.—There is as yet no specific cure for ulcerative colitis. The following drugs are often useful :—

(*a*) Phenobarbitone, $\frac{1}{2}$ gr. three times a day, is very useful for allaying the anxiety and nervous tension seen in these patients.

(*b*) Codeine and belladonna are useful to relieve the abdominal colic. Hot stupes and hot-water bottles also help to relieve abdominal pain.

(*c*) Iron is given for the anæmia.

(*d*) Vitamins. The diet should contain all the necessary vitamins, but if necessary extra supplies of vitamins should be given. Vitamins B and K are particularly likely to be deficient.

(e) Salazopyrin, a combination of a sulphonamide with salicylates, is often helpful, prescribed as one or two tablets three times a day. Antibiotics, such as chloramphenicol, are sometimes of value.

4. BLOOD TRANSFUSIONS.—For some unknown reason blood transfusions may in some cases bring about a dramatic remission of symptoms. Transfusions may, therefore, be tried in severe cases not responding to the other measures mentioned above.

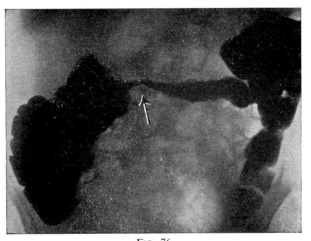

FIG. 76

X-ray (barium enema) showing an obstruction with narrowing of the gut in the region of the hepatic flexure of the colon, due to a carcinomatous stricture.

5. CORTISONE AND ALLIED DRUGS.—In very severe attacks which have not responded to the above measures, cortisone or allied drugs such as prednisone or prednisolone may succeed in bringing about a remission. Hydrocortisone given in the form of an enema is sometimes helpful, but the patient must be taught to retain the enema for several hours. This enema can be repeated daily.

6. SURGICAL MEASURES.—Surgery is indicated :—

(a) Where medical treatment, after adequate trial, has failed.

(b) In cases complicated by multiple polyposis (because of the danger of carcinoma developing).

(c) In cases of intestinal obstruction due to strictures formed in healing of the ulcers.

LOW RESIDUE DIET

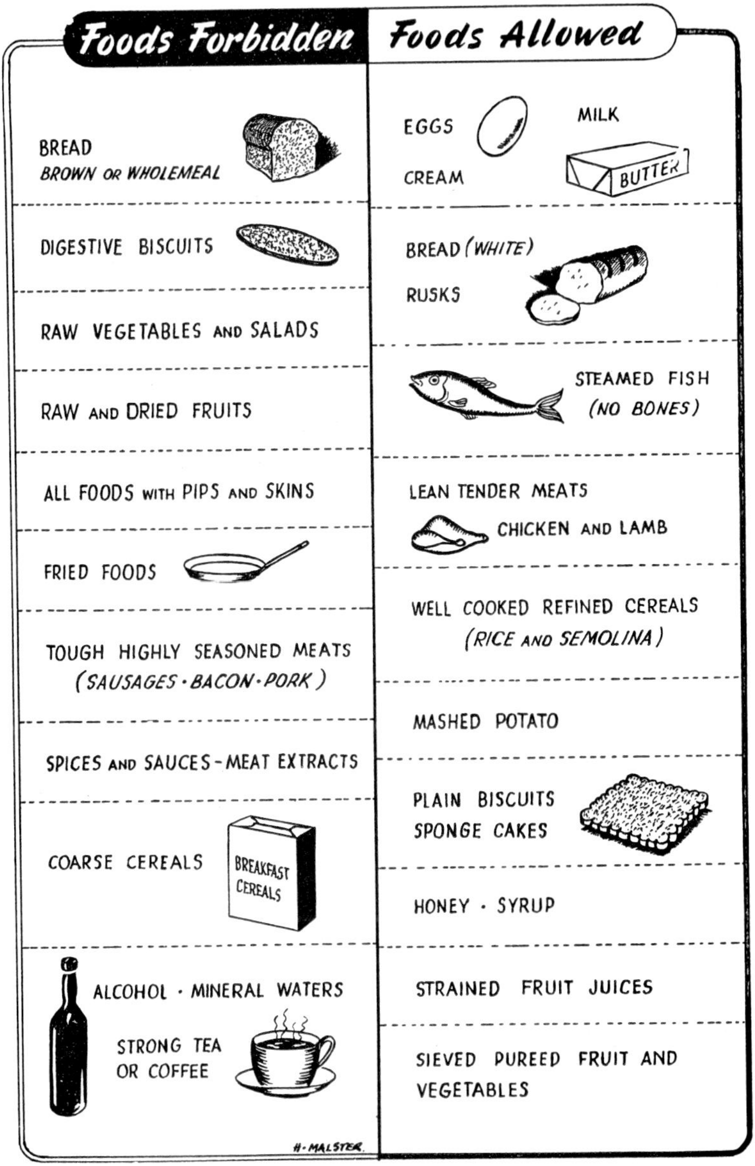

Foods Forbidden | Foods Allowed

Foods Forbidden	Foods Allowed
BREAD *BROWN OR WHOLEMEAL*	EGGS MILK CREAM BUTTER
DIGESTIVE BISCUITS	BREAD (*WHITE*) RUSKS
RAW VEGETABLES AND SALADS	STEAMED FISH (*NO BONES*)
RAW AND DRIED FRUITS	
ALL FOODS WITH PIPS AND SKINS	LEAN TENDER MEATS CHICKEN AND LAMB
FRIED FOODS	WELL COOKED REFINED CEREALS (*RICE AND SEMOLINA*)
TOUGH HIGHLY SEASONED MEATS (*SAUSAGES · BACON · PORK*)	MASHED POTATO
SPICES AND SAUCES - MEAT EXTRACTS	PLAIN BISCUITS SPONGE CAKES
COARSE CEREALS BREAKFAST CEREALS	HONEY · SYRUP
ALCOHOL · MINERAL WATERS STRONG TEA OR COFFEE	STRAINED FRUIT JUICES
	SIEVED PUREED FRUIT AND VEGETABLES

H · MALSTER

FIG. 77

The surgical treatment usually carried out is removal of the affected portion of the colon (*colectomy*), leaving the patient with a permanent ileostomy.

7. GENERAL MEASURES.—Owing to the chronic and relapsing nature of the illness and the anxiety factor which is usually present, patients with ulcerative colitis demand all the understanding and continual reassurance which the doctor and the nurse can give. A sympathetic and kindly nurse can do much to help these patients through a tiresome and trying illness.

CARCINOMA OF THE COLON

Carcinoma of the colon is usually dealt with in full in textbooks on surgery, but as the condition may be seen in medical wards during the preliminary stages of investigation, a brief word on the disease is advisable here.

Carcinoma of the colon is most frequently seen in middle-aged or elderly people, but it can arise in young people.

Symptoms and Signs.—The main symptom is an increasing degree of constipation which characteristically alternates with bouts of diarrhœa. Abdominal colic is usually present. If the growth is in the rectum or sigmoid colon, bright red blood may be passed with the motion. If the carcinoma is higher up, the blood in the fæces is not usually visible to the naked eye, but may be detected by a chemical examination for occult blood.

In some patients the first sign of an intestinal growth may be an attack of acute intestinal obstruction with vomiting, absolute constipation, abdominal distension and pain. In advanced cases of carcinoma of the colon, wasting and anæmia are present.

Diagnosis.—This is usually made on the symptoms of alternating constipation and diarrhœa, abdominal colic and, in many cases, the presence of visible or occult blood in the fæces. If the carcinoma is in the rectum a digital examination will reveal a palpable hard mass. A sigmoidoscopy will detect a growth situated in the pelvic or sigmoid colon.

An X-ray examination (**barium enema**) is most useful in confirming the diagnosis, and the barium is usually held up at the site of the growth.

The treatment of carcinoma of the colon is surgical, consisting of removal whenever possible.

SPRUE AND CŒLIAC DISEASE (STEATORRHŒA)

Sprue and cœliac disease are two conditions in which the clinical features are very similar. Sprue, however, occurs in adults and cœliac disease in young children. Neither disease is very common, but both give rise to complications, such as anæmia, rickets, tetany, etc., which have been discussed in the different sections dealing with these conditions. In view of the importance of these complications it is worth saying a few words about sprue and cœliac disease, and for the sake of convenience both diseases will be dealt with as one—sprue.

Cause.—The exact cause of sprue and cœliac disease is unknown, but there is a deficient absorption of fats, mineral salts and vitamins. In cœliac disease it has recently been shown that the primary defect is an intolerance of or idiosyncrasy to gluten, the protein of wheat.

Symptoms and Signs.

1. A characteristic feature is a chronic diarrhœa with very large, bulky, pale, offensive stools. The appearance of the stools is due to the large excess of fat which they contain.

2. The patients are undernourished, wasted and easily fatigued. Loss of appetite is a marked feature.

3. Many complications may arise which are best described according to their specific cause :—

   (*a*) Deficient absorption of folic acid and vitamin B_{12}, resulting in a pernicious (macrocytic) type of anæmia.

   (*b*) Deficient absorption of *iron*, causing a hypochromic anæmia.

   (*c*) Deficient absorption of *vitamins* :—

      (i) Of vitamin D—causing rickets in children and osteomalacia in adults. The vitamin D deficiency is also responsible, in conjunction with a deficient absorption of calcium, for the tetany seen in sprue.

      (ii) Of vitamin B complex—causing a sore tongue (glossitis) and peripheral neuritis.

      (iii) Of vitamin K—resulting in prothrombin deficiency and hæmorrhagic manifestations.

   (*d*) Deficient absorption of *calcium*, causing tetany and softening of the bones (osteoporosis).

(e) The combination of the deficient absorption of fats, carbohydrates, minerals and vitamins causes the lack of growth
and infantilism seen in children with cœliac disease.

Treatment.—During the active stages of the disease, bed rest is
essential to rapid recovery. Diet is of the utmost importance. In
cœliac disease the main essential is to exclude the wheat protein,
gluten, and this is achieved by cutting out from the diet all articles
made with wheat flour and by using instead corn flour or soya bean
flour. When gluten is excluded from the diet, children with cœliac
disease are able to tolerate fat in the diet to a much greater degree.
In sprue, it has not yet been proved that a gluten-free diet is as
beneficial as in cœliac disease.

The diet in sprue and cœliac disease should contain a high
protein, low starch and low fat content as well as excluding gluten.
All the missing vitamins must be given, especially A, D, B complex
and K. Calcium should also be added to the diet. Food is best
given in small amounts at frequent intervals, the amount being
gradually increased as the condition improves.

Folic acid (and in some cases vitamin B_{12}) is most useful,
especially when a macrocytic anæmia is present. If a hypochromic
anæmia is present this denotes a deficiency of iron, and ferrous
succinate or ferrous gluconate will be given.

ACUTE INTUSSUSCEPTION

Acute intussusception (which almost invariably arises in infants)
is described in surgical textbooks, but mention is made of the
condition here because it can be mistaken for acute bacillary
dysentery in infants. In intussusception, part of the intestine
becomes invaginated into the intestine immediately below it. The
invaginated part of the intestine can then travel onwards for a
considerable distance in the gut. The result of intussusception is
to produce an acute intestinal obstruction. An intussusception
usually starts in the region of the lower end of the ileum near the
ileocæcal valve.

Symptoms and Signs.

1. Breast-fed infants under one year are usually affected.
2. The onset is sudden with abdominal colic, the infant having
attacks of screaming and drawing up its legs.
3. Vomiting starts early and is severe and repeated.

4. After the first motion the infant passes only pure blood and mucus from the bowel—the " red-currant jelly " stool.

5. A typical sausage-shaped tumour is usually palpable in the abdomen. This tumour is the invaginated portion of the intestine. On rectal examination the lower end of the invaginated bowel may in some cases be felt. The finger when withdrawn will be covered in blood.

Diagnosis and Treatment.—Intussusception must be distinguished from the other acute illnesses in infants in which blood and mucus are passed in the stools. Acute bacillary dysentery (usually due to the Sonne bacillus) is the condition which is most likely to be confused with acute intussusception. In the dysentery cases, however, the vomiting and the screaming attacks of colic are slight or absent and an abdominal tumour is not felt.

The treatment of intussusception is immediate operation to relieve the obstruction. The invaginated portion of intestine is " milked back," great care being needed to prevent the bowel tearing. If, as happens in some cases, the bowel is gangrenous, then resection of the gangrenous part is necessary.

TUBERCULOSIS OF THE INTESTINES

Tuberculosis of the intestines falls more conveniently into the same section as tuberculous peritonitis (p. 269).

REGIONAL ILEITIS (Crohn's Disease)

Regional ileitis or Crohn's disease is an inflammation of unknown origin which usually affects the terminal portion of the ileum and also the cæcum. In the acute stage it gives rise to abdominal pain and many cases are, as a result, operated on as cases of acute appendicitis.

In the normal course, however, the acute symptoms will subside although attacks of abdominal pain and diarrhœa recur. The general health of the patient becomes affected, with loss of weight and energy and the development of anæmia.

In the acute stages, rest in bed with a full high protein and low residue diet (similar to that outlined in Ulcerative Colitis) is necessary. There is no specific treatment, but for some patients sulphonamides or antibiotics may be of benefit. For the chronic stages, surgery may be needed with excision of the affected portion of the bowel.

9 A

MEGACOLON

Megacolon, which is also known as *Hirschsprung's* disease, is a relatively rare condition. It occurs both in children (when, for some unknown reason, it is nearly always boys who are affected) and adults. In megacolon, due to disturbance in the nerve supply, part of the colon in the recto-sigmoid region becomes narrowed and thickened with the result that the bowel above the contracted segment becomes enormously dilated.

The cardinal signs of megacolon are extreme constipation and abdominal distension. In children the symptoms date from soon after birth, and in severe cases the abdomen becomes enormously distended with coils of bowel visible through the abdominal wall. Evacuation of the bowel may take place only at intervals of weeks, and in these severe cases death can ensue from toxæmia and intestinal obstruction. X-ray examination (barium enema) reveals the grossly distended large bowel.

Treatment of megacolon consists of resection of the narrowed segment of the colon (recto-sigmoidectomy).

INTESTINAL WORMS (Helminths)

Worms often inhabit the intestinal tract. Those most commonly found in Western countries are :—

        1. Threadworms.
        2. Roundworms.
        3. Tapeworms.

In tropical countries there are many other types of worms as well which cause serious ill health, with severe anæmia as a particular feature.

1. Threadworms.

Threadworm infection is extremely common, especially in children, the tiny white worms being seen in the fæces or around the anus. Marked perianal itching is present. The child becomes infected by swallowing the eggs (ova). Continuous reinfection takes place through the child scratching the anus and thereby infecting the hands.

Treatment.—As most of the children and even adults in the family are usually infected with threadworms at the same time, it is most important for all members of the family to be examined and for those infected to be treated together : failing this, reinfection will take place.

(*a*) ERADICATION OF THE WORMS.—A suitable anthelmintic (drug which kills worms) is given after the bowels have been well opened by a mild purgative. Piperazine is at present the drug of choice. Piperazine citrate (antepar) is given in doses of 50 to 75 mgm. for each kilogram of body-weight daily for seven days. The maximum dose for an adult is 1 gm. twice daily. With piperazine adipate (entacyl) the usual dose is 200 mgm. for each year of age up to a maximum of 1,200 mgm. daily for patients over the age of 6. Alternatively piperazine may be given in one single large dose of 3 gm. for a child aged 2 to 5 years. A useful preparation for this purpose is piperazine combined with senekot (pripsen).

(b) PREVENTION OF REINFECTION.—This is most important. The anal region must be properly cleansed after each motion and mercury ointment applied. The hands must be washed after visiting the toilet. The child's nails must be cut short, whilst painting with iodine will prevent the fingers being sucked and so causing reinfection. Wearing gloves at night also helps to prevent scratching. The underclothes, night attire and linen should be boiled after all infected members of the family have been treated.

2. **Roundworms** (*Ascaris lumbricoides*).

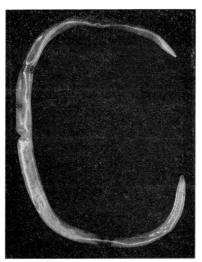

FIG. 78
Roundworm.

Roundworm infection results from eating or drinking contaminated food (particularly raw vegetables and salads) or water.

The worms mainly inhabit the intestines, but occasionally invade the bile ducts, liver or trachea. In adults the main symptoms are abdominal pain, diarrhœa or constipation, whilst in infants, enuresis (bed-wetting) and convulsions are common. With many patients the first sign is the presence of the worms in the motions. Piperazine is usually given in a single large dose up to a maximum of 3 gm. for an adult.

3. Tapeworms.

Tapeworm infection occurs in both adults and children. There are two common types : *Tænia saginata* derived from infected cattle

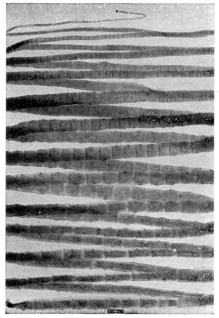

Fig. 79
Tapeworm.

and *Tænia solium* from infected pigs. Man becomes infected through eating infected meat or pork which has been insufficiently cooked. Adequate cooking of meat and pork destroys the worms.

Tapeworms grow to a length of many feet. The worm, which has a flat white appearance, is made up of a head and individual small segments which usually drop off in turn and are passed in the fæces. The symptoms of tapeworm infection are slight, usually consisting of excessive appetite, mild abdominal colic and perhaps some loss of weight.

Treatment.—Mepacrine (atebrin, quinacrine) is considered to be one of the best drugs available for the treatment of tapeworm infection. For the day before treatment the patient is kept on a light diet and a saline purgative is given in the evening. The patient takes no food except fluids on the morning of treatment when two doses of 0·5 gm. of mepacrine are given by mouth or by duodenal tube during a one-hour period. Two hours after the mepacrine a saline purgative (½ oz. sodium or magnesium sulphate) is given. All the motions passed on the day of treatment must be carefully examined to identify the head of the worm. Instead of mepacrine, filix mas (male fern) in three doses of 30 minims each may be used.

Diclorophen (anthiphen) is another anthelmintic, which has given good results in the treatment of tapeworm infestation. It has the great advantage that dietary restriction or the administration of purgatives are not necessary, whilst side-effects are slight, mainly colic and mild diarrhœa. The dose is 0·5 gm. per 16 lb. body-weight.

DISEASES OF THE PERITONEUM

PERITONITIS

Inflammation of the peritoneum (peritonitis) is often seen as the result of a spread of infection from the intestinal tract or pelvic organs. Most cases of acute peritonitis are caused by such surgical conditions as acute appendicitis, perforated peptic ulcer or acute salpingitis (inflammation of the Fallopian tubes). Rarer types of acute peritonitis are those due to perforation of a typhoid ulcer in the intestines and the primary pneumococcal peritonitis usually resulting from a generalised blood-stream infection.

Apart from the above forms of acute peritonitis, which are mainly surgical problems, there remains tuberculous peritonitis, which is essentially a medical condition and is, therefore, dealt with in more detail.

TUBERCULOUS PERITONITIS

Tuberculous peritonitis is often seen in children as a result of the drinking of infected milk. The bovine tubercle bacilli penetrate the intestinal wall to reach the mesenteric lymph glands, whereupon the tuberculous glands frequently set up a tuberculous peritonitis by direct spread of the infection.

In adult women, tuberculous peritonitis is not uncommonly caused by the spread of infection from tuberculosis of the Fallopian tubes (tuberculous salpingitis).

Symptoms and Signs.—Tuberculous peritonitis varies in its onset from a slow gradual process to a much more acute attack.

1. Abdominal pain and signs of general ill health are the main features in the early stages. Loss of weight and appetite with a persisting low-grade fever are usually present.

2. Constipation often alternating with diarrhœa occurs.

3. The abdomen may be distended owing to the presence of a large amount of fluid in the peritoneal cavity (*ascites*). This form of tuberculous peritonitis is spoken of as the ascitic type. In other cases the abdomen is not distended with fluid but is characteristically described as doughy to the touch, whilst the enlarged mesenteric glands may be felt (adhesive type).

Course and Treatment.—The majority of cases of tuberculous peritonitis, especially in children, recover. In those patients, however, where there is extensive tuberculous disease of other organs, *e.g.*, the lungs, the outlook is not so good.

Treatment, as in all forms of tuberculosis, consists of rest and a prolonged course of chemotherapy. The general treatment is as outlined on page 93.

The ascites seldom becomes so great that a paracentesis abdominis has to be performed to relieve the distension.

ASCITES

Ascites is the presence of fluid in the peritoneal cavity, and may be caused by many different types of disease bearing little relation to each other. It is convenient, therefore, to summarise the main types of ascites according to the causative diseases.

Causes of Ascites.

1. **Congestive Heart Failure.**—This is the commonest cause of an ascites and the fluid present is part of a general œdema. Œdema of the legs and a " sacral pad " are also present. The ascites in heart failure may require tapping (paracentesis abdominis), when the fluid removed will be clear yellow in colour.

2. Diseases of the Peritoneum.

(*a*) Tuberculous Peritonitis. The ascites is accompanied by a general wasting, fever and diarrhœa. The fluid seldom needs tapping.

(*b*) Secondary carcinoma of the peritoneum caused by spread (metastases) from other organs, particularly the ovaries, stomach and intestines. Malignant peritonitis causes a rapid and large ascites that needs frequent tapping. The general condition of the patient is poor, severe wasting and anæmia being present. The outlook is, of course, hopeless.

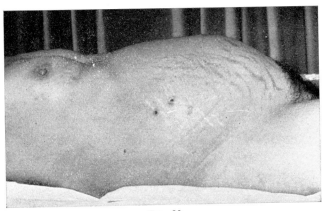

Fig. 80

Ascites. The abdomen is grossly distended. The two puncture marks from the paracentesis can be clearly seen.

3. Diseases of the Liver.

(*a*) Carcinoma of the liver, usually the result of spread from other organs such as the lungs, stomach or intestines.

(*b*) Cirrhosis of the liver. Ascites is present in the late stages of most cases of cirrhosis. It is caused by pressure on the portal vein from the fibrous tissue in the liver. Enlarged veins are often present in the abdominal wall (caput medusæ).

4. Nephritis.—Ascites, as part of a general œdema, is sometimes present in cases of nephritis, particularly in the œdematous forms of chronic nephritis.

CHARACTER OF THE STOOLS IN DISEASE

1. **Number.**—The number of stools passed in the day varies from person to person. On an average the bowels are opened once a day,

but constipation is not necessarily present if the bowels are not opened daily. Frequent motions which are also semi-formed or watery are seen in diarrhœa.

2. **Colour.**—Normal stools are dark brown owing to the presence of stercobilin (altered bilirubin).

   (*a*) *Pale Stools* are seen :—

> (i) When no bile reaches the intestine, *e.g.*, the clay-coloured stools of obstructive jaundice.
>
> (ii) If excessive fat is present, *e.g.*, in sprue and cœliac disease.
>
> (iii) In patients on a purely milk diet.

   (*b*) *Black Stools* are due to :—

> (i) Administration of iron, bismuth or charcoal.
>
> (ii) Altered blood from bleeding in the upper intestinal tract, *i.e.*, the black tarry stools of melæna.

   (*c*) *Green Stools.*—The stools may be green in colour when there is severe acute diarrhœa due to inflammation of the small intestine. Green stools are particularly characteristic of the acute infective gastro-enteritis of infants.

3. Consistency and Formation.

   (*a*) In constipation the stools are hard, dry and often in the shape of round balls.

   (*b*) In all types of diarrhœa the stools are unformed, whilst in extreme cases the stools are watery and contain little fæcal matter. For instance, in the tropical disease, cholera, where diarrhœa is intense, the stools are watery, colourless and contain mucus—the " rice-water " stools of cholera.

   (*c*) Stools containing a great deal of mucus are " slimy " in appearance.

   (*d*) Ribbon-shaped stools are seen in intestinal obstruction, *e.g.*, in carcinoma of the bowel.

   (*e*) In typhoid fever the stools are characteristically described as " pea-soup " stools.

4. Abnormal Substances in the Stools.

   (*a*) *Undigested Food and Curds.*—In diarrhœa undigested particles of food may appear in the stools. During infancy, curds may be seen when the protein or fat is not properly digested. Protein curds are yellow or white in colour and large and hard—sinking in water. Fat curds are also yellow or white, but are smaller and softer—floating in water. In patients on a milk diet, curds due to undigested protein may appear in the stool; if so, citrate should be added to the milk or the amount reduced.

(b) *Blood.*—The appearance of the stool with blood in it varies according to the site of the bleeding in the gastro-intestinal tract and also, of course, according to the amount of blood present.

(i) A large hæmorrhage from the upper part of the gastro-intestinal tract (usually due to peptic ulcer) produces black tarry stools—*melæna*. A small hæmorrhage from the upper gastro-intestinal tract causes little change that is visible to the naked eye and chemical tests are necessary to detect the presence of blood (*occult blood*).

(ii) Blood from the large intestine is usually bright red in colour. If the bleeding is in the upper part of the large intestine the blood may be partially mixed with fæcal matter. Bleeding from the rectum (usually due to hæmorrhoids, carcinoma or anal fissure) produces a streaking of the outside of the motion.

(iii) Blood accompanied by mucus or pus is seen in severe inflammation of the intestines, *e.g.*, in dysentery and ulcerative colitis. In very severe cases no fæcal matter may be present, the stools consisting of blood and muco-pus only.

(iv) Pure blood and mucus with no fæcal matter are passed in acute intussusception in infants, producing the " red-currant jelly " stool characteristic of intussusception.

(c) *Mucus.*—The presence of mucus in the fæces indicates disease, usually an inflammation in the large bowel. Mucus, which gives the stool a " slimy " appearance, may be on the outside of the motion or mixed with it. Mucus may be present alone in less severe degrees of inflammation of the large bowel, but it is usually accompanied by blood in such diseases as ulcerative colitis and dysentery. As already stated the " red-currant jelly " motion of acute intussusception consists of pure blood and mucus.

(d) *Pus.*—Pus, either as pure pus or muco-pus, is present in the stools in severe inflammation and ulceration of the large bowel, *i.e.*, in severe cases of dysentery and ulcerative colitis.

(*e*) *Parasites.*—The commonest parasites found in the fæces in Western countries as opposed to tropical countries are the intestinal worms, especially threadworms, roundworms and tapeworms.

SUMMARY OF SOME ROUTINE PROCEDURES UNDERTAKEN IN DISEASES OF THE ALIMENTARY SYSTEM

1. **Fæces Examination.**

   (*a*) For occult blood.

    (i) In peptic ulcer, to exclude hæmorrhage and to follow progress of healing in cases of hæmorrhage.

    (ii) In all suspected cases of bleeding from the gastro-intestinal tract, especially carcinoma of stomach and bowel.

   (*b*) Bacteriological examination.

    In cases of acute diarrhœa, particularly when the presence of enteric, food-poisoning and dysentery organisms is suspected.

   (*c*) For parasites.

    In cases of intestinal worms.

   (*d*) Fat estimation.

    In diseases with upset in fat digestion and absorption, such as cœliac disease and sprue. (In normal people the daily excretion of fat in the stools seldom exceeds 5 gm.).

2. **X-ray Examination.**

   (*a*) Barium swallow, to exclude any disease of the œsophagus, particularly when dysphagia is a symptom.

   (*b*) Barium meal, in cases of dyspepsia, to confirm or exclude peptic ulcer, carcinoma of stomach and pyloric stenosis.

   (*c*) Barium enema, to diagnose particularly carcinoma of the intestines ; also in cases of colitis, diverticulitis, persistent chronic diarrhœa and constipation.

3. **Test Meal.**

   (*a*) In peptic ulcer, where excess of acid is usually present.

   (*b*) In carcinoma of the stomach, where an achlorhydria is common and blood may be present in the gastric specimens.

   (*c*) In the diagnosis of certain anæmias, especially pernicious and simple achlorhydric anæmias, wherein achlorhydria is always present.

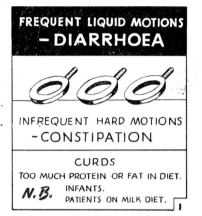

FREQUENT LIQUID MOTIONS – DIARRHOEA

INFREQUENT HARD MOTIONS – CONSTIPATION

CURDS

TOO MUCH PROTEIN OR FAT IN DIET.

N.B. INFANTS.
PATIENTS ON MILK DIET. 1

BLACK STOOLS
ALTERED BLOOD – MELAENA

BLEEDING FROM UPPER G.I.T
(PEPTIC ULCER. CARCINOMA)

IRON OR BISMUTH COLOUR STOOLS BLACK 2

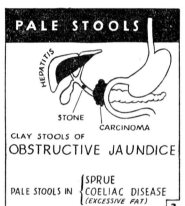

PALE STOOLS

HEPATITIS
STONE
CARCINOMA

CLAY STOOLS OF
OBSTRUCTIVE JAUNDICE

PALE STOOLS IN { SPRUE
COELIAC DISEASE
(EXCESSIVE FAT) 3

GREEN STOOLS

FREQUENT WATERY GREEN STOOLS IN INFANTS
ACUTE GASTRO-ENTERITIS
URGENCY · ISOLATE

BRIGHT RED BLOOD
STREAKING THE MOTION
CARCINOMA
HAEMORRHOIDS 4

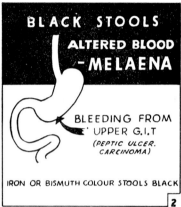

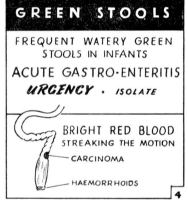

BLOOD & MUCUS

INFLAMMATION & ULCERATION OF BOWELS

ACUTE   BACILLARY DYSENTERY
AMOEBIC DYSENTERY

E. HISTOLYTICA

CHRONIC ULCERATIVE COLITIS
(RECURRENT DIARRHOEA WITH BLOOD & MUCUS.)

INTUSSUSCEPTION IN INFANTS

INVAGINATED INTESTINE

RED CURRANT JELLY STOOLS
(BLOOD & MUCUS) 5

H.MALSTER.

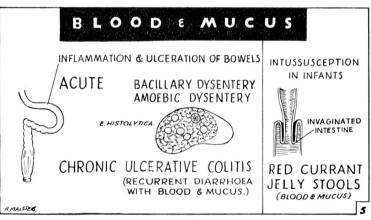

FIG. 81
Characteristics of the stools in various diseases.

(*d*) To estimate the amount of resting juice and delay in emptying in cases of suspected pyloric stenosis.

4. Sigmoidoscopy.

In the diagnosis of chronic diarrhœa, particularly in cases of ulcerative colitis and carcinoma of the lower colon.

5. Œsophagoscopy.

(*a*) In the diagnosis of dysphagia, especially to exclude carcinoma of the œsophagus.

(*b*) To remove a foreign body lodged in the œsophagus.

6. Gastroscopy.

(*a*) In the diagnosis of gastric ulcer and gastric carcinoma.

(*b*) In the diagnosis of anastomatic ulcer.

SUMMARY OF IMPORTANT DRUGS USED IN DISEASES OF THE ALIMENTARY SYSTEM

1. **Alkalis** (aluminium hydroxide, aluminium glycinate, magnesium trisilicate, calcium carbonate, etc.).

   Peptic ulcer.
   Dyspepsia.

2. **Anthelmintic Drugs.**

   (*a*) Piperazine.
   Threadworms.
   Roundworms.
   (*b*) Mepacrine.
   Tapeworms.
   (*c*) Dichlorophen (anthiphen).
   Tapeworms.
   (*d*) Filix Mas.
   Tapeworms.

3. **Antispasmodic and Anticholinergic Drugs** (atropine, belladonna, probanthine, etc.).

   Peptic ulcer.
   Dyspepsia.

4. **Cortisone and allied Drugs.**

   Ulcerative colitis.

5. **Eumydrin.**

Congenital pyloric stenosis.

6. **Folic Acid.**

Sprue.

7. **Isoniazid.**

Tuberculosis of the intestines.
Tuberculous peritonitis.

8. **Kaolin.**

Chronic diarrhœa.

9. **Neomycin.**

Gastro-enteritis.
Pre-operatively in intestinal diseases.

10. **Para-aminosalicylic Acid (P.A.S.).**

Tuberculosis of the intestines.
Tuberculous peritonitis.

11. **Penicillin.**

Vincent's infection.

12. **Purgatives and Aperients.**

Constipation.

13. **Pylostropin.**

Congenital pyloric stenosis.

14. **Streptomycin.**

Tuberculosis of the intestines.
Tuberculous peritonitis.

15. **Sulphonamides.**

Colitis.
Dysentery.
Pre-operatively in intestinal diseases.

16. **Vitamin B_{12}.**

Sprue.

CHAPTER VIII

DISEASES OF THE LIVER AND BILIARY TRACT

ANATOMY AND PHYSIOLOGY.—Both anatomically and physiologically the liver and biliary systems are intimately connected. The liver, which is situated beneath the right leaf of the diaphragm, is composed of two main types of cells :—

1. The hepatic cells, which are the main excretory cells of the liver.
2. The Kupffer cells, which are entirely different from the hepatic cells and belong to the specialised system known as the reticulo-endothelial system.

Running between the liver cells are the small bile capillaries which merge together to form larger ducts which ultimately form one large duct—the common hepatic duct. The common hepatic duct joins with the cystic duct from the gall-bladder to form the common bile duct which opens into the duodenum. The gall-bladder acts as a reservoir where the bile can be stored and where it is also concentrated.

MAIN FUNCTIONS OF THE LIVER

1. Bile Metabolism.

(*a*) BILE PIGMENTS.—The red blood cells have a normal life of about 120 days, after which they become worn out and are destroyed by the reticulo-endothelial system. In the course of their destruction bile pigments are formed of which the pigment *bilirubin* is the most important. This bilirubin is excreted by the hepatic cells of the liver into the biliary tract and eventually emptied into the duodenum. In the intestine the bilirubin is, in a changed form, known as stercobilin, and gives the fæces their normal dark brown colour. In the absence of stercobilin the fæces are pale. In addition to being excreted in the fæces a small amount of the biliary pigment stercobilin is reabsorbed back into the blood stream from the intestines to be partially excreted in the urine. This small amount of pigment which is excreted in the urine is given the name urobilin, although it is in fact identical with stercobilin. In normal health the amount of urobilin present in the urine is too small to be found on ordinary routine examination.

(*b*) BILE SALTS.—These are formed by the hepatic cells, and

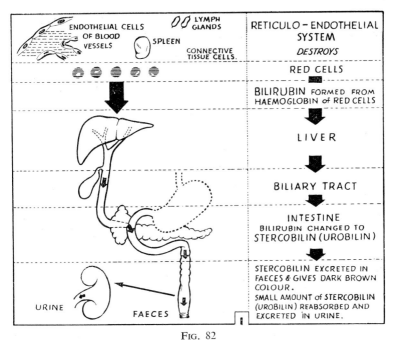

FIG. 82

A diagram showing normal bile pigment formation and circulation.

together with the bile pigments pass into the common hepatic duct, are stored in the gall-bladder and are eventually emptied into the duodenum. The bile salts are most important in aiding the proper absorption and digestion of fats and also in the absorption of vitamin K.

2. Metabolism of Carbohydrates.

The liver plays a very important role in the metabolism of carbo-hydrate foodstuffs, as it stores glucose in the form of glycogen to be used as necessary by the body. The liver is thus a great store-house of energy, as glucose is one of the most important foodstuffs for providing energy.

3. Metabolism of Protein.

The liver plays an important role in the metabolism of proteins, during which process urea is formed. Urea is excreted as a waste product by the kidneys.

4. Storage of Vitamin B_{12}.

The liver is the main storage place for vitamin B_{12}, which is essential for the proper formation of the red blood cells.

5. Formation and Storage of Prothrombin.

Vitamin K which is present in certain foods and also manufactured by bacteria in the bowel is absorbed from the intestines to form prothrombin in the liver. Prothrombin is essential for the proper clotting of blood.

JAUNDICE

Before discussing individual diseases affecting the liver and biliary tract it is advisable to explain the main causes and types of jaundice. This is because jaundice is a very common and frequently the predominating sign in most diseases of the liver and biliary tract. Jaundice is the term given to the yellow discoloration of the skin and conjunctiva caused by an excess of bile pigment in the blood stream. This yellowish colour is the clinical sign of jaundice.

Types of Jaundice.—Jaundice can be divided into two main types, according to the manner in which the excess of bile pigment develops in the blood :—

(A) Obstructive Jaundice (Regurgitation Jaundice).
(B) Hæmolytic Jaundice (Retention Jaundice).

(A) OBSTRUCTIVE JAUNDICE (Regurgitation Jaundice)

In this type excess of bilirubin occurs in the blood stream owing to a blockage or disease in some part of the liver or biliary passages. As the bile cannot pass down its normal channel it is reabsorbed back into the blood stream, thereby giving rise to jaundice.

Causes.

1. Obstruction in the Ducts.

Gall-stones.
Stricture.

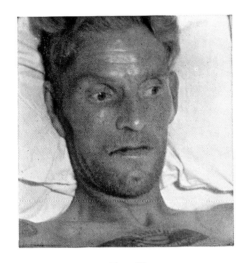

FIG. 83
Jaundice.

[*To face page* 280

2. Obstruction and Pressure on the Ducts from Outside.

Carcinoma of the head of the pancreas.
Secondary carcinoma in the lymph glands.

3. Obstruction or Disease in the Liver.

Inflammatory diseases, *i.e.*, hepatitis.
Toxic drugs and poisons.
Cirrhosis of the liver.
Carcinoma of the liver.

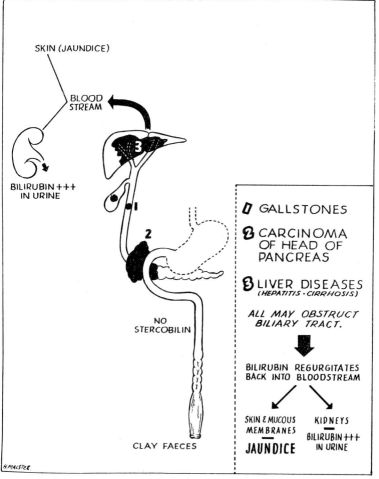

FIG. 84
A diagram showing the main causes and features of obstructive jaundice.

Symptoms and Signs.

1. The jaundice is usually very deep and easily recognisable. It is generally first noticed in the conjunctiva.

2. The fæces are pale. This is because the bilirubin is not reaching the intestine owing to the obstruction. As a result the normal dark brown colour of the fæces which is due to the bile pigment is replaced by a clay colour.

3. The urine is dark brown in colour owing to the presence of bilirubin.

4. Pruritus or itching of the skin. The well-marked itching of the skin seen in obstructive jaundice is caused by the accumulation of the bile salts in the blood.

5. In long-standing cases of obstructive jaundice the absence of bile salts, which prevents the absorption of vitamin K from the bowel, leads to prothrombin deficiency. This deficiency causes a prolonged blood clotting time. Prothrombin deficiency is the cause of the excessive bleeding sometimes seen in operations on cases of obstructive jaundice.

(B) HÆMOLYTIC JAUNDICE (Retention Jaundice)

In hæmolytic jaundice the excess of bile pigments in the blood, which gives rise to the jaundice, is not due (as in obstructive jaundice) either to disease in the liver or to obstruction in the biliary passages but to excessive destruction (hæmolysis) of the red cells.

Jaundice does not necessarily develop with hæmolysis of the red cells because the liver can cope with a certain excess of bile pigments. When the hæmolysis goes beyond a certain level, however, the overworked liver cannot deal with the resultant large excess of bile pigment and therefore the bile accumulates in the blood and jaundice develops.

The causes of hæmolysis of the red blood cells which may give rise to hæmolytic jaundice are fully discussed under Hæmolytic Anæmias (p. 376).

Symptoms and Signs.—The factor common to both obstructive and hæmolytic jaundice is the presence of excess bile pigment in the blood giving rise to staining of the skin and conjunctiva. There are, however, several differences between the two types of jaundice apart from the different causes. In hæmolytic jaundice :—

1. As there is no obstruction either in the liver or biliary tracts the bile pigment, stercobilin, is present in the fæces, which are not

therefore clay-coloured as in obstructive jaundice. Indeed, as there is an excess of bile formed the stools are often darker than usual.

2. Bile salts do not accumulate in the blood as in obstructive jaundice and therefore itching of the skin does not arise. (As the bile salts are formed in the liver and there is no obstruction they are excreted in the normal way.)

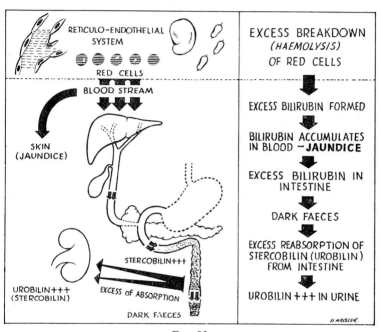

FIG. 85

A diagram showing the mechanism of hæmolytic jaundice.

3. As there is an excess of the bile pigment, stercobilin (urobilin), in the intestine, there is also a great increase in the amount of stercobilin (urobilin) absorbed from the intestine and excreted in the urine. In hæmolytic jaundice, therefore, excess of urobilin is found in the urine.

It is convenient to note here that the commonest causes of jaundice seen in clinical practice are :—

1. Gall-stones.
2. Acute infective hepatitis.
3. Carcinoma, especially carcinoma of the head of pancreas.

INDIVIDUAL DISEASES OF THE LIVER

HEPATITIS

Hepatitis means inflammation of the liver and can be caused by a variety of agents, such as infections, toxic drugs and poisons.

Types.

1. Acute Infective Hepatitis (most common).
2. Weil's Disease.
3. Hepatitis due to Drugs and Poisons (arsenic, benzene and cinchophen).

ACUTE INFECTIVE HEPATITIS

Acute infective hepatitis, the most common form of hepatitis, is caused by a virus. The disease is not very infectious, but large epidemics do occur from time to time. The virus usually spreads by the intestinal route, as the virus is excreted in the fæces. A very similar type of virus hepatitis is transmitted by transfusions of serum or by the use of inadequately sterilised syringes—*homologous serum jaundice.*

Symptoms and Signs.—The onset is usually gradual over a matter of days, with marked loss of appetite and nausea as the predominating symptoms, the sight of food, especially fats, being enough to cause nausea or even vomiting. There is a general feeling of being off-colour, with headache and slight pyrexia.

After a few days of these symptoms the urine becomes dark owing to the presence of bile, and the fæces clay-coloured. The conjunctiva and skin become yellow.

The severity of the attack varies; usually it is mild, but in a small percentage of cases the attacks are severe and fulminating, with delirium, high fever and intense jaundice. These cases are exactly the same as those of acute yellow atrophy, where severe liver necrosis is present.

Diagnosis and Course.—The diagnosis is usually simple. The absence of any severe pain or history of previous attacks of pain usually distinguishes it from the common type of jaundice caused by gall-stones.

Various liver function tests are available which can show whether the jaundice is caused by damage and obstruction in the liver, as in cases of hepatitis, or by obstruction outside the liver, *e.g.*, gall-stones

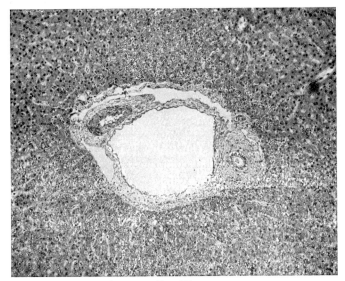

FIG. 86
Section through a normal liver.

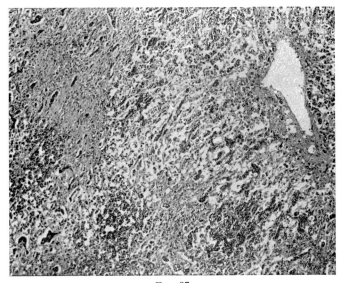

FIG. 87
Hepatitis. The liver cells have been destroyed and their
normal orderly pattern disarranged.

or carcinoma of the head of the pancreas, in which case there is no actual damage to the liver itself. The drawback with these tests is that the liver has to be fairly severely damaged before the tests are positive. Recently it has been found that with liver damage, as in hepatitis, the pyruvic transaminase level (S.G.P.T.) in the blood is markedly raised and this should therefore prove a sensitive liver function test.

Usually the jaundice subsides in a matter of weeks. Complete recovery occurs in most cases, but in a small minority the jaundice may persist for months or years. In these patients damage to the liver is usually so severe that complete recovery is impossible and death takes place within a few years.

Treatment.

1. Even in the mildest cases the patient should be put to bed, because rest in bed lessens the damage to the liver and hastens convalescence.

2. As the patient has almost a complete loss of appetite, especially for fats, it will be found in practice that in the early stages only a light diet will be tolerated. Plenty of fluids with abundant glucose are essential. As soon as the patient can be induced to eat more a high protein diet should be given. Protein appears to hasten the recovery of the damaged liver. Animal protein in the form of meat, fish, milk and eggs is particularly valuable.

The problem of whether to exclude fats from the diet, and if so for how long, is often raised. In practice it will be found that the patients will not eat fats for some time, and when they feel like doing so again there is no reason why dairy fats (butter, milk and eggs) should be excluded from the diet. The important factors in the dietary regime are a high protein content, abundant glucose and as full a diet as the patient will take. Alcohol must be avoided for at least several months after recovery.

3. Drugs play a small part in the treatment. If severe itching is present the antihistamine drugs (phenergan, sandosten, etc.) are useful.

WEIL'S DISEASE (Leptospirosis)

Weil's disease is uncommon except in people whose work brings them in contact with rats (*e.g.*, workers in sewers, miners and fish curers), as the responsible organism, a spirochæte, is excreted in the urine of infected rats. Infection in man may occur by contamination of food or through abrasions in the skin.

Symptoms and Signs.

1. The disease varies in severity from moderately severe attacks to acute fulminating cases which gravely damage the liver, *i.e.*, acute yellow atrophy.

2. Signs of severe fever with prostration and, in some cases, delirium are present. Severe conjunctivitis is often a feature.

3. An obstructive form of jaundice, with pale stools and dark urine, develops about the fourth day. In addition to the bile in the urine heavy albuminuria is also usually present.

4. In severe cases hæmorrhages from the nose, bowel, kidneys or into the skin (purpura) develop. These hæmorrhages are often so predominant that Weil's disease is also known as *infective hæmorrhagic jaundice*.

Treatment is on the lines of that for Acute Infective Hepatitis, with copious fluids and abundant glucose. In addition, the tetracycline antibiotics and penicillin have been found effective in some cases.

ACUTE YELLOW ATROPHY (Acute Hepatic Necrosis)

This condition is relatively rare, except in tropical countries, but mention is made of it here because sometimes it is caused by the severe fulminating forms of acute infective hepatitis or by severe attacks of Weil's disease. In acute yellow atrophy there is severe damage to the liver with necrosis of the cells, the liver becoming shrunken and atrophied. The liver also becomes yellow, hence the name.

Any severe infection, poison or drug that severely damages the liver can cause acute yellow atrophy. The commonest causes are :—

1. Severe fulminating acute infective hepatitis.
2. Severe Weil's disease.
3. Toxæmia of pregnancy.
4. Severe arsenical, cinchophen (atophan) or benzene poisoning.

Symptoms and Signs.—The patient is usually seriously ill with a high swinging temperature, sweating and rigors. Jaundice is present and, in some cases, hæmorrhages. The patient is quite frequently delirious, may lapse into unconsciousness and in a high percentage of cases death occurs.

Treatment.—Unfortunately there is no specific treatment. As the patients are usually severely ill they are kept on a very light diet, with an abundance of glucose. Intravenous glucose saline infusions are often given. In all cases of severe acute liver failure, especially if the patient is in hepatic coma, protein must be excluded from the diet until the patient has started to recover.   Convalescence is likely to be a matter of many months at least.   Many patients may, however, never be fully restored to health owing to permanent liver damage.

CIRRHOSIS OF THE LIVER

In cirrhosis of the liver there is a degeneration of the liver cells and also a dense infiltration of the liver by fibrous tissue, so that the

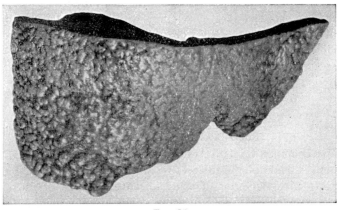

FIG. 88

Cirrhosis of the liver showing the typical granular appearance resulting from the excessive fibrous tissue.

liver cells become strangled and die.   The process is usually slowly progressive until in the end the liver ceases to function and death ensues.   There are several types of cirrhosis :—

1. Portal (Alcoholic) Cirrhosis.
2. Biliary Cirrhosis (due to long-standing obstruction in the bile ducts).
3. Syphilitic Cirrhosis (rare).

Portal or alcoholic cirrhosis is the commonest type and will therefore be described in full.

PORTAL (ALCOHOLIC) CIRRHOSIS

Portal cirrhosis is the form which is associated with chronic alcoholism.   The exact nature of the disease is not fully understood and some other factor is probably involved apart from the alcoholic poisoning.

Symptoms and Signs.—Most of the symptoms and signs are the result of the obstruction of the various parts of the liver and biliary tract by the contracting fibrous tissue. This may obstruct :—

1. THE PORTAL VEIN : causing

    (*a*) Ascites.

    (*b*) Congestion of the veins in the intestinal tract (especially those in the stomach and rectum), leading to a hæmatemesis or to the development of hæmorrhoids.

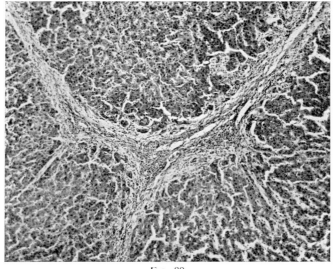

FIG. 89

Cirrhosis of the liver. Section of the liver to show the dense strands of fibrous tissue present. The liver cells are beginning to degenerate.

2. THE BILE DUCTS, causing an obstructive jaundice. The intensity of the jaundice is, however, usually slight.

The patients often complain of severe dyspepsia. Hæmorrhage, most often in the form of hæmorrhoids or a hæmatemesis, is common. The general health is affected and in the late stages the patients become confused in mind and wasted in body. Ascites is a characteristic feature of the disease.

Once the condition has advanced beyond the early stages the patients become progressively worse, eventually bed-ridden and die in coma from liver failure.

Treatment.—In the early stages if the patient can be persuaded to give up alcohol a complete cure can result. A full diet with a high protein and carbohydrate content is most important. Due to the accompanying alcoholic gastritis the patients usually have a very poor appetite, so that every effort must be made to persuade them to eat enough.

In the advanced stages, ascites can be treated by diuretics such as chlorothiazide or mersalyl, sometimes with the addition of aldactone. These diuretics are so successful in disposing of retained fluid that paracentesis is not often necessary. To avoid absorption of toxic material from the bowel, which the diseased liver is unable to detoxicate, the bowel is sterilised by giving neomycin. Hæmatemesis, due to congested veins in the œsophagus, can sometimes be controlled by injections of pitressin.

CARCINOMA OF THE LIVER

Carcinoma of the liver is very common because malignant growths in various organs of the body very often spread to the liver,

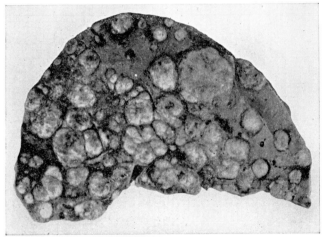

Fig. 90
Secondary carcinomatous deposits in the liver from a primary
growth in the stomach.

so causing a secondary carcinomatosis of the liver. A *primary* carcinoma of the liver (*i.e.*, where the growth starts in the liver) is, however, rare.

Symptoms and Signs.—With most patients there is a history or evidence of the primary growth. For instance, in cases due to spread from carcinoma of the stomach a history of epigastric pain, vomiting and loss of appetite is usual; in cases of carcinoma of the bronchus of the lung there is usually a cough and perhaps hæmoptysis. By the time the primary growth has spread to involve the liver the progress of the illness is rapid and death is not far off.

The specific signs of liver involvement are:—

1. An enlarged, stony-hard liver, palpable in the abdomen.
2. Ascites, which may need frequent tapping; the fluid withdrawn is serous or bloodstained.
3. Obstructive jaundice.

Treatment.—This is purely palliative as the outlook is hopeless. Sedatives for any pain are necessary. Tapping the ascites, as already mentioned, is often necessary.

DISEASES OF THE BILIARY TRACT

CHOLECYSTITIS AND GALL-STONES

Cholecystitis occurs in both acute and chronic forms and with most patients gall-stones are present. **Acute cholecystitis** causes severe pain in the right side of the upper abdomen in the region of the gall-bladder, and it characteristically radiates around the lower costal margin. Fever, nausea and vomiting accompany the pain. Acute cholecystitis is one of the causes of an " acute abdomen " and is more fully discussed in surgical textbooks.

Chronic cholecystitis is one of the causes of chronic dyspepsia, with recurrent flatulence, heartburn, nausea and pain in the epigastrium as the main symptoms. Gall-stones are commonly present and may give rise to attacks of **biliary colic.** Here severe agonising pain occurs in the epigastrium, radiating around

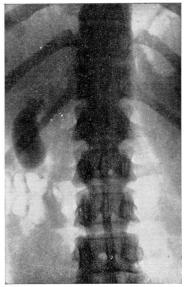

Fig. 91
X-ray (cholecystogram) of the
normal gall-bladder.

to the back, and often referred to the tip of the right shoulder. Sweating and vomiting accompany the pain.

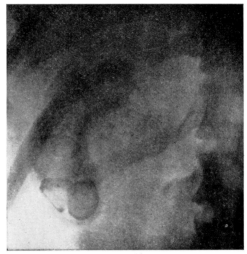

FIG. 92

Gall-stones.   In this case the stones were radio-
opaque and were visualised on a straight X-ray.

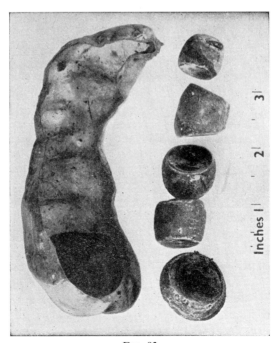

FIG. 93

A large distended chronically inflamed gall-bladder
filled with gall-stones (same patient as Fig. 92).

In addition to biliary colic, gall-stones may cause obstructive jaundice by blocking the common bile duct.

Diagnosis.—In the diagnosis of chronic cholecystitis and gall-stones an X-ray examination is usually performed. As most gall-stones are radio-opaque a plain film of the gall-bladder may reveal the presence of the stones. In some cases it is, however, necessary first to give a dye which is excreted in the bile and thus outlines the gall-bladder (*cholecystogram*). By this means it is possible to see whether the gall-bladder is functioning properly and also to determine whether or not stones are present.

Treatment.—In all cases in which gall-stones are causing symptoms an operation to remove the stones is necessary. If obstructive jaundice is present, vitamin K is given before the operation to prevent hæmorrhage.

Cases of chronic cholecystitis in which gall-stones are not present may respond to medical treatment. The patients are put on a diet similar to that used in the after-treatment of peptic ulcer, especial care being taken to omit all fried fatty and rich carbohydrate foods.

TUMOURS

Tumours of the gall-bladder and bile ducts are rare and cause a progressive obstructive jaundice, cachexia and death. A progressive obstructive jaundice is, however, frequently caused by a carcinoma of the head of the pancreas, which obstructs the common bile duct as it passes through the head of the pancreas.

The progressive nature of the obstructive jaundice in carcinoma of the head of the pancreas may be contrasted with the cases due to gall-stones, in which the obstructive jaundice is intermittent and accompanied by biliary colic.

CHAPTER IX

DISEASES OF THE CENTRAL NERVOUS SYSTEM

ANATOMY AND PHYSIOLOGY.—Nowhere else in medicine is knowledge of the relevant anatomy and physiology so important in understanding diseases of the part as in the central nervous system. The nurse should, therefore, before reading this chapter on Diseases of the Nervous System refresh her knowledge of the anatomy and physiology. It is intended here merely to outline briefly the main parts of the nervous system which are especially important in understanding neurological diseases.

The central nervous system can be divided into the following parts :—

I. Motor System. III. Sensory System.
II. Reflexes. IV. Special Senses.

I. MOTOR SYSTEM

The motor system can be conveniently divided into two main parts—the upper and lower motor neurone. A neurone is a nerve cell and the fibre which arises from it.

1. UPPER MOTOR NEURONE.—The starting point of the motor pathway is the nerve cell (Betz cell) in the motor cortex of the parietal lobe of the cerebrum. It is called the motor cortex because all the motor cells which supply motor power to all the muscles of the body are situated here. The nerve fibres originating in the Betz cells travel downwards in a compact bundle or tract called the **pyramidal tract,** which is therefore the great main motor tract of the nervous system.

The pyramidal tract passes downwards through the internal capsule, mid-brain, pons and into the medulla. Here the pyramidal tract from the right side crosses over to the left side to travel downwards in the lateral part of the spinal cord, ending opposite the second lumbar vertebra. The pyramidal tract from the left cerebral motor cortex similarly crosses over in the medulla to the right side. Because the motor fibres cross over in this way a disease in the right motor cortex or right pyramidal tract above the point of crossing of the tracts produces its effects on the left side of the body.

Individual fibres continually leave the pyramidal tract in its

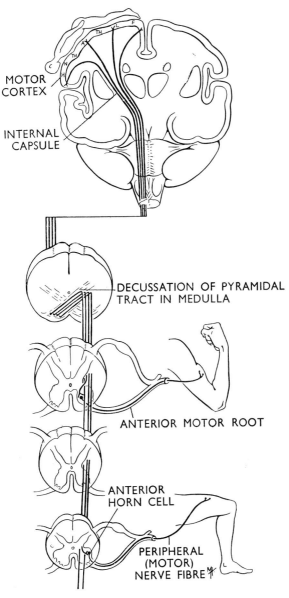

MOTOR
CORTEX

INTERNAL
CAPSULE

DECUSSATION OF PYRAMIDAL
TRACT IN MEDULLA

ANTERIOR MOTOR ROOT

ANTERIOR
HORN CELL

PERIPHERAL
(MOTOR)
NERVE FIBRE

FIG. 94
The motor system.

passage through the spinal cord, and these fibres end around the anterior horn cells situated in the central grey matter of the cord. The upper motor neurone consists therefore of the nerve cell in the motor cortex and its fibre, which passes down in the pyramidal tract to its termination around the anterior horn cell. The

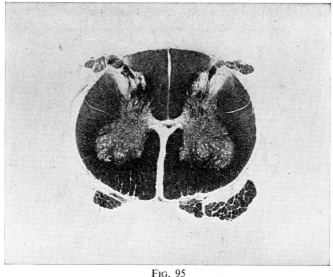

FIG. 95

Section of a normal spinal cord. The central mass of grey matter (nerve cells) can be clearly distinguished from the surrounding white matter.

pyramidal tract is thus made up of individual upper motor neurone fibres.

2. LOWER MOTOR NEURONE.—The lower motor neurone fibres (known as the anterior motor roots) start in the anterior horn cells and leave the spinal cord to join up with the posterior roots. The latter are sensory fibres which end around the posterior horn cells. The combined motor and sensory fibres form what are known as the peripheral nerves, which leave the vertebral canal through the intervertebral foramina to end in whatever part they supply.

We shall see later that this division of the motor system is extremely important, in that a disease affecting the upper motor neurone produces a different set of signs from those produced by a disease affecting the lower motor neurone. This difference in the signs helps in clinical practice to locate the exact site of the disease in the nervous system. Before, however, we can understand the difference between an upper and lower motor neurone lesion it is necessary to consider the reflexes.

II. THE REFLEXES

The reflexes are peculiar motor actions which usually occur without any conscious effort. There are many different types of

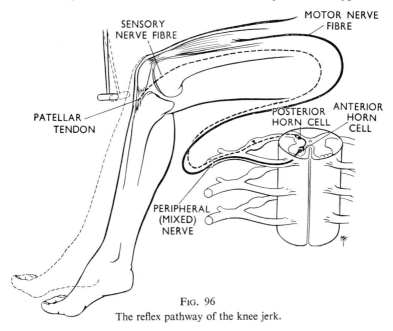

FIG. 96

The reflex pathway of the knee jerk.

reflex, but especially important are the deep tendon reflexes and the superficial reflexes.

1. DEEP TENDON REFLEXES :—

Knee jerk.   Ankle jerk.   Arm jerks.

To explain the deep tendon reflex action we shall consider the knee jerk. When the tendon over the knee is tapped an impulse travels up the sensory fibre in the peripheral nerve supplying the knee tendon, enters the spinal cord through the posterior sensory root and so into the posterior horn cell. From here the impulse (unlike all non-reflex sensory impulses which go up towards the brain) travels directly across the spinal cord to the anterior horn cell, thence out in the anterior motor root and down the motor

IO A

fibre of the peripheral nerve to the quadriceps muscle. This motor impulse causes the quadriceps muscle to contract and the typical jerk of the knee results.

The important point in this reflex pathway is that the impulse goes only through the *lower* motor neurone and does not use the *upper* motor neurone pathway. As a result, as we might expect, loss of the deep tendon reflexes occurs only in diseases affecting the lower motor neurone pathway.

2. SUPERFICIAL REFLEXES.—These reflexes are as important in the study of neurological disease as the deep reflexes, but they are very complex actions, and it is proposed only to mention the main types and the changes that affect them as a result of disease in the central nervous system.

The **abdominal reflexes** are elicited by stroking or scratching the skin of the abdominal wall, when a flickering of the underlying abdominal muscle occurs. These reflexes, unlike the deep tendon reflexes, use the *upper* motor neurone in their reflex arc. For this reason loss of the abdominal reflexes is seen only with lesions affecting the upper motor pathway.

The **plantar reflex** is a most important reflex which like the abdominal reflexes uses the *upper* motor pathway for its reflex arc. It is elicited by stroking the sole of the foot, when normally the big toe will turn downwards (flex). In diseases of the upper motor pathway this reflex is altered and the big toe turns upwards (extends). The abnormal response therefore is called an extensor response. It is also commonly called *Babinski's* sign, after the discoverer of this change in the plantar reflex.

Common Symptoms and Signs in Diseases of the Motor Pathway.

We have so far discussed the path taken by the motor impulses which activate the various muscles and organs of the body so that the body can perform the various actions required in everyday life. We have also described the important reflexes which use this motor pathway. We are therefore in a position to understand the common symptoms and signs which occur in diseases affecting the motor system.

First, it must be repeated that the motor path is divided into two main divisions and that according to which part is affected so a different set of signs is produced. These differences in the effects produced by diseases affecting the upper motor neurone and those affecting the lower motor neurone are of great importance to the doctor, as they enable him to approximately locate the site of the disease in the nervous system. It is also of value to the nurse to understand the principal signs of neurological diseases, as she will every day in the course of her ward duties see the doctor examining the nervous system by testing reflexes, noting the power in the muscles and also observing the tone, *i.e.*, whether they are stiff (spastic) or limp (flaccid).

TABLE VII

CHANGES IN THE AFFECTED LIMBS.	IN UPPER MOTOR NEURONE DISEASE.	IN LOWER MOTOR NEURONE DISEASE.
1. Paralysis (loss of power)	Present, often not complete. Tends to affect *whole* limbs.	Present, usually complete. Affects *groups of muscles* in a limb or limbs.
2. Tone of muscles .	Stiff and rigid (spastic).	Limp (flaccid).
3. Wasting of muscles	Usually slight.	Usually marked.
4. Tendon reflexes .	Present (usually exaggerated).	Absent.
5. Abdominal reflexes	Absent.	Present.
6. Plantar reflex .	Extensor response (Babinski's sign present).	Normal flexor response.
7. Sensation . .	Usually only slightly disturbed.	Sensory disturbances more evident.

The main differences between an upper motor neurone disease and a lower motor neurone disease are in the reflexes and in the tone and degree of wasting of the muscles. As pointed out above, because the deep tendon reflexes use only the lower motor pathway, upper motor neurone lesions do not abolish these reflexes as do the lower motor neurone lesions. On the other hand, the two important superficial reflexes, the abdominal and the plantar, use the upper motor neurone and so are affected in the upper motor neurone lesions only.

The more severe wasting and loss of tone in the lower motor lesions are due to the more complete interference with the motor and the muscle tone fibres which occurs in lower, as opposed to upper, motor neurone lesions.

Common Types of Paralysis.

We have just seen that the main effect of a lesion in the motor pathway is a paralysis (loss of power), which varies in form according to the site of the disease. In addition, however, to the differences between the types of paralysis produced respectively by upper and lower motor neurone lesions, the extent of the paralysis will also vary according to the actual site and severity of the disease in either the upper or lower motor pathway.

The following are the common types of paralysis with their main causes:—

1. *Upper Motor Neurone Types.*

(*a*) HEMIPLEGIA.—This is a paralysis of one side of the body, and when complete includes the lower half of the face, arm and leg. A complete hemiplegia is caused by disease affecting all the motor fibres in one pyramidal tract which supply the opposite side of the body. In the disease known as apoplexy (stroke) a hæmorrhage, thrombosis or embolism frequently affects the brain in the region known as the *internal capsule*, where the pyramidal tract lies. The most frequent result of a stroke therefore is a hemiplegia. Other diseases which commonly affect the pyramidal tract to cause a hemiplegia include disseminated sclerosis and cerebral tumour.

In a hemiplegia the paralysis is spastic in form with increased deep tendon reflexes because the upper motor pathway is affected.

(*b*) PARAPLEGIA.—Paralysis of both the lower limbs is called a paraplegia. In most cases of paraplegia the paralysis is spastic and is caused by a disease which affects both pyramidal tracts. The diseases disseminated sclerosis and general paralysis of the insane (one form of syphilis affecting the brain) are frequently associated with a spastic paraplegia. Again, pressure on the spinal cord by tumours or by tuberculous disease of the spine (Pott's disease) also often causes a spastic paraplegia.

Injuries to the spine, especially fracture dislocations, may give rise to a paraplegia. In these cases the damage to the spinal cord is usually very severe and involves most of the tracts in the spinal cord, including both the upper and lower motor and sensory pathways. The resulting paraplegia is usually a complete flaccid paralysis, with extensive sensory loss accompanied by disturbances in bladder function (retention or incontinence of urine).

(*c*) MONOPLEGIA.—Paralysis of the whole of one limb is called a monoplegia. In apoplexy the lesion may not be sufficiently extensive to cause a complete hemiplegia, and in these cases a monoplegia is often the form of paralysis present.

2. *Lower Motor Neurone Types.*

(*a*) INDIVIDUAL PERIPHERAL NERVE PARALYSES.—Lesions of the individual nerves are usually seen as a result of wounds or other injuries. The resultant paralysis is a typical example of a lower motor neurone lesion, with complete loss of power in the part affected, loss of deep reflexes, loss of sensation and severe wasting. Common examples of this form of peripheral nerve lesions are paralysis of the radial nerve (causing dropped wrist), paralysis of the ulnar nerve and brachial plexus birth injuries in infants.

(b) MULTIPLE PERIPHERAL NERVE PARALYSES.—Paralysis of several peripheral nerves is usually termed *peripheral* or *multiple neuritis*. The commonest causes are poisons and infections, especially alcohol, arsenic, diabetes and diphtheria. The paralysis is usually symmetrical, affecting both arms or legs, and is of the classical lower motor neurone type.

In addition to the above types of lower motor neurone paralysis there is another common form caused by the disease, acute anterior poliomyelitis, where the lesion is in the actual anterior motor horn cell. This causes a paralysis of various muscles or groups of muscles in one or more limbs.

III. SENSORY SYSTEM

There are various forms of sensation such as touch, pain and the feeling of heat and cold. The sense of position of a limb or joint is also important. The different sensory impulses arise in the skin, muscles and joints, and are carried backwards (upwards) in the sensory fibres which run together with the motor fibres in the peripheral nerves. The sensory fibres enter the spinal cord through the posterior spinal root (sensory root) and end around the posterior horn cell, which is situated in the grey matter of the spinal cord. From here start a new set of sensory fibres which run upwards in the spinal cord in many different tracts (sensory tracts) to end in cells in different parts of the brain. The main sensory cells are grouped together in the sensory cortex in the parietal lobe of the cerebrum, just behind the motor cortex. The sensory fibres cross over as do the motor fibres.

Disturbances in sensation are much more prominent in lesions of the peripheral nerves than in lesions of the brain. Such disturbances of sensation include :—

Anæsthesia. Loss of sensation of touch.
Analgesia. Loss of sensation of pain.
Hyperæsthesia. Increased sensation of touch, causing tenderness.
Paræsthesia. Sensation of pins and needles.

IV. SPECIAL SENSES

The special senses include sight, speech, hearing, smell and taste. Special areas exist in the brain which deal with the specialised reception and interpretation of these sensations. For instance, the sight areas are in the occipital lobes and hearing in the temporal lobes. Speech is different from the other senses in that it has centres on the *left* side of the brain only. Therefore only diseases affecting the left side of the brain produce speech disturbances. The term *aphasia* is used to describe disturbances in speech resulting from a brain lesion.

CONTROL OF THE BLADDER

Control of micturition in adults is a complex act which is often disturbed in diseases of the central nervous system. Sensory fibres convey pain and a sense of distension upwards to the brain, where these sensations are interpreted and controlled by the person's will. If it is desired to empty the bladder impulses travel downwards to relax the sphincter muscles and contract the detrusor (expelling) muscles. Disturbance of this voluntary control of bladder action is often present in central nervous diseases.

Incontinence of urine, often with incontinence of fæces, is present in most cases of coma, whatever the cause. When the patient becomes conscious, bladder control is usually quickly regained. In elderly people incontinence of urine may also arise in any severe illness and may persist for some time.

Instead of incontinence of urine, retention of urine may be seen in cases of coma. Spinal cord injuries, especially where caused by fracture-dislocation of the spine, are commonly accompanied by retention of urine, which may persist for weeks or months.

It should be noted that in some cases of retention an *overflow* dribbling of urine may occur which may be mistaken for a simple incontinence without retention. The importance of distinguishing between the two must be stressed because an unrelieved retention of urine can cause severe and lasting damage to the kidneys. In cases of overflow dribbling of urine caused by retention of urine the distended bladder can be felt and often seen as a firm round swelling in the midline of the abdomen just above the pubes.

It must be realised that local disease in the bladder and prostate also frequently causes incontinence or retention of urine. Indeed an enlarged prostate is the commonest cause of retention.

The importance of the care of the bladder will be dealt with under the different diseases affecting this organ.

SUMMARY OF THE COMMON SYMPTOMS AND SIGNS IN NEUROLOGICAL DISEASES

The exact site of the disease in the central nervous system determines the part to be affected. Also, according to whether it is mainly a motor, sensory or special sense area involved, so the signs will be mainly motor, sensory or " special sense " in type. Certain of the more common symptoms and signs seen in central nervous system diseases will be briefly summarised.

1. Diseases affecting the motor pathway produce loss of power (paralysis) as the predominating sign. The paralysis varies in extent, depending on the site and severity of the disease. Common forms of paralysis include hemiplegia, paralysis of one side of the body; paraplegia, paralysis of both lower limbs; and monoplegia, paralysis of one limb.

2. Changes in the muscles, such as wasting and in tone, either spastic or flaccid, are important signs of motor lesions. The exact degree and type of change depends, as described earlier, on whether the upper or lower motor neurone is affected.

3. Changes in the reflexes, especially the deep (tendon) reflexes and the abdominal and plantar reflexes, occur in lesions of the motor pathway. Again, the type of change in the reflex depends on whether an upper or lower motor neurone lesion is present.

4. Disturbances in sensation are common, particularly in diseases of the peripheral nerves. Changes in the sensation of touch (anæsthesia and hyperæsthesia) and in the sensation of pain (analgesia) are common disturbances. Paræsthesia in the form of " pins and needles " is also frequently met with.

5. Disturbances in sight, hearing, speech and other special senses depend on lesions directly affecting the specialised areas and nerves in the brain which deal with these senses.

6. Control of the bladder is often affected in certain neurological diseases, leading to incontinence of urine or to retention.

7. Other signs common to many neurological diseases include :—

(a) TREMORS.—These are disordered rapid movements of muscles leading to a shakiness of the parts affected. There are many different types of tremor, such as *intention tremor* where the tremor occurs only when the affected limb performs or intends to perform any action. Fine tremors also occur in toxic diseases as well as in neurological diseases, as in thyrotoxicosis and alcoholism. In diseases of the nervous system the tremors are usually coarse and very obvious. Such diseases as paralysis agitans, disseminated sclerosis and general paralysis of the insane are usually associated with obvious tremors.

Nystagmus is a tremor of the eyeballs which causes a to-and-fro movement of the eyes, which is especially marked when the patient looks to one or other side. It occurs in such conditions as disseminated sclerosis and diseases affecting the cerebellum.

(*b*) TROPHIC LESIONS.—When the sensation of pain is lost, ulceration of the skin and damage to the joints commonly follow. Perforating ulcers on the feet are seen in tabes dorsalis (one form of syphilitic disease of the nervous system). In the disease known as syringomyelia, where loss of pain is a marked feature, severe ulceration of the fingers is a prominent sign.

Charcot's joints, where gross arthritis and derangement of the joints are present, are most frequently seen in tabes dorsalis and syringomyelia. This is because injury to a joint which has lost the sense of pain passes unheeded and therefore eventually with continued use or with repeated injuries, however trivial, gross destruction of the joint develops.

Pressure sores, which are a form of trophic lesion, are liable to occur in cases of paralysis but, as will be stressed in the nursing of a paralysed patient, can be prevented in most patients by careful nursing.

(*c*) ATAXIA.—This term means inco-ordination of movement and particularly applies to the gait or walking. Various types of gait characteristically occur in different neurological diseases. A patient with the disease known as paralysis agitans can be at once picked out by means of the typical shuffling, short-step gait present. The patient with tabes dorsalis walks with a wide, stamping, staggering gait, usually aided with sticks. The gait in the common form of paralysis, hemiplegia (wherein one half of the body is affected), is also typical. Here the patient drags one leg, and the arm on the paralysed side does not swing but is held close to the side.

(*d*) REACTION OF DEGENERATION.—When muscles are paralysed certain changes develop in their reaction to stimulation with an electrical current. These changes, the reaction of degeneration, are often used for diagnosis and also to estimate the possibility of recovery in paralysed muscles.

DISEASES OF THE MENINGES

MENINGITIS

Meningitis (inflammation of the meninges) is the most common and important disease affecting the meninges.

Types.

1. Pyogenic meningitis. This includes several types of meningitis, of which the commonest are meningococcal, pneumococcal, influenzal, streptococcal and staphylococcal meningitis, caused by various pus-forming organisms.

2. Tuberculous meningitis.

3. Virus meningitis.

4. Syphilitic meningitis (rare).

Symptoms and Signs.—Most of the symptoms and signs are the same in all forms of meningitis, and are due to the inflammation of the meninges causing increased intracranial pressure. These common symptoms and signs will be given first, and afterwards the special features of the different types will be mentioned.

1. ONSET.—This is in most cases sudden, with the one exception of the tuberculous type. The patient is severely ill and toxic, with a high fever. The pulse is relatively slow in relation to the height of the temperature.

2. HEADACHE.—This is very constant and persistent. It comes on early and is associated with

3. VOMITING.—The combination of severe headache and vomiting is always suggestive of an intracranial lesion.

4. The patient is drowsy and irritable, and often delirious. He lies in a characteristic attitude, curled up in bed and turned away from the light, as photophobia (dislike of light) is present. He resents being touched or disturbed and, if a child, cries with a high-pitched cry.

5. CONVULSIONS OR FITS.—These are common, especially in infants.

6. NECK RIGIDITY.—There is a marked stiffness of the neck, and any attempt to flex the head is strongly resisted. This rigidity of the neck muscles is due to the inflamed meninges. As bending the neck stretches the meninges and so causes pain the patient holds the neck rigid to prevent this pain.

7. KERNIG'S SIGN.—This is the resistance met with on attempting to straighten the flexed knee, as here again straightening the

flexed knee by stretching the inflamed meninges in the spinal cord causes pain.

Special Features of the Individual Types.

1. MENINGOCOCCAL MENINGITIS.—This is the most common form of pyogenic meningitis and is also known as cerebrospinal fever. It is acute in onset and often very severe. Meningococcal meningitis often occurs in epidemics.

2. PNEUMOCOCCAL AND INFLUENZAL MENINGITIS.—Both these types are very acute and severe in their onset and course.

3. STREPTOCOCCAL AND STAPHYLOCOCCAL MENINGITIS.—In many cases of these types of meningitis there is often evidence of infection in the ear (otitis media), mastoid (mastoiditis) or sinuses (sinusitis), the meningitis developing as a result of spread of the infection to the meninges.

4. TUBERCULOUS MENINGITIS.—Tuberculous meningitis differs from all the other types in that the onset is gradual, often one or two weeks elapsing before the characteristic picture of meningitis appears. After the meningococcal form it is the most common type met with.

5. VIRUS MENINGITIS.—This type of meningitis is usually less severe than the pyogenic forms.

Course.—If untreated the patient lapses into coma, becomes delirious and incontinent and death usually supervenes, except in virus meningitis. In pyogenic meningitis chemotherapy has, however, dramatically improved the outlook. In tuberculous cases recovery, when it occurs, is much slower, taking many months.

Diagnosis.—The symptoms and signs of meningitis are in most cases so definite that the condition will be at once suspected. To confirm the diagnosis a **lumbar puncture** will be done. Here a special needle with stilette is inserted, *under the strictest aseptic technique*, between the fourth and fifth or third and fourth lumbar vertebræ, piercing the dura mater and passing into the subarachnoid space. On the withdrawal of the stilette the cerebrospinal fluid flows through the needle. A normal cerebrospinal fluid comes out drop by drop at a certain pressure (which can be measured by a special manometer, such as Greenfield's) and, most important, normal fluid is always crystal clear.

In all types of meningitis the fluid, being under pressure, spurts out and is definitely cloudy. In all pyogenic types of meningitis the fluid is not only cloudy but usually frankly purulent, and at once the diagnosis of meningitis can be made. By examining the fluid in the laboratory and culturing the organism the exact type of meningitis—meningococcal, pneumococcal, influenzal, etc.—can be ascertained. With a purulent cerebrospinal fluid, treatment is immediately started as for a pyogenic meningitis without waiting for the result of the culture.

In the early stages of tuberculous meningitis the fluid is only slightly cloudy, and therefore the diagnosis of meningitis may not

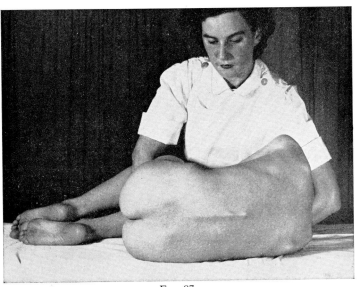

FIG. 97

The position of the patient for lumbar puncture. The spine
must be fully flexed.

be obvious from the naked-eye appearance of the cerebrospinal fluid. Confirmation may therefore have to await the results of the laboratory examination. In any case, tuberculous meningitis being much more subacute there is not the same urgency to commence treatment as in pyogenic meningitis.

Treatment of Meningitis.

1. NURSING.—Patients with meningitis are severely ill and toxic, thus requiring the most skilled nursing. They resent all interference, so that great patience on the part of the nurse is needed in order to make sure that the patient gets sufficient fluids. In the early stages

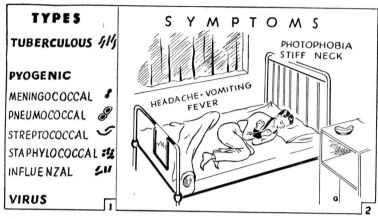

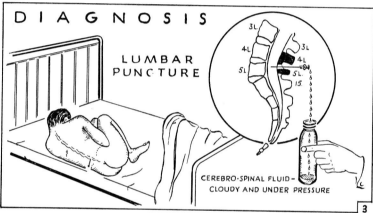

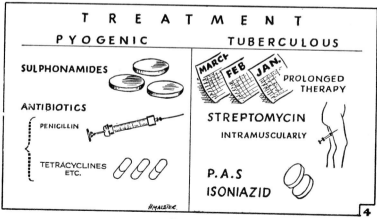

FIG. 98
Meningitis.

the patient will be able to take only fluids with glucose, but as soon as specific treatment has had effect light diet will be possible. The patient is best nursed in a subdued light on account of the photophobia. Quietness is essential as noise is badly tolerated.

2. SPECIFIC TREATMENT.

(a) *Pyogenic Meningitis.*—The introduction of the sulphonamide drugs and antibiotics has completely changed the outlook in pyogenic meningitis. Before these drugs were used the majority of cases of meningitis died. Now the vast majority recover. Sulphonamides, such as sulphadiazine, sulphatriad or sulphadimidine, are very effective, particularly in meningococcal meningitis. In the more fulminating and resistant cases, however, especially the pneumococcal and influenzal types, one of the antibiotics is usually given in addition to the sulphonamides. The tetracycline antibiotics or penicillin are frequently used with very good effect in most cases. Penicillin (10,000 to 20,000 units) is sometimes given by the intrathecal route, but great care is necessary if penicillin is used in this way owing to the irritating effect of concentrated doses of penicillin on the meninges.

(b) *Tuberculous Meningitis.*—Before the introduction of streptomycin and isoniazid all patients with tuberculous meningitis died. Chemotherapy has, however, resulted in the complete recovery of many patients, especially when treatment is started early. Streptomycin and isoniazid are given in a prolonged course lasting for at least six months. Isoniazid appears to be a very valuable drug in tuberculous meningitis as it easily penetrates the cerebrospinal fluid. Intrathecal streptomycin is seldom given nowadays.

VASCULAR DISEASES OF THE BRAIN

APOPLEXY (Stroke)

Causes.—Apoplexy is an extremely common disease and may be caused by three different lesions in the cerebral arteries, all of which produce a similar clinical picture, so that they can be conveniently grouped together.

1. **Cerebral Thrombosis.**—Thrombosis in a cerebral artery occurs as a result of two main diseases which affect the artery, arteriosclerosis (atherosclerosis) and syphilis. Arteriosclerosis is much the

more frequent cause and accounts for most of the cases of stroke seen in elderly people. Syphilitic cerebral thrombosis is much less common and attacks a younger age group.

2. **Cerebral Hæmorrhage.** — Hypertension frequently causes rupture of a cerebral artery, producing hæmorrhage into the brain and the clinical picture of apoplexy. Cerebral hæmorrhage from hypertension and cerebral thrombosis from arteriosclerosis are the two commonest causes of stroke.

3. **Cerebral Embolism.**—An embolus, or detached clot, may lodge in one of the cerebral arteries and produce apoplexy. This variety of stroke is seen in diseases where a clot forms on the left side of the heart and is carried up in the blood stream to lodge in one of the cerebral vessels. The diseases which most frequently cause a clot in the left side of the heart are :—

(a) Mitral stenosis with auricular fibrillation.

(b) Subacute bacterial endocarditis.

(c) Coronary thrombosis.

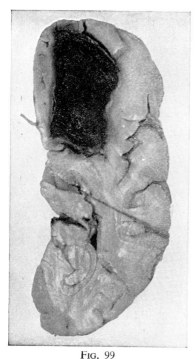

FIG. 99

Section of the brain showing a large cerebral hæmorrhage. The patient had severe hypertension.

Symptoms and Signs.

1. The symptoms and signs of cerebral thrombosis, hæmorrhage and embolism are all exactly the same except for the *onset*. In thrombosis this is a matter of hours or even days, while in embolism the onset is very sudden. In hæmorrhage the onset is also fairly sudden, over a few hours only. There is usually a history of preceding hypertension in cases of cerebral hæmorrhage, whilst in cases of embolism the patient may be under treatment for mitral stenosis, coronary thrombosis or bacterial endocarditis.

2. In mild cases, which are usually due to cerebral thrombosis, the first sign of apoplexy may be the onset of the paralysis

without unconsciousness, but in most cases the patient becomes drowsy and lapses into *coma* or alternatively goes into coma with extreme suddenness. While the patient is unconscious the breathing is usually very deep and stertorous and the pupils dilated; incontinence of urine and fæces is also present.

3. The patient in severe cases may die without regaining consciousness. In other cases when the patient regains consciousness paralysis is usually present, generally taking the form of a

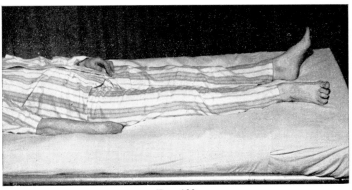

FIG. 100

Right hemiplegia. The leg is externally rotated and the foot is dropped. The paralysed arm is adducted and the hand curled under the body.

complete **hemiplegia** (*i.e.*, paralysis of one side of the body, including the face, arm and leg). The degree of paralysis may, however, vary from a complete hemiplegia to a monoplegia, where only one limb is affected.

The nurse may wonder why nearly all cases of apoplexy due to such lesions as a thrombosis, hæmorrhage or embolism result in a hemiplegia. The reason is that by far the commonest site for a thrombosis, hæmorrhage or embolism is one particular area known as the internal capsule, through which the pyramidal (motor) pathway runs. Why this area (the internal capsule) is nearly always picked out is not known.

4. If the site of the lesion is on the right side of the brain the paralysis occurs on the left side of the body, because as already mentioned the pyramidal motor tracts cross over in the medulla to supply the opposite side of the body. If the lesion is on the left side of the brain the speech centre may be involved, with resulting disturbances of speech (*aphasia*).

Course.—If the patient remains in a coma for over two days recovery is unlikely. In other cases the patient often regains some power of movement in the paralysed limbs. The degree of recovery, which varies considerably, may be almost complete with one patient and extremely limited with another. In the latter case the patient becomes bed-ridden for the remainder of his life, with the ever constant danger of pneumonia, pressure-sores or urinary infections which threaten all paralysed patients.

Treatment of Apoplexy.

1. NURSING.—During the stage of coma the nursing of the patient is of the utmost importance. As in any case of coma with paralysis certain dangers are very prone to arise which, if possible, must at all costs be prevented.

(*a*) A clear airway must be maintained so that the patient does not become asphyxiated through the paralysed tongue falling back in the mouth. The patient's head is best put on the side, and if necessary an airway should be inserted. If there is any difficulty over drainage of the mouth secretions, the patient is best nursed in the prone or semi-prone position. The nurse will recognise asphyxia by the presence of cyanosis.

(*b*) Pressure sores are very liable to develop in any prolonged coma, especially in elderly people, and particularly if paralysis is also present. In apoplexy the vast majority of the patients are elderly, and as paralysis is nearly always present, pressure-sores are extremely liable to occur. For this reason preventive measures, such as attention to the skin over the pressure areas and frequent changing of the patient's position, are particularly important. A rubber mattress is also most useful and every effort should be made to maintain a " dry bed."

(*c*) Frequent changing of the patient's position, which must be done with great care and gentleness, will also help to avert another prevalent danger—pneumonia. If pneumonia should develop, penicillin or one of the other antibiotics will be given.

(*d*) Careful watch on the bladder is necessary. As has already been stated, either incontinence of urine (which is more usual) or in some cases retention of urine with a distended bladder may occur. In cases of retention when the bladder becomes grossly distended an overflow dribbling of urine can occur. A large distended bladder is felt as a tense rounded tumour in the midline of the abdomen above the pelvis. Catheterisation, under the strictest

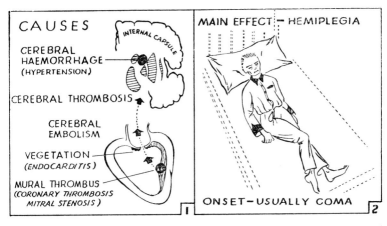

CAUSES

CEREBRAL
HAEMORRHAGE
(HYPERTENSION)

INTERNAL CAPSULE

CEREBRAL THROMBOSIS

CEREBRAL
EMBOLISM

VEGETATION
(ENDOCARDITIS)

MURAL THROMBUS
(CORONARY THROMBOSIS
MITRAL STENOSIS)

1

MAIN EFFECT — HEMIPLEGIA

ONSET — USUALLY COMA

2

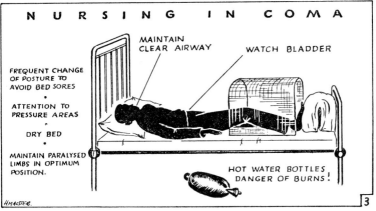

N U R S I N G   I N   C O M A

MAINTAIN
CLEAR AIRWAY

WATCH BLADDER

FREQUENT CHANGE
OF POSTURE TO
AVOID BED SORES
•
ATTENTION TO
PRESSURE AREAS
•
DRY BED
•
MAINTAIN PARALYSED
LIMBS IN OPTIMUM
POSITION.

HOT WATER BOTTLES
DANGER OF BURNS!

H.M.ALSTER.

3

FIG. 101
Apoplexy.

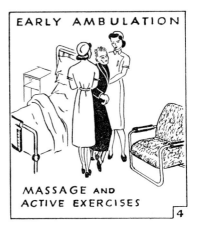

EARLY AMBULATION

MASSAGE AND
ACTIVE EXERCISES

4

asepsis (as, of course, in all catheterisations), will then be needed. These patients are very liable to develop urinary infections, such as cystitis or pyelitis, which can have a serious effect. For this reason the most careful aseptic technique in catheterisation is needed.

(*e*) The question of providing warmth to the patient will naturally arise and, as with all unconscious patients, the greatest care must be taken with hot-water bottles to ensure that they do not burn the patient. All patients are apt to be restless when recovering from the coma, and the covers of hot-water bottles can be easily kicked

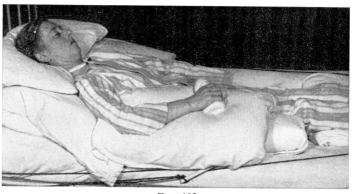

FIG. 102

The correct positioning of the upper limb in hemiplegia. The pillow prevents adduction of the arm and the hand-roll keeps the fingers and thumb opposed to each other.

off, with resulting burns. It is best, therefore, not to use hot-water bottles with any comatose patient and to supply any necessary warmth with sufficient bed-clothes.

(*f*) When the patient has recovered consciousness fluids can be given by mouth; later, when the patient's condition has improved, light diet is given.

(*g*) If the hemiplegia is on the right side, speech disturbance (*aphasia*) is very likely to be present. Patients so affected are greatly distressed to find that they cannot speak and therefore the nurse must take great care to reassure the patient and make sure she understands all the patient's wants. Speech therapy, under the supervision of a speech therapist, will be required for many patients with aphasia.

2. TREATMENT OF THE PARALYSED LIMBS.

(*a*) All weight must be taken off the paralysed limbs by bed-cradles.

(*b*) The paralysed limbs must be put in the best position for the prevention or minimisation of deformities. The affected leg should be prevented from rotating outwards by the proper use of sandbags or firm pillows. The leg should be in a position of extension with

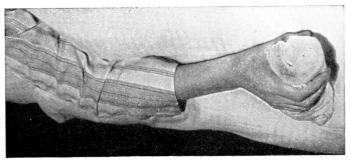

FIG. 103

Close-up view of the hand with the hand-roll in place to show the proper positioning of the fingers, thumb and wrist.

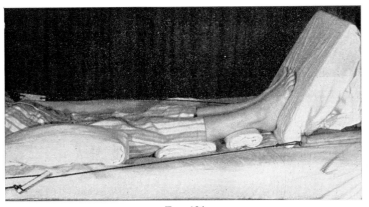

FIG. 104

The correct positioning of the lower limb in hemiplegia. The large firm pillow against the thigh prevents external rotation of the whole leg. The pillow just below the knee slightly flexes the knee and relaxes the muscles. The small pillow under the ankles prevents pressure on the heels and the foot-board overcomes the foot-drop.

the knee slightly flexed to relax the muscles. A small pad or pillow, placed under or just below the knee, helps to maintain this position. To prevent pressure on the heels a small flat pillow should be placed under the ankles. On no account must heel rings be used to prevent pressure sores as they themselves cause pressure. A foot-board or pillow at the end of the bed will help to prevent foot-drop.

A small pillow should be placed in the axilla on the affected side to prevent adduction of the arm and to relax the muscles. To prevent flexion of the fingers a soft rubber sponge or firm roll of cotton-wool should be placed in the hand so that the fingers and the thumb are opposed to each other. The sponge or hand-roll acts as a useful resistance against which the patient can later undertake active movements.

(c) It is essential to put the paralysed limbs through a full range of passive movements several times a day from the very start of the illness. Passive movements help to prevent arthritis and fixation of the joints.

(d) Soon after the patient has regained consciousness active movements and exercises must be undertaken and massage given, preferably by a skilled masseuse.

The patient must be encouraged to get out of bed as soon as possible. If patients with apoplexy are allowed to lie in bed indefinitely with no active exercises and massage, many of those who otherwise might have been able to get about and do a good deal for themselves are inevitably condemned to a bed-ridden existence for the rest of their lives.

CEREBRAL ANEURYSM (Spontaneous Subarachnoid Hæmorrhage)

Hæmorrhage into the subarachnoid space of the brain is usually caused by extensive cerebral hæmorrhage (apoplexy). Injury to the brain, especially a fracture of the skull, may also cause sub-arachnoid hæmorrhage. In addition, a *spontaneous* subarachnoid hæmorrhage may arise, and in these cases rupture of an unsuspected cerebral aneurysm is usually the cause. Small aneurysms of the cerebral arteries are not uncommon and are a result of congenital weakening of the arterial wall. These aneurysms may never give rise to symptoms unless they rupture.

Symptoms and Signs.

1. The patient is either a young adult or in the middle span of life. For this reason the condition is often referred to as the apoplexy of young people.

2. The onset is usually sudden with intense headache and vomiting. If the hæmorrhage is large the patient may be comatose and convulsions may be present.

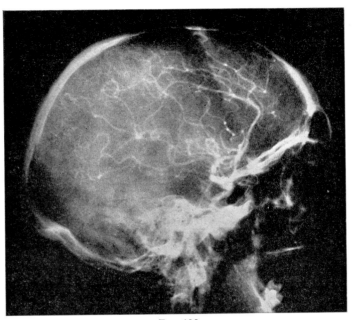

Fig. 105

Cerebral angiogram in a normal person. The opaque dye is injected into the carotid artery so that the carotid artery and cerebral blood vessels are clearly outlined.

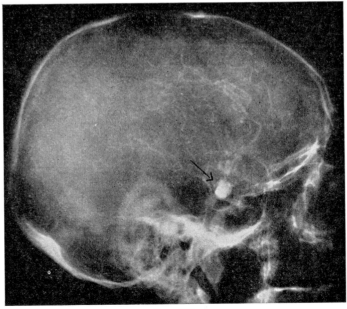

Fig. 106

Cerebral angiogram showing a large aneurysm.

3. The pulse is slow.   Neck rigidity is a characteristic feature.

4. The urine often contains a heavy deposit of albumin and sugar.

5. In some cases paralysis, often of the cranial nerves, may develop.

Diagnosis.—The picture of intense headache, vomiting, neck rigidity and slow pulse resembles that of a meningitis except for the absence of fever.   A lumbar puncture, however, will establish the diagnosis, as in subarachnoid hæmorrhage the cerebrospinal fluid is heavily bloodstained and not purulent as in meningitis.

Angiography is also very helpful in the diagnosis and localisation of a cerebral aneurysm and is always done before any operative procedure.   A radio-opaque dye is injected into the carotid artery and an X-ray of the skull then taken.   The dye outlines the blood vessels and may show up the aneurysm.   (Angiography is also used in the diagnosis and localisation of cerebral tumours (see p. 330).)

The subarachnoid hæmorrhage due to apoplexy occurs as a rule in older people and hypertension is usually present.

Treatment.—At the present time it is believed by many that the best hope of a cure lies in immediate surgery after angiography has been carried out to localise the aneurysm.   Either the carotid artery is ligatured or the aneurysm is removed if it is accessible.

Patients treated medically must be nursed at complete rest, everything being done for them to eliminate the least possible strain. The patient remains in bed for about six weeks.   Recurrence of rupture of the aneurysm is not uncommon and often takes place two to three weeks after the initial attack.

DISEASES OF THE PERIPHERAL NERVES

Lesions of the peripheral nerves are frequently seen.   Wounds or other injuries often produce a paralysis of the radial, ulnar or peroneal nerves.

Birth injuries are dealt with on page 349.   The remaining common disease affecting the peripheral nerves is known as peripheral neuritis.

PERIPHERAL NEURITIS (Multiple Neuritis, Polyneuritis)

Causes.

1. Poisons (arsenic, mercury, gold, benzol, etc.).

2. Chronic alcoholism.

3. Diabetes mellitus.
4. Vitamin B deficiency.
5. Acute infective polyneuritis.
6. Carcinoma, especially carcinoma of the bronchus.
7. Diphtheria.

Symptoms and Signs.

1. Usually the larger nerve trunks of the arms and legs are affected, resulting in diminution of power or even a complete paralysis. The typical result of this loss of motor power is a dropped wrist or foot. The muscles affected show some wasting.

2. Sensory disturbances are present usually in the form of pins and needles in the hands and feet. In some cases, however, severe pains in the arms and legs may occur with marked tenderness of the muscles. Alternatively, there is usually some degree, varying from mild to severe, of loss of sensation to pain and touch.

3. The tendon reflexes both in the legs (knee and ankle jerks) and the arms are absent. This is because the reflex arc has been interrupted. In fact all the signs present are typical of a lower motor neurone lesion, with severe loss of power, marked sensory disturbances, wasting of muscles and loss of the deep tendon reflexes.

4. In some cases the cranial nerves, such as the facial, are affected.

Features of the Different Types.

1. ALCOHOLIC NEURITIS.—This mainly affects the legs, causing dropped feet and ataxia (inco-ordination) of gait. Sensory disturbances are common and the muscles of the legs are very tender to the touch.

2. DIABETIC NEURITIS.—Diabetic neuritis is seldom very severe, and mainly causes slight pins and needles in the legs with loss of the knee jerks.

3. DIPHTHERITIC NEURITIS.—This causes a very characteristic type of paralysis which includes the following :—

(*a*) Paralysis of the soft palate, resulting in regurgitation of fluids through the nose and the voice becoming " nasal."

(*b*) Paralysis of the accommodation muscles of the eyes with consequential difficulty in reading.

(*c*) Paralysis of the limbs, causing typical peripheral neuritis as described above.

4. ACUTE INFECTIVE POLYNEURITIS (Guillain Barre Syndrome).—
The cause of this form of peripheral neuritis is unknown but appears
to be an infection, with all the usual symptoms of fever, headache
and malaise, which is followed by paralysis of the arms and legs.
In some cases the paralysis may spread to affect the respiratory
muscles with the danger of asphyxia developing. The cranial nerves
may also be involved, particularly the seventh, causing a facial
paralysis.

Treatment of Peripheral Neuritis.

1. In all but the mildest cases the patient is put to bed. Care
must be taken to avoid injury to the affected limbs, and in this
respect bed-cradles are very valuable. Particular attention to the
skin and pressure areas is most important to prevent pressure sores.

2. The foot-drop usually present must be corrected by the use
of a foot-board or pillow against the feet, or, alternatively, well-
padded light splints may be used. Passive movements to prevent
fixation of the joints must be started from the onset.

3. If the case is acute, with a good deal of tenderness and pains in
the muscles, active massage and movements will be postponed until
the symptoms subside. Analgesics for the relief of pain are usually
needed, and in cases with severe pains hot packs may be useful.

4. All the appropriate specific measures will be taken, such as
the giving of vitamin B in the vitamin deficiency cases, control of
the diabetes and the withdrawal of any poisons.

5. The use of a respirator will be necessary in those cases of
respiratory paralysis due to acute infective polyneuritis. Cortisone
and allied steroids are said to have effect in some patients and may
be used.

SCIATICA

The term *sciatica* is given to the common pain which occurs
along the distribution of the sciatic nerve.

Causes.

1. In between each of the vertebræ is a small disc, which acts as
a cushion or shock absorber to prevent jarring of the spine. One of
these discs, usually in the lumbar region of the spine, may become
dislodged and protrude backwards into the spinal canal to press
on the nerves. A displaced disc in the lumbar region usually presses
on the sciatic nerve roots, so producing the sciatic syndrome. This

condition is known as a **ruptured** (or **prolapsed**) **intervertebral disc.**

A ruptured intervertebral disc is generally due to an injury which can, however, be quite trivial.

2. Malignant tumours of the vertebræ or the pelvic organs can press on the sciatic nerve so as to give rise to sciatica.

3. Arthritis of the lumbar spine or pelvic joints can cause sciatica.

4. A primary peripheral neuritis may also affect the sciatic nerve, but this is rare.

Symptoms and Signs.—The characteristic symptom in sciatica is pain occurring along the distribution of the sciatic nerve. The pain is thus felt in the back and down the back of the thigh to the ankle. Anything that causes stretching of the sciatic nerve produces the pain, so that lifting the leg makes the pain worse. The ankle jerk is usually absent, and in some cases there is loss of sensation in the area supplied by the sciatic nerve.

Treatment.—Sciatica caused by a ruptured disc is treated by complete rest, the patient lying flat on his back. Bed-boards placed under the mattress give an added support to the back and help to relieve the pain. In addition, analgesic drugs (aspirin with phenacetin, codeine, etc.) will probably be required, at least in the early stages. The patient is usually kept lying flat for several weeks after which, if the pain has gone, he is allowed to get up gradually. Active exercises for the spinal muscles are then given.

For many patients, after the initial period of strict rest, a special belt is needed to give adequate support to the back. For the minority of patients who do not respond to medical treatment, or in cases of recurring sciatica, surgical removal of the displaced disc is necessary.

Treatment of sciatica caused by malignant disease is purely palliative, consisting of rest and drugs to relieve the pain.

It is perhaps convenient to mention here that another common site for a ruptured or prolapsed intervertebral disc to occur is in the cervical region of the spine—**prolapsed cervical disc.** There is usually severe pain in the neck, often radiating into the arms; limitation of neck movements is present. Also there may be pressure from the displaced disc on the large nerve tracts in the spinal cord, causing severe paralysis of the limbs or even paraplegia. The term *cervical spondylosis* is often used to describe the various pressure signs caused by a prolapsed cervical disc.

COMMON DISEASES OF THE CRANIAL NERVES

The cranial nerves, which arise from the brain and run their course almost entirely within the skull, are frequently affected by diseases affecting the brain, especially any lesion which causes pressure in the skull. Only the more common and important diseases affecting the cranial nerves will be discussed.

THE OPTIC NERVE

The optic nerve conveys the visual impulses from the retina of the eye back to the sight centre in the occipital lobe of the brain. The optic nerve is of extreme importance in the diagnosis of certain diseases of the central nervous system because it is the one nerve which can actually be seen. By means of an instrument called an ophthalmoscope a clear picture of the whole of the retina of the eye, including the actual optic nerve (optic disc), can be obtained.

Normally, the optic disc is seen as a white circular area with a distinct margin. In cases of increased intracranial pressure, however, œdema or swelling of the optic nerve (**papillœdema**) develops and the optic disc becomes swollen and the margins blurred. Papillœdema is a most valuable sign of increased intracranial pressure.

Optic Neuritis.

A neuritis of the optic nerve may be caused by excessive alcohol and tobacco. Syphilis and disseminated sclerosis also cause an optic neuritis. The symptoms are those of dimness of vision or in severe cases, partial blindness.

Optic Atrophy.

Atrophy, or wasting, of the optic nerve fibres may follow a severe papillœdema or optic neuritis. Syphilis is especially prone to cause this effect. Total blindness results from complete optic atrophy.

Examination of the eye with an ophthalmoscope is of importance not only in disease of the central nervous system but in certain other diseases too which may show characteristic changes in the retina. Hypertension frequently causes hæmorrhages and white spots (exudates) in the retina, and also œdema of the optic disc. Diabetes and chronic nephritis also produce similar changes.

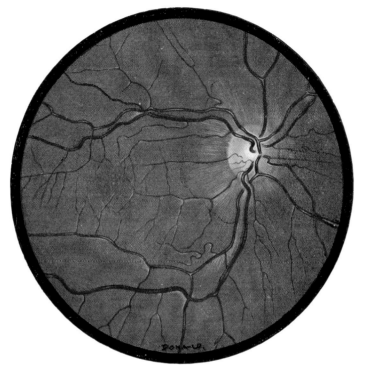

FIG. 107

The normal fundus of the eye as seen through an ophthalmoscope. The clear-cut white disc is the papilla or head of the optic nerve (optic disc).

[*To face page* 322

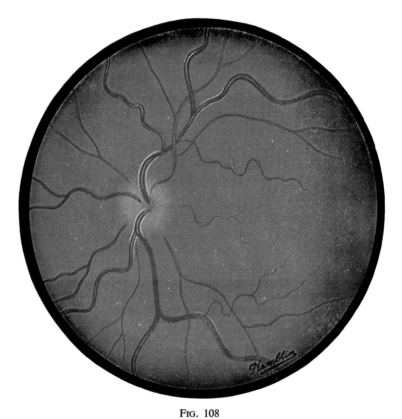

FIG. 108

Papillœdema. The optic disc is swollen and the clear-cut edges can no longer
be seen. The vessels are markedly swollen. The patient had a malignant
cerebral tumour (glioma).

THE OCULAR NERVES

The third, fourth and sixth cranial nerves supply the muscles of the eyes responsible for the movement of the eyeball. The iris muscle of the eye, which causes contraction and dilatation of the pupils, is also supplied by these nerves.

In addition, these nerves supply the muscle which raises the upper eyelid.

Diseases which affect the ocular nerves can produce any of the following signs :—

1. Drooping of the upper eyelids known as *ptosis*.
2. Squint (*strabismus*), often associated with seeing double (diplopia).
3. Unequal pupils.

The diseases which most commonly affect these nerves to produce the above signs include syphilis, brain tumours and aneurysms, encephalitis (inflammation of the brain) and myasthenia gravis.

THE FIFTH NERVE (Trigeminal)

A lesion of the fifth nerve which is sometimes met with is **trigeminal neuralgia,** where paroxysms of extremely severe pain occur in the distribution of the fifth nerve, *i.e.*, over the jaw, cheek and forehead. The slightest touch in these areas may bring on an attack.

Treatment of trigeminal neuralgia is often difficult. Bad teeth or sinus infection must be attended to if present. Analgesic drugs to relieve the pain are necessary during an attack. In severe cases section of the nerve root or an injection of alcohol into the nerve has to be carried out.

THE SEVENTH NERVE (Facial)

A paralysis of the facial nerve is frequently seen as part of a hemiplegia, of which the most common cause is apoplexy. In a hemiplegia, only the lower half of one side of the face is paralysed. In contrast to this, paralysis of the whole of one side of the face including the forehead is often seen in the condition known as **Bell's palsy.**

The exact cause of Bell's palsy is not known, but it usually follows exposure to cold and is supposed to be due to inflammation or neuritis of the facial nerve. The condition usually clears up in a few weeks without any special treatment. The eyelid cannot be

closed owing to the paralysis so that the eye must be guarded against
any injury.

A facial paralysis is sometimes seen after operations on the
mastoid owing to injury to the nerve during the operation.   Finally,

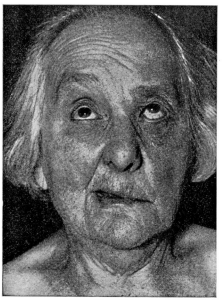

FIG. 109
Left-sided facial paralysis (Bell's palsy).

a transitory facial paralysis may arise in infants owing to a birth
injury, especially in cases of forceps delivery.

THE EIGHTH NERVE
(Auditory)

The eighth nerve has two main functions, one dealing with hearing
and the other with the maintenance of equilibrium and proper posture
of the body.   Diseases of the auditory, or hearing, part of the
nerve commonly cause deafness and buzzing in the ears
(*tinnitus*).   Diseases of the division of the nerve dealing with
equilibrium cause severe attacks of giddiness, during which all
objects may appear to spin around.   In severe attacks the patient
may fall and vomiting may also occur.   These attacks are known as
vertigo.   Motion sickness (sea-sickness, car-sickness) with its nausea,

vomiting and vertigo is probably caused by the undue motion affecting the eighth nerve.

Tumours of the eighth nerve causing deafness and tinnitus are common and are removed by operation. **Ménière's disease** is seen in elderly people: it causes severe vertigo, tinnitus and progressive deafness. The exact cause of Ménière's disease is unknown.

THE TWELFTH NERVE (Hypoglossal)

The twelfth nerve supplies the muscles of the tongue. Paralysis of the tongue is generally seen as part of a hemiplegia. Here, when the tongue is protruded from the mouth, the unaffected half of the tongue pushes the tongue over to the paralysed side, *e.g.*, in cases of paralysis of the right side of the tongue, the tongue is pushed over to the right side when it is protruded.

COMMON DISEASES OF THE NERVOUS SYSTEM

DISSEMINATED SCLEROSIS

Disseminated sclerosis is one of the commonest diseases of the nervous system met with in medicine. The cause of the disease is unknown. It produces scattered areas of degeneration throughout the brain and spinal cord, causing widespread and varied symptoms.

Symptoms and Signs.

1. Young adults in their twenties are usually affected, but, as will be seen later, it takes many years for the disease to run its course. The most common mode of onset is a paralysis, often a hemiplegia or monoplegia. This paralysis usually clears up completely after a time, only to return at a later date.

2. Eye symptoms, such as the patient's seeing double or dimness of vision from an optic neuritis, are very common.

3. Disturbances of bladder function, such as difficulty in micturition and incontinence or retention of urine, may occur.

4. Nystagmus, the to-and-fro movement of the eyes, is very constant.

5. Intention tremor. This is a marked tremor (usually most clearly seen in the arms) which occurs on movement but not at rest.

6. Scanning speech, the peculiar staccato voice, is a feature of the late stages.

Course.—Disseminated sclerosis tends to run a characteristic

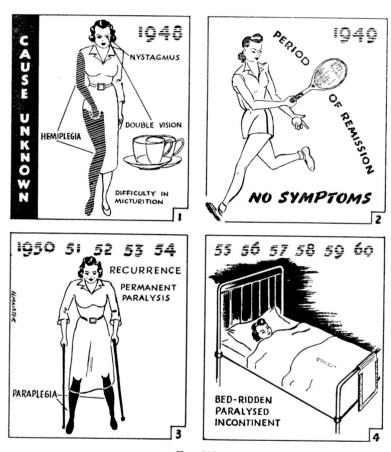

FIG. 110
Disseminated sclerosis.

course with prolonged remission of symptoms in the early stages. In a young adult recurrent paralysis, often a hemiplegia, with or without dimness of vision and disturbances of micturition, is suggestive of the disease; particularly so if in between the attacks the patient appears to be all right. Eventually, after some years, the

the
it cε
mea
and
skul

paralysis returns and remains for good. At this stage the paralysis is usually predominant in both legs (paraplegia) : the result is a marked ataxia (inco-ordination of the gait). At first the patient may be able to get about with the aid of sticks, but with progression of the disease he ultimately becomes severely paralysed and bed-ridden. The whole course of the disease, from the onset to the stage where the patient becomes bed-ridden, may take ten to fifteen years.

Treatment.—There is no specific treatment, and most patients eventually die of pressure sores, pneumonia or urinary infection. The important thing in the early stages is to keep the patients up and about as much as possible with the aid of exercises and massage. If they are kept in bed for any long period it is very difficult to get them back on their feet again.

CEREBRAL TUMOUR

(A) Primary.

Tumours of the brain are fairly common and often occur in people younger than those affected by tumours of other parts of the body. There are many types of primary tumours of the brain which include :—

1. Glioma, which tends to be very malignant and rapidly fatal.
2. Meningioma. This is a tumour growing from the meninges on the surface of the brain and is not malignant.

Cerel
arter

3. Pituitary tumour. This grows from the pituitary gland and in many cases can be successfully removed. It causes endocrine disturbances as well as pressure changes.
4. Auditory nerve tumour, which is seen in older people and is of slow growth.

(d
a con
(e
(J
increε
sign.
(g
memc
cases.

(B) Secondary.

Secondary cerebral tumours are due to spread from a primary growth somewhere else in the body, usually the bronchi or stomach. Secondary brain tumours are more common than primary.

Symptoms and Signs.—Tumours of the brain cause symptoms and signs in two main ways :—

1. Symptoms and signs due to the increased intracranial pressure.

2. LOCALISING SIGNS.—These depend on the area of the brain which is affected by the tumour. As has been seen earlier, different parts of the brain deal with different functions, and a lesion in a particular area will affect the functions of that area, enabling the lesion to be localised. However, there are many areas in the brain which are known as silent areas, *i.e.*, as far as is known they have no definite functions. A lesion in these areas tends to produce no definite localising sign. Some common localising signs of tumours in the non-silent areas are :—

(*a*) *In the Motor Cortex.*—Fits are very common and in many cases they tend to cause localising convulsive movements of the face, arm or leg. These fits are called *Jacksonian epilepsy*. In addition, a weakness or paralysis in the form of a monoplegia is common.

(*b*) *In the Occipital Cortex.*—A tumour in this area tends to cause early blindness as the sight centre is situated here.

(*c*) *Of the Auditory Nerve.*—Deafness, giddiness and vertigo are common and predominant.

(*d*) *In the Pituitary Gland.*—Disturbances in the endocrine function of the gland, leading to such conditions as gigantism and acromegaly, are often present (see p. 430).

Diagnosis.—The diagnosis is made from the symptoms and signs of increased intracranial pressure with the help of any localising signs present. The occurrence for the first time of fits in an adult is very suggestive of a brain lesion such as a tumour.

X-rays of the skull may be of value, especially after injection of air or of an opaque substance such as myodil, into the ventricles of the brain (*ventriculography*). The injection of air or myodil outlines the shape of the ventricles and any abnormality in their shape or size caused by pressure from a tumour may then be seen.

Angiography (see p. 318) may also be used in the diagnosis of cerebral tumours (or aneurysms). The radio-opaque dye outlines the cerebral blood vessels and any distortion or displacement of the vessels due to a tumour can be seen.

Lastly, an *electro-encephalogram* (see p. 338) may also help in the diagnosis and localisation of brain tumours (and cerebral abscesses) as it may reveal abnormal waves over the site of the tumour.

Treatment.—This depends on the type of tumour present. Secondary tumours are, of course, hopeless, as are many of the more malignant types of primary tumours. Many of the less malignant types have, however, been successfully removed by operation. The meningiomas and auditory nerve and pituitary tumours offer the best hope for surgical cures.

CEREBRAL ABSCESS

Cerebral abscess is usually caused by spread of infection from septic disease in the ears, mastoid cells or nasal sinuses. A cerebral abscess can also result from a septic embolus lodging in the brain, particularly in cases of bronchiectasis.

Symptoms and Signs.—These are essentially the same as for cerebral tumours. There will be the signs of increased pressure and also the localising signs according to the site of the abscess in the brain. Signs of infection, like fever and raised white cell count both in the blood and the cerebrospinal fluid, help to distinguish abscess from tumour. Evidence of septic ear disease or bronchiectasis also helps in the diagnosis.

Treatment.—Sulphonamides, penicillin or the tetracycline antibiotics are of great value, but, in addition, operation to evacuate the abscess may be necessary. Penicillin and streptomycin may be injected locally into the abscess cavity after evacuation of the abscess. The primary focus of infection (ear, mastoid, etc.) must also be dealt with by the appropriate measures.

ACUTE ANTERIOR POLIOMYELITIS (Infantile Paralysis)

Cause.—Although acute anterior poliomyelitis is an acute infectious disease, it is more conveniently considered under Diseases of the Nervous System. The disease is caused by a virus infection which specifically attacks the anterior (motor) horn cells in the spinal cord. It may also, however, affect the brain, especially the mid-brain, producing what is called *encephalitis*. (An encephalitis is an inflammation of the cells in the brain and may arise from several causes, *e.g.*, as a complication of certain infectious fevers, especially measles and whooping cough. It may, in rarer instances, follow vaccination.) The encephalitis caused by the poliomyelitis virus is known as *polioencephalitis*. Acute anterior poliomyelitis tends to occur in epidemics in the autumn.

Spread of Infection.—Infection arises in two ways: it may occur via the respiratory tract or, alternatively, as is shown by the fact that the virus has been found in the fæces, the virus may be ingested.

Incubation Period.—Seven to fourteen days.

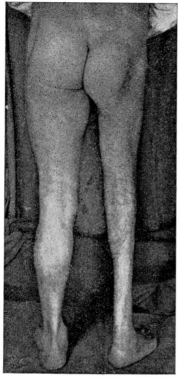

FIG. 113

Poliomyelitis, late stage of the disease, showing permanent wasting of the muscles of the right leg.

Symptoms and Signs.

1. Children and young adults are most commonly affected, but the incidence of the disease varies in different epidemics; in recent years the age of the patients has risen. The onset is sudden, with fever, headache and the general feeling of malaise.

2. Stiffness of the neck with pain in the back are common early symptoms.

In some patients the disease may progress no further than this stage, which is known as the **pre-paralytic stage.** Such cases are known as abortive attacks and are frequently only definitely diagnosed during an epidemic.

3. All other cases go on to the stage of paralysis. Here one or more limbs or the trunk muscles may become paralysed. The areas most commonly affected are the legs, shoulder girdle muscles (especially the deltoid), intercostal muscles or diaphragm. Any part of the body may, however, be affected.

The paralysed part is limp and the deep tendon reflexes are lost. Wasting of the muscles is an early and prominent feature. This is, in fact, a typical example of a lower motor neurone paralysis.

4. Pain in the affected muscles is usually present and in some cases may be very pronounced. The muscles are usually tender to touch in the acute stage.

5. In cases where the brain cells are affected (polioencephalitis)

paralysis of some of the cranial nerves, such as the seventh (facial) nerve, with a resulting weakness of one side of the face, occurs. More important, however, is the paralysis of the vital centres (*bulbar paralysis*) which may develop. Paralysis of the respiratory centre, with marked dyspnœa and cyanosis, is a common form of bulbar paralysis. Respiratory failure in poliomyelitis may, however, also be caused by paralysis of the intercostal muscles and diaphragm.

Pharyngeal paralysis is another most important result of bulbar paralysis. Pharyngeal paralysis causes difficulty in swallowing with consequential accumulation of secretions in the throat which may lead to choking and asphyxia.

Diagnosis and Course.—The sudden onset after a few days of fever, during an epidemic, of a flaccid paralysis of a limb or part of a limb allows the diagnosis to be readily made. The diagnosis may be confirmed by examination of the cerebrospinal fluid, which will show an increase in the number of the white cells.

The paralysis usually reaches its maximum in the first few days, after which it remains stationary. Slow gradual improvement usually takes place over the next few months, but it may take as long as a year before the maximum recovery has been effected. In some cases complete recovery may take place, but in others residual paralysis with severe wasting of the muscles remains.

Treatment of Poliomyelitis.

1. PREVENTIVE.—During an outbreak of poliomyelitis crowded places (*e.g.*, cinemas) should be avoided, as the disease is more rapidly spread in crowds. (During some epidemics schools and swimming baths may be closed on the instructions of the Medical Officer of Health.) It is also important to wash the hands thoroughly after defæcation as the virus may be present in the fæces and thus food may become contaminated through unclean hands.

Active Immunisation.—Active immunisation against poliomyelitis is now carried out on a large scale and appears to be most effective in preventing the disease. At least three inoculations are necessary to afford good protection and all young people should receive these injections.

2. CURATIVE.

(*a*) The patient is nursed at complete rest and full isolation procedure as outlined on page 39 is carried out. Masks should be worn and the fæces must be handled with care and disposed of promptly.

(b) The affected limbs must be placed in a position of optimum rest. It is most important that paralysed muscles should not be stretched as permanent damage may result. (See p. 314 for the proper care of paralysed limbs and the prevention of pressure sores.)

Passive movements are started from the onset, and it is for this reason that any splints used should be capable of easy removal.

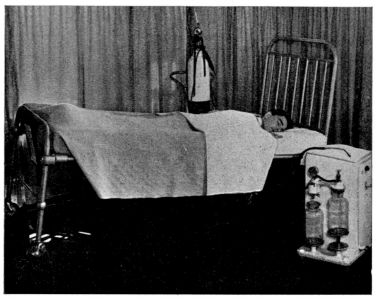

Fig. 114

The correct position for nursing a patient with pharyngeal paralysis. The prone (or semi-prone) position with the head on one side and elevation of the foot of the bed allow the maximum drainage of the mouth secretions. The patient should be turned frequently from side to side.

Prolonged rigid fixation of a limb in heavy splints must at all cost be avoided. As soon as the pains and the acute tenderness of the muscles subside active exercises are started, preferably under the supervision of a skilled physiotherapist. Baths are very useful in that active exercises of the muscles are carried out with greater ease in water. Physiotherapy may have to be continued for months or even years to ensure the maximum degree of recovery possible.

Special orthopædic appliances, like walking calipers, may be necessary, and in some cases operations may be performed to aid movement in the paralysed parts.

(c) If the respiratory muscles (intercostals and diaphragm) are affected respiratory failure may develop, and for these cases special apparatus known as a respirator (" iron lung ") is available to tide the patient over the acute phase.   Several different types of respirator

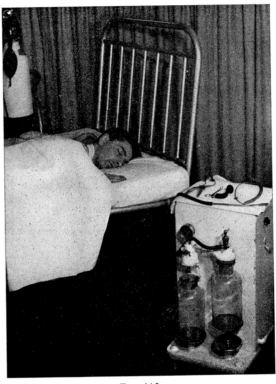

FIG. 115

The various instruments, suction apparatus and oxygen necessary for nursing a patient with pharyngeal paralysis. They must always be available at the bedside.

are used and all require the utmost skill in management.   Patients who have to be placed in a respirator are naturally very apprehensive and often terrified.   Constant reassurance and explanation of the benefits to be gained from the use of the respirator are therefore needed to allay this anxiety.

In the bulbar form of poliomyelitis pharyngeal paralysis may be present causing an inability to swallow which can lead to choking and asphyxia as a result of the accumulation of secretions in the throat.   A suction apparatus must therefore always be available at the bedside to remove the mouth secretions.   Postural drainage helps to prevent the accumulation of secretions in the throat and so these patients are best nursed in the prone or semi-prone position with the foot of the bed elevated.

The bulbar form of poliomyelitis with its pharyngeal paralysis and also paralysis of the respiratory centre, calls for the greatest care and constant attention to ensure that a clear airway is at all times maintained. Tracheotomy is being increasingly used in poliomyelitis to maintain a clear airway. Patients with respiratory and bulbar paralysis must never be left unattended.

(d) Finally, it should be realised how apprehensive are patients suffering from poliomyelitis. Every encouragement must be given to them and they must be continually reassured that they will recover a great deal of the lost power in their limbs. As progress may be very slow and take many months or years the need for continued sympathy, understanding and encouragement for these patients must be stressed.

CONVULSIONS (Fits)

Convulsions or fits are commonly seen in a wide variety of diseases and tend to occur more frequently in infants and children than in adults ; a fit or convulsion in an infant often takes the place of a rigor in an adult.

We can classify fits under two main heads :—

(A) Symptomatic.   (B) Idiopathic (Epilepsy).

(A) Symptomatic Fits.

Symptomatic fits are those in which there is some underlying discoverable cause. In contrast to symptomatic fits, idiopathic fits (or epilepsy) are those recurring fits without any obvious cause which are frequently seen in children and adults. Symptomatic fits are much more frequent than idiopathic epilepsy, so they will be described first. Again, for the sake of convenience, we can divide symptomatic fits into (1) in infants and children, and (2) in adults.

1. COMMON CAUSES OF FITS IN INFANTS AND CHILDREN.—Fits or convulsions are very commonly seen in infants. Any severe general illness or fever in an infant may start with a convulsion. Rigors do not occur in young children, being replaced by a convulsion. Whooping-cough, measles, pneumonia and otitis media commonly cause convulsions in infants.

Gastro-intestinal disturbances are another frequent cause of fits, especially in the first year of life; gastro-enteritis and intestinal worms may be associated with convulsions. Simple digestive upsets, especially in the teething stage, may also cause fits.

Diseases of the central nervous system (such as meningitis, cerebral tumours, hydrocephalus and the various forms of paralyses due to maldevelopment or injury which are so often seen in infants) are especially liable to cause repeated fits.

2. COMMON CAUSES OF FITS IN ADULTS.—The following is a brief list of the more common conditions in adults in which convulsions occur :—

(*a*) Following severe head injury.
(*b*) Uræmia (renal failure).
(*c*) Severe hypertension (hypertensive encephalopathy).
(*d*) Toxæmias of pregnancy (eclampsia).
(*e*) Cerebral tumours.
(*f*) Neuro-syphilis, especially general paralysis of the insane.
(*g*) Hysteria.

(B) Idiopathic Fits—Epilepsy.

The term *idiopathic fits*, or *epilepsy*, is given to the frequently seen recurring fits without obvious underlying cause. Epilepsy usually begins in childhood, rarely occurring for the first time in adult life. Fits which do start for the first time in adult life therefore usually have some definite underlying cause and so come into the category of symptomatic fits.

There are two main forms of idiopathic epilepsy :—

1. Major Epilepsy (Grand Mal).
2. Minor Epilepsy (Petit Mal).

1. *Major Epilepsy.*—In this form fits occur with loss of consciousness and usually in well-defined stages.

(*a*) The Warning. This takes different forms in different people, *e.g.*, a peculiar sensation, an odd taste or smell, a sense of nausea, etc.

(*b*) Tonic Stage. In this stage the patient falls unconscious, often with an epileptic cry. All the muscles go rigid, the breathing ceases and the patient goes blue in the face. The tongue is frequently bitten.

(*c*) Clonic Stage. Spasms of the muscles occur, resulting in violent movements of the limbs. Frothing at the mouth and incontinence of urine and fæces are also usually present.

(*d*) Stage of Coma. After the clonic spasms the patient remains in a coma, which, however, quickly passes into a deep ordinary sleep if the patient is not awakened. The duration of the fit is hardly ever more than two minutes and may be much less. In severe cases, fit may succeed fit, causing the condition of **status epilepticus.** This may go on for hours and, if the fits are not controlled, death from exhaustion can occur.

2. *Minor Epilepsy.*—Minor fits are much more common than major fits and may occur separately or in a patient also suffering from major fits. The attacks are much briefer and often more numerous. The fit consists of a transient loss of consciousness, perhaps lasting only for a second or two. This loss of consciousness may be so brief that the patient feels only " dazed " and onlookers may not notice anything wrong. The patients often describe their attacks as " blackouts." No convulsions occur, the patient merely staying still with a vacant expression and ceasing any action he may be carrying out.

Post-epileptic Automatism.—Post-epileptic automatism is a peculiar state which may follow epileptic fits. It may last for several hours, and while in this state the patient appears normal even to carrying out any work. There is no recollection, however, on the part of the patient of what has been done. The importance of this state is that the patients may perform actions which can have serious legal consequences. The term *psychomotor epilepsy* is used to describe the disorders of behaviour often associated with loss of memory (amnesia) where this is due to epilepsy.

Course and Diagnosis.—The diagnosis is made by ruling out all the other possible causes of fits as outlined in symptomatic convulsions. Examination of the urine and blood pressure, blood urea estimation and the Wassermann test are all routine procedures. A specialised test known as an **electro-encephalogram,** which measures in graph form the electrical waves given off by the brain, is often done. In idiopathic epilepsy typical waves are seen which are helpful in the diagnosis. (As mentioned on page 330 an electro-encephalogram is also used in the diagnosis and localisation of cerebral tumours and abscesses.)

Many cases of epilepsy tend to lessen in severity when adult life is reached, and in some patients the fits may cease completely. Some severe cases may, however, be associated with mental deterioration, and these patients are best treated in special epileptic colonies or homes.

Treatment of Epilepsy.

1. TREATMENT OF THE FIT.—The patient should be prevented

from injuring himself; all tight clothing should be loosened, especially around the neck, and a spatula (or handle of a spoon) should be put between the teeth to prevent the tongue being bitten. The fit seldom lasts more than two minutes so nothing further needs to be done at the time, except in cases of status epilepticus. Here urgent measures to stop the recurring fits are necessary. Injections of phenobarbitone intramuscularly, 1 to 3 gr. according to age, are valuable. If this is not successful paraldehyde, chloral hydrate or other sedative is usually tried.

2. PREVENTION OF THE FITS.—The following drugs are in common use in the treatment of epilepsy, either alone or in combination:—

(*a*) Phenobarbitone (luminal). This drug is most frequently used and is given in doses of ½ to 1½ gr. three times a day, according to the patient's age and the severity of the fits. Phenobarbitone is the most valuable drug available in the treatment of epilepsy.

(*b*) Phenytoin sodium (epanutin, dilantin) is given in capsules of 1½ gr. each, usually up to a maximum of 3 daily. It is often combined with phenobarbitone when phenobarbitone alone does not succeed in controlling the fits.

In addition to the above drugs several more have recently been introduced in the treatment of epilepsy:—

(*a*) Primidone (mysoline) is used in the treatment of major attacks. The initial dose is usually 0·25 gm. daily which is gradually increased to an average dose of 1 to 1·5 gm. daily.

(*b*) Methoin (mesontoin) is an effective anticonvulsant for major seizures. Fifty to 100 mgm. are usually given as an initial dose, which is then increased to an average daily dose of 300 to 400 mgm. Toxic effects include dermatitis, severe anæmia and agranulocytosis.

(*c*) Troxidone (tridione) (capsules of 4½ gr.) is very effective in controlling minor epileptic attacks but has no effect in major epilepsy. The drawback with tridione is its toxic reactions which include photophobia and, more important, depression of the bone marrow, with agranulocytosis and severe anæmia.

(*d*) Paramethadione (paradione) is used in the treatment of minor epilepsy. The average daily dose is 0·9 gm. Toxic reactions include bone marrow depression with agranulocytosis and anæmia.

(*e*) Phenacemide (phenurone) is used in the treatment of both major and minor epilepsy. The initial dose is 0·5 gm. three times a day increasing to an average dose of 2 to 3 gm. daily. Toxic reactions include agranulocytosis and anæmia.

Operative measures may be carried out in some cases of severe

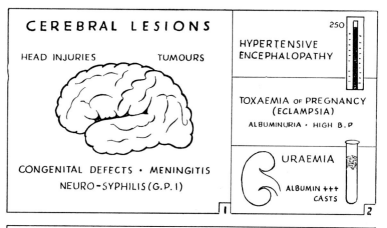

CEREBRAL LESIONS

HEAD INJURIES   TUMOURS

CONGENITAL DEFECTS · MENINGITIS

NEURO-SYPHILIS (G.P. I)

HYPERTENSIVE ENCEPHALOPATHY   250

TOXAEMIA OF PREGNANCY (ECLAMPSIA)

ALBUMINURIA · HIGH B.P

URAEMIA

ALBUMIN +++
CASTS

1

2

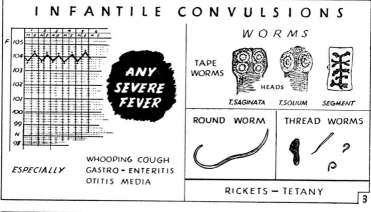

INFANTILE CONVULSIONS

F 105
104
103
102
101
100
99
N
98

ESPECIALLY   WHOOPING COUGH
GASTRO-ENTERITIS
OTITIS MEDIA

ANY SEVERE FEVER

WORMS

TAPE WORMS   HEADS

T. SAGINATA   T. SOLIUM   SEGMENT

ROUND WORM   THREAD WORMS

RICKETS — TETANY

3

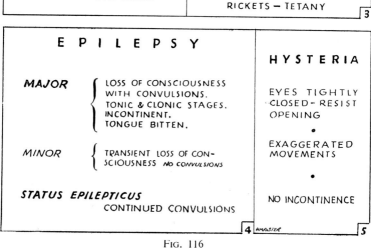

EPILEPSY

MAJOR { LOSS OF CONSCIOUSNESS WITH CONVULSIONS.
TONIC & CLONIC STAGES.
INCONTINENT.
TONGUE BITTEN.

MINOR { TRANSIENT LOSS OF CON-
SCIOUSNESS *NO CONVULSIONS*

STATUS EPILEPTICUS
CONTINUED CONVULSIONS

HYSTERIA

EYES TIGHTLY
·CLOSED- RESIST
OPENING

•

EXAGGERATED
MOVEMENTS

•

NO INCONTINENCE

4   HMALSTER   5

FIG. 116

Some common causes of convulsions.

epilepsy to remove a focal abnormality in the brain. Removal of part of the temporal lobe, in what is called temporal lobe epilepsy, is the most common operative treatment at present performed.

PARALYSIS AGITANS
(Parkinson's Disease)

Cause.—The cause of paralysis agitans is unknown. It is a degenerative lesion in the brain which occurs in late life and is more common in men than women. It is also called Parkinson's disease.

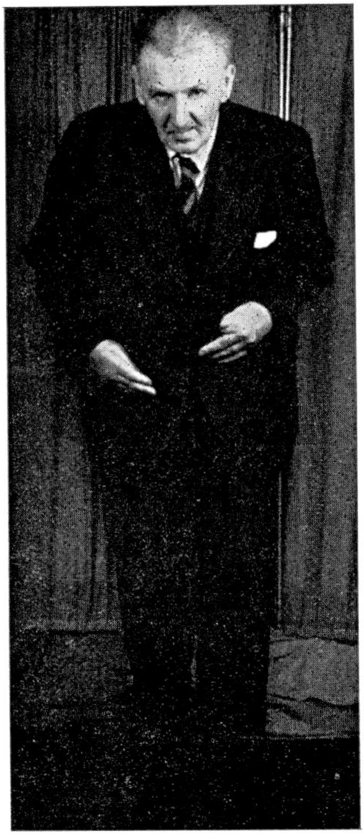

Symptoms.

1. There is the characteristic rigidity of appearance and movement. The face tends to be mask-like, showing very little emotion. The patient walks in a characteristic manner with short shuffling steps; the arms are pressed to the sides and do not swing on walking.

2. Tremor. This is very common and is usually most marked in the hands. There is the constant movement of the fingers which has been given the name of " pill-rolling." The tremor may be very severe in some cases, affecting the arms and the head too. The tremor is usually made worse by emotion, but tends to stop when performing any definite action.

3. The paralysis is seldom severe and mainly results in a general slowness of movement.

FIG. 117

Paralysis agitans. The fixed rigid attitude of the patient and lack of emotional expression are characteristic of the disease.

Diagnosis.—The diagnosis is usually obvious on looking at the patient from his typical appearance, walk and tremor.

Treatment.—There is no specific cure for this condition, which slowly progresses over many years. The most useful drug at present available to reduce the tremor and rigidity is benzhexol hydrochloride (artane), 2 to 5 mgm. three times a day. Drugs of the belladonna group (atropine, stramonium, hyoscine), either one or more, are also frequently used; they have to be given in large doses to produce an effect. Antihistamine drugs, such as benadryl, have been found effective in some patients.

POST-ENCEPHALITIC PARKINSONISM

The picture of paralysis agitans, with some modifications, is sometimes seen in much younger patients. In these it is a late complication (often many years later) of a form of encephalitis known as *encephalitis lethargica*, or, as it is often called, sleepy sickness. This disease, now rare, occurred in an epidemic form in the nineteen-twenties.

Post-encephalitic Parkinsonism, in addition to the general picture of paralysis agitans, also produces a marked tremor of the eyes and tongue with excessive salivation. Mental deficiency, which may necessitate treatment in a mental hospital, is also frequently present in these patients.

CHOREA

Chorea, which occurs in young children, causes irregular purposeless movements as the characteristic feature. It is allied to rheumatic fever, as many children who have suffered from chorea later on develop signs of rheumatic heart disease. For some unknown reason this form of chorea never occurs in adults except during pregnancy.

Symptoms and Signs.

1. There are the characteristic choreiform movements. These are sudden, changing, purposeless movements which occur in the face, arms and legs, so that the child appears to be continually fidgeting and grimacing. He tends to drop articles held in the hands.

2. There is a clumsiness of movement which is due to the involuntary movements described above and also to the general weakness of the muscles.

3. The child is often nervous and emotional.

4. There may be evidence of acute rheumatic heart disease, such as a rapid and perhaps irregular pulse.

5. Chorea, when it occurs in women during pregnancy, may take a very severe course with violent movements and mental confusion often bordering on acute mania.

Treatment.—The child must be nursed with absolute rest as in acute rheumatic fever, so as to avoid any strain on a possibly damaged heart. For the same reason the child must not do anything for itself, but must be fed and washed. As these patients are inclined to be nervous and emotional the carrying out of all the necessary details in these cases will call for utmost patience and skill.

The clothing should be light and warm, and as the clothing may get thrown off during the choreiform movements a sleeping suit and bedsocks are useful in severe attacks. Care must be exercised in the choice of feeding utensils as these may get broken as a result of the violent movements. The child must be prevented from injuring itself in severe attacks by suitable padding of the bed.

There is no specific treatment as yet available. Sodium salicylate is usually given in 10 to 20 gr. doses as in cases of rheumatic fever. If the choreiform movements are severe, sedatives, such as phenobarbitone ($\frac{1}{2}$ gr. two or three times a day), are useful.

When all active signs of the disease have gone, *i.e.*, when the choreiform movements have ceased, or almost so, when the pulse rate is normal and there are no abnormal signs in the heart, the child is gradually allowed to get up. Convalescence, as in cases of acute rheumatic fever, must be prolonged. Constructive toys help the child to regain co-ordinated movements and, in addition, keep him amused.

HERPES ZOSTER

Herpes zoster is a very common disease caused by a virus infection of a posterior nerve root. It may affect any nerve. It is often known as *shingles.*

Symptoms and Signs.—At first there is pain along the course of the affected nerve, which is followed soon after by the characteristic eruption. This takes the form of small blebs, or vesicles, scattered along the line of the nerve so that they map out the path of the affected nerve. The vesicles dry up to form crusts.

The pain, particularly in elderly patients, may be most severe and persistent, lasting perhaps for many weeks or months after all signs of the eruption have gone. The pain may be so severe as to lead to marked mental depression.

Two nerves are commonly the site of herpes zoster infections :—

1. The ophthalmic division of the fifth cranial nerve with resultant pain and eruption above the affected eye. The cornea of the eye may also be affected, leading to corneal ulceration.

2. The intercostal nerves, when pain and the typical eruption occur in a girdle fashion around one side of the chest.

Treatment.—In severe cases with a lot of pain the patient is best treated in bed. A light dusting powder, such as zinc oxide, is used for the eruption. Sedatives, *e.g.*, aspirin, phenacetin or codeine, are usually needed to relieve the pain.

In the cases affecting the eye particular attention must be paid to prevent or minimise corneal ulceration. Hyoscine or atropine drops are instilled into the eye to dilate the pupil; hot bathing may also be useful.

SYPHILIS OF THE NERVOUS SYSTEM

Syphilitic disease of the central nervous system, often known as neuro-syphilis, is a common disease. There are three main types :—

    (A) Meningo-vascular.
    (B) Tabes Dorsalis.
    (C) General Paralysis of the Insane.

(A) MENINGO-VASCULAR SYPHILIS

Particularly in the second stage of syphilis changes can occur in the meninges and the vessels of the brain. A rare cause of meningitis not previously mentioned is syphilis. The symptoms and signs of **syphilitic meningitis** are exactly the same as those in other acute forms.

In differentiating between syphilitic and other types of meningitis the Wassermann test is most helpful as it is usually strongly positive in syphilitic meningitis.

Cerebral thrombosis is the main syphilitic lesion of the blood vessels. Syphilitic cerebral thrombosis tends to occur in a younger age group than is affected by the common form of cerebral thrombosis due to cerebral arteriosclerosis. The signs and symptoms of cerebral thrombosis caused by syphilis are similar to those described under Apoplexy.

Treatment is given on page 312.

(B) TABES DORSALIS (Locomotor Ataxia)

Pathology.—The form of neuro-syphilis known as tabes dorsalis occurs in the tertiary stage of syphilitic infection from five to fifteen years after the primary stage. The main lesions are in the posterior columns of the spinal cord, and as these carry sensory impulses the early predominating symptoms tend to be sensory.

Symptoms and Signs.—Men are more commonly affected, usually in middle life. A juvenile form of tabes, however, is seen in congenital syphilis.

1. The earliest symptoms are the characteristic *lightning pains*, so called because they last for a few brief seconds, shooting up and down or through the legs. They are often likened to the effect of pins

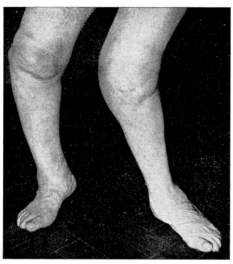

Fig. 118

Charcot's joints in a case of tabes. The knee joints are grossly swollen and deformed with painlessly abnormal mobility.

being stuck into the limb. The patients may refer to the pains as "rheumatism." The pains come on in periodic attacks which may last several hours.

2. Disturbances of bladder function occur early, usually consisting of difficulty in holding the urine or, in other cases, retention of urine.

3. The gait is very typical, there being a well-marked ataxia present. This is often so predominant that the other name for tabes dorsalis is *locomotor ataxia.* The patient tends to fall about, especially when the eyes are closed or in a dark room. The patient characteristically walks with the feet wide apart and

with marked stamping of the feet. The difficulty in walking gets progressively worse, and eventually getting about even with the aid of sticks is impossible and the patient becomes bed-ridden.

4. Owing to the loss of the sensation of pain, trophic changes in the joints, such as gross swelling, marked destruction and deformity, develop. Extreme abnormal mobility without pain is the typical result of these changes. Similar trophic joint changes, which are commonly known as *Charcot's joints*, can and do occur in any neurological disease where the sensation of pain in a joint is lost. The absence of the sensation of pain allows repeated trivial injuries to effect the destructive changes in the joints.

Other frequently seen trophic lesions are perforating ulcers on the feet, especially on the ball of the big toe.

5. Sudden acute severe abdominal pain with vomiting may occur, which may give the appearance of an acute abdomen. This attack is known as a *gastric crisis* of tabes. Similar crises may affect other parts, *e.g.*, the larynx, causing difficulty in breathing owing to spasm of the laryngeal muscles, or the rectum, causing pain and the constant desire to defæcate.

6. Characteristic eye changes, known as Argyll Robertson pupils, occur in tabes dorsalis as in all forms of neuro-syphilis. These changes are absolutely diagnostic of syphilis and so form an extremely valuable sign. The complete eye changes as described by Argyll Robertson are :—

(*a*) Unequal pupils.
(*b*) Very small pupils with irregularity of outline.
(*c*) Failure of the pupils to contract like normal pupils on exposure to light. The reaction to accommodation is, however, normal.

7. The deep tendon reflexes, especially the ankle and knee jerks, are absent from an early stage.

Diagnosis.—The lightning pains, marked ataxic gait and the presence of Argyll Robertson pupils are usually sufficient for diagnosis. A lumbar puncture is, however, usually done in most cases to confirm the diagnosis, when changes such as an increase in cells and in the protein in the cerebrospinal fluid are found to be present. The Wassermann test on the spinal fluid is usually but not always positive.

(C) GENERAL PARALYSIS OF THE INSANE
(Dementia Paralytica)

General paralysis of the insane, like tabes, arises in the tertiary stage of syphilis. It affects the higher centres of the brain and also the pyramidal motor tracts. The name is descriptive, emphasising the predominant changes, *i.e.*, a paralysis associated with insanity.

Symptoms and Signs.

1. Mental changes. The earliest symptoms are usually a deterioration of intellect and abnormal behaviour on the part of the patient, particularly as regards personal appearance and moral conduct. Eventually complete dementia sets in.

The grandiose form, with ideas of grandeur and delusions of power and wealth, is nowadays much less frequently seen.

2. Paralysis. This mainly affects the legs, causing a paraplegia (paralysis of both lower limbs). This paralysis may progress so that getting about becomes so difficult that the patient becomes bed-ridden and incontinent.

3. Convulsions or fits are frequent.

4. Well-marked fine tremors of the lips and tongue are a feature of this disease.

5. Argyll Robertson pupils are often present, as in other types of neuro-syphilis.

6. Lastly, tabes dorsalis and general paralysis of the insane may occur in the same patient (*Tabo-paresis*).

Diagnosis.—The mental changes combined with paralysis and often with fits, together with the Argyll Robertson pupils, give a characteristic picture. Lumbar puncture to obtain a specimen of the cerebrospinal fluid is usually performed, and the fluid always shows a positive Wassermann reaction. A Wassermann test of the blood will also be positive.

Treatment of Neuro-syphilis.

1. The specific treatment for neuro-syphilis, as for all types of syphilitic infection, is large doses of penicillin. At least ten million units are given over a period of approximately fourteen days. A second course may be necessary. Injections of bismuth and artificial fever therapy are rarely used nowadays in the treatment of neuro-syphilis owing to the efficacy of penicillin therapy.

2. TABES DORSALIS.—Re-educational exercises to improve the

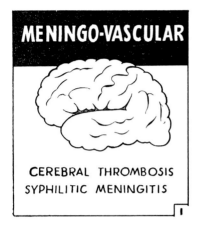

MENINGO-VASCULAR

CEREBRAL THROMBOSIS
SYPHILITIC MENINGITIS

1

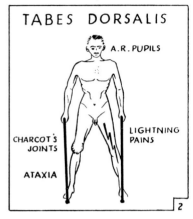

TABES DORSALIS

A.R.PUPILS

CHARCOT'S
JOINTS

LIGHTNING
PAINS

ATAXIA

2

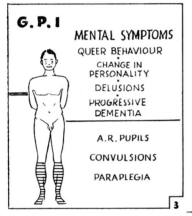

G.P.I

MENTAL SYMPTOMS

QUEER BEHAVIOUR
·
CHANGE IN
PERSONALITY
·
DELUSIONS
·
PROGRESSIVE
DEMENTIA

A.R. PUPILS

CONVULSIONS

PARAPLEGIA

3

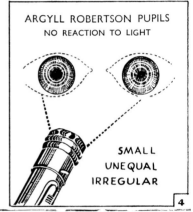

ARGYLL ROBERTSON PUPILS
NO REACTION TO LIGHT

SMALL
UNEQUAL
IRREGULAR

4

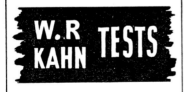

W.R
KAHN TESTS

USUALLY POSITIVE
IN BLOOD AND C·S·F
IN MOST CASES
OF NEURO-SYPHILIS

5

Fig. 119
Syphilis of the
nervous system.

walking are extremely useful and may enable a patient to get about who otherwise would be bed-ridden. As with patients with disseminated sclerosis, the tabetic patient must be encouraged to keep up and about as much as possible.

Sedatives and analgesics, such as aspirin or codeine, are necessary for the lightning pains. Phenobarbitone and chloretone are the most useful drugs for the crises.

For a Charcot's joint supportive splints will be needed.

Occlusive dressings should be applied to any ulcer present.

Finally, a careful watch on the urine for any sign of infection of the urinary tract is essential, and if infection develops it should be treated with sulphonamides or suitable antibiotics.

DISEASES OF THE NERVOUS SYSTEM IN INFANTS AND CHILDREN

BIRTH INJURIES

1. Facial Paralysis.

A facial paralysis, usually due to forceps delivery, often occurs, but is of little importance as it always clears up completely.

2. Brachial Plexus Injuries.

The brachial plexus is the main network of nerves which supplies the upper limb. This plexus may be injured at birth in cases of difficult labour.

Two main forms of paralysis occur: **Erb's Palsy,** where the shoulder girdle muscles are particularly involved, and the upper limb takes up a characteristic attitude known as the " porter's tip " position, with the palm of the hand facing backwards and outwards; and **Klumpke's Palsy,** where the hand and forearm are mainly involved, giving rise to marked wasting and the typical " claw hand."

Treatment consists of applying light splints to relax the affected muscles and massage is started early. Active movements are encouraged as far as possible. Operative measures may have to be undertaken if the paralysis has not improved after six months.

3. Intracranial Hæmorrhage.

In cases of difficult labour, such as may result from disproportion or a difficult forceps delivery, trauma to the brain may lead to cerebral hæmorrhage which if severe is usually fatal. In some cases the meninges may be torn and adhesions may then form which block the flow of the cerebrospinal fluid. This leads to the development of **hydrocephalus,** which in infancy is accompanied by gross enlargement of the head.

Severe birth injury, such as intracranial hæmorrhage, may also give rise to paralysis, *e.g.*, a hemiplegia, and, in addition, may be responsible for the development of epileptic fits and mental deficiency.

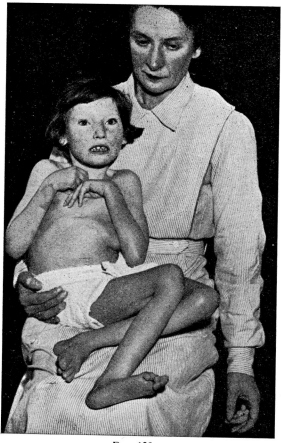

FIG. 120

Spastic diplegia (Little's disease) showing the character-istic position of the spastic limbs. The child was mentally defective and suffered from fits.

PARALYSIS IN CHILDREN

1. Owing to failure of the brain to develop properly various forms of paralysis may arise. Hemiplegias or paraplegias are the most common. As the lesions are in the brain the paralysis is spastic owing to the involvement of the upper motor neurone. The term *Little's disease* is given to a common form of spastic diplegia (paralysis of both sides of the body) seen in infancy. Here the legs are so spastic and rigid that the child has great difficulty in walking, and does so with the legs crossed over each other—" scissors gait."

2. A birth injury, as stated, can lead to paralysis, usually from intracranial hæmorrhage. Premature infants are particularly liable to be affected by paralysis caused by birth injuries.

3. Later on in infancy hemiplegia may occur as a complication of some of the acute infectious fevers, such as whooping-cough or measles. Congenital syphilis may also cause various forms of paralysis.

4. All the diseases considered so far produce a spastic type of paralysis because the upper motor neurone is affected. These spastic palsies are very often associated with other complications such as mental deficiency and convulsions.

Diseases affecting the lower motor neurone are also common in children, the most frequent being *acute anterior poliomyelitis*, or infantile paralysis, which has been fully described already. Peripheral neuritis is rare in children except when caused by diphtheria.

5. Diseases affecting the muscles (myopathies) occur in children, leading to marked weakness of power. These are described later.

HYDROCEPHALUS

Interference with the circulation of the cerebrospinal fluid leads to distension of the brain, and in children this is also accompanied by enlargement of the skull itself. The enlarged head of a hydrocephalic infant or child is at once apparent. It is globular or rounded in outline and the forehead bulges forward over the eyes.

Causes.

1. CONGENITAL.—Failure of the brain to develop properly is a frequent cause of hydrocephalus. Congenital hydrocephalus is often associated with other abnormal developmental changes such as hare-lip, cleft palate and spina bifida.

2. BIRTH INJURIES. — Intracranial hæmorrhage is another common cause of hydrocephalus. Difficult labour, especially with forceps delivery, may give rise to intracranial hæmorrhage.

3. MENINGITIS.—Adhesions resulting from meningitis may block the circulation of the cerebrospinal fluid and so lead to hydrocephalus.

4. CEREBRAL TUMOURS.—A short-lived hydrocephalus is often seen as a result of a cerebral tumour.

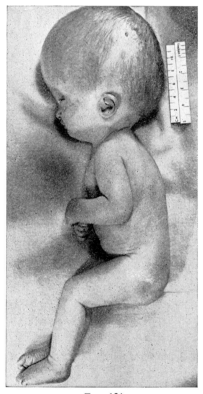

FIG. 121
Hydrocephalus.

As with many serious intracranial diseases in early childhood, convulsions and mental deficiency are often present with hydrocephalus. Treatment is of little avail in most cases.

MENTAL DEFICIENCY

Mental deficiency can be associated with a wide variety of diseases. It is proposed to give here a brief list of the more common forms of mental defect.

Cases of severe mental deficiency are usually classed as *idiots*, those with lesser degrees of deficiency as *imbeciles*, and cases of the mildest forms as *feeble-minded* or *morons*.

1. Failure of the central nervous system to develop properly during fœtal life results in mental deficiency, and usually physical

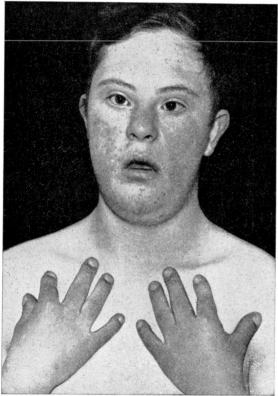

FIG. 122

Mongol, showing the characteristic slanting eyes
and the small incurving little fingers.

defects like an abnormally small skull (microcephaly); hydrocephalus or various types of paralysis, *e.g.*, spastic diplegia of Little's disease, are also present.

2. *Injury* at or immediately after birth is a common cause of mental deficiency, particularly with severe injuries like intracranial hæmorrhage.

3. *Mongolian idiocy* is frequently met with and is due to a

12

chromosomal defect of the ovum at the time of conception. Here the infant has typical Mongolian features, with slanting eyes, small skull, broad flat nose and thick fissured tongue. The hands are also characteristic in that the little finger is abnormally small and curved inwards. Congenital heart lesions are commonly associated with mongolism. Mongols are usually happy bright children but have a severe degree of mental deficiency.

4. *Cretinism*, due to diminished function of the thyroid gland,

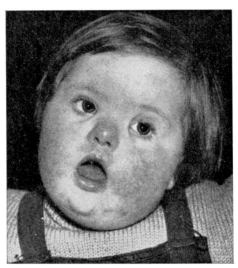

FIG. 123

A second case of mongolism showing the thick
protruded tongue.

causes marked retardation of growth resulting in dwarfism and also idiocy. Cretinism is fully described on page 443.

Many cases of mental deficiency, especially where there is some physical defect as well, are accompanied by convulsions. Another feature is the occasional presence of peculiar [writhing snake-like movements of the limbs, to which the name *athetosis* is given.

Severe cases of mental deficiency have to be looked after in a mental hospital, but less severe cases can often be trained to some useful occupation and even become self-supporting.

MYOPATHIES (Muscular Dystrophies)

Diseases which primarily affect the muscles, leading to profound weakness and wasting, are called myopathies. They usually occur, or start, in childhood and differ in type according to the particular muscles affected. For example, in the *facio-scapulo-humeral* form the face, shoulder girdle and upper arms are mainly involved, with marked wasting (atrophy) and weakness of power in these parts. The child has a typical look, the normal facial expression being absent, and there is inability to raise the arms above the head. If the distal parts of the arms and legs are mainly affected it is often known as the *distal type* of myopathy.

One striking form does occur which differs from the others in that the wasted muscles are replaced by fat, and so look larger than normal instead of wasted. This form is known as the **pseudo-hypertrophic type.** It usually affects boys, and starts about the age of 4 or 5. The shoulder and pelvic girdle muscles are particularly involved, and these muscles become enlarged. In addition, the calf muscles too are enlarged. The child has difficulty in getting about and has a waddling gait. One characteristic feature is the peculiar way in which the child rises from the lying-down position. The child has to roll over on to his face, and then on to his hands and knees, and gradually " works up " the legs with the hands—the so-called " climbing up his knees " position. Many of these children become bed-ridden in later childhood. Mild cases, however, may live in fair health for many years. So far no treatment is of any real benefit.

SOME RARER CENTRAL NERVOUS SYSTEM DISEASES

Apart from the many different diseases of the central nervous system so far discussed, there remain many more which, however, are less common and so of less importance to the nurse. These rarer neurological diseases are mostly seen in special neurological hospitals or centres.

It is proposed here to mention only the names and the most predominant symptoms and signs of these diseases and any specific treatment.

SUBACUTE COMBINED DEGENERATION OF THE CORD

This disease is associated with pernicious anæmia, and early cases respond to treatment with vitamin B_{12}, but NOT folic acid. It causes a spastic paralysis of both lower limbs (paraplegia), with marked sensory disturbances such as numbness, pins and needles and sensory loss in the legs; the gait is usually very ataxic.

SYRINGOMYELIA

This peculiar malady is due to a distension of the central canal in the spinal cord, which becomes progressively larger and presses on the various tracts in the spinal cord. It usually starts in early adult life and slowly progresses till the patient becomes totally paralysed.

The main distinguishing features of syringomyelia are a slow paralysis starting usually in the arms and spreading to the lower limbs, with profound wasting of the hands. There is also the characteristic *dissociated anæsthesia* where pain, heat and cold sensations are lost, but touch sensation is retained. This is due to the peculiar crossing of the sensory tracts in the spinal cord which allows the touch sensory tracts to escape damage in syringomyelia. These patients frequently burn themselves from holding cigarettes or matches and also develop ulcers from injuries which they do not feel. Charcot's joints are frequently present.

Treatment is of no avail.

Progressive Muscular Atrophy (Motor Neurone Disease)

Slow progressive degeneration of the anterior (motor) horn cells in the grey matter of the spinal cord, the cause of which is unknown, leads to profound wasting and paralysis of the affected limbs. The disease usually occurs in adults and often starts in the anterior horn cells supplying the muscles of the hands, causing severe wasting of the hands—" claw hands." Eventually most of the muscles of all limbs become affected, resulting in complete paralysis, by which time the patient has a skeleton appearance.

The wasting muscles show typical twitchings or tremors known as *fibrillation*. The pyramidal tracts may be affected in some cases, leading to a spastic paralysis, usually of the legs. It is characteristic of this disease that no sensory changes develop because only the motor tract or anterior motor horn cells are damaged.

All treatment so far used is of little avail, and ultimately the patients become bed-ridden and incontinent.

Transverse Myelitis (Compression of the Spinal Cord)

The term *transverse myelitis* is often used to describe severe damage to the spinal cord, usually caused by lesions pressing on the cord. The term *myelitis* is therefore in most cases a misnomer as inflammatory lesions are seldom responsible for the disease.

Compression of the spinal cord leads to marked motor and sensory disturbances below the level of the lesion, which is usually in the lumbar region of the cord. There is complete loss of sensation in the legs and in part of the trunk, associated with a paralysis of the affected area. Incontinence or retention of urine is present. Trophic ulcers and pressure sores are very prone to develop, due to the sensory loss.

The causes of compression of the cord can be conveniently divided into the acute (sudden) and the slow and progressive. In the acute forms the sensory loss and degree of paralysis are much more complete and severe than in the slow onset types. Fracture-dislocations of the spine, usually in the cervical region, account for most of the acute cases. Hæmorrhage and thrombosis in the spinal cord, due to hypertension or syphilis, are more rarely responsible.

Slow compression of the cord is usually due to one of two main causes: firstly, to tuberculous disease of the spine (Pott's caries) seen in young people, and secondly, to malignant tumours of the spine in older people.

In all cases nursing calls for a great deal of skill to prevent pressure sores and urinary infections. Most patients are treated by immobilising the spine in a plaster-bed for many months. Suitable cases may be operated on, as in tuberculous caries when a bone graft is done. Cases due to malignant tumours are hopeless and only palliative treatment can be given.

MYASTHENIA GRAVIS

Myasthenia gravis is a slow progressive disease usually met with in adults and rare before the age of puberty. It causes a most peculiar form of paralysis, which tends to get worse with fatigue or use of the affected muscles and to improve with rest. Characteristically, therefore, the paralysis is minimal in the morning and worst at night. The disease most often affects the eye, facial and shoulder girdle muscles and, less often, the legs. Paralysis of the eye muscles (ophthalmoplegia), leading to squints and double vision, is present. Drooping of the eyelids (ptosis) and weakness of the face muscles cause the peculiar lack of expression and typical myasthenic (snarling) smile. Gradual loss of voice with prolonged speech or difficulty in chewing during the course of a meal are also frequent complaints. Weakness of the arms, especially in combing the hair or lifting anything, may be complained of.

Myasthenia responds to the drugs neostigmine (prostigmin) and pyridostigmine (mestinon) and a profoundly weak patient may be dramatically improved on taking these drugs. Nevertheless, in many cases the disease gradually progresses, and after many years death may occur owing to involvement of the respiratory muscles. Recently some cases have been greatly improved by removal of the thymus gland (thymectomy) which for some unknown reason tends

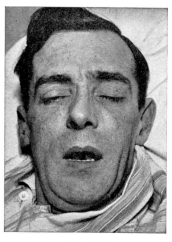 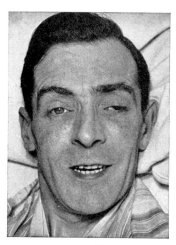

FIG. 124   FIG. 125

Fig. 118—Myasthenia gravis, patient cannot open his eyes or fully close his mouth.
Fig. 119—Myasthenia gravis after an injection of prostigmin showing a marked improvement. The typical " snarling " smile still remains, however.

to be enlarged in most cases of myasthenia. If, however, an actual tumour (thymoma) of the thymus gland is present the outlook is much graver. Myasthenia associated with a thymoma is best treated with deep X-ray therapy first, and afterwards by thymectomy.

SUMMARY OF SOME ROUTINE PROCEDURES UNDERTAKEN IN DISEASES OF THE CENTRAL NERVOUS SYSTEM

1. Lumbar Puncture.

(a) For diagnosis :—

(i) In meningitis to confirm the diagnosis and to isolate the particular organism. The fluid shows typical changes : increased pressure, turbidity from increased cells and a rise in the protein.

(ii) In cases of subarachnoid hæmorrhage due to cerebral hæmorrhage (apoplexy) and ruptured cerebral aneurysm. Blood is present in the cerebrospinal fluid.

(iii) In acute anterior poliomyelitis, where the cells in the fluid are raised, thus confirming the diagnosis.

(iv) In neuro-syphilis, where the cells and protein in the cerebrospinal fluid are raised and the Wassermann reaction is usually positive.

(v) In all cases of undiagnosed coma.

(vi) In some cases of suspected cerebral tumour.

(b) For treatment :—

(i) Occasionally for intrathecal injection of penicillin in some resistant types of pyogenic meningitis.

(ii) To reduce excessive intracranial pressure in cases of hypertensive encephalopathy.

(iii) To relieve excessive intracranial pressure in some cases of ruptured cerebral aneurysm.

2. Wassermann Test.

This is carried out in neuro-syphilis to confirm the diagnosis, and in all cases of obscure diseases of the central nervous system to exclude neuro-syphilis as a possible cause.

N.B.—The Wassermann test is frequently performed in diseases of many different systems which can be affected by syphilis. The latter must be excluded as a possible cause of disease where there is the slightest suspicion that syphilis can be responsible.

3. Examination of the Fundus (Retina) of the Eye.

(a) In increased intracranial pressure, where papillœdema (swelling of the optic disc) is usually present.

(b) In hypertension and chronic nephritis, when hæmorrhages and exudate are often seen.

(c) In neuro-syphilis, when optic atrophy may be present.

4. Electro-encephalogram (E.E.G.).

(a) In the diagnosis of epilepsy, where characteristic alterations in the electrical waves from the brain are present.

(b) To localise cerebral tumours and abscesses.

5. **Ventriculography.**

In the diagnosis of cerebral tumours, when distorted or displaced ventricles may be present.

6. **Angiography (Arteriography).**

(a) In the diagnosis of cerebral aneurysm and especially before any operative procedure.

(b) In the diagnosis and localisation of cerebral tumours, when distortion and displacement of the cerebral arteries may be present.

SUMMARY OF IMPORTANT DRUGS USED IN DISEASES OF THE CENTRAL NERVOUS SYSTEM

1. **Anticonvulsants** (phenobarbitone, phenytoin sodium, troxidone, methoin, primidone, etc.).

Epilepsy.

2. **Atropine (or belladonna).**

Paralysis agitans.

3. **Benzhexol** (artane).

Paralysis agitans.

4. **Chloramphenicol** (chloromycetin).

Pyogenic meningitis.
Cerebral abscess.

5. **Demethylchlortetracycline** (ledermycin).

Pyogenic meningitis.
Cerebral abscess.

6. **Ephedrine.**

Myasthenia gravis.

7. **Isoniazid.**

Tuberculous meningitis combined with streptomycin.

8. **Neostigmine** (prostigmin).

Myasthenia gravis.

9. **Oxytetracycline** (terramycin).

   Pyogenic meningitis.
   Cerebral abscess.

10. **Para-aminosalicylic acid (P.A.S.).**

    Tuberculous meningitis, combined with streptomycin or isoniazid.

11. **Penicillin.**

    Pyogenic meningitis.
    Neuro-syphilis
    Cerebral abscess.

12. **Pyridostigmine** (mestinon).

    Myasthenia gravis.

13. **Streptomycin.**

    Tuberculous meningitis combined with isoniazid or P.A.S.

14. **Sulphonamides.**

    Pyogenic meningitis.

15. **Tetracycline** (achromycin, tetracyn).

    Pyogenic meningitis.
    Cerebral abscess.

16. **Vitamin B$_1$.**

    Peripheral neuritis.

17. **Vitamin B$_{12}$.**

    Subacute combined degeneration of the cord.

CHAPTER X

DISEASES OF THE BLOOD

P *HYSIOLOGY.*—Blood is composed of the following parts :—
1. Cells.
  (*a*) Red blood cells with their hæmoglobin.
  (*b*) White blood cells.
  (*c*) Tiny little bodies much smaller than the red cells which are called platelets.

2. A clear yellow fluid which is known as plasma. Plasma contains the following important substances :—

(*a*) Certain substances like prothrombin and fibrinogen which are important in the mechanism of blood clotting.
(*b*) Various salts, such as calcium, sodium, etc., sugar and also proteins, all of which are essential for the proper nutrition of the body.
(*c*) Certain waste products from the various organs, such as urea.
(*d*) Certain substances known as antibodies which play their part in the important problems of immunity and resistance against infection.

The Function of the more important Components of the Blood.

1. RED BLOOD CELLS.—The primary function of the red blood cells is to carry oxygen, by means of the hæmoglobin that they contain, from the lungs throughout the body to the various organs and tissues. It must be stressed that this is the all-important function of the blood, and it will be seen that both the red cells and the hæmoglobin play their part.

2. WHITE BLOOD CELLS.—It will be seen later that there are various types of white blood cells. Their main function, however, is as a defensive mechanism in the body's fight against invasion by bacteria and other organisms that cause infection.

3. THE PLATELETS.—These little bodies function as one means of controlling bleeding. Even when a small prick is made in the skin, without some mechanism to control the bleeding it can be realised that the person could lose an enormous quantity of blood. One of the ways of controlling bleeding is by these platelets. Another way is by a constriction of the blood vessels (vasoconstriction).

4. PROTHROMBIN AND FIBRINOGEN.—These substances are also concerned with blood clotting. If the skin is cut or whenever blood is shed it will be found that the blood instead of remaining fluid clots into a solid mass. This is another of the body's mechanisms to control the loss of blood from the body, and prothrombin and fibrinogen each play a part in causing the blood to clot. Diseases affecting the prothrombin and fibrinogen are dealt with later.

5. THE SALTS, SUGAR AND PROTEINS.—These are necessary for the maintenance of proper health. Various diseases occur which alter their concentration in the blood, and these diseases are discussed in the appropriate sections (Diabetes, Addison's Disease, Tetany, etc.).

6. ANTIBODIES.—These have been discussed under Immunity (p. 29).

Normal Blood Formation.

Before discussing the diseases that may affect the blood we must first see how blood is normally formed and what constitutes a normal blood count.

1. *Red Blood Cells.*—These are formed in the red marrow which in adults is found in the flat bones, such as the sternum and skull, and in the ends of the long bones. The red cells in the marrow are all in different stages of formation, from the early immature cells to the completely developed mature red cells such as are found in the peripheral blood. Normally only the completely mature red cells pass into the circulation, all the immature cells remaining in the marrow. In certain diseases, however, these immature red cells may pass out into the circulation.

FACTORS NECESSARY FOR THE NORMAL FORMATION OF RED CELLS.—In order that the red cells may become completely mature and adequate in number various factors are necessary, of which the following are the most important :—

(a) **Vitamin B_{12}** (Cyanocobalamin).—This substance is present in various foods, especially liver, meat, milk, eggs and cheese.

(b) **The Intrinsic Factor.**—This is an enzyme normally formed by certain cells in the stomach. The intrinsic factor is essential for the proper absorption of vitamin B_{12}.

Vitamin B_{12}, which is absorbed into the body when the intrinsic factor is present, is stored in the liver and released to the bone marrow as required. Vitamin B_{12} is essential for the production of adequate numbers of fully mature red cells. If vitamin B_{12} is missing, the bone marrow will not produce sufficient numbers of red cells, whilst, moreover, many of the red cells produced will be immature. They will tend to be larger than normal (macrocytes) and many of them will contain a nucleus (megaloblasts).

(c) **Folic Acid.** Folic acid is part of the vitamin B complex. It has an action very similar to that of vitamin B_{12}, i.e., it is essential for the development of adequate numbers of fully mature red cells. In the absence of folic acid a macrocytic anæmia will develop.

2. *Hæmoglobin.*—Hæmoglobin is the essential component of the red cells and it is by means of this that oxygen is carried in the red cells. Hæmoglobin is mainly composed of iron, and if for any reason iron is not available there will be a reduction in the amount of hæmoglobin in each red cell, and, as we shall see later, this is one cause of anæmia. This lack of iron can be caused in several different ways :—

(a) By insufficient iron in the diet. For instance, the diet of normal infants is mainly composed of milk, which contains little iron, with the result that infants commonly suffer from an iron deficiency anæmia in the first year of life.

(b) Diseases of the stomach and intestines may prevent the proper absorption of iron from the intestinal tract. We shall see later that there are several diseases which are associated with a deficient absorption of iron and so cause anæmia.

3. *White Blood Cells.*

4. *Formation of Prothrombin.*

5. *Formation of Platelets.*

The formation of the white cells, prothrombin and platelets is more conveniently discussed under the diseases which affect them.

The Normal Blood Count.

The normal blood count in an adult is :—

Red blood cells : 5,000,000 per c.mm.

Hæmoglobin : 14·5 gm. per 100 ml. of blood (usually expressed in percentage).

White blood cells : 5,000 to 10,000 per c.mm.

Platelets : 200,000 per c.mm. approximately.

The red cells are small round discs which are coloured red

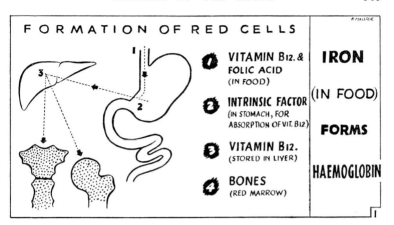

FORMATION OF RED CELLS

1 VITAMIN B12 & FOLIC ACID (IN FOOD)

2 INTRINSIC FACTOR (IN STOMACH, FOR ABSORPTION OF VIT. B12.)

3 VITAMIN B12. (STORED IN LIVER)

4 BONES (RED MARROW)

IRON (IN FOOD) FORMS HAEMOGLOBIN

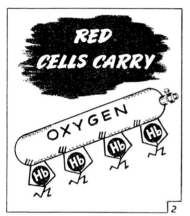

RED CELLS CARRY

OXYGEN

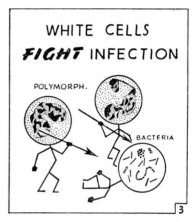

WHITE CELLS **FIGHT** INFECTION

POLYMORPH.

BACTERIA

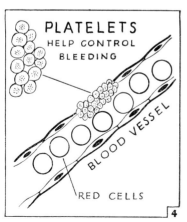

PLATELETS HELP CONTROL BLEEDING

BLOOD VESSEL

RED CELLS

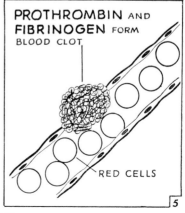

PROTHROMBIN AND FIBRINOGEN FORM BLOOD CLOT

RED CELLS

FIG. 126

The formation and function of various components of the blood.

because of the hæmoglobin they contain. Normally when the hæmoglobin is 100 per cent. they are completely filled with this substance.

DISEASES AFFECTING THE RED CELLS AND HÆMOGLOBIN

Anæmia is the term used for a reduction in the number of red blood cells and in the amount of hæmoglobin. Whether the reduction is primarily in the number of red cells, or primarily in the amount of hæmoglobin will depend on the type and cause of anæmia present. Apart from the decrease in the number of red cells, alterations in the shape and size also occur. Anæmias are often classified according to these changes and the following terms are used :—

TABLE VIII

TYPE OF ANÆMIA.	ALTERATION IN RED CELLS.	ALTERATION IN HÆMOGLOBIN.	CAUSE.
Hyperchromic macrocytic.	Larger than normal (macrocytes).	Hæmoglobin content less reduced than number of the red cells (hyperchromic).	Lack of vitamin B_{12} or folic acid.
Hypochromic microcytic.	Smaller than normal (microcytes).	Severe reduction in the hæmoglobin content, more so than the reduction in the number of the cells.	Deficiency of iron.
Normocytic.	Normal in size.	Reduced in the same proportion as the red cells.	Acute hæmorrhage.

We shall see later, however, that it is more convenient to classify anæmias according to their causes.

GENERAL EFFECTS (SYMPTOMS AND SIGNS) OF ANÆMIA

Anæmia, no matter what the type or cause, produces certain general effects. These are known as the common symptoms and signs of anæmia. They will be described here before the individual anæmias with any of their more particular signs are dealt with.

Many of the symptoms and signs of anæmia are brought about by the deficiency in oxygen supply caused by shortage of the red

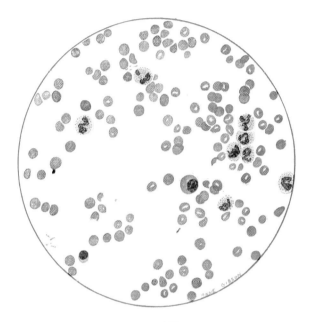

Fig. 127

Blood film showing the appearance of the normal red blood
cells and the polymorphonuclear and lymphocytic white
blood cells.

[*To face page* 366

cells and hæmoglobin. The red cells and hæmoglobin are the vital agents in the transport of oxygen throughout the body for the supply of all tissues and organs.

1. Pallor of the skin and mucous membranes. This is especially seen in the mucous membranes of the lower eyelid and the lips.

2. Weakness, giddiness and fainting. In women, amenorrhœa is commonly present.

3. Increased heart rate (tachycardia). To compensate for the deficiency in the amount of oxygen transported, which is caused by the reduction in the red cells and hæmoglobin, the heart quickens its rate. This, by making the existing red cells and hæmoglobin do more work, may overcome the oxygen deficiency in the tissues and organs in the less severe degrees of anæmia.

4. Dyspnœa and œdema of the ankles. These important signs are seen in severe cases where the heart fails to compensate for the reduction in the carriage of oxygen and so, as a result, heart failure develops. As in all cases of heart failure, from whatever cause, dyspnœa is the earliest symptom and is most marked on exertion.

5. If the anæmia is both rapid in onset and also severe, all the above symptoms (pallor, weakness, fainting and dyspnœa) will be very pronounced. In addition, the condition of shock may be present (see p. 368). On the other hand, if the anæmia is more gradual in onset, symptoms may continue to be slight (mainly fatigue and loss of energy) until a profound degree of anæmia is present.

6. Blood examination. This will naturally reveal reductions both in the number of red cells and in the amount of hæmoglobin to varying extents according to the particular type of anæmia present. Furthermore, in addition to the reduction in the number of the red cells and the amount of hæmoglobin the size, shape and colour of the red cells are in most cases altered. Either macrocytic (large) or microcytic (small) cells may be present, according to the type of anæmia, whilst the cells may be highly coloured (hyperchromic) or pale (hypochromic).

Classification of the Anæmias.—Anæmias are very common and have many different causes, and to understand the subject it is best to have some form of classification. One can classify anæmias according to the type, that is as hyperchromic macrocytic or hypochromic microcytic, or according to their cause. The usual classification is according to the cause and this will be the one used here, the rarer causes being omitted.　Anæmias may be divided into three main groups :—

(A) Hæmorrhagic Anæmias, due to Blood Loss.

(B) Dyshæmopoietic Anæmias, due to Decreased Blood Formation.

(C) Hæmolytic Anæmias, due to Increased Blood Destruction.

(A) HÆMORRHAGIC ANÆMIAS

Hæmorrhagic anæmias are probably those most frequently encountered in clinical practice.　As can be readily appreciated, any sudden **acute** loss of blood is likely to result in a reduction in the red cells and hæmoglobin.　According to the size of the hæmorrhage, it may take several weeks or more before the body can replace this loss in both red cells and hæmoglobin.　In medical diseases acute hæmorrhage is most frequently seen as a hæmatemesis due to peptic ulcers, and as a hæmoptysis from chronic chest conditions, especially tuberculosis and carcinoma.　Acute hæmorrhage is also commonly seen in maternity and surgical diseases such as post-partum hæmorrhage, abortions, injuries, etc.

It is only when a sufficient quantity of blood, usually over one pint, has been lost that any appreciable anæmia occurs.　In most cases of acute sudden loss of large quantities of blood there is also an associated condition of **shock** which calls for proper treatment. The exact causes producing the clinical symptoms and signs associated with shock are not fully appreciated, but they are certainly in some way caused by actual loss of fluid from the circulation, which leads to failure of the peripheral circulation.　When the blood volume is severely reduced the blood pressure falls, and if the fall is too great the vital centres are affected and shock results.　Therefore in severe acute hæmorrhage fluid is vitally needed to restore the blood volume and raise the blood pressure.　In addition, it is also essential to replace the severe deficiency in the red cells and hæmoglobin as otherwise the tissues will lack oxygen.　The fluid lost to the circulation and the red cells and hæmoglobin can all be replaced by transfusions of whole blood, which is the ideal therapy.　Blood transfusions are indeed essential in all cases of severe acute hæmorrhage.　A fall in systolic blood pressure to below 100 mm. of mercury is a definite indication that a blood transfusion is required in acute hæmorrhage. In these cases the patient is restless, with marked pallor and a cold clammy skin.　The pulse is very rapid, usually in the region of 110, and it may be difficult to feel owing to the low pressure. There is also a marked reduction in output of urine.

It might be convenient at this stage to mention that the condition of shock with a low blood pressure may occur owing to severe injuries without actual hæmorrhage. In these cases, too, it is essential to correct the low blood pressure by transfusions, but here transfusions with plasma instead of with whole blood may be

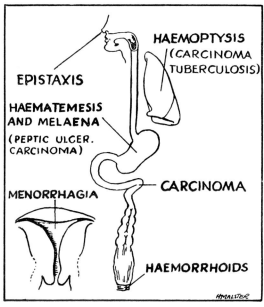

FIG. 128
Some causes of hæmorrhagic anæmias.

sufficient. Transfusions with saline are useless to restore the blood pressure in severe acute hæmorrhage and shock as saline is rapidly poured out of the circulation.

Chronic blood loss also leads to anæmia, and in these cases the hæmoglobin is reduced more than the red cells because the red cells can be replaced much more quickly than the hæmoglobin. The conditions which most commonly give rise to anæmia due to chronic blood loss are chronic hæmorrhoids, severe menorrhagia, chronic peptic ulcer and carcinoma. The anæmia is treated by clearing up the cause of the chronic blood loss and by giving large doses of iron to manufacture hæmoglobin. The red marrow usually replaces the red cells without special treatment.

(B) ANÆMIAS DUE TO DECREASED BLOOD FORMATION

This second group of anæmias includes some very common and important types. In our earlier discussion on the red cells and the hæmoglobin it was seen that several factors were essential for their

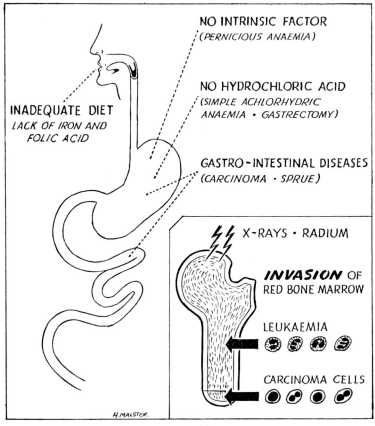

NO INTRINSIC FACTOR
(PERNICIOUS ANAEMIA)

NO HYDROCHLORIC ACID
(SIMPLE ACHLORHYDRIC ANAEMIA · GASTRECTOMY)

INADEQUATE DIET
LACK OF IRON AND FOLIC ACID

GASTRO - INTESTINAL DISEASES
(CARCINOMA · SPRUE)

X-RAYS · RADIUM

INVASION OF RED BONE MARROW

LEUKAEMIA

CARCINOMA CELLS

H.MALSTER.

Fig. 129
Anæmias due to decreased blood formation—some of the causes.

proper formation, vitamin B_{12} and folic acid in food and the intrinsic factor in the stomach being essential for the formation of the red cells, and iron being the essential component of hæmoglobin. It can therefore be realised that either lack of or deficient absorption of any of these factors could lead to deficient blood formation.

Again, from the earlier statements on normal blood formation, it was seen that the blood is formed in the red bone marrow.

Diseases of the bones, therefore, could interfere with the formation of the blood in the marrow, and in clinical practice we meet with several forms of anæmia due to bone diseases.

On the basis of the above remarks we can classify the more important types of anæmia due to decreased blood formation as follows :—

1. Pernicious Anæmia. Lack of the intrinsic factor.
2. Simple Achlorhydric Anæmia. Deficient absorption of iron and probably lack of iron in the diet.
3. Nutritional Anæmia of Infants. Lack of iron in the diet.
4. Anæmias of Pregnancy. Increased demands for iron and deficiency of folic acid.
5. Anæmias associated with Diseases of the Gastro-intestinal Tract.

   (a) Cœliac disease and sprue. Deficient absorption of folic acid, vitamin B_{12} and iron.
   (b) Carcinoma of the stomach.

6. Anæmias due to Interference with the Red Marrow in the Bones.

   (a) Drugs and toxic poisons (gold, troxidone, chloramphenicol, benzol, chronic infections, X-rays and radio-active substances).
   (b) Mechanical interference (anæmias of leukæmia and carcinomatosis of bones).
   (c) Primary failure of the marrow (aplastic anæmia).

Some of the more important of these forms of anæmia will now be discussed in more detail.

PERNICIOUS ANÆMIA

Pernicious anæmia is the commonest form of anæmia caused by lack of vitamin B_{12}. As mentioned earlier (p. 363), vitamin B_{12} is necessary both for the formation of adequate numbers of red blood cells and also for the red cells to become fully mature. In pernicious anæmia, for some unknown reason, the intrinsic factor normally secreted by the stomach is absent with the result that vitamin B_{12} is not absorbed from the gastro-intestinal tract.

Symptoms and Signs.

1. This anæmia is commonest after the age of forty and affects both sexes equally. The onset is gradual and typical remissions occur when the anæmia improves of its own accord.

2. General symptoms and signs of anæmia, as outlined earlier, are present, including pallor and weakness. Their severity naturally varies with the degree of anæmia, but usually they are marked.

3. The patient often complains of soreness of the tongue, which is smooth and inflamed (glossitis).

4. The skin may have a slightly yellowish tint due to a mild degree of jaundice (of the hæmolytic type) which combined with the pallor gives the pale lemon-yellow colour of pernicious anæmia.

5. Symptoms and signs of involvement of the nervous system may be present, including difficulty in walking (ataxia) and pins and needles in the hands and feet. These are due to the characteristic neurological complication of *subacute combined degeneration of the cord* met with only in pernicious anæmia.

6. Examination of the patient will often reveal an enlarged spleen. Test-meal examination shows a complete *achlorhydria*, no free hydrochloric acid being present even after a histamine test meal. (Histamine is the most powerful stimulant for the production of hydrochloric acid in the stomach.)

7. There is a characteristic blood picture in pernicious anæmia, which is always a hyperchromic macrocytic (large cell) anæmia. Immature cells often appear in the peripheral blood and the white cells are reduced in number (leucopenia).

If the blood picture is not absolutely typical, examination of the red marrow is carried out, when in all cases a characteristic picture with numerous megaloblasts is obtained, thus giving a definite diagnosis. (Megaloblasts are abnormal immature red cells.) This examination is known as a marrow puncture. As it is often performed from the marrow of the sternum it is also called a *sternal puncture*. A special needle (Salah's) is needed.

Diagnosis.—The diagnosis of anæmia is readily made on the pallor, fatigue and other general signs of anæmia. The diagnosis of pernicious anæmia is made from the typical blood picture, the complete achlorhydria and, if necessary, by a sternal puncture.

Carcinoma of the stomach or intestinal tract often gives rise to effects similar to those of pernicious anæmia, so that careful examination of the gastro-intestinal tract by barium X-rays and examination of the fæces for occult blood are necessary in any doubtful case.

Treatment of Pernicious Anæmia.

1. The essential aim in treatment is to supply the missing VITAMIN B$_{12}$ (cyanocobalamin). In the early stages of treatment when there

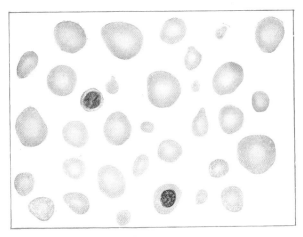

Fig. 130

Blood film from a case of pernicious anæmia showing the characteristic large red cells (macrocytes) and one immature nucleated red cell (megaloblast).

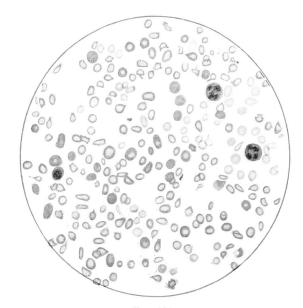

Fig. 131

Blood film from a case of iron deficiency anæmia (simple achlorhydric anæmia) showing the characteristic small pale red cells.

[*To face page* 372

is severe anæmia, 100 micrograms of vitamin B_{12} are injected intramuscularly once or twice a week until the number of red blood cells and the amount of hæmoglobin return to normal. Thereafter a maintenance dose of vitamin B_{12} of 50 to 100 micrograms every two to four weeks is given as the patient will relapse if vitamin B_{12} is stopped. The patient must be warned that vitamin B_{12} will be necessary for the rest of his life. This point is of importance. At periodic intervals a blood count is done to ensure that adequate vitamin B_{12} therapy is being given.

If subacute degeneration of the spinal cord is present much larger doses of vitamin B_{12} are necessary; usually 100 micrograms are given weekly for at least six to twelve months and then followed by the usual maintenance doses mentioned above.

Liver extracts are hardly ever used nowadays in the treatment of pernicious anæmia.

2. BLOOD TRANSFUSIONS.—In desperately ill patients with signs of heart failure owing to an extremely severe degree of anæmia blood transfusions with fresh blood are necessary to IMMEDIATELY improve the blood count. In these desperate cases the red cell count is often in the region of 1 million per c.mm. instead of the normal 5 million. The blood should be given very slowly to prevent reactions, and 2 to 3 pints are often necessary. In addition to the transfusion vitamin B_{12} is started at once. It is only in very rare instances, however, that blood transfusions are required.

SIMPLE ACHLORHYDRIC ANÆMIA
(Idiopathic Hypochromic Anæmia)

This very common form of iron-deficiency anæmia is usually confined to middle-aged women. There are the general symptoms and signs of anæmia, and achlorhydria is always present. The nails may be cracked and spoon-shaped. The most typical feature revealed by a blood count is the severe deficiency of hæmoglobin. The exact cause of this anæmia is not definitely known. It is probably a combination of a diet poor in iron, a lack of hydrochloric acid causing a deficiency in iron absorption and in some cases menorrhagia causing blood loss.

Treatment.—The treatment of any iron-deficiency anæmia, of which simple achlorhydric anæmia is a good example, is to give large doses of iron. The most frequently used preparation of iron is one of the ferrous salts, given orally, such as ferrous sulphate, ferrous gluconate or ferrous succinate. One or two tablets (3 to 5 gr. each) is usually given three times a day.

Oral therapy is usually effective, but occasionally parenteral

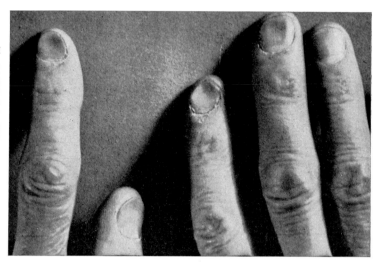

FIG. 132
Spoon-shaped nails (koilonychia) from a case of simple
achlorhydric anæmia.

iron therapy is needed if the anæmia fails to respond to oral treatment or in cases where iron by mouth causes nausea or diarrhœa.

For intravenous iron therapy, saccharated iron oxide (ferrivenin, iviron) is used, the initial dose being 1 to 2 ml. (20 to 40 mgm.). If there are no toxic reactions (nausea, fainting) the dose is increased to 5 ml. on alternate days.

A full mixed diet is important as in many iron-deficiency anæmias the diet is often inadequate.

NUTRITIONAL ANÆMIA OF INFANTS

Milk, which is relatively poor in iron content, forms practically the entire diet during the first months of life. An iron-deficiency anæmia, therefore, frequently occurs in infants and is called the nutritional anæmia of infants. Premature infants are particularly likely to suffer from anæmia.

In the milder cases the anæmia usually corrects itself at the end of the first year. In more severe cases, however, iron is needed.

ANÆMIAS OF PREGNANCY

During pregnancy an iron-deficiency anæmia is often seen. Various factors combine to bring about this anæmia, including the demands of the fœtus for iron and also a deficiency of iron in the diet.

Less frequently an anæmia similar in type to that of pernicious anæmia (the macrocytic anæmia of pregnancy) is met with. The exact cause of this form of anæmia is unknown, but the anæmia seems to respond best to folic acid therapy.

ANÆMIAS ASSOCIATED WITH DISEASES OF THE GASTRO-INTESTINAL TRACT

In discussing the anæmias due to blood loss it was seen that a common cause of anæmia was hæmorrhage from a bleeding peptic ulcer or from a carcinoma. Apart from these causes there are various other gastro-intestinal conditions which may be accompanied by anæmia.

1. In cœliac disease and sprue, in which chronic diarrhœa is a feature, lack of absorption of vitamin B_{12} or folic acid may lead to a macrocytic anæmia similar to that of pernicious anæmia. Alternatively an iron-deficiency anæmia may develop from deficient absorption of iron.

2. Carcinoma of the stomach usually causes an iron-deficiency anæmia due to chronic bleeding, but sometimes it also causes a macrocytic anæmia similar to pernicious anæmia owing to interference with the formation of the intrinsic factor in the stomach. A similar anæmia may also arise after the stomach has been removed (gastrectomy) in the treatment of carcinoma or a large gastric ulcer.

Again, removal of large portions of the intestines (colectomy), as carried out for carcinoma or chronic ulcerative colitis, may interfere with the absorption either of iron or of vitamin B_{12} to cause anæmia.

ANÆMIAS DUE TO INTERFERENCE WITH THE RED MARROW IN THE BONES

Many different diseases have as a predominant feature an anæmia which in all cases has the same underlying cause, *i.e.*, interference with the formation of blood in the red bone marrow. Blood formation may be depressed by chemical poisons like benzol or arsenic or by drugs such as chloramphenicol, phenylbutazone, troxidone or gold salts. In addition such conditions as chronic sepsis, rheumatic fever, chronic nephritis and uræmia are often accompanied by an anæmia due to depression of blood formation.

Over-exposure to X-rays, radium and some radioactive substances may cause a very severe anæmia. This is so important that people like radiologists and radiographers, who are constantly in contact with X-rays, have a blood examination at periodic intervals. The anæmia due to X-rays and radioactive substances is typically associated with a depression of the white cells. This fact is often made use of in treating such conditions as leukæmia, where there is a great increase in the white cells. Here deep X-rays are often of value.

Another cause of interference with the bone marrow, resulting in depression of blood formation, is extensive disease in the bones. Anæmias due to widespread secondary carcinomatous deposits in the bones are of this type. Also the disease leukæmia by crowding the red marrow with gross over-production of white cells can depress red cell formation. Anæmia is very constantly present in all forms of leukæmia.

In some cases the marrow may become atrophied (*aplastic*) and a very severe and often fatal anæmia may result. This form of anæmia, known as aplastic anæmia, may be secondary to any of the above poisons (drugs, infections or X-rays), but a primary type of unknown cause also occurs.

(C) HÆMOLYTIC ANÆMIAS

The third main group of anæmias is that due to an increased destruction of the red cells. Normally a red cell has a life of about 120 days, after which it is worn out and destroyed by certain types of cells present in the spleen, liver and the connective tissues, known as the reticulo-endothelial system of cells. The hæmoglobin is broken down into the pigment bilirubin, which is then excreted by the liver through the biliary passages into the intestines.

In some diseases an over-destruction of the red cells takes place with the result that an anæmia occurs, known as hæmolytic anæmia. One of the features of a hæmolytic anæmia, in contrast to the other types, is that it is usually associated with a form of jaundice called **hæmolytic jaundice.** It has just been stated that the hæmoglobin of the broken-down red cell is turned into bile pigment, bilirubin. Excess of bile pigment accumulating in the blood stream causes jaundice. Therefore in hæmolytic anæmias, where there is an excess of bile pigment owing to the excessive breakdown of the red cells, hæmolytic jaundice often occurs. In mild hæmolytic anæmias, however, the jaundice may be slight or even absent as the body is able to deal with a small excess of bile pigment without jaundice developing.

Causes of Hæmolytic Anæmias.

1. Severe Infections, especially septicæmias.
2. Toxic Chemicals and Drugs.
3. Incompatible Blood Transfusions.
4. Hæmolytic Disease and the Rhesus Factor.
5. Congenital Hæmolytic Anæmias (Acholuric Jaundice).

1. Severe Infections.

Some infectious diseases, especially where the organisms actually grow in the blood stream, cause a hæmolytic anæmia. Such diseases are streptococcal septicæmias, malaria and also gas gangrene infection.

2. Toxic Chemicals and Drugs.

Certain chemicals, *e.g.*, lead, cause hæmolysis of the red cells. The poisonous venom of some snakes also has this effect. Again sulphonamide drugs may produce this form of anæmia.

3. Incompatible Blood Transfusions.

Whilst anæmia is not commonly caused by incompatible blood transfusions, there are other important reactions from giving a patient the wrong blood group and it is convenient to discuss the subject here.

Blood can be divided into four main groups. Blood from one group can be given to another person of the same group without ill effect. However, if blood of one group is given to a person of a different group the red cells of the donor's blood may be immediately destroyed. Agglutinins in the recipient's plasma act on the donor's red cells causing agglutination or clumping of these cells. Severe hæmolytic jaundice results, and in severe cases death occurs.

It is therefore essential to ensure before any blood is given to an

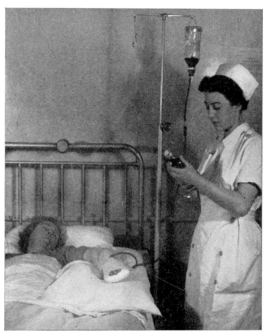

FIG. 133

The nurse is checking the particulars on the bottle of blood to make sure that it is the correct blood to give to the patient.

individual that it is of the correct type. This is known as **blood grouping.** There are four main blood groups :—

    1. Group O (or Group IV) often written as O/IV.
    2. Group A (or Group II) often written as A/II.
    3. Group B (or Group III) often written as B/III.
    4. Group AB (or Group I) often written as AB/I.

In addition to being able to give blood from one person in one group to another person of the same group, it is also possible to give group O/IV blood to all the other groups. For this reason people with Group O/IV blood are known as *universal donors*. Group AB/I can receive blood from any other group and so are known as *universal recipients*. Group A/II blood can be given only to the same group or to Group AB/I. Similarly, Group B/III blood can be given only to the same group or to Group AB/I.

Having tested the blood group before a blood transfusion is given a second check must be made. Some of the recipient's blood is withdrawn and allowed to clot. The serum (clotted plasma) thus obtained is mixed with a small amount of the proposed donor's blood, and if the donor's blood is suitable, *i.e.*, of the right group, no agglutination or clotting should occur. This is known as *direct cross-matching*.

If, through some mistake or failure to carry out these essential preliminaries, the wrong blood is given the result is serious destruction (hæmolysis) of the transfused red cells with jaundice, as stated above. This is often spoken of as an incompatible or *mis-matched transfusion*. Another effect seen in mismatched trans-fusions is that the clumped red cells may block the kidneys, when renal failure (uræmia) may result, which is often fatal.

In incompatible blood transfusions the patient becomes restless and has a severe rigor, whilst there is a rise in pulse rate and temperature. There is usually pain in the chest and back. In severe cases anuria and jaundice develop after a few hours. The nurse must keep a close watch on all patients having a blood transfusion, particularly at the start of each new bottle of blood, so that the transfusion can be immediately stopped if any untoward reactions (severe rigor, pain in the back and rise in temperature) occur.

After all blood transfusions, the transfusion bottle must not be washed out but returned (with the small drop of blood remaining in the bottle) to the laboratory. This is so that further compatibility tests may be done if any adverse reactions have occurred.

4. Hæmolytic Disease and the Rhesus (Rh) Factor.

In addition to the four blood groups mentioned above there is another factor present in the blood of some people which can also cause serious hæmolysis and jaundice. This is known as the Rh factor. Eighty-five per cent. of people are supposed to have this factor and are said to be *Rh positive* ; the remaining 15 per cent. of people lack this factor and are *Rh negative*. If Rh positive blood is given to an Rh negative person, even though it may be the right blood group (that is, O or A, etc.), Rh antibodies are produced in the Rh negative person which may destroy the Rh positive blood. It is necessary, therefore, in giving transfusions to ascertain not only the normal blood group of the person but also the Rh factor, and if this is Rh negative to give only Rh negative blood.

At this point it is convenient to discuss the diseases seen in infants due to this Rh factor.

Even though a pregnant woman may be Rh negative the fœtus's blood may be Rh positive because it may have inherited this Rh positive factor from the father. The Rh positive factor of the child can give rise to antibodies (agglutinins) in the mother's blood, and in the course of time sufficient antibodies may be produced in the mother's blood to destroy the baby's red cells. In severe cases the child may be born dead with severe anæmia and jaundice. In many cases, however, for some unknown reason the crisis develops only as the child is born. As a result, as soon as it is born the baby may become jaundiced and anæmic owing to the destruction of its blood by the Rh antibodies produced in the mother's blood. In mild cases the effect may not be too serious, but in severe cases it can lead to rapid death, or after a few months may give rise to serious changes in the brain with mental deficiency (*kernicterus*).

Various names are used to describe the effects on infants of the Rh factor. In the most severe cases the infant is born dead, and is also usually macerated and very œdematous; the condition of *hydrops fœtalis* is then said to be present. In the most common cases, where the infant becomes deeply jaundiced immediately after birth, the name *icterus gravis* is used. Lastly, where the main effect is a severe anæmia with slight jaundice the term *congenital hæmolytic anæmia* is used. All these effects are different degrees of the same underlying condition, *i.e.*, hæmolytic disease due to the Rh factor. The name *erythroblastosis fœtalis* is also used as well as hæmolytic disease of the newborn.

Treatment of Hæmolytic Disease of the Newborn.—Nowadays it is the commonly accepted practice to blood-group all women during pregnancy and also ascertain their Rh factor. If it is found that they are Rh negative and that antibodies have already developed in their blood premature labour is induced and a replacement transfusion of the child's blood may be done. Here as much of the infant's blood as possible is taken off and replaced by Rh negative blood. In many cases this leads to a complete cure. In milder cases a simple transfusion with Rh negative blood instead of a replacement transfusion is sufficient.

Finally, it must again be stressed that when blood transfusions are necessary, especially in women, the Rh factor must be determined. If the patients are Rh negative then only Rh negative blood must be used. If not antibodies may be produced in the woman's blood, and if at a later date (even after several years) she becomes pregnant these antibodies can destroy her infant's blood if the latter is Rh positive.

5. Congenital Hæmolytic Anæmias (Acholuric Jaundice).

This form of hæmolytic anæmia is due to a congenital defect in the red cells which makes them more fragile than normal and so more easily destroyed. The disease is chronic and usually recognised in childhood, although mild cases may be missed for many years. Recurrent attacks of jaundice of the hæmolytic type, with anæmia, are the main features. The spleen is usually enlarged.

The diagnosis of the disease can be confirmed by performing a fragility test, when the abnormally increased fragility of the red cells will be evident.

In mild cases treating the anæmia with iron or liver may be sufficient, but in any severe case the only effective remedy is to remove the spleen. This increases the life of the red cells and so decreases the amount of red cell destruction. (The function of the spleen as one of the main parts of the reticulo-endothelial system is normally to destroy the worn-out red cells.)

THE HÆMORRHAGIC DISEASES

We saw earlier, in the discussion on the functions of the various components making up human blood, that there were several factors present which had to do with controlling hæmorrhage. We saw that the platelets were concerned with this and that the substances prothrombin and fibrinogen were important in causing blood to clot and so controlling hæmorrhage. The blood vessels themselves also play an important role in controlling hæmorrhage, and contraction of the blood vessel (vasoconstriction) usually takes place when a blood vessel is injured.

The hæmorrhagic diseases are a large group which have as a predominating feature the presence of hæmorrhages. These hæmorrhages may occur into the skin to give rise to purple spots which do not fade on pressure and are called *purpuric* hæmorrhages (small purpuric hæmorrhages are usually known as petechiæ). In addition to purpuric hæmorrhages into the skin, bleeding may occur from the mucous membranes, *e.g.*, from the nose (epistaxis), from the bowels (melæna), or from the kidneys (hæmaturia).

The commoner hæmorrhagic diseases can be roughly classified according to the type of underlying interference with the normal mechanism for the control of bleeding :—

(A) Damage to the Wall of the Blood Vessels (Vascular Purpura).

(B) Diminished Platelets (Thrombocytopenic Purpura).

(C) Prothrombin Deficiency.

(D) Hæmophilia and Christmas Disease.

(E) Fibrinogen Deficiency.

(A) DAMAGE TO THE WALLS OF THE BLOOD VESSELS
(Vascular Purpura)

This group comprises by far the most common causes of purpura, and can be divided into the following types :—

1. **Infections.**—Many infections are associated with purpuric hæmorrhages caused by damage to the vessel wall. In some cases small emboli actually containing bacteria cause the purpuric or petechial spots. This is seen in *meningococcal meningitis* (also called *spotted fever* owing to the occurrence of purpuric spots) and *bacterial endocarditis*, another cause of embolic purpura, where the petechial spots occur in the skin and also under the nails.

In the severe hæmorrhagic forms of such acute infectious fevers as measles, scarlet fever or smallpox the purpuric spots are caused by damage to the walls of the blood vessels.

2. **Drugs.**—Belladonna, quinine and sulphonamides may cause purpura ; also the heavy metals used in medicine, *e.g.*, gold.

3. **Vitamin C Deficiency.**—The classical sign of vitamin C deficiency is hæmorrhage due to alteration in the vascular wall.

4. **Allergic Diseases.**—Purpura is sometimes associated with various allergic manifestations, such as urticaria, œdema of the skin and joint pains. The underlying factor is damage to the lining of the vascular wall which allows leakage of blood and fluid. *Henoch's purpura*, with abdominal pain and melæna, occurs in children. *Schonlein's purpura* is seen in young adults, with pain and swelling of the joints in association with the purpuric spots.

5. **Purpura Simplex.**—This is the commonest type of purpura and is found most often in elderly people, recurrent purpuric spots

appearing in the skin. There is little or no upset in the general health and the purpura is of little significance.

(B) DIMINISHED PLATELETS (Thrombocytopenic Purpura)

One of the functions of the small round bodies known as the platelets (or thrombocytes) is to seal off any lesions or openings in the small blood vessels (capillaries) and so prevent undue loss of blood from a slight injury. The platelets are formed in the bone marrow and, like the red cells, are destroyed by the spleen. Most of the causes, therefore, of this group of hæmorrhagic diseases (purpuras) are diseases affecting the blood, the bone marrow and the spleen.

1. **Leukæmia,** by crowding the marrow with abnormal white cells, may depress the formation of platelets in exactly the same way as it may cause anæmia. Purpura, including bleeding from the mucous membranes, may be a feature of some severe cases of leukæmia.

2. **Secondary Carcinomatosis of the Bones** acts like leukæmia in causing purpura in that the widespread invasion of the bone marrow by the malignant cells decreases the formation of the platelets. We have already seen that carcinomatosis of the bones causes an anæmia in the same fashion.

3. **Aplastic Anæmia** is due to atrophy of the marrow by poisons, toxins, drugs or unknown causes. Severe purpura with bleeding from the mucous membranes caused by depression of the platelets is often a feature of aplastic anæmia.

4. **Drugs,** such as quinine, quinidine, sulphonamides and sedormid, may cause purpura associated with a deficiency of platelets.

5. **Primary Thrombocytopenic Purpura (Purpura Hæmorrhagica).** —Having dealt with the above causes of purpura with diminished platelets we are left with one further type. This is seen most commonly in women and is associated with severe bleeding from the mucous membranes (nose, bowel, kidneys) and into the skin. Anæmia is present, and the spleen is nearly always enlarged. Before diagnosing the primary type of thrombocytopenic purpura careful search for any of the other causes mentioned above must be made. The treatment depends on the severity of the condition, and in mild cases treating the anæmia only may suffice. In cases of severity, however, the spleen is usually removed. Blood transfusions to control any severe hæmorrhage may be necessary. Cortisone or

allied steroids have also proved of value in bringing about either a complete remission or a temporary improvement and so making the patient fit for splenectomy.

(C) PROTHROMBIN DEFICIENCY

Coagulation of Blood.—At the beginning of this chapter the roles of various components of the blood were discussed. It was stated that the substances prothrombin and fibrinogen were concerned with the coagulation of blood. Blood coagulation or clotting plays a major part in the control of hæmorrhage, and although the actual mechanism of blood coagulation is, indeed, very complex and not yet fully understood a simple version should enable the nurse to understand the various diseases which involve blood coagulation. The process of blood clotting can most easily be described as follows:—

1. Prothrombin + Thromboplastin + Calcium = Thrombin.
2. Thrombin + Fibrinogen = Fibrin (clot).

The substance thromboplastin is liberated from injured tissues and also from platelets to convert the prothrombin in the blood into thrombin. Calcium, normally present in the blood, assists in this process. The thrombin thus formed quickly acts on the fibrinogen (which is also normally present in blood) to form fibrin. Fibrin is a solid tough fibre network which is the actual blood clot.

A deficiency in prothrombin is the only condition which commonly arises as a result of interference with this clotting mechanism of the blood. (The disease hæmophilia, which is also associated with a prolonged clotting time, is much rarer. It is discussed later.)

To understand the various diseases which occur owing to prothrombin deficiency it is necessary to understand how this substance is normally formed in the body. Prothrombin is produced in the liver by vitamin K. This vitamin is present in certain foods, such as spinach, cabbage and egg yolk. Those bacteria which are normally present in the bowel can also manufacture vitamin K. For the proper absorption of vitamin K bile salts are necessary.

Causes of Prothrombin Deficiency.

1. **Obstructive Jaundice.**—Here the absence of bile salts leads to deficient absorption of vitamin K and so, after a matter of six to eight weeks, to a fall in the prothrombin level in the blood. When this is severe, hæmorrhages occur. Jaundiced patients are often known to bleed very readily at an operation, and in former years

this was supposed to be due to lack of calcium. It is now known that it is not the calcium but vitamin K that is lacking.

In any operation on a patient with obstructive jaundice the

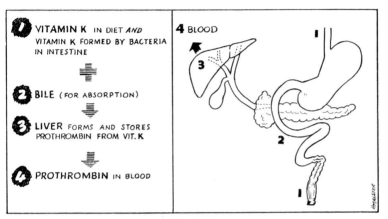

FIG. 134
The formation of prothrombin.

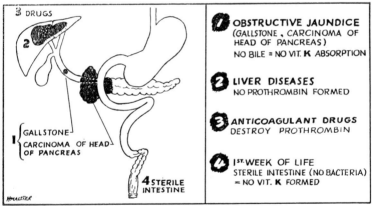

FIG. 135
The causes of prothrombin deficiency.

prothrombin level should be estimated, and if below normal vitamin K must be given.

2. **Hæmorrhagic Disease of the Newborn.**—Occasionally during the first week of life hæmorrhages, such as epistaxis or melæna, may occur giving rise to the condition known as hæmorrhagic disease of the newborn. The cause is prothrombin deficiency brought about by

13

a shortage of vitamin K received from the mother, combined with the inability of the infant during the first week to manufacture vitamin K itself. The newborn infant's bowel is sterile, and the absence of bacteria is thus the cause of the infant's inability to form vitamin K.

Premature infants are especially lacking in prothrombin and should be given vitamin K after birth as a routine.

3. **Diseases of the Liver.**—Diseases of the liver may be associated with prothrombin deficiency as prothrombin is manufactured and stored in the liver. Prothrombin deficiency with its resulting hæmorrhages is mainly seen in cases of acute liver damage such as occurs in acute yellow atrophy, and less often in chronic conditions such as cirrhosis of the liver.

4. **Chronic Diseases of the Gastro-intestinal Tract.**—Those chronic intestinal diseases which cause severe and persistent diarrhœa may lead to a deficiency in vitamin K absorption, resulting in some cases in so severe a prothrombin deficiency that actual hæmorrhages may occur. Such intestinal diseases include chronic ulcerative colitis and sprue.

5. **Anticoagulant Drugs.**—Anticoagulant drugs are used in the prevention and treatment of thrombosis and embolism, especially thrombosis of the veins and of the coronary arteries. Anticoagulant drugs destroy the prothrombin and thus cause a prolonged blood clotting time. The aim in treatment is to prolong the clotting time of the blood so that thrombosis does not occur or, if already present, does not spread; the risk of a complicating embolism is thus greatly reduced.

An overdosage of anticoagulant drugs may cause too great a prolongation of the clotting time so that hæmorrhages occur. Hæmaturia, epistaxis and severe bruising of the skin are those most frequently seen.

In all patients on anticoagulant drugs frequent estimation of the prothrombin time is essential to control the treatment. Daily routine examination of the urine for red cells, whose presence may give forewarning of a more massive hæmaturia, is also valuable.

The anticoagulant drugs most commonly used at present include phenindione (Dindevan), marcoumar, nicoumalone (sinthrome), dicoumarol, and warfarin sodium (marevan).

Treatment of Prothrombin Deficiency.—In all cases of prothrombin deficiency, except those due to liver disease and to overdosage with anticoagulant drugs, treatment with injections of vitamin K (menaphthone or synkavit), 10 to 15 mgm., leads to a rapid and complete cure. In infants with hæmorrhagic disease of the new-born, only 1 mgm. of synkavit is necessary, as larger doses may cause a toxic hæmolytic anæmia. In liver disease there is usually only a partial response. In overdosage with anticoagulant drugs, vitamin K_1 (5 to 20 mgm.) is needed to restore the prothrombin level to normal. If any appreciable hæmorrhage is present transfusions with fresh blood, 1 to 2 pints, are needed.

(D) HÆMOPHILIA AND CHRISTMAS DISEASE

Hæmophilia is a rare disease in which severe hæmorrhages into the joints are the predominant feature. The hæmorrhages are usually brought on by some injury which may be no more than trivial, such as the patient knocking himself. Hæmophilia is seen only in men and is a hereditary disease passed down in certain families from generation to generation. It is passed on through the females who are, however, never themselves affected by the disease. Hæmophilia is caused by the lack of a factor which is essential for the proper clotting of blood, namely, antihæmophilic globulin. Consequently, there is in hæmophilia a markedly prolonged blood clotting time leading to hæmorrhages.

Treatment.—There is no really satisfactory cure for this condition. Blood transfusions are the mainstay of treatment or, alternatively, injections of antihæmophilic globulin itself.

Christmas disease gives a very similar clinical picture to that of hæmophilia with severe hæmorrhages into the joints. The cause of Christmas disease is lack of a factor which is normally present in blood and necessary for blood coagulation. This factor has been called the Christmas factor. If severe bleeding occurs blood transfusions are necessary.

(E) FIBRINOGEN DEFICIENCY

In recent years the condition of acquired fibrinogen deficiency has been increasingly recognised. It arises during pregnancy and is usually associated with such complications as accidental hæmorrhage, abortions and intra-uterine death of the fœtus. Very severe hæmorrhage from the uterus develops and the condition is one of extreme emergency, necessitating transfusions of concentrated dried plasma or injections of fibrinogen to restore the fibrinogen content of the blood.

POLYCYTHÆMIA

Polycythæmia is a rare disorder of the blood wherein there is a marked increase in the number of red blood cells and in the volume of the blood. Instead of the normal count of approximately 5 million red cells per c.mm., the number of red cells may be as high as 7 million or more per c.mm. The condition may arise as a compensatory mechanism in diseases where there is incomplete oxygenation of the blood, *e.g.*, severe chronic diseases of the heart and lungs, especially congenital heart diseases. Certain drugs may also produce this condition.

A primary form of the disease, of unknown cause, *polycythæmia vera*, is more rarely seen. This form is usually treated with radio-active phosphorus (P^{32}), which diminishes the number of red cells. An alternative therapy is by X-ray irradiation.

THE WHITE BLOOD CELLS

There are three main types of white cell in the blood :—

1. Polymorphonuclear white cells or granulocytes (so called because they have granules present). There are three forms of polymorphonuclear white cells; neutrophils, eosinophils and basophils.
2. Lymphocytes.
3. Monocytes.

The main function of the white cells is to help defend the body against infection, and for this purpose the polymorphonuclear cells are the most important. In most infections caused by bacteria the number of polymorphonuclear cells is increased to combat the infection, and this increase in white cells is known as a **leucocytosis.** The presence of a leucocytosis in cases of infection is a good sign as it means that the body is responding to overcome the infection.

In certain chronic inflammations not due to pyogenic (pus-forming) organisms, *e.g.*, tuberculosis, syphilis and certain virus infections, the number of polymorphonuclear cells is not increased but the monocytes quite frequently are.

A reduction in the white cells below normal is called a **leucopenia.** For some unknown reason a leucopenia occurs in some infections, especially typhoid fever.

Formation of White Cells.—The polymorphonuclear cells, the main white cells in the body, are formed in the red marrow of the bones and the lymphocytes in the lymphoid tissues   The monocytes are formed in the specialised system of cells which includes the endothelial cells, the bone marrow and the spleen (reticulo-endothelial system).

Normal White Cell Count.—The normal total white cell count is between 5,000 and 10,000 per c.mm. in an adult. The polymorphonuclear cells form 65 per cent. of this total, the lymphocytes 30 per cent. and the monocytes 5 per cent.

DISEASES OF THE WHITE BLOOD CELLS

LEUKÆMIA

In leukæmia the white cells are greatly increased in number, and immature forms appear in the blood. Any type of white cell may be affected :—

1. The polymorphonuclear cells (myeloid leukæmia).
2. The lymphocytes (lymphatic leukæmia).
3. The monocytes (monocytic leukæmia).

The symptoms of all three types of leukæmia are usually similar, differing only in one or two respects. The actual type of cell affected is usually easily seen by examining the blood and if necessary examining the marrow itself by doing a sternal puncture.

It should be emphasised again that leukæmia is actually a disease of the cells, of unknown cause, which leads to a great increase in the number of cells. Leucocytosis is an increase in the number of white cells as the result usually of infection by organisms such as bacteria. It is the natural response of the body to overcome the infection.

General Symptoms and Signs of Leukæmia.

1. The disease may be acute, and this is especially likely in children when the whole course may last only a few weeks or months. In adults it is usually more chronic and runs a course lasting several years.

2. There are the general symptoms of anæmia, including fatigue and loss of energy. Leukæmia causes anæmia through interference with the formation of the red blood cells in the marrow as the enormous number of white cells in the marrow " crowd out " the red cells.

3. Hæmorrhages into the skin and mucous membranes (that is, purpura) very commonly occur in leukæmia, especially in the acute

forms. We have seen earlier that this purpura is due to a deficiency in the formation of platelets, which are normally formed in the marrow, but are " crowded out " in the same way as the red cells.

4. When the blood is examined it will be seen that the white cells have greatly increased, perhaps up to 100,000 or 200,000 per c.mm. In some rare forms the white cells may not have increased in the peripheral blood, but if the marrow is examined it will be found that the whole increase in white cells has occurred in the marrow, so that it is completely packed with white cells. This rarer form is called *aleukæmic* leukæmia.

Special Features of the Different Types.—In myeloid leukæmia the spleen is enlarged and the lymph glands slightly so. In lymphatic leukæmia, on the other hand, the lymph glands are usually relatively more enlarged than the spleen. In monocytic leukæmia, which is rarer than the other two types, the spleen is not greatly enlarged and the lymph glands only slightly so. A characteristic feature of monocytic leukæmia is severe bleeding and swelling of the gums.

Diagnosis.—Any anæmia associated with purpura and a greatly enlarged spleen or enlarged lymph glands is suggestive of leukæmia. A blood count will usually settle the diagnosis, and in many cases will also establish the exact type of leukæmia. In the rarer forms, when the cells in the blood are not increased, a sternal puncture will be necessary for a definite diagnosis.

Treatment.—There is no complete cure for leukæmia, and some of the acute forms are rapidly fatal. In the more chronic types deep X-ray therapy to the spleen and lymph glands often relieves the symptoms and prolongs life for many years. Irradiation with radio-active phosphorus (P^{32}) may be used instead of deep X-rays.

In recent years many different drugs have become available which have a temporary effect on leukæmia and are often used if irradiation therapy is not available.

At present busulphan (myleran), 4 mgm. daily, appears to be the best drug available for chronic myeloid leukæmia, but mercapto-purine (2·5 mgm. per kilogram of body-weight) and the nitrogen mustards are also used. For chronic lymphatic leukæmia, tretamine and the nitrogen mustards are most often given.

In acute leukæmia, irradiation therapy is never used as it exacerbates the disease. Blood transfusions are usually necessary at first. Cortisone or prednisone may sometimes induce a remission. Mercaptopurine or aminopterin (0·5 to 1 mgm. daily) may also be of temporary benefit. The ultimate prognosis is always, however, fatal.

AGRANULOCYTOSIS

The term *agranulocytosis* is used to denote either the complete absence of the granular cells (or polymorphonuclear cells as they are more often called) or a severe reduction in their number, combined with clinical symptoms and signs due to this deficiency. It must be stressed that a leucopenia means a reduction in the white cells which does not necessarily cause harmful results and is not the same condition as agranulocytosis.

Causes.—The usual cause of agranulocytosis is some toxic depression of the bone marrow, as a result of which the polymorphs are not formed in adequate numbers. Drugs are the commonest cause of this toxic depression, especially the sulphonamides, anti-thyroid drugs (thiouracil and neo-mercazole), phenylbutazone, chloramphenicol, gold salts and troxidone.

In view of the frequent use of sulphonamides and antithyroid drugs, with their special liability to give rise to agranulocytosis, it is absolutely essential that the early symptoms and signs of this condition should be watched for. Whenever sulphonamides are given for a prolonged period, frequent examinations of the white cells should be made to ensure that they have not been abnormally reduced.

Symptoms and Signs.

1. The commonest early symptom is one of sore throat, which may be very severe, with marked œdema and exudate in the throat. The sore throat is so invariable that the disease is often given the name *agranulocytic angina.*

2. The temperature rises, and if it is already above normal it usually rises further.

3. The patient becomes toxic and lethargic. The pulse is rapid.

Diagnosis.—The complaint of a sore throat with fever in a patient on sulphonamides or antithyroid drugs should immediately raise the suspicion of agranulocytosis. The drugs must at once be stopped until a white cell count is done and the presence of agranulocytosis confirmed or not.

Treatment.—Penicillin is given in large doses, usually 100,000 to 200,000 units six-hourly. This is to combat any infection that is present or likely to arise. Penicillin is non-toxic to the white cells so that it can be given with safety.

SUMMARY

1. Blood is composed of red and white cells suspended in a clear yellow fluid called plasma. Plasma contains various salts and the sugar necessary for the proper nutrition of the body. In addition, various substances (prothrombin and fibrinogen) are present in the plasma which are concerned with the coagulation (clotting) of blood. Blood clotting is one of the methods whereby undue loss of blood is prevented when a blood vessel is cut.

2. The red cells are formed in the red marrow of the bones. Vitamin B_{12} normally present in liver, meat, milk, eggs, is one of the essential factors for the proper formation of mature red cells. Vitamin B_{12} is stored in the body in large quantities in the liver. The intrinsic factor secreted by the cells in the gastric mucosa is necessary for the proper absorption of vitamin B_{12}. The red cells contain hæmoglobin, which is mainly composed of iron. In addition to vitamin B_{12}, the intrinsic factor and iron, folic acid, which is part of the vitamin B complex, is also necessary for the normal development of the red blood cells.

The function of the red blood cells is to carry oxygen by means of their hæmoglobin throughout the body.

3. Anæmia is a reduction in the number of red cells and in the amount of hæmoglobin. In general, lack of vitamin B_{12} (and less frequently of folic acid) causes a type of anæmia which mainly affects the red cells, which become altered in size, shape, and colour as well as being reduced in number. The red cells in this type of anæmia are often described as macrocytic (large) and hyperchromic (hæmoglobin in each cell not reduced). On the other hand, anæmias due to lack of iron mainly reduce the hæmoglobin content of the red cells, which therefore become hypochromic and usually microcytic (small in size).

This differentiation of anæmias into macrocytic hyperchromic and microcytic hypochromic is of value in treatment. Macrocytic anæmias usually require to be treated with vitamin B_{12} or folic acid. On the other hand, in hypochromic anæmias the main essential is iron. Of course in all anæmias the cause, wherever possible, must be dealt with.

4. Anæmias can be brought about in many different ways. Hæmorrhagic anæmias are due to loss of blood from the body. In medicine, hæmatemesis or melæna (from peptic ulcer or carcinoma of the stomach) and hæmoptysis (from pulmonary tuberculosis or carcinoma of the lung) are the common causes of acute loss of blood and, therefore, of an anæmia. Repeated epistaxis, bleeding hæmorrhoids, menorrhagia and carcinoma of the intestinal tract are frequent causes of chronic hæmorrhagic anæmia.

In the treatment of massive acute hæmorrhage or very severe anæmias blood transfusions are often necessary. Before giving a blood transfusion it is essential to see that the donor's blood is compatible with the patient's. This is done by determining which of the four blood groups (O, A, B, AB) the patient belongs to and then giving him blood from that same group or instead from the " universal donor " blood group O. In addition, especially when giving blood transfusions to a woman of child-bearing age, it is necessary to determine the Rhesus factor of the patient, and if it is Rh negative only Rh negative blood of the right group is transfused. The importance of the Rh factor is in connection with hæmolytic disease of the newborn.

5. Decreased blood formation, through interference with any of the many

factors essential for normal blood development mentioned above, is a common cause of anæmia. Pernicious anæmia is one of the main anæmias of this type and is due to absence of the intrinsic factor in the stomach. Lack of iron in the diet and deficient absorption of iron from the gastro-intestinal tract are other frequent and important causes of anæmia (simple achlorhydric anæmia).

6. Another way in which disordered blood formation can lead to anæmia is through disease affecting the marrow of the bones. X-rays and radioactive substances can depress blood formation in the red marrow. Severe infections, toxic drugs and some diseases, especially nephritis, may have a similar effect on the marrow. In addition, extensive carcinomatous deposits in the bones will " crowd out " the red cells in the marrow and cause anæmia. In a similar fashion, leukæmia, by invasion of the marrow by enormous numbers of white cells, causes anæmia.

7. In addition to anæmias caused by blood loss and by disordered blood formation, there remains one further main group of anæmias which are the result of undue destruction of the red cells—hæmolytic anæmias. Toxic infections, poisons, the Rhesus factor and congenital abnormal fragility of the red cells are all causes of hæmolytic anæmia. A feature of hæmolytic anæmias is hæmolytic jaundice, because the hæmoglobin of broken-down red cells is converted into bile pigment which, when present in the blood in excess, causes hæmolytic jaundice (yellow discoloration of the skin).

8. Many diseases of the blood have one common feature—hæmorrhage. The hæmorrhage is usually into the skin (when it causes purpuric (hæmorrhagic) spots) and also from the mucous membranes, e.g., epistaxis, melæna or hæmaturia. The causes of these hæmorrhagic diseases can be roughly divided into five groups.

(a) Damage to the walls of the blood vessels as caused by severe toxic infections, certain drugs, vitamin C deficiency and allergic diseases.

(b) Diminished platelets, caused by interference with the formation of the platelets in the red marrow of the bones as a result of diseases affecting the marrow, e.g., carcinomatosis of the bones and leukæmia. In the disease known as primary thrombocytopenic purpura the hæmorrhages into the skin and from the mucous membranes are due to a diminution in the platelets from an unknown cause.

(c) Prothrombin deficiency. In this third group of hæmorrhagic diseases neither the vessel walls nor the platelets are at fault ; instead, there is a deficiency of prothrombin in the blood. Prothrombin is essential for the coagulation of the blood which is necessary to prevent excessive hæmorrhage, such as may arise when a blood vessel is injured. Vitamin K, present in certain foods and also manufactured by those bacteria normally present in the bowel, is necessary for the formation of prothrombin which is then stored in the liver. In addition, bile salts are necessary for the proper absorption of vitamin K. Obstructive jaundice, hæmorrhagic disease of the newborn (due to the sterile intestinal tract), disease of the liver and anticoagulant therapy, may all be associated with prothrombin deficiency. (Anticoagulant drugs destroy the prothrombin in the blood.) If this deficiency is severe, hæmorrhage, especially hæmaturia, melæna, epistaxis and purpura, may occur.

(d) In the hereditary diseases, hæmophilia and Christmas disease, which practically always occur in males but are transmitted by females, hæmorrhages, especially into the joints, are the predominant feature.

(e) Finally, during pregnancy, accidental hæmorrhage abortion or death of the foetus may cause a deficiency of the fibrinogen content of the blood leading to massive hæmorrhage from the uterus.

13 A

9. The white cells (leucocytes) in the blood help to combat infections, and particularly important are the polymorphonuclear (granular) cells. A leucocytosis means an increase of white cells (usually the polymorphs) and normally occurs as part of the body's defence against infections. Leucopenia, a reduction in the number of white cells, is found in some diseases, e.g., typhoid fever. Leukæmia is a disease directly affecting the white cells which results in an enormous increase in their number and also in the presence of immature white cells in the blood. Leukæmia, which may be acute or chronic in its course, is invariably fatal.

Finally, the disease agranulocytosis may arise where there is a marked reduction in the number of the granular white cells. Agranulocytosis is most commonly seen as a result of overdosage of or idiosyncrasy to certain drugs or poisons, particularly sulphonamides, phenylbutazone and antithyroid drugs.

SUMMARY OF SOME ROUTINE PROCEDURES UNDERTAKEN IN DISEASES OF THE BLOOD

1. **Examination of Blood Film, Hæmoglobin Estimation and Red Cell Count.**

   (a) In all cases of suspected anæmias, for diagnosis of the exact type of anæmia and to observe results of treatment.

   (b) Following hæmorrhage, to estimate the severity of the resulting anæmia. Also to follow progress and make sure that the hæmorrhage has ceased, particularly in cases of internal hæmorrhage.

2. **White Cell Count.** (This also applies to diseases of other systems.)

   (a) In all cases of anæmias, particularly to exclude leukæmia as a cause.

   (b) In all cases of acute and chronic inflammation, where a leucocytosis is nearly always present. Especially important in acute abdominal disease where a leucocytosis denotes an inflammatory lesion and so the probable necessity for operation.

   (c) In typhoid fever, where a leucopenia may be present and is of diagnostic value.

   (d) In whooping-cough, where a marked leucocytosis is usually present.

   (e) In all cases of sore throats developing while the patient is on such drugs as antithyroid drugs, sulphonamides, phenylbutazone and gold, to exclude agranulocytosis.

3. **Blood Grouping.** (This also applies to diseases of other systems.)

   In all patients before a blood transfusion is given or where a transfusion might be necessary, e.g., before major operations, in cases of severe anæmias and in all cases of severe hæmorrhage.

4. Cross-matching.

In all cases before a blood transfusion is given.

5. Determination of the Rhesus Factor.

(*a*) In all cases before blood transfusion.

(*b*) In pregnancy.

6. Prothrombin Clotting Time.

(*a*) In all patients on anticoagulant drugs.

(*b*) In obstructive jaundice.

(*c*) In liver diseases.

(*d*) In hæmorrhagic disease of the newborn.

(*e*) In all cases of obscure unexplained bleeding.

7. Test Meal.

In the diagnosis of certain anæmias, particularly pernicious and simple achlorhydric anæmias.

8. Coagulation and Bleeding Times.

(*a*) In all patients on heparin.

(*b*) In purpura.

(*c*) In hæmophilia.

9. Sternal Puncture.

(*a*) For the diagnosis of obscure anæmias.

(*b*) In leukæmia.

10. Red Cell Fragility Test.

In the diagnosis of congenital hæmolytic anæmia (acholuric jaundice).

SUMMARY OF IMPORTANT DRUGS USED IN DISEASES OF THE BLOOD

1. Aminopterin.

Acute leukæmia.

2. Antihæmophilic globulin.

Hæmophilia.

3. **Busulphan** (myleran).

   Chronic myeloid leukæmia.

4. **Cortisone and Allied Drugs** (prednisone, prednisolone, dexamethasone, ACTH).

   Acute leukæmia.
   Primary thrombocytopenic purpura.

5. **Fibrinogen** (or concentrated dried plasma).

   Fibrinogen deficiency associated with pregnancy.

6. **Folic Acid.**

   In some macrocytic anæmias, especially the macrocytic anæmia of pregnancy, cœliac disease and sprue.

7. **Iron** (ferrous gluconate, ferrous succinate, ferrous sulphate, saccharated iron oxide).

   Chronic hæmorrhagic anæmias.
   Simple achlorhydric anæmia.
   Iron deficiency anæmias of pregnancy, sprue, cœliac disease, premature infants, etc.

8. **Mercaptopurine** (puri-nethol).
   Chronic myeloid leukæmia.
   Acute leukæmia.

9. **Nitrogen Mustards.**

   Chronic leukæmia.

10. **Penicillin.**

    Agranulocytosis.

11. **Radioactive Phosphorus.**

    Polycythæmia vera.

12. **Tretamine.**

    Chronic lymphatic leukæmia.

13. **Vitamin B$_{12}$** (cyanocobalamin).

    Pernicious anæmia.
    All anæmias of the macrocytic type.

14. **Vitamin K.**

Prothrombin deficiency in obstructive jaundice.
Hæmorrhagic disease of the newborn.
Liver diseases.

15. **Vitamin K$_1$** (Konakion).

Overdosage with anticoagulant drugs.

CHAPTER XI

DISEASES OF THE SPLEEN AND LYMPH GLANDS

THE SPLEEN

T*HE FUNCTIONS OF THE SPLEEN.*—The spleen acts as a reservoir for blood in times of need and, in addition, forms part of the widespread system of cells called the reticulo-endothelial system. This system includes specialised cells in the spleen, lymph glands, liver, blood vessels and many other parts of the body. Among the functions of the reticulo-endothelial system are the breaking down of worn-out red cells, the destruction of invading organisms and parasites and the formation of antibodies.

The lymphoid tissue of the spleen, like all other lymphoid tissues, manufactures the lymphocytes.

SPLENOMEGALY (Enlargement of the Spleen)

Disease seldom starts in the spleen as a primary condition, but the spleen is often affected in the course of a wide variety of ailments, including acute and chronic infective diseases and also blood diseases.

An enlarged spleen is a most important finding in medicine for the diagnosis of many diseases. A brief list of the more important causes of an enlarged spleen is therefore given.

1. **Acute Infections.**—The acute infective diseases which in Great Britain most commonly give rise to an enlarged spleen are enteric fever, subacute bacterial endocarditis and miliary tuberculosis. In tropical countries an enlarged spleen is a most frequent finding, usually as a result of acute and chronic malarial infection. Typhus fever and undulant fever (brucellosis) are also common causes of splenomegaly in the tropics.

2. **Chronic Infections.**—Malaria is by far the commonest cause of splenomegaly due to chronic infection. Other causes include syphilis and tuberculosis.

3. **Blood Diseases.**—It is in this group of diseases that greatly enlarged spleens are met with. Leukæmia, especially the myeloid

type, is one of the commonest causes. The rare type of purpura called primary thrombocytopenic purpura is often associated with enlargement of the spleen.

In congenital hæmolytic anæmia (acholuric jaundice) too a splenomegaly is usually present.

One other anæmia, not so far mentioned, is characterised by a marked enlargement of the spleen. This disease (which also shows a low white count—leucopenia) is called splenic anæmia or **Banti's disease.** It usually starts in young people, and a feature of the disease (apart from the anæmia and enlarged spleen) is recurrent hæmorrhage, usually in the form of a hæmatemesis. The disease eventually affects the liver, causing a cirrhosis, which leads to obstruction of the portal system. At this stage recurring ascites and cachexia are the main features. Treatment is unsatisfactory, although in the early stages, before cirrhosis of the liver develops, splenectomy is of benefit in some cases.

THE LYMPH GLANDS

The lymph glands form part of the reticulo-endothelial system and, in addition, manufacture the white blood cells known as the lymphocytes. The lymph glands, with their lymphatic ducts, form a " drainage system " throughout the body which, amongst other things, acts as a filter to remove such foreign bodies as organisms and malignant cells.

LYMPHADENOPATHY (Enlargement of the Lymph Glands)

Generally, when disease affects the lymph glands the glands become enlarged. For the sake of convenience we can divide such enlargement into local and general.

1. **Local.**—Localised enlargement of one group of lymph glands is commonly due to septic inflammation of the tissues drained by those lymph glands. For instance, a septic finger often causes an enlarged axillary gland, while inflammation of the throat may give rise to enlarged cervical glands.

Apart from inflammatory lesions, tumour cells often spread along the lymphatics to cause enlargement of the lymph glands draining the area, *e.g.*, carcinoma of the breast giving rise to enlarged axillary glands.

Another frequent cause of localised lymph gland enlargement is tuberculosis, which very commonly affects the cervical glands.

2. **General.**—The most common causes of a generalised enlargement of the lymph glands include:—

   (*a*) Lymphatic leukæmia.
   (*b*) Glandular fever.
   (*c*) Hodgkin's disease.
   (*d*) Syphilis (secondary stage).

As lymphatic leukæmia and syphilis have been discussed elsewhere only glandular fever and Hodgkin's disease will be dealt with here.

GLANDULAR FEVER (Infectious Mononucleosis)

Glandular fever is caused by infection with a virus which usually affects children and young adults.

Symptoms and Signs.

1. A sore throat is very common at the onset, and in some cases the tonsils may be covered with heavy exudate almost resembling a diphtheritic membrane. Fever, with its usual symptoms (headache, malaise and loss of appetite), is present. A measles type of rash may develop.

2. The lymph glands are enlarged, especially the cervical groups, but usually all groups, axillary, inguinal, etc., are affected to some degree.

3. Characteristic changes occur in the white blood cells. A raised white count (leucocytosis) is present, the numbers of lymphocytes and monocytes being increased. Abnormal types of these cells appear in the blood.

4. The diagnosis may be confirmed by doing an agglutination test called the Paul-Bunnell test, which is positive in some cases.

Course and Treatment.—Practically all cases recover, although it may take several weeks or months before normal health is restored. The patients should be nursed in bed whilst any fever is present. Treatment is entirely symptomatic as there is as yet no specific remedy available.

HODGKIN'S DISEASE

Cause.—Unknown.

Symptoms and Signs.

1. The disease is commonest in the twenty to forty age group, but it may arise at any age. The first sign of the disease is often an enlargement of one group of lymph glands.

2. Any group (or groups) of lymph glands may be affected. Usually the cervical glands in the neck or the axillary or inguinal glands are involved. In some cases, however, the deep internal lymph glands in the thorax or abdomen may be the first to be affected, and here the diagnosis of the condition is often difficult till the superficial palpable lymph glands also become enlarged.

3. The general health may be little affected at first, but as the disease advances weakness, anæmia and loss of weight develop. A characteristic feature of many cases is the recurrent pyrexia, which

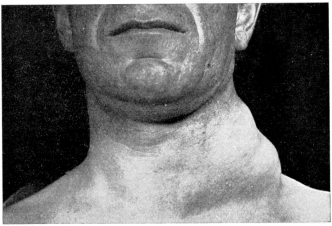

FIG. 136
Hodgkin's disease showing enlarged glands in the neck.

typically comes in waves lasting ten to fourteen days and then subsides only to rise again. This undulating type of fever is called the Pel-Ebstein fever.

4. Enlargement of the thoracic lymph glands can give rise to the pressure symptoms of cough and dyspnœa, while the enlarged abdominal glands may cause abdominal distension or ascites.

Diagnosis.—The disease has to be distinguished from the other causes of enlargement of the lymph glands. Lymphatic leukæmia, which also causes a generalised enlargement of the lymph glands, is differentiated by the diagnostic gross increase in the white cells accompanied by the presence of abnormal types of white cells. Tuberculosis of the lymph glands remains confined to one group only, and the affected glands become matted together and may break down to form a chronic sinus. Hodgkin's glands remain mobile and do not adhere to the skin or break down. Malignant disease of the lymph glands, which is usually due to secondary invasion, gives rise to very hard fixed glands and the primary growth is usually easily found.

Course and Treatment.—The average duration is about two years, and all cases ultimately die. Some cases may, however, live for as long as ten years. The most successful treatment to date in slowing down the progress of the disease is deep X-ray therapy, which has to be repeated at periodic intervals. The only drugs found to have any effect in arresting the disease are the nitrogen mustards which are given by a course of injections. Nitrogen mustards are of benefit where the facilities for deep X-ray therapy are not available.

SARCOIDOSIS

Cause.—The cause of sarcoidosis is not known. It chiefly arises in young adults between the ages of twenty and forty. The disease bears a close resemblance to tuberculosis and indeed in a certain percentage of patients tuberculosis supervenes.

Symptoms and Signs.—Although most organs and tissues may be affected and infiltrated by the typical sarcoid lesions, the skin, lymph glands, lungs and bones are those mainly affected.

1. **Skin.**—Nodular eruptions of yellow-purple colour occur, usually on the face, chest and abdomen. They do not ulcerate.

2. **Lymph Glands.**—Enlargement of lymph glands in the neck, mediastinum, axillary and inguinal regions is present. The glands, unlike tuberculous glands, do not break down.

3. **Lungs.**—The commonest lesion is a diffuse fine miliary infiltration of the lung tissue. The appearances on X-ray are very similar to those of miliary tuberculosis.

4. **Bones.**—Typical " punched out " areas are seen on X-ray of the hands and feet.

Eye lesions (conjunctivitis and iritis), parotid swelling and facial paralysis are also common signs which may develop.

Course and Treatment.—The disease runs a variable course often with remissions but after many months or even years the majority of patients recover. For a small percentage active tuberculosis may supervene and is treated with chemotherapy. So far there is no specific treatment for sarcoidosis but steroids may be given.

CHAPTER XII

DISEASES OF THE URINARY SYSTEM

ANATOMY.—The urinary system consists of :—

A 1. The Kidneys. These lie in the posterior abdomen on each side of the spinal column. They consist essentially of millions of tubules which start around the small blood capillaries known as the glomeruli, and after a tortuous course within the kidneys enter the pelvis of the kidney. The pelvis of the kidney leads into the

2. Ureter, which is a long narrow tube which enters the

3. Bladder. This is a hollow muscular organ which acts as a reservoir for the secretion of the kidneys, *i.e.*, the urine. The bladder is under the control of the nervous system. When it becomes distended impulses travel to the brain to record this sense of distension. The bladder is emptied by means of motor impulses which travel down from the brain to contract the muscles of the bladder and relax the sphincters. In early infancy control of the bladder does not exist and emptying takes place merely by in-voluntary action. In diseases of the nervous system this nervous control of the bladder is very often upset, with either retention of urine or incontinence as a result (see p. 302).

Physiology.—The essential function of the kidney is to remove from the body waste products formed during metabolism. One of the commonest waste products thus removed is urea.

In addition to this function, the kidneys, by excreting certain salts and retaining others, maintain the acid-alkali reaction of the blood at a fairly constant level. Again, the kidneys are an important factor in regulating fluid balance in the body. If there is too much fluid the kidneys will excrete more and *vice versa*.

The glomeruli in the kidneys through which all the blood flows act as filters, and one of the most important functions of glomerular filtration is to prevent the proteins in the blood from leaking through. Thus in health no albumin (the main type of protein in the blood) is present in the urine. Another very important function of the kidneys is to regulate the level in the blood of such substances as glucose; for instance, if the sugar in the blood reaches above a certain level or " threshold," sugar, which normally is not present in the urine, starts to be excreted.

403

THE URINE

Examination of the urine is one of the most important routine examinations made, not only in renal diseases but in *all* diseases. *It must never be omitted.* Certain tests are always carried out (such as those for albumin and sugar), whilst others, *e.g.*, for bile and pus, are done only in specific diseases.

Full examination of the urine includes the following tests :—

1. Volume and Reaction.

The amount of urine passed varies with many factors, especially the amount of fluid drunk and also the amount lost in perspiration. The average normal twenty-four hour quantity is usually in the region of 1,500 ml. (50 oz.). An increased output of urine is usually spoken of as a *polyuria*, a diminished output as *oliguria* and a complete suppression of urine as *anuria*.

With all patients a careful check should be kept on the daily output of urine and, if there is any reason to suspect that the patient is not passing an adequate amount, an output chart must be kept. A severe reduction in the amount of urine passed is always a serious matter and calls for prompt attention. In the first instance, especially in acutely ill and elderly patients, it must be ascertained that the patient is drinking enough.

The reaction of the urine is normally slightly acid so that it turns blue litmus paper red ; alkaline urine turns red litmus paper blue.

2. Specific Gravity.

The specific gravity of urine (which is measured by a urinometer) varies principally with the amount passed. The larger the amount the lower the specific gravity and vice versa. The average normal range is usually 1,012 to 1,024.

Certain substances in the urine have a profound effect on the specific gravity, especially sugar, which raises the specific gravity to the very high figure of 1,035 or more.

3. Normal Deposits.

(*a*) URATES.—Urates may form a sediment in urine when it is cold, but they dissolve on heating. They are usually a brownish or salmon pink colour.

(*b*) PHOSPHATES.—Phosphates usually appear when the urine is neutral or alkaline in reaction. They are white in colour and dissolve when acetic acid is added.

(c) Mucus.—Mucus, especially in non-catheter specimens, is often present as a transparent fluffy deposit, easily recognised.

4. Tests for Proteins (Albumin).

This examination is always made in all diseases.

As mentioned earlier, normal healthy glomeruli of the kidney do not allow the protein in the blood to filter through into the tubules. One of the first and most constant signs of damage to the kidneys (from whatever cause) is the presence of protein (albumin) in the urine, and, conversely, if no albumin is present it is a good indication in most cases of the absence of a serious kidney lesion. Testing for albumin is therefore of great clinical importance in establishing whether or not damage to the kidneys is present.

Cold (a) Salicyl-sulphonic Acid Test.—Eight drops of salicyl-sulphonic acid are added to approximately 5 ml. of urine in a test-tube. If albumin is present a white cloud forms. This is the simplest and most reliable test for albumin. *1st Dilute acetic acid may be added if not acid.*

Hot (b) Boiling Test.—Urine is boiled in a test-tube, and a turbidity which does not clear when dilute acetic acid is added will form if albumin is present. A turbidity that clears after the addition of acetic acid is not due to albumin but to phosphates.

(c) Albustix Test.—This is a rapid and fairly reliable test for protein in urine although it is not so sensitive or reliable as the salicyl-sulphonic acid test.

The test end of the albustix strip is dipped in the urine and then removed. The colour compared with the colour scale provided shows the amount of protein present, if any.

Quantitative Estimation of Albumin.—The actual amount of albumin present in the urine may be estimated by means of *Esbach's albuminometer*. First, however, the urine must be clear; if not it is necessary to filter it. If the specific gravity is 1,010 or more the urine is diluted to 1,008. Finally, acetic acid must be added if the urine is alkaline in reaction. The urine is then poured into the albuminometer up to the mark U. Esbach's reagent is added up to the mark R. The tube, closed with a rubber bung, is gently inverted several times to mix the fluids, and is then left to stand in a vertical position for twenty-four hours. The amount of albumin present is estimated by the height of the precipitate on the graduated scale marked on the tube. This scale is expressed in grammes of albumin per litre of urine. The amount of albumin may be expressed as a percentage by dividing by 10.

Causes of Albuminuria.—Because one of the earliest signs of kidney damage from whatever cause is the presence of albumin in the urine, the causes of albuminuria are many and varied; the most important causes include the following:—

(*a*) Any acute febrile disease.   (*e*) Pyelitis and cystitis.
(*b*) Congestive heart failure.   (*f*) Toxæmias of pregnancy.
(*c*) Prolonged coma.   (*g*) Tumours of the kidney.
(*d*) Nephritis—all stages.   (*h*) Tuberculosis of the kidney.

5. Tests for Sugar.

This examination is always made in all diseases.

(*a*) The *Clinitest* is a simple and convenient test for sugar on similar lines to Benedict's test, but external heat is not required. Five drops of urine from a standard dropper are placed in a clean test-tube and 10 drops of water are then added. One special Clinitest reagent tablet is dropped into the test-tube whereupon a boiling reaction takes place. Fifteen seconds after boiling has ceased (not before) the tube is shaken. If sugar is present the fluid will change colour, turning green, orange or dark brown according to the amount of sugar present. If sugar is not present the fluid remains blue.

The reagent tablets readily absorb moisture, which turns them blue, so that care must be taken to keep them dry. It is essential to use only white reagent tablets in the test; never use a tablet that has turned blue. Also, as the reagent tablets contain caustic soda they should be handled with care.

(*b*) *Benedict's* test may be used instead of the Clinitest. Five millilitres of Benedict's reagent, which is a clear blue colour, are placed in a test-tube to which 8 drops of urine are added. The mixture is then boiled for two minutes. It is important that adequate boiling be carried out as, if not, small amounts of sugar will be missed. A green, yellow, orange or brick-red precipitate forms, according to the amount of sugar present. A brick-red precipitate denotes a large quantity of sugar.

(*c*) The *Clinistix* test is a specific test for glucose in urine. It merely shows, however, whether sugar is present or not as it is not a quantitive test like the Clinitest or Benedict's. To carry out the test the test end of the Clinistix strip is dipped in the urine, or alternatively the end is moistened with a drop of urine. If sugar is present the moistened end turns blue in about one minute. If a blue colour does not develop, sugar is absent.

The presence of any appreciable amount of sugar in the urine is in most cases due to the disease diabetes mellitus. In the early stages of diabetes, however, the symptoms may not be characteristic and suggestive of the disease, although sugar is usually present in the urine. Failure to make a routine test for sugar in all patients may therefore mean that the diagnosis of diabetes will be missed.

6. Tests for Ketone Bodies.

Ketone bodies (acetone and diacetic acid) usually occur in the urine in the following conditions :—

(a) Diabetes mellitus (and are always present in diabetic coma).
(b) Excessive vomiting.
(c) Acute febrile states in children.
(d) Starvation.

TEST FOR ACETONE (Rothera's Test).—To 5 to 10 ml. of urine in a test-tube about an inch of ammonium sulphate crystals is added and the mixture thoroughly shaken. After all the ammonium sulphate has dissolved, more is added until some excess remains, i.e., until there is a saturated solution. To this solution are added one or two crystals of sodium nitro-prusside. The mixture is then thoroughly shaken to dissolve the crystals. Lastly, strong ammonium is added, and if acetone is present a mauve or purple colour (which takes a few minutes to develop fully) will appear.

TEST FOR DIACETIC ACID.—Gerhardt's ferric chloride test is used. To 5 ml. of urine ferric chloride is added, drop by drop. If diacetic acid is present a deep port wine or claret colour develops. This colour, however, may also develop if substances like aspirin or salicylates are present. To distinguish therefore between the presence of diacetic acid and that of drugs such as aspirin, a second sample of urine is boiled for two minutes and ferric chloride then added. Boiling destroys any diacetic acid present, and the claret colour, if originally due to diacetic acid, will therefore not be present in the second heated specimen of urine. Boiling does not, however, destroy the colour due to aspirin or salicylates.

ACETEST.—This is an alternative, simple and reliable test for acetone. One of the special acetest reagent tablets is placed on a clean, dry surface. One drop of urine is carefully dropped on to the tablet. If the urine contains acetone the tablet will change colour within thirty seconds, the result varying from lavender to deep purple according to the amount of acetone present. If, at the end of thirty seconds, the colour of the tablet remains unchanged, the urine does not contain acetone.

7. Tests for Blood.

If blood is present in any quantity it is obvious to the naked eye as it colours the urine red. Lesser amounts of blood produce a typical *smoky* appearance. If only small amounts of blood are present the colour of the urine, while dark, may not be diagnostic. The most reliable test for blood is therefore by microscopic examination, when the actual red cells may be seen.

Occultest.—This is a simple reliable test for blood in the urine. One drop of urine is placed on a piece of filter paper and the special reagent occultest tablet is put in the centre of the moist area. Two drops of water are now placed on the tablet and if the paper immediately surrounding the tablet turns blue within two minutes the test is positive for blood in the urine.

Blood in the urine is called **hæmaturia.** Causes of hæmaturia include the following :—

(*a*) Calculi (stones) in the kidney, ureter or bladder.

(*b*) Acute nephritis (where the urine is usually smoky).

(*c*) Trauma.

(*d*) Tumours of the renal tract.

(*e*) Infection.

(*f*) Bacterial endocarditis (when the hæmaturia is the result of emboli in the kidneys).

(*g*) Overdosage with anticoagulant drugs (phenindione, warfarin, marcoumar, tromexan, dicoumarol, etc.).

(*h*) Sulphonamide crystals.

(*i*) Purpura and scurvy.

8. Test for Pus.

The only satisfactory examination for the presence of pus in the urine is examination under the microscope, when the pus cells can be recognised.

Pus is usually present in the urine in cases of inflammation of the renal tract, especially pyelitis, cystitis and urethritis. Tuberculosis is a less common cause.

9. Tests for Bile.

(*a*) BILE PIGMENTS.—Bilirubin is present in the urine in cases of obstructive jaundice. Urine containing bile is dark with a yellow or greenish colour. One of the simplest methods of detecting bilirubin is to shake the urine in a test-tube and if the froth is yellow bilirubin is present. Normally, in the absence of bile, the froth is white.

Ictotest.—Five drops of urine are placed on a test mat and one ictotest tablet put in the centre of the moist area. Two drops of water are placed on the tablet. If bilirubin is present in the urine, a bluish-purple colour appears on the mat around the tablet within thirty seconds. A pink or red colour is of no significance.

Apart from the bile pigment bilirubin, which is present in the urine in obstructive jaundice, another bile pigment called *urobilin* is found in the urine in cases of hæmolytic jaundice. The detection of urobilin is a more complicated procedure and is not usually performed in the ward.

(*b*) BILE SALTS.—Bile salts are usually present in the urine together with bilirubin in obstructive jaundice.

Hay's Test.—Powdered sulphur is sprinkled on the surface of the urine, and if bile salts are present the sulphur will sink to the bottom of the tube. If bile salts are not present the sulphur does not sink.

RENAL FUNCTION TESTS

Many tests have been devised in order to find out how capable the kidneys are of performing their functions. These tests, on the whole, are not extremely accurate so that often several tests are done on the same patient.

1. **Blood Urea Estimation.**—Normally the urea content of the blood remains at a fairly constant level, between 20 and 40 mgm. per cent. One of the main functions of the kidneys is to excrete urea, which is the waste product of protein. In any kidney disease urea may accumulate in the blood giving higher values than the normal. The drawback to estimation of blood urea as a kidney function test is that the kidney has to be fairly severely damaged before the blood urea rises. Nevertheless, it is a very important investigation and is carried out in most renal diseases as a measure of renal function.

2. **Urea Concentration Test.**—This test is fairly easily carried out and measures the ability of the kidneys to concentrate urea in the urine. The patient has nothing to drink from 10 P.M. on the night before the test is carried out. At 6 A.M. the next morning the bladder is completely emptied and 15 gm. of urea are given to the patient to drink. At 7, 8 and 9 A.M. the bladder is emptied completely; the specimens of urine are then clearly labelled 1, 2 and 3 and sent to the laboratory for estimation of the urea content. Normally the

concentration of urea should be 2 per cent. or above in at least one specimen.

3. **Urea Clearance Test.**—This is a more refined test of kidney function, but if it is to have any value the necessary specimens must be collected with great care. For this test the urine is collected at the end of each of two consecutive one-hour periods and a sample of blood is taken for urea estimation, *e.g.*,

9 A.M.   Bladder emptied *completely* and urine discarded.

10 A.M.   Bladder emptied *completely* and the whole of the specimen of urine sent to the laboratory.

11 A.M.   Repeat as for 10 A.M.

Blood urea taken between 10 and 11 A.M.

It is essential that the complete urine specimens with the exact time at which they were passed be sent to the laboratory. From the urea content of the blood and urine and the volume of urine passed a measure of the renal function can be estimated, the results being usually expressed as percentages of normal.

4. **Urine Concentration and Dilution Test.**—This is a fairly simple test of the ability of the kidneys to concentrate and dilute, and is relatively accurate. The patient has nothing to eat or drink from the previous evening, and at 7, 8 and 9 A.M. the next day complete specimens of urine are collected. Two pints of water are given at 9 A.M., and the complete specimens of urine passed at 10 and 11 A.M. and 12 mid-day are then also collected. Normally the specific gravity of the earlier specimens should be high (1,020 or above), showing that the kidneys can retain water in the body when the patient is fasting. Conversely, when the 2 pints of water are given, normal kidneys should excrete the excess water, thereby producing a dilute urine with a low specific gravity in the region of 1,005.

NEPHRITIS

Nephritis, or Bright's disease, is a very common disease of the kidneys. It is an inflammatory disease of which the exact cause is unknown, but it usually follows a streptococcal infection, so that generally there is a history of acute tonsillitis, scarlet fever or other streptococcal lesion before the onset of acute nephritis.

Types.—Nephritis can be divided into two different types or stages :—

          (A) Acute.   (B) Chronic.

(A) ACUTE NEPHRITIS

Symptoms and Signs.

1. The patient is generally a child or young adult, and quite

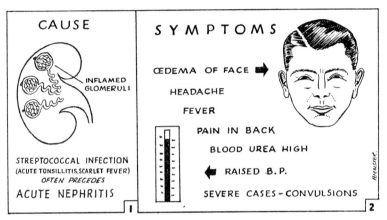

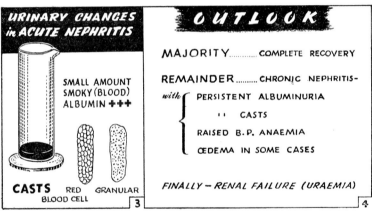

Fig. 137
Acute nephritis.

often has had a sore throat or an attack of scarlet fever about seven to ten days before. The onset is fairly sudden with :—

    (*a*) Fever.   (*c*) Pain in the back.
    (*b*) Headache.   (*d*) Vomiting.

2. The presence of **œdema** is typical, particularly in the face (especially around the eyes) and in the ankles. It tends to be worse

in the morning and better in the evening. (This œdema should be contrasted with the œdema of heart failure, which never occurs in the face and is worse in the evening and better in the morning.) The œdema gives the patient a characteristic bloated appearance.

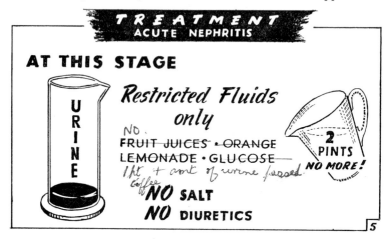

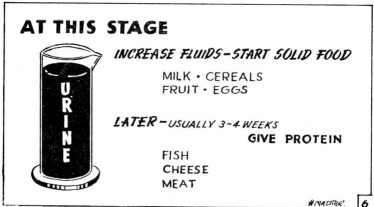

FIG. 138

In severe cases fluid may accumulate in the pleural cavity (pleural effusion) or the peritoneal cavity (ascites).

3. URINARY CHANGES.—These are fairly constant, and are most important as they denote the degree and severity of the kidney damage.

(*a*) There is diminished output of urine (oliguria). In very severe cases very little urine may be passed.

(*b*) The urine is dark, concentrated and often smoky in colour from the presence of blood (hæmaturia).

(*c*) Albumin is always present, usually in very heavy amounts.

(*d*) Casts (which can be seen under the microscope) are present. Red blood cells and granular casts are the types of cast most frequently present in the acute stage of nephritis. Casts, when present in any number, are always evidence of severe kidney disease, particularly nephritis.

4. The blood pressure is usually raised, and in severe cases may

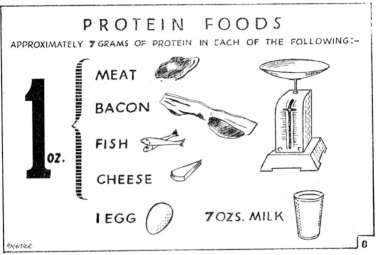

Fig. 139

be extremely high, with severe headaches, vomiting and perhaps convulsions (*hypertensive encephalopathy*).

Course.—Most patients with acute nephritis recover completely, but a small percentage become chronic. In the majority of cases of chronic nephritis, however, there is no history of an acute attack, the cases presenting themselves as chronic from the start.

Treatment of Acute Nephritis.

1. REST.—The patient is nursed at complete rest in a warm well-ventilated room. Bed rest is continued until all the symptoms have gone and the urine is free of red blood cells and, if possible, of albumin also. As, however, in some patients the albumin persists indefinitely in the urine (the acute nephritis going on into the chronic stage) it may not be possible to keep all patients in bed till the urine is completely normal.

2. DIET.—Because of the need to rest the diseased kidneys as much as possible, perhaps the most important item in the treatment of acute nephritis is the diet. As most of the work of the kidneys consists of excreting the waste products of protein, as little protein as possible is given in the vital early days. In addition, owing to the presence of œdema, fluids and salt are restricted.

To carry out these principles of diet an initial period of starvation is necessary, when only 1 pint a day of sweetened orange juice, lemon juice or barley water is given, with perhaps some toffee. Nothing else is given until the kidneys begin to recover, the signs of this being an increased output of urine and the lessening or disappearance of blood from the urine. In most cases a *diuresis* sets in after a few days and the diet can then be increased by the addition of bread, butter, cereals, milk and puddings. Eggs, fish, cheese and meat are gradually added later with the continued improvement of the patient.

It is important to realise that an initial starvation period followed by a very limited protein diet (usually in the region of 40 gm.) is of the utmost value in resting the kidneys; if, however, there is no improvement in the urinary findings after two or three weeks this low protein diet must be increased in order to supply sufficient protein (70 to 90 gm.) to build up the patient's general nutritional state.

An *intake and output chart* must be kept for all patients, and the urine examined daily for albumin, red cells and casts. The bowels are kept open by means of a suitable aperient, but excessive purgation does no good and only distresses the patient.

3. COMPLICATIONS.—The convulsions seen in severe cases are treated by sedatives such as chloral hydrate, paraldehyde or barbiturates. If the blood pressure is very high the rapid withdrawal of a pint of blood is often very useful in relieving the strain on the heart.

4. INFECTIVE FOCI.—As stated earlier, acute nephritis often follows a streptococcal infection (tonsillitis, scarlet fever, otitis media, etc.) and therefore penicillin may be given to treat the infection.

TYPE I AND TYPE II ACUTE NEPHRITIS

These terms are often used to distinguish between two forms of acute nephritis. Type I acute nephritis is most commonly seen in young children after a streptococcal infection. The course of the illness is abrupt with marked general symptoms and obvious hæmaturia and œdema at the onset. The prognosis of this type of acute nephritis is very good and most patients recover completely. In contrast, in Type II acute nephritis, there is an insidious onset; a preceding streptococcal infection is often absent, and hæmaturia is minimal. Œdema, however, is often a marked feature and persists. In this type of acute nephritis the outlook is not as good and most patients develop chronic nephritis.

(B) CHRONIC NEPHRITIS

The minority of cases of acute nephritis which do not completely clear up pass on into the chronic stage of nephritis, wherein permanent renal damage is present. As mentioned earlier, however, many cases of chronic nephritis are met with in which there is no history of a previous acute attack.

Symptoms and Signs.—The course of chronic nephritis is extremely variable as the disease may show itself in various ways.

1. THE LATENT STAGE.—In this type the presence of chronic nephritis may be discovered by a routine examination of the urine, which reveals the presence of albumin and casts. There may be no symptoms or merely a general feeling of being run down. Anæmia is a fairly constant feature, and in many cases the blood pressure is raised.

2. ŒDEMATOUS STAGE.—Many cases of chronic nephritis have œdema at some stage or other. In some patients the œdema may be very mild and escape notice, while in others the œdema is a predominating feature (nephrotic form of chronic nephritis). The œdema occurs in the face and legs, and in very severe cases a pleural effusion and ascites may also be present. In addition, very heavy albuminuria is a constant finding in the œdematous stage of chronic nephritis, and it is this continued loss of protein from the blood that mainly accounts for the massive œdema.

3. STAGE OF RENAL FAILURE.—Here the symptoms are those of chronic uræmia, with weakness, vomiting, drowsiness and eventually coma. The blood urea is extremely high as is also the blood pressure. Uræmia is more fully described later (p. 417).

Treatment.

1. IN THE LATENT STAGE.—Here, where there are few or no symptoms and there is no evidence of renal failure, *e.g.*, the blood urea is normal, no very active measures are called for. The patient is encouraged to carry on with his normal work as far as possible, although excessive fatigue and exposure must be avoided. A normal well-balanced diet is given, with perhaps a slight restriction in the amount of protein. Fruit and vegetables should be taken in sufficient quantities to supply the necessary vitamins and minerals. The anæmia must be treated with iron.

2. IN THE ŒDEMATOUS STAGE.—If this is at all severe the patient

is best nursed in bed until the œdema has completely or almost completely disappeared. The diet in this stage is very important.

(*a*) Salt must be curtailed as much as possible as salt tends to retain water in the body and thus to increase the œdema.

(*b*) In the œdematous stage there is a continued loss of protein in the urine, which plays a large part in causing the œdema. For this reason a moderately high (100 to 125 gm.) protein diet is often given. It is possible to give a high protein diet in most cases in

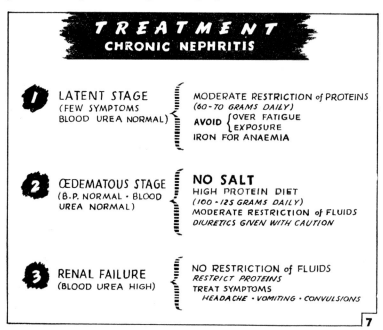

FIG. 140

the œdematous stage of chronic nephritis because the blood urea is normal, showing that there is no gross evidence of renal failure.

If the œdema does not respond to a low salt and high protein diet, diuretics are given. Chlorothiazide (saluric) is a most valuable diuretic as it is potent, can be given by mouth and, unlike the mercurial diuretics (mersalyl), does not cause renal damage. Saluric is given in 0·5 to 1 gm. doses twice daily for three to five days a week.

Instead of chlorothiazide, similar preparations such as hydro-chlorothiazide or hydroflumethiazide may be used, but in smaller doses of 25 to 50 mgm. as they are much more potent. A careful watch must be kept for signs of the salt depletion syndrome (see p. 461) and for potassium deficiency (see p. 462). Mercurial diuretics are not used as they can cause renal damage.

(c) If the œdema does not diminish with the above treatment, cortisone or allied drugs (prednisone, prednisolone or ACTH), which have yielded good results in some patients, may be tried.

3. STAGE OF RENAL FAILURE.—At this stage palliative treatment to relieve the symptoms (headache, vomiting, convulsions) only is possible. As the blood urea is high the protein in the diet must be restricted (40 gm. daily), but since there is usually little or no œdema fluids are not limited.

Chronic nephritis usually runs a prolonged course. The most essential factors in the treatment are, therefore, provision of a suitable diet varying, as described above, according to the stage of nephritis present; the avoidance, as far as possible, of intercurrent infections which may cause an acute exacerbation of the nephritis and appropriate modification of the patient's daily work to suit his state of health.

HYPERTENSIVE KIDNEY DISEASE

In discussing Hypertension (p. 128) it was noted that whilst the majority of cases of hypertension end in congestive heart failure or cerebral hæmorrhage a small number develop uræmia. Severe kidney damage, ending in uræmia, is particularly common in the very severe and rapidly progressive form of essential hypertension known as *malignant* hypertension (to distinguish it from the more common form called *benign* hypertension). The treatment of renal failure due to hypertension is as outlined under Uræmia.

URÆMIA

Uræmia is the term used to describe the condition of renal failure. Uræmia can be conveniently divided into two forms: (A) Chronic Renal Failure and (B) Acute Renal Failure.

(A) CHRONIC RENAL FAILURE

Causes.

1. Chronic nephritis.

2. Hydronephrosis, due to chronic obstruction of the renal tract. This obstruction may take the form of:—

(a) Enlarged prostate.   (b) Bilateral calculi.

(c) Urethral stricture.

3. Hypertensive kidney disease.

14

Symptoms and Signs.

1. The onset of symptoms in chronic uræmia is usually very gradual, and in the early stages the main features are a general fatigue and exhaustion usually accompanied by anæmia. As the renal failure progresses the patient becomes increasingly and excessively drowsy and more acute symptoms develop.

2. Vomiting and diarrhœa are frequently present and *hiccoughing* is often a predominant feature.

3. The drowsiness lapses into a coma in the terminal stages, and twitchings developing into convulsions may occur.

4. The breathing is usually laboured, and in the late stages the waxing and waning type of respiration (Cheyne-Stokes) is usually present.

5. The total output of urine is usually normal or even increased. Albumin is usually present to some extent, thus denoting the presence of a kidney lesion, but in some cases the amount may be small.

6. Well-marked changes in the retina of the eye (*retinitis*) are present in most cases of uræmia, and the patients usually complain of dimness of vision. White patches (exudates), hæmorrhages and swelling of the optic disc are the common findings when the retina is examined by an ophthalmoscope.

7. In most cases the blood pressure is raised.

8. The blood urea is markedly elevated and the presence of a high blood urea in conjunction with the above symptoms confirms the diagnosis.

Treatment.—As there is no cure for chronic uræmia, treatment is entirely palliative.

(B) ACUTE RENAL FAILURE (Acute Anuria)

Although the outlook in most cases of established chronic renal failure is extremely bad and any treatment is merely palliative, this is far from being the case with acute renal failure.

Causes.

1. Severe toxic poisons causing acute intense damage to the kidneys. Mercurial poisons are especially prone to cause severe kidney damage.

2. Acute obstruction within the kidney tubules resulting from the deposit of crystals during sulphonamide therapy.

3. Mismatched blood transfusions.   The agglutinated (clumped) red cells obstruct the kidney tubules.

4. Severe shock.   Here the blood pressure may fall so low that the blood flow through the kidneys practically ceases, and as a

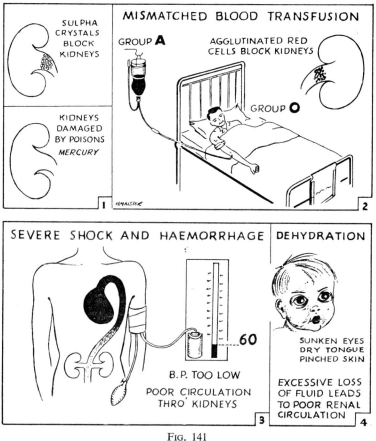

SULPHA CRYSTALS BLOCK KIDNEYS

MISMATCHED BLOOD TRANSFUSION

GROUP **A**

AGGLUTINATED RED CELLS BLOCK KIDNEYS

GROUP **O**

KIDNEYS DAMAGED BY POISONS MERCURY

HMALSTER

SEVERE SHOCK AND HAEMORRHAGE

DEHYDRATION

60

B. P. TOO LOW

POOR CIRCULATION THRO' KIDNEYS

SUNKEN EYES DRY TONGUE PINCHED SKIN

EXCESSIVE LOSS OF FLUID LEADS TO POOR RENAL CIRCULATION

FIG. 141

The causes of acute renal failure (acute anuria).

result little or no urine is formed.   The severe shock may be caused by injury (serious crushing injuries are for some reason especially liable to cause acute renal failure), by severe hæmorrhage or by overwhelming toxic infections.

5. Severe dehydration, with its excessive loss of fluid from the body, may result in markedly reduced blood circulation

through the kidneys, with a consequential cessation of urinary secretion.

The fundamental change resulting from all the causes of acute renal failure is a sudden cessation of urinary output. In all cases the kidneys, previously normal, are suddenly prevented from performing their prime function of secreting urine in order to excrete the waste products of metabolism.

Symptoms and Signs.—The cardinal sign of acute renal failure is thus the complete, or almost complete, suppression of urine—**anuria.** In the early stages the few ounces of urine passed may contain frank blood, especially in the cases caused by mismatched transfusions and sulphonamides. In the severe cases complete anuria develops and may last for as long as seven to ten days, after which time the kidneys in many cases recover and begin to secrete urine. If after ten to fourteen days urinary secretion does not recommence sudden death is likely to occur.

In the first few days of the anuria the patient may have few symptoms and the general condition may remain good. After five or six days, however, vomiting usually starts and the patient's general condition slowly deteriorates, with perhaps increasing drowsiness and in some cases twitching and convulsions. With the sudden onset of diuresis the patient will make a rapid recovery or, alternatively, with no diuresis may die.

Treatment of Acute Anuria.

1. *Prevention.*

(*a*) Sulphonamide Cases.—The importance of adequate fluid intake (4 to 6 pints) in all patients on sulphonamides has been repeatedly stressed. A sudden fall in urinary output or the occurrence of hæmaturia calls for the immediate stoppage of the drug.

(*b*) Mismatched Transfusions.—The carrying out of all the essential preliminaries before giving a blood transfusion will prevent these cases. Blood grouping, giving blood of the same group and, in addition, cross-matching the patient's serum against the donor's red cells are the essential preliminaries to all blood transfusions.

When a blood transfusion is started a very close watch must be kept on the patient to make sure that there are no severe reactions. If by mistake incompatible blood is given, as little as an ounce of such blood may be enough to make the patient complain of severe shivering, restlessness, nausea and pain in the back. The skin is cold, the pulse and temperature rise and the patient becomes shocked. In the presence of any of these symptoms, the transfusion must immediately be stopped and the doctor notified.

It must be stressed that giving correctly matched blood to every

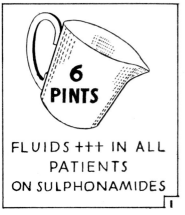

FLUIDS +++ IN ALL
PATIENTS
ON SULPHONAMIDES

1

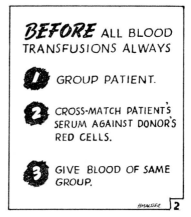

BEFORE ALL BLOOD
TRANSFUSIONS ALWAYS

1 GROUP PATIENT.

2 CROSS-MATCH PATIENT'S SERUM AGAINST DONOR'S RED CELLS.

3 GIVE BLOOD OF SAME GROUP.

HMALSER 2

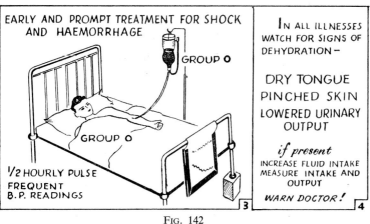

EARLY AND PROMPT TREATMENT FOR SHOCK AND HAEMORRHAGE

GROUP O

GROUP O

½ HOURLY PULSE
FREQUENT
B. P. READINGS

3

IN ALL ILLNESSES
WATCH FOR SIGNS OF
DEHYDRATION —

DRY TONGUE
PINCHED SKIN
LOWERED URINARY
OUTPUT

if present
INCREASE FLUID INTAKE
MEASURE INTAKE AND
OUTPUT

WARN DOCTOR! 4

FIG. 142
The prevention of acute anuria.

patient is the only way to prevent transfusion reactions (see p. 377).

(*c*) SHOCK.—In all cases of shock, with its low blood pressure and diminished blood circulation to the organs and tissues, early and adequate transfusions with blood (or serum) will prevent acute renal failure. The essential aim in cases of shock is to raise the blood pressure enough (at least above a systolic reading of 100 mm.

of mercury) to ensure an adequate circulation of blood to all organs and tissues.

(*d*) DEHYDRATION.—The provision of an adequate fluid intake in all illness has been repeatedly mentioned. With severely ill patients, especially children and elderly people, the nurse must not only provide adequate fluids but see that the patient takes them. Accurate measurement of the urinary output, which should reach 40 to 50 oz. a day, will enable the nurse to see whether sufficient fluids are, in fact, being taken. In addition, the presence of a dry tongue and pinched skin (in infants the sunken fontanelle and sunken eyes are further signs) means that sufficient fluids are not being taken.

2. *Curative.*—Once anuria has developed it means that the kidneys are severely damaged and the aim in treatment is to rest the kidneys as much as possible until recovery begins. As there is no chronic damage to the kidneys, if the patient can be tided over the acute phase the outlook is good.

DIET AND FLUIDS.—To rest the kidneys as completely as possible protein is reduced to an absolute minimum whilst the fluid intake too is kept at the lowest level necessary for metabolism. Sufficient fluid is given to counterbalance the loss from the skin and lungs (about 500 to 800 ml.) with, in addition, a further amount of fluid equal in quantity to any urine passed. Usually about one pint of water is given with 200 to 300 gm. of glucose. If possible this amount of fluid and glucose is given by mouth, if necessary by an intragastric drip. If, however, persistent vomiting prevents the required amount of fluid and glucose from being taken by mouth, then it must be given intravenously. As so large a concentration of glucose will inevitably cause thrombosis in a small vein, a polythene tube is passed into a large vein like one of the venæ cavæ.

Saline is not given unless blood tests (estimation of the blood chlorides) reveal that the sodium chloride (salt) in the blood is depleted. The excessive vomiting which may be present can lead to a dangerous fall in the blood chlorides. On the other hand, to give salt, either by mouth or intravenously as saline, if there is no depletion of the salt in the body, will give rise to œdema of the lungs and tissues. Salt depletion requiring the administration of salt by mouth is likely to arise in the post-anuric period when large amounts of salt may be lost in the urine.

Frequent estimations of blood potassium are necessary throughout the course of the illness. In the anuric stage, potassium may accumulate in the blood giving rise to signs of potassium intoxication (marked lethargy, weakness and heart damage as revealed by a slow and irregular pulse : a careful watch must always therefore be kept on the pulse). If potassium intoxication occurs glucose and insulin are usually given. Ion-exchange resins, which absorb potassium from the intestines, are also often tried.

In patients not responding to this treatment, hiccough, lethargy, vomiting and even convulsions are ominous signs of uræmia. Recourse may now be made to the artificial kidney, and the patients have to be moved to special hospitals for this purpose. Blood is taken from the patient and is anticoagulated to prevent clotting. The blood is now passed through the artificial kidney apparatus which by a process of dialysis removes urea, potassium and other toxic substances before the blood is returned to the patient.

PYELITIS

Inflammation of the pelvis of the kidney, called pyelitis, is a common disease. In some cases the inflammation may spread to involve the kidney substance itself, whereupon the term *pyelonephritis* is used.

Causes.—The inflammation is usually due to infection by *B. coli* organisms. Less often it is caused by streptococci and staphylococci. Any obstructing lesion in the renal tract is likely to increase the liability to infection and so to pyelitis. Pyelitis also tends to occur commonly in infancy and during pregnancy.

Symptoms and Signs.

1. The onset is most sudden, with pyrexia, shivering attacks (rigors) and headache.

2. Acute severe pain is felt in the loin of the affected side. The pain sometimes radiates downwards and forwards to the groin as in renal colic.

3. Frequency of and pain on micturition are fairly constantly present.

4. The urine always shows albumin and pus cells. Culture of the urine reveals the infecting organism.

Treatment.

1. The patient is nursed in bed and all the routine measures as for an acute fever are carried out. The diet should be light, but abundant fluids are necessary, especially as the patient is usually

treated with sulphonamides. If rigors occur tepid sponging should be performed.

2. DRUGS.—The specific treatment of pyelitis is to give sulphonamides, which are very effective with most patients. Sulphadimidine (sulphamezathine), sulphatriad or sulphamethizole (urolucosil) are all very useful and are given as described on page 575. In a few resistant cases additional therapy may be required to eradicate the infection. In these cases, sensitivity of the infecting organism to the various antibiotics is tested in the laboratory and the appropriate antibiotic is then given. Streptomycin, chloramphenicol, the tetracycline antibiotics and nitrofurantoin (furadantin) are frequently used in the treatment of pyelitis which has proved resistant to sulphonamide therapy.

CYSTITIS

Inflammation of the bladder is called cystitis, and is frequently due to organisms similar to those causing pyelitis. Cystitis is more frequently seen in females (where the infection often spreads from inflammation of the pelvic organs). Cystitis is also especially likely to arise where there is any obstruction or other disease in the bladder, such as stones, tumours or enlarged prostate. In diseases of the central nervous system, paralysis, causing incontinence or retention of urine, is very prone to set up infection in the bladder. Repeated catheterisation, necessary in cases of retention, is particularly liable to cause cystitis. Finally, such specific diseases as gonorrhœa and tuberculosis may cause a cystitis.

The symptoms of cystitis are chiefly pain and frequency of micturition; the urine contains albumin, pus and the infecting organisms. In the acute stage fever and rigors may be present.

The treatment is similar to that of pyelitis with sulphonamides or antibiotics. In addition, any primary disease predisposing to cystitis must be dealt with. The need for the utmost care in achieving adequate asepsis in carrying out all catheterisations must be stressed.

One of the commonest complications causing death in a case of paralysis with retention of urine is an infection of the bladder which spreads to the kidneys (*pyelonephritis*).

TUBERCULOSIS OF THE URINARY SYSTEM

Tuberculosis may affect one or both kidneys and the infection may spread to involve the bladder. In advanced cases of renal tuberculosis large, multiple, tuberculous abscess cavities develop.

Symptoms and Signs.—The most common symptom is frequency of micturition, which is usually very severe and persistent. The patients pass urine in very small amounts throughout the day and night. Hæmaturia is also commonly present. Pain in the loins and on micturition is often complained of. There are usually general symptoms, including malaise, loss of appetite and fever.

The diagnosis is usually made by finding the tubercle bacilli in the urine. For this a twenty-four hour specimen of urine must be collected as the organisms are present in very scanty numbers. X-ray examination (*pyelography*) may show some deformity of the kidneys, such as distortion of the outline of the calyces.

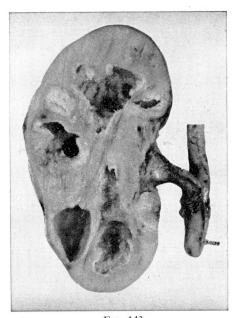

Treatment.—When the disease is localised in one kidney surgical removal of the affected organ is usually carried out. Before and after operation chemotherapy with streptomycin, isoniazid and para-aminosalicylic acid is given. In bilateral renal tuberculosis, surgery is not usually possible,

FIG. 143

Tuberculosis of the kidney. The progressive caseation has produced widespread cavitation.

and for these patients only chemotherapy and the usual general measures to build up the patient's resistance are possible.

NON-SPECIFIC URETHRITIS (Reiter's Syndrome)

Cause.—Unknown.

Incidence.—Fairly common; usually occurs in young adult males. The disease may occur in association with bacillary dysentery.

Symptoms and Signs.—There are three distinct groups of symptoms:—

1. Urethritis, with a purulent urethral discharge.

2. Arthritis. The joint changes are very similar to those of rheumatoid arthritis. The ankles, knees and hands are chiefly affected.

3. Eye lesions. Conjunctivitis is usually present but occasionally iritis may develop.

Course and Treatment.—Pyrexia and general malaise usually accompany the above signs. After several weeks the disease usually clears up without any specific treatment.

RENAL CALCULI

Renal calculi, or stones, are very common, but as they are usually fully described in surgical textbooks only a brief mention is necessary here.

Renal calculi may remain silent in the kidney and cause no

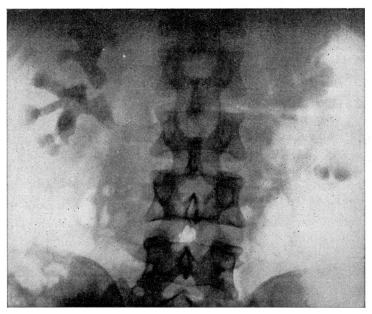

FIG. 144
Renal calculus. Typical staghorn stone in the right kidney.

symptoms; on the other hand, they may move and give rise to **renal colic.** Here severe pain occurs causing restlessness, sweating and vomiting. The pain characteristically starts in the loin and

Fig. 145

Hydronephrosis of the kidney showing the dilatation of the pelvis and calyces. The multiple stones causing the obstruction and consequent dilatation can be seen.

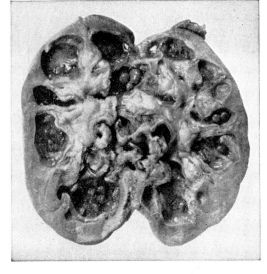

Fig. 146

Retrograde pyelography. The calyces and pelvis of the right kidney are normal. In the left kidney a large tumour has caused marked distortion of the calyces and pelvis.

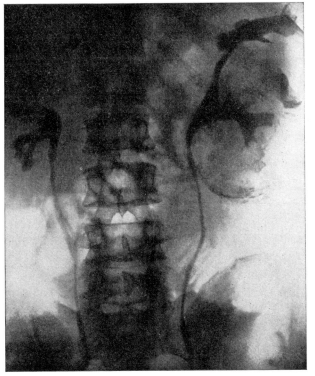

radiates downwards and forwards to the groin. The urine usually contains albumin and blood.

Renal calculi in addition to causing colic can obstruct the kidney and so lead to dilatation and distension (**hydronephrosis**). If the hydronephrosis is severe the kidney loses its power to function properly. (Not only calculi but also any obstruction, such as an enlarged prostate, can cause hydronephrosis.)

X-ray examination after administration of an opaque dye (pyelography) usually reveals the dilated hydronephrotic kidney.

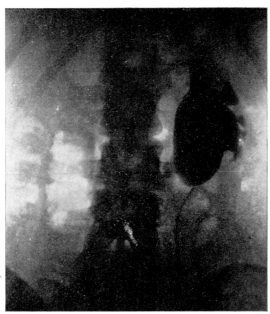

Fig. 147
Hydronephrosis of the left kidney, outlined
by retrograde pyelography.

The treatment of renal calculi, where these are causing symptoms, is operative removal. Small stones, however, are frequently passed in the urine. In cases where there is a severe hydronephrosis with a poorly functioning kidney the affected kidney is usually removed (nephrectomy), the fact that the opposite kidney is normal having first been established.

CHAPTER XIII

DISEASES OF THE DUCTLESS GLANDS

T HE name *ductless glands* is given to a series of small glands which are situated in various parts of the body and form specific secretions which are poured directly into the blood stream. These glands are also called the endocrine glands.

The specific secretions of these glands are called **hormones,** and any alteration in the amount of a hormone produced has in many cases a profound effect on the body. Some of these glands are extremely important and are commonly the site of disease.

The main endocrine glands which are frequently affected by disease and which produce important effects on the body are the :—

      (A) Pituitary Gland.
      (B) Thyroid Gland.
      (C) Adrenal Glands.
      (D) Parathyroid Glands.
      (E) Pancreas.
      (F) Ovaries and Testes.

(A) PITUITARY GLAND

Anatomy and Physiology.—This gland is often known as the *master gland* as various of its secretions, of which it has very many, directly affect the functions of many of the other glands. The pituitary is a small gland situated within the skull and is divided into two main divisions, or lobes, the anterior and the posterior.

The Hormones of the Anterior Lobe.

1. THE GROWTH HORMONE.—An excess of this hormone gives rise to gigantism in young people and acromegaly in older people. Lack of the growth factor causes various forms of dwarfism.

2. SEX HORMONES.—There are various hormones which have a direct effect on reproduction which is also intimately linked with ovarian function.

3. ADRENOCORTICOTROPHIC HORMONE (ACTH).—This hormone stimulates the cortex of the adrenal glands. Deficiency of ACTH is seen in Simmonds' disease of the pituitary. Many of the features of

Simmonds' disease are similar to those of Addison's disease of the adrenal cortex, in which there is a deficiency of cortisone.

4. THYROTROPHIC HORMONE.—This hormone stimulates the activity of the thyroid gland. Deficiency of the thyrotrophic hormone occurs in Simmonds' disease of the pituitary, and for this reason many of the signs of Simmonds' disease resemble those seen in thyroid deficiency (myxœdema).

DISEASES OF THE PITUITARY

GIGANTISM

If overactivity or an actual tumour of the cells of the anterior pituitary which produce the growth hormone develops in childrɛn before the epiphyses of the bones unite, the result is the formation of giants. Several instances of giants reaching 8 or 9 ft. are known. In many cases, however, these giants lose their excessive strength and develop signs of increased intracranial pressure (headaches, vomiting, blindness and coma) from growth of the tumour.

ACROMEGALY

Oversecretion of the growth hormone arising after the epiphyses of the bones have united leads to the condition known as acromegaly. There is no increase in height, but nevertheless characteristic changes occur in the bones, *i.e.*, the lower jaw becomes massive and the whole contour of the face broadened, whilst the hands and feet become excessively wide, usually being described as spade-like. In addition to the above changes, the skin becomes thick and coarse and the tongue hypertrophied.

If a tumour is responsible for the acromegaly, signs of increased intracranial pressure may gradually develop as a result of growth of the tumour. In these cases surgical removal may be carried out. In cases of acromegaly with no signs of tumour there is no specific treatment of any value.

SIMMONDS' DISEASE

Simmonds' disease is also known by several other names, *e.g.*, pituitary cachexia, Sheehan's syndrome and pituitary dwarfism.

The underlying lesion is a deficiency of most of the pituitary hormones: this leads to disordered function of many of the other ductless glands, especially the adrenal and thyroid glands. As a result many of the symptoms of Simmonds' disease are

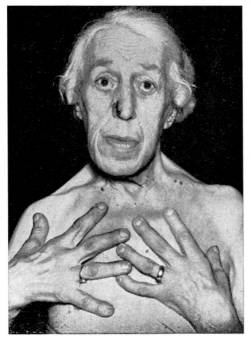

FIG. 148
Acromegaly showing the enlargement of the
lower jaw and hands.

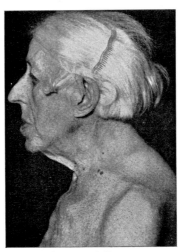

FIG. 149
Acromegaly showing the enlargement
of the lower jaw.

very like those of deficiency of the adrenal gland (Addison's disease) or of the thyroid gland (myxœdema).

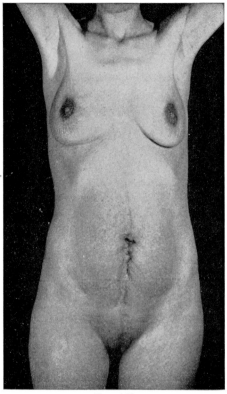

FIG. 150

Simmonds' disease showing the lack of axillary and pubic hair.

Causes.

1. Post-partum necrosis of the pituitary. Thrombosis or hæmorrhage of the pituitary are most often seen in cases of difficult labour—usually those associated with severe hæmorrhage. This form of Simmonds' disease is by far the commonest.

2. Tumour.

3. Injury.

Symptoms and Signs.

1. Wasting. In very severe cases wasting is very marked, but in milder cases (which are the more common) wasting is not always a noticeable feature.

2. Loss of sexual functions with amenorrhœa and atrophy of the genital organs.

3. Marked loss of energy with dull, sluggish mentality. In advanced cases mental changes supervene.

4. Dry, wrinkled skin and loss of axillary and pubic hair. The appearance is one of premature senility, particularly in young people.

5. Very low blood pressure and basal metabolism.

Diagnosis.—In advanced cases, especially the post-partum cases where there is a history of difficult labour with hæmorrhage, the diagnosis is usually obvious owing to the wasting, appearances of senility and loss of axillary and pubic hair. In less severe cases the clinical picture of Simmonds' disease may resemble that of Addison's disease or myxœdema.

Treatment.—Treatment of Simmonds' disease is not always satisfactory, but cortisone, in small doses by mouth (12·5 to 50 mgm.) has produced a marked improvement in many patients. In addition to cortisone, other hormone therapy is often needed, such as thyroid, œstrogens and testosterone.

CUSHING'S DISEASE

Cushing described a syndrome of obesity, excessive growth of hair of masculine distribution, purple striæ on the abdomen (similar to those seen in pregnancy), amenorrhœa in women and hypertension. In Cushing's first cases the cause of this syndrome was ascribed to a tumour of the basophil cells of the pituitary. It is now known that a picture very similar to that of Cushing's disease is caused by tumours or hyperfunction of the adrenal cortex and by tumours of the ovaries or testes. Indeed, the majority of cases are due to adrenal cortical hyperplasia or tumours (see p. 449).

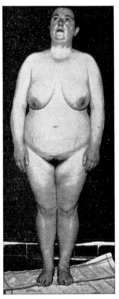

Fig. 151

Cushing's syndrome showing the typical obesity.

DWARFISM

Dwarfism (or infantilism as it is also called) may be due, as already mentioned, to a lack of the hormones of the anterior lobe of the pituitary, resulting usually from tumours or unknown causes. Various types of dwarfism occur owing to pituitary lesions, such as Fröhlich's syndrome, of which the main features are those of obesity and sexual under-development. Prematurely senile dwarfs (Simmonds' disease of children) is another variety.

It should be realised, however, that pituitary diseases account for only a minority of the causes of dwarfism and it is convenient here to classify briefly the main causes of dwarfism.

1. Chronic Infections in Early Childhood.

    (*a*) Congenital syphilis.   (*b*) Chronic nephritis.

2. Metabolic and Deficiency Diseases.

    (*a*) Rickets (deficiency of vitamin D).

    (*b*) Cœliac disease (disordered fat metabolism).

3. Bone Diseases.
   (a) Achondroplasia (" clowning circus dwarf ").
   (b) Microcephaly (under-development of the brain and skull).
4. Ductless Gland Diseases.
   (a) Pituitary diseases.
   (b) Cretinism (lack of thyroid hormone in infants).
5. Congenital Heart Disease.
6. Unknown Causes.
   Dwarfism due to unknown causes includes the common type of dwarfism seen in circus dwarfs, who appear to be perfectly normal except for the stunted growth.

DISEASES OF THE POSTERIOR LOBE

The only disease commonly recognised as being due to changes in the posterior lobe of the pituitary is **diabetes insipidus.** One of the main secretions of the posterior lobe of the pituitary is the antidiuretic hormone. In diabetes insipidus there is a lack of this hormone with the result that these patients pass tremendous quantities of urine which is characteristically very pale and of a low specific gravity. These patients commonly complain of thirst. It should be noted that in diabetes insipidus, as opposed to the other form of diabetes, diabetes mellitus, the urine does not contain any sugar.

Treatment.—The deficient hormone is given either by injection (vasopressin) or in the form of a nasal snuff.

(B) THYROID GLAND

Anatomy and Physiology.—The thyroid gland is situated in the neck and comprises two lobes, one on each side of the trachea, joined by a middle portion called the isthmus. It is made up of cells which produce one important hormone called thyroxine. The main function of this hormone is to control metabolism in the body. Excess of the hormone leads to a general overactivity of bodily function and produces the condition of thyrotoxicosis (hyper-thyroidism).

In most cases of thyrotoxicosis the thyroid gland becomes enlarged, and the term *goitre* is used to describe such enlargement. in addition, however, to toxic goitre, *i.e.*, goitre associated with thyrotoxicosis, enlargement of the thyroid without oversecretion of the thyroid hormone also occurs—non-toxic goitre.

Undersecretion of the thyroid hormone causes a lowering of bodily function, which in adults causes the disease myxœdema and in children cretinism.

One of the main substances required for the manufacture of the thyroid hormone is iodine.

DISEASES OF THE THYROID GLAND

GOITRE

There are various forms of goitre or enlargement of the thyroid :—

1. SIMPLE (NON-TOXIC) GOITRE.—This form of goitre is not associated with oversecretion of the thyroid hormone and there-fore there are no signs of thyrotoxicosis.

2. TOXIC GOITRE.—This type of goitre is accompanied by signs of overactivity of the thyroid hormone. It takes two forms :—

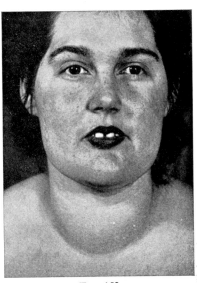

(a) Primary diffuse toxic goitre (exophthalmic goitre or Graves' disease).

(b) Nodular toxic adenoma.

3. MALIGNANT GOITRE.

1. Simple (Non-toxic) Goitre.

This is a common con-dition, especially in some areas where it is almost endemic. It is believed that in these areas this type of goitre is due to lack of iodine in the water.

FIG. 152
Simple (non-toxic) goitre.

It is very prevalent in Switzer-land, parts of America and in certain regions of England, such as Derbyshire. It is also commonest at certain periods of life, e.g., at puberty and during pregnancy. In most cases little treatment is needed as the goitre usually subsides of its own accord. Preventive treatment has been used in many endemic areas and has definitely succeeded in lowering the incidence of this type of goitre. The treatment consists of adding a small quantity of iodine to ordinary table salt.

In some cases, however, a non-toxic goitre may persist and eventually cause trouble. It may grow so large that it is unsightly: or it may cause pressure symptoms, such as difficulty in breathing and stridor: or it may become toxic in later life and so cause damage, particularly to the heart; whilst finally, there is the possibility of these long-standing non-toxic goitres becoming malignant.

Whenever non-toxic goitre persists into later life the question of its removal by operation must be considered. Any signs of the development of toxic symptoms or, of course, of pressure symptoms will call for operation.

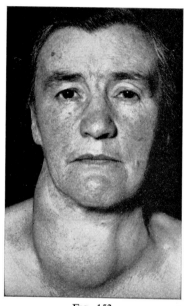

Fig. 153

Non-toxic goitre. The goitre was removed because it was causing pressure symptoms.

2. Toxic Goitre (Thyrotoxicosis).

When swelling of the thyroid gland (goitre) appears in conjunction with oversecretion of the thyroid hormone it is known as toxic goitre. There are two main types of toxic goitre, but the symptoms of toxicity are practically the same in both. The primary diffuse type (which is also known as *Graves' disease* or *exophthalmic goitre*) occurs in younger people and causes generalised diffuse enlargement of the gland. In the nodular toxic adenomatous type (which usually occurs in older people) the gland is not diffusely enlarged: instead, one or more adenomata develop causing a nodular goitre. Toxic adenomatous goitre in particular (probably because it affects older people) damages the heart.

Symptoms and Signs of Toxic Goitre (Thyrotoxicosis).—Thyrotoxicosis is due to oversecretion of the thyroid hormone, the general effect of which is to increase metabolism throughout the body. The symptoms and signs of thyrotoxicosis are as follows :—

(*a*) Patients usually complain of general nervousness, irritability, being on edge and a feeling of anxiety.

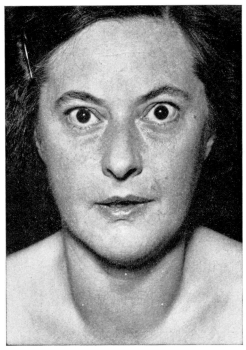

FIG. 154

Primary toxic goitre (Graves' disease) showing the characteristic staring, apprehensive expression and the enlarged thyroid.

(*b*) There is usually continuous loss of weight although the patient has a good appetite. This is an important point, as most diseases which cause loss of weight are associated with a poor appetite. (The only other common cause of severe loss of weight with a good appetite is diabetes mellitus.)

(*c*) Sweating is usually a marked feature and the patient normally dislikes hot weather.

(*d*) There is a fine tremor of the fingers, best seen when the hands are outstretched.

(*e*) Exophthalmos. This is a term used for the characteristic protrusion or prominence of the eyes which is most often caused by thyrotoxicosis, and especially by the primary type (Graves' disease). A characteristic " staring " expression is often present. Lagging of the upper eyelid on looking down is also a useful sign.

(*f*) Tachycardia. A persistently fast pulse rate is one of the marked features of thyrotoxicosis. In most cases the heart rate is

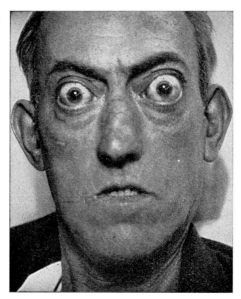

FIG. 155
Severe exophthalmos in a case of primary
toxic goitre (Graves' disease).

regular, but auricular fibrillation commonly occurs in elderly patients suffering from the toxic nodular form of goitre. In severe cases heart failure may develop, and thyrotoxicosis is in fact one of the known common causes of congestive heart failure.

(*g*) Attacks of diarrhœa and vomiting may occur in the more severe cases. The enlarged thyroid gland can usually be seen or felt in the neck.

Diagnosis.—In the presence of such typical symptoms as wasting, sweating, tremor, exophthalmos and tachycardia, together with enlargement of the thyroid gland, the diagnosis is easy. In less obvious cases a *basal metabolism test* is often performed to confirm the diagnosis. This is a measure of the amount of oxygen the body uses up when at rest and is markedly increased in thyrotoxicosis.

In addition, radioactive iodine (I^{131}) is used in the diagnosis of thyrotoxicosis (as also in myxœdema). A small tracer dose of radioactive iodine is given and all the urine passed for the next forty-eight hours carefully collected. In thyrotoxicosis the amount of iodine excreted in the urine is very low as the overactive gland takes up so much iodine. The converse is true in myxœdema, where there is an abnormally high output of radioactive iodine in the urine.

Treatment.—Treatment can be divided into two main groups—medical and surgical.

MEDICAL TREATMENT.

(*a*) *Antithyroid Drugs.*—These drugs reduce the activity of the thyroid gland and are therefore frequently used in the treatment of toxic goitre. The drugs in most frequent use are carbimazole (neo-mercazole) and thiouracil. Carbimazole is less toxic than thiouracil and is given in initial doses of 10 mgm. three times a day and in maintenance doses of 5 to 15 mgm. daily. Thiouracil is given in initial doses of 200 to 400 mgm. and in maintenance doses of 50 to 100 mgm. daily. Potassium perchlorate may also be used, usually at a dose of 800 mgm. daily.

The main toxic reactions from antithyroid drugs are :—

(i) Agranulocytosis, where there is a marked reduction in the number of polymorphonuclear white blood cells. In severe forms this may prove fatal.

(ii) Marked increase in the size of the goitre.

(iii) Drug rashes, often resembling measles.

The main danger is agranulocytosis, and if a patient who is on antithyroid drugs complains of a sore throat the drug must be stopped immediately and a white blood cell count performed to confirm the diagnosis. A sore throat is an early symptom of agranulocytosis (see p. 391).

Antithyroid drugs are most useful in patients with thyrotoxicosis where the gland is small and smooth.

(*b*) *Radioactive Iodine.*—Treatment with radioactive iodine is usually very successful. As, however, it is not certain that after such treatment malignancy will not develop in the gland after a period of 15 to 20 years, radioactive iodine is at present usually given only to patients with toxic adenoma who are over the age of

45 and not fit to undergo surgery. Radioactive iodine is also used in the treatment of malignant goitre. Complicated apparatus for adjusting the dose of radioactive iodine is required, so that this treatment is possible only at special hospitals.

SURGICAL TREATMENT.—Surgical treatment is probably best in all cases of toxic adenoma (as opposed to Graves' disease). It is also necessary in all cases which have been treated medically and have failed to respond, and in cases where the goitre is causing pressure symptoms.

The aim of surgical treatment is to remove the larger portion of the gland, leaving only enough to prevent the development of myxœdema.

Except for very mild cases, patients with toxic goitre are usually given a short pre-operative course of carbimazole so as to reduce toxicity. Alternatively, Lugol's iodine may be used. Unlike carbimazole, however, Lugol's iodine loses its effect after a few weeks so that it is only used as a pre-operative measure and has no part in long-term medical treatment.

When carbimazole is used as a pre-operative measure the drug must be discontinued two weeks before the operation and replaced by Lugol's iodine, 5 minims twice a day. If carbimazole is not discontinued before the operation excessive hæmorrhage from the gland during the operation is liable to occur.

3. Malignant Goitre.

Some cases of toxic goitre, particularly the toxic adenoma, may become malignant. In these cases the goitre is very hard and often painful. Malignant goitre is very likely to cause local pressure symptoms, such as dyspnœa, stridor and dysphagia. Thyroid carcinoma is also liable to spread and so cause secondary growths, which are especially common in the bones.

The treatment is surgical removal of all the thyroid if possible. Treatment by radioactive iodine is sometimes usefully combined with surgical removal of the thyroid gland.

DISEASES DUE TO DEFICIENCY OF THE THYROID HORMONE

It has already been stated that the main function of the thyroid hormone is to control metabolism in the body and that oversecretion of the hormone causes a great increase in metabolism with well-marked physical changes (thyrotoxicosis). Similarly, undersecretion of the thyroid hormone causes a lowering of bodily function which is seen in two diseases, myxœdema in adults and cretinism in infants and young children.

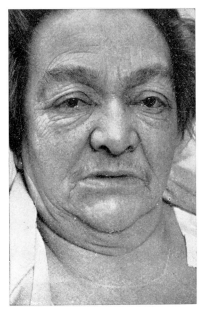

FIG. 156

Myxœdema showing the characteristic puffy and bloated appearance. The condition developed after thyroidectomy for a toxic goitre. (The scar in the neck is still visible.)

MYXŒDEMA

Causes.

1. Removal of the thyroid gland in the treatment of thyrotoxic and malignant goitre.

2. Primary atrophy of the gland, of unknown cause.

Symptoms and Signs.

1. A general increase in weight is an early and fairly constant feature and extreme obesity may eventually develop.

2. Skin changes, with coarse thickening of the skin and a puffiness almost like that due to œdema, are very common. The

skin, however, although very puffy does not actually pit on pressure as in true œdema.

3. The hair tends to fall out.

4. The pulse is usually slow.

5. The patients have a very dull and sluggish mentality and often a defective memory. They easily become tired.

6. Constipation is a marked feature.

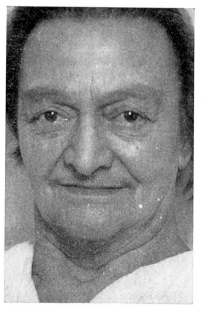

FIG. 157

Myxœdema after thyroid therapy showing the marked improvement. (Same patient as Fig. 156.)

The whole appearance of the patient—an obese person, with puffy bloated face, dry skin and scanty hair and of dull sluggish mentality—is fairly characteristic, especially in advanced cases. A basal metabolism test will reveal a marked lowering of the basal metabolic rate, thus confirming the diagnosis.

A radioactive iodine excretion test (see p. 439) is also helpful in the diagnosis of myxœdema.

Treatment.—Thyroxin or thyroid extract is given orally. The dose of thyroxin is 0·1 mgm. or less initially, and this is gradually increased as necessary. Signs of overdosage with thyroid extract are excessive loss of weight, tachycardia, sweating and diarrhœa.

CRETINISM

Causes.—Cretinism is usually due to an atrophy of the thyroid gland which is itself of unknown cause. It is especially common

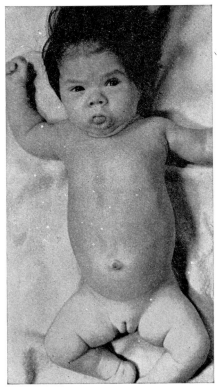

FIG. 158

Cretin, aged 8 months. The appearance with the thick protruding tongue is typical, as is also the umbilical hernia.

in districts where goitre is very frequently found, and in many cases the mother has a goitre. Lack of iodine is undoubtedly a factor.

Symptoms and Signs.

1. The infant is usually normal at birth, but symptoms begin to appear within six months.

2. There is a failure of growth, both physical and mental. If the condition is allowed to continue unrecognised and untreated the child becomes a mentally deficient dwarf.

3. The infant is of very ugly appearance, with a flat depressed

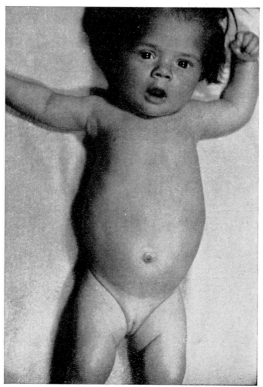

FIG. 159
Same patient as Fig. 158. Three months after
starting thyroid therapy.

nose, dry skin and scanty hair. The hands become thick and spade-like. The tongue is very thick, coarse and wide, and is constantly protruded through the open mouth.

4. The abdomen is usually distended (pot belly) and an umbilical hernia is often present.

Diagnosis.—Cretinism must be distinguished from the other causes of mental deficiency and stunted growth (see Dwarfism, p. 433).

Treatment.—It is most important that cretinism should be recognised as early as possible as early treatment can result in a complete cure. If, however, treatment is delayed too long then some permanent mental deficiency may remain. As in myxœdema,

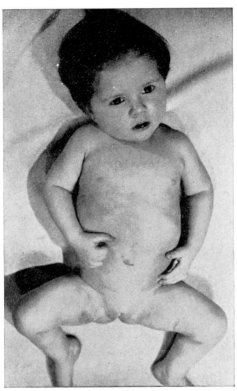

Fig. 160

Same patient as Fig. 158. Eleven months after starting treatment: the child's health is now normal.

thyroxin is prescribed though naturally in much smaller doses applicable to a child.

(C) ADRENAL GLANDS

Anatomy and Physiology.—The adrenal or suprarenal glands are divided into two main parts, the cortex and medulla.

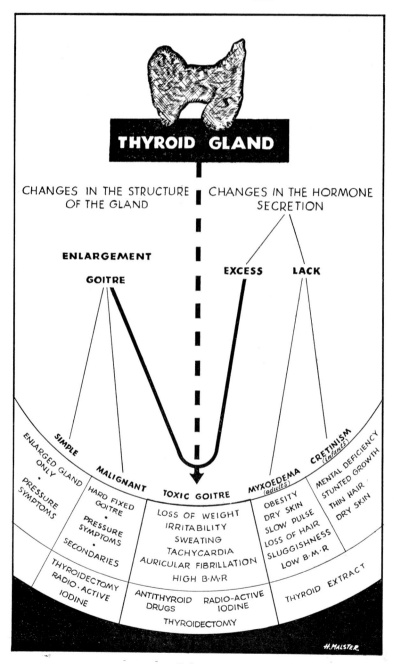

FIG. 161

Diagram showing the main symptoms and signs and treatment
in diseases of the thyroid gland.

THE CORTEX.—The adrenal cortex secretes many different hormones, which can be classified as follows :—

1. Hormones affecting carbohydrate metabolism. These are cortisone and hydrocortisone. They raise the blood sugar level by converting protein into glucose.

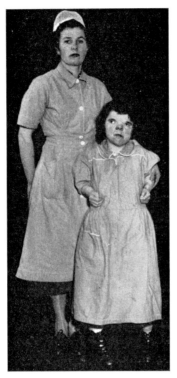

FIG. 162
Untreated cretin, aged 36 years.
She was an idiot.

2. Hormones regulating mineral metabolism. The main hormone of this group is aldosterone, which causes the retention of sodium and chloride and thereby the retention of water. It also causes the excretion of potassium. (Deoxycortone acetate is a synthetic hormone which has a similar action.)

3. Sex hormones. These include the various androgenic hormones, which have a masculinising effect and also tend to cause bodily growth. The other main sex hormones are the œstrogens.

Corticotrophin (ACTH) is the pituitary adrenocorticotrophic hormone which stimulates the adrenals to produce cortisone and allied hormones.

THE MEDULLA.—The medulla secretes two hormones, adrenaline and noradrenaline, which have very powerful effects and are used in the treatment of several diseases (see p. 586).

DISEASES OF THE ADRENAL CORTEX

1. Addison's disease, which leads to lack of the several hormones which deal especially with the regulation of the various salts in the blood.

2. Hyperplasia or tumours, which lead to overproduction of the hormones.

ADDISON'S DISEASE

Causes.

1. Tuberculous disease producing wide destruction of the gland.

2. Atrophy of the gland of unknown cause.

Symptoms and Signs.

1. There is profound weakness which, in later stages, may be so severe that the patient is unable to get about. Wasting is also a fairly early feature.

2. There is a characteristic pigmentation of the skin and mucous membranes. Dark purplish patches are often seen on the lips, in the mouth and around the nipples. The pigmentation may also be more generalised and brownish in colour.

3. Nausea, with attacks of diarrhœa and vomiting, is very frequent.

4. A diagnosis of Addison's disease is not usually made with a systolic blood pressure reading of over 100 mm. of mercury.

5. When the blood is examined it will be found that there are many typical changes present. The amount of sodium and chloride is usually diminished and the potassium raised, especially during the acute stages. The fasting blood sugar is often low.

6. Estimation of the amount of 17-hydroxcorticoids excreted in the urine is usually performed and is helpful in the diagnosis. 17-hydroxcorticoids are hormones produced in the adrenal glands and normally excreted in the urine. In Addison's disease, the urinary excretion of 17-hydroxcorticoids is very low in men and almost absent in women.

Course.—Remissions occur when, for no apparent reason, the patient's symptoms subside, but nevertheless untreated cases usually die in a few years. Severe exacerbations or " crises " occur from time to time. Crises are usually precipitated by exposure to cold, by even a mild infection or by taking drugs. During a crisis there is usually a high fever, severe vomiting, profound weakness and signs of dehydration and shock. The patient may die during a crisis.

Treatment.

1. Many patients with Addison's disease can be maintained in good health on small doses of cortisone or hydrocortisone; 12·5 to 37·5 mgm. of cortisone or 10 to 30 mgm. of hydrocortisone daily are usual doses.

2. In some patients 0·1 mgm. of fludrocortisone (florinef) can be taken daily in addition to cortisone to maintain normal salt metabolism.

3. TREATMENT OF AN ACUTE ADRENAL CRISIS.—The patient is put on an hourly pulse chart and frequent blood pressure readings are taken. The foot of the bed should be raised. Intravenous hydrocortisone is given as soon as possible: 100 mgm. eight-hourly the first day and 50 mgm. six-hourly the second day. This dose is gradually reduced. An intravenous saline drip is usually necessary in the initial stages because of the severe vomiting: food by mouth is not usually tolerated, but as soon as the patient can take food a light diet is given.

The prevention of adrenal crisis is most important and the patient should be warned to avoid chills if possible and to obtain prompt treatment for even the mildest infection.

ADRENAL CORTICAL HYPERPLASIA AND TUMOURS

Both hyperplasia of the adrenal cortical cells and cortical tumours cause an oversecretion of the various hormones produced by the adrenal cortex. As mentioned earlier (p. 447) some of these hormones affect carbohydrate and mineral (salt and water) metabolism, whilst others regulate sexual characteristics. The clinical picture of hyperfunction or oversecretion of the adrenal cortex will vary according to which of these hormones predominate. The following syndromes are chiefly seen :—

1. Cushing's Syndrome.
2. Adrenogenital Syndrome (Virilism).

15

1. Cushing's Syndrome.

In this syndrome there is an excessive production of cortisone and, to a lesser extent, of sex hormones.

(*a*) The condition is most commonly seen in women. The predominant change is a peculiar obesity which mainly affects the trunk and face (" moon face ") but spares the limbs. Purple striæ develop on the abdomen and thighs.

(*b*) Marked weakness occurs and mental changes such as depression are frequent.

(*c*) Diabetes may develop with sugar in the urine. The blood pressure is usually raised.

(*d*) Increased growth of hair on the face (*hirsutism*), acne of the skin and amenorrhœa are all commonly seen.

(*e*) Softening of the bones (osteoporosis) causing fractures is not unusual.

Diagnosis.—When cortisone is produced in the body by the adrenal cortex, it is eventually broken down and excreted in the urine as 17-hydroxcorticoids. In Cushing's disease there is a marked increase (above 20 mgm. in twenty-four hours) of 17-hydroxcorticoids measurable in the urine.

Treatment.—Operative treatment is usually carried out in most cases of Cushing's syndrome. If a tumour is present it is removed ; if hyperplasia is present, bilateral subtotal or total adrenalectomy is usually done, often with very good results.

2. Adrenogenital Syndrome (Virilism).

Here, there is chiefly an excessive secretion of the sex hormones, although the other adrenal cortical hormones may also be affected. For this reason a " mixed " picture of Cushing's syndrome and the adrenogenital syndrome is often met with.

(*a*) The most predominant signs are seen in women, who develop masculine characteristics with excessive growth of hair on the face (hirsutism). The voice deepens and muscular development resembles that of a man. The sex organs undergo striking changes, with enlargement of the clitoris. Amenorrhœa is present and acne of the skin is also a feature.

(*b*) In adult males there may be few striking changes, but generally the picture is similar to that described under Cushing's syndrome.

(c) In young boys there is very early sex development with growth of hair on the face, enlargement of the penis and pronounced muscular growth—pseudo-sexual precocity.

(d) If excessive adrenal activity occurs in intrauterine life it produces in girls the picture of virilism plus pseudo-hermaphroditism with abnormality of the urogenital organs. The child may be mistaken for a boy. Pre-natal adrenal cortical oversecretion in boys causes marked enlargement of the external genitalia.

Diagnosis.—The various tests as outlined under Cushing's syndrome are usually carried out and similar findings are noted.

Treatment depends on whether an actual tumour or merely hyperplasia is present. Tumours, which are more likely to be present in adults than in children, are removed. If hyperplasia only is present, as is probable in young children, cortisone is given and this will suppress the activity of the adrenals.

DISEASES OF THE ADRENAL MEDULLA

PHÆOCHROMOCYTOMA (Paraganglioma)

The only disease known to affect the adrenal medulla is a tumour called a phæochromocytoma. This tumour produces an excess of the normal secretion of the medulla—adrenaline. The main effect of this overproduction of adrenaline is severe hypertension, which characteristically occurs in paroxysmal attacks. During these attacks the patient complains of very severe headaches, sweating and vomiting, and the blood pressure is markedly raised.

In the diagnosis of phæochromocytoma, phentolamine (rogitine) is injected intravenously and if a tumour is present a marked drop in blood pressure usually occurs, whereas in essential hypertension no marked reduction occurs. In phæochromocytoma there is also a marked increase in the urinary excretion of catecholamines (adrenaline and nor-adrenaline), and estimation of the catecholamines in the urine is most helpful in the diagnosis of this disease.

Treatment consists of removal of the tumour.

(D) PARATHYROID GLANDS

Anatomy and Physiology.—The parathyroid glands are four in number and are situated behind the thyroid gland. The main function of the parathyroids is the regulation of the calcium and phosphorus content of the bones and blood. Therefore, to understand the changes that arise as a result of diseases of the parathyroids, it is necessary to appreciate the role that calcium plays in the body in health. The main functions of calcium are :—

1. The formation of bone. (Any disturbance in the level of calcium can lead to improper development of and deformities in the bones.)

2. The control of the irritability of muscles and nerves.

3. As a factor in the proper clotting of blood.

The proper absorption and usage of calcium is regulated in two main ways :—

1. Vitamin D controls the absorption of calcium from the bowel. Most of the calcium absorbed goes to the bones to help in their proper formation and calcification. Lack of vitamin D, as one would expect, leads to marked changes in the bones (rickets in children and osteomalacia in adults).

2. The parathyroid hormone (parathormone) regulates the flow of calcium between the bones and the blood. Excessive secretion of the hormone causes a withdrawal of calcium from the bones into the blood with the result that the bones become soft, spongy, deformed and liable to fracture. On the other hand, deficiency of parathormone leads to a low level of calcium in the blood, which causes one form of the clinical syndrome known as *tetany*. (As there are many different factors which cause tetany this disease will be described later.)

DISEASES OF THE PARATHYROID GLANDS

1. Tumours.

2. Injuries during Operations on the Thyroid Gland.

1. TUMOURS

Tumours of the parathyroid gland are rare. They lead to over-secretion of the parathyroid hormone which produces a very characteristic clinical picture known as **osteitis fibrosa cystica** or **hyperparathyroidism.**

Symptoms and Signs.

These may be divided into three main groups due to :—

(*a*) Excessive Calcium in the Blood.

(*b*) Changes in the Bones.

(*c*) Increased Excretion of Calcium by the Kidneys into the Urine.

(*a*) EXCESSIVE CALCIUM IN THE BLOOD.—This usually causes weakness and loss of appetite and weight. Generalised muscle and joint pains are common. In severe cases there may be nausea and vomiting.

(*b*) CHANGES IN THE BONES.—Owing to the excessive removal of calcium from the bones as a result of the overactivity of the parathyroid hormone the bones become soft, deformed and liable to fracture. Large cysts may occur in the bones.

(*c*) EXCRETION OF CALCIUM INTO THE URINE.—Because of the presence of excessive calcium in the urine renal calculi develop, and in severe cases blockage of the kidneys may occur with signs of renal damage and uræmia.

Diagnosis.—The diagnosis is usually made on the above symptoms and signs and by estimating the amount of calcium in the blood, which is markedly raised above normal.

Course and Treatment.—Unless the condition is treated the patients usually become bed-ridden owing to the bony deformities, and they usually die from renal failure. The treatment is to explore the parathyroid glands and remove the tumour. If this is done early a complete cure can be effected.

2. INJURIES DURING OPERATION ON THE THYROID GLAND

The condition which most commonly affects the parathyroid glands is accidental injury or removal of the parathyroids during operations on the thyroid gland. The main effect is to produce a deficiency of parathyroid hormone which results in tetany. In most cases, however, the tetany is transient and responds to large doses of calcium which raise the blood calcium level.

TETANY

In the discussion on the action of the parathyroid hormone we saw that undersecretion of this hormone can lead to a low blood calcium level and so to the condition of tetany. Tetany presents a clinical picture with characteristic symptoms and signs that develop owing to lowering of the blood calcium ; it can be caused in several different ways :—

1. By Undersecretion of Parathyroid Hormone.—This cause is rare and is usually the result of injury to or accidental removal of the parathyroids during operations on the thyroid gland.

2. By Lack of Vitamin D.—It was mentioned previously that

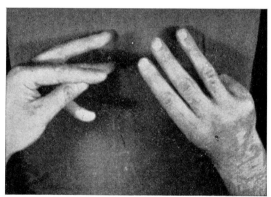

Fig. 163
Tetany showing the characteristic position of
the hands in carpopedal spasm.

vitamin D is necessary for the control of absorption of calcium from the bowel. If vitamin D is lacking, various diseases result, especially the condition known as rickets, which may also be associated with tetany.

3. By Alkalosis.—Normally, the reaction of the blood is kept at a constant level. If the blood should become too alkaline the calcium becomes altered and is not available to the body, i.e., a deficiency of calcium results with consequential development of tetany. Alkalosis can arise in several ways, e.g.,

(a) From loss of acid owing to persistent vomiting in cases of pyloric stenosis. The gastric secretion contains hydrochloric acid and if this is continuously depleted by persistent vomiting alkalosis can result.

(*b*) Excessive overbreathing leads to loss of the acid, carbon dioxide, and a resulting alkalosis with tetany. This type of tetany is commonest in hysteria.

(*c*) Excessive administration of large doses of alkalis (especially sodium bicarbonate).

Symptoms and Signs.

1. Painful cramps occur in the hands and feet. The hands take up a characteristic attitude with the thumbs pressed into the palms and the fingers hyperextended. This attitude is known as *carpopedal spasm.* Pressure on the arms will bring on the carpopedal spasms and this reaction is referred to as Trousseau's sign.

2. Convulsions, which are particularly common in children.

3. Laryngeal spasm. Sudden spasm of the larynx occurs causing cyanosis and stridor. This laryngeal spasm is called *laryngismus stridulus* and is particularly seen in the tetany of rickets.

4. Chvostek's sign. Tapping on the branches of the facial nerve in the face produces twitching of the muscles of the face. This is due to the irritability of the nerves which is present in tetany.

5. There are the signs of the disease, *e.g.*, rickets in children, pyloric stenosis and hysteria, which is associated with the tetany.

Treatment.—The immediate aim is to raise the blood calcium level and then to treat the cause of the tetany. In mild cases it is usually sufficient to give calcium by mouth in the form of calcium lactate tablets. In more severe cases calcium has to be given intramuscularly or intravenously as calcium gluconate, 5 to 10 ml.

THYMUS GLAND

The thymus gland is normally very large in infancy and becomes atrophied in adult life. The exact function of this gland is not known. Diseases of the thymus gland are rare and imperfectly understood. Sudden death in infants, accompanied by stridor and asthma, has often been ascribed to an enlarged thymus, but it is doubtful if this was the cause. The rare disease known as myasthenia gravis is often associated with an enlarged thymus or thymic tumour. Removal of the thymus is sometimes performed for myasthenia.

SUMMARY OF SOME ROUTINE PROCEDURES UNDERTAKEN
IN DISEASES OF THE DUCTLESS GLANDS

1. **Basal Metabolic Rate.**

   (a) To confirm the diagnosis of thyrotoxicosis, wherein the basal metabolic rate is raised.

   (b) To confirm the diagnosis of myxœdema, wherein the basal metabolic rate is lowered.

2. **Blood Calcium.**

   (a) In all cases of tetany, where a low blood calcium is often present.

   (b) Parathyroid tumours, where a high blood calcium is present.

3. **Blood Cholesterol.**

   In cases of myxœdema, where a high blood cholesterol can confirm the diagnosis.

4. **Blood Sodium.**

   In Addison's disease low sodium content confirms the diagnosis.

5. **Estimation of 17-hydroxycorticoids and Ketosteroids in the Urine.**

   Increased excretion of these hormones in the urine is found in some tumours and in hyperplasia of the adrenal glands.

6. **Estimation of Catecholamines in Urine.**

   In the diagnosis of phæochromocytoma, where there is a marked increase in urinary output of catecholamines.

7. **Radioactive Iodine Urinary Excretion Test.**

   (a) In the diagnosis of thyrotoxicosis where there is a marked reduction in the excretion of radioactive iodine in the urine after a test dose.

   (b) In the diagnosis of myxœdema, where there is an increased excretion of radioactive iodine in the urine after a test dose.

SUMMARY OF IMPORTANT DRUGS USED IN DISEASES OF
THE DUCTLESS GLANDS

1. **Calcium.**

   Tetany.

2. **Carbimazole** (Neo-mercazole).

   Thyrotoxicosis.

3. **Cortisone, Hydrocortisone and Fluorohydrocortisone.**

Addison's disease.
Adrenal hyperplasia.
Simmonds' disease.

4. **Deoxycortone Acetate (DCA).**

Addison's disease.

5. **Lugol's Iodine.**

Before thyroidectomy.

6. **Œstrogens.**

Simmonds' disease.

7. **Phentolamine** (Rogitine).

Phæochromocytoma.

8. **Radioactive Iodine.**

Thyrotoxicosis.
Carcinoma of the thyroid.

9. **Salt.**

Addison's disease.

10. **Testosterone.**

Simmonds' disease.

11. **Thiouracil.**

Thyrotoxicosis.

12. **Thyroid Extract.**

Cretinism.
Myxœdema.

13. **Vasopressin** (Pitressin).

Diabetes Insipidus.

CHAPTER XIV

METABOLISM AND ITS DISORDERS

BEFORE considering the specific diseases which affect the metabolism of the body it is first necessary to understand a little about normal metabolism and how it can be upset.

The term *metabolism* is used to define the various changes which continuously take place in the body in everyday life. An example of these changes is the breakdown of foods into suitable substances which can be used by the body for the provision of energy and the repair of tissues. The metabolism of the body requires very many different factors if normal health is to be maintained.

THE ESSENTIALS OF NORMAL METABOLISM

1. Carbohydrates.
2. Fats.
3. Proteins.
4. Mineral salts.
5. Vitamins.
6. Hormones.
7. Water.
8. Normal Gastro-intestinal Tract.
9. Normal Liver and Bile.

CARBOHYDRATES

The carbohydrates are the " sugar " foods and in most normal diets form the main items eaten. The chief carbohydrates in a normal diet are :—

1. Starches (bread, cereals and potatoes).
2. Cane sugar.
3. Milk sugar.
4. Fruit.

The carbohydrates are digested to glucose by the various juices in the saliva, stomach and intestines, and it is in the form of glucose that carbohydrates are absorbed into the blood. Glucose is stored in the liver and muscles in the form of glycogen, and is reconverted into glucose when needed to supply fuel and energy for the body.

Control of Carbohydrate Metabolism.

In health the level of blood sugar is kept fairly constant. The control of carbohydrate metabolism depends on various factors, including :—

1. INSULIN.—Insulin, which is a secretion of the islets of Langerhans of the pancreas, plays a most important part in ensuring the proper use of glucose in the body. Insulin

enables the glucose both to be stored in the liver and muscles in the form of glycogen and also to be utilised as necessary.

With a deficiency of insulin, such as is met with in the disease *diabetes mellitus*, glucose is neither utilised nor stored, so that it accumulates in the blood and is excreted in the urine (glycosuria). On the other hand, too much insulin causes a fall in blood sugar, which, if severe, produces coma (insulin coma).

2. Normal liver function is essential for the proper storage of glucose (as glycogen). In some diseases of the liver the metabolism of glucose is upset.

3. Certain of the ductless glands, especially the thyroid and pituitary, play a part in glucose metabolism. Thus with overactivity of the thyroid gland, *e.g.*, in thyrotoxicosis, an excess of glucose may occur in the blood, to be excreted in the urine.

FATS

The fats, next to the carbohydrates, form the chief energy foods. The principal fats eaten in the average diet are :—

1. Butter and margarine.
2. Cream.
3. Oils and lard, as used in cooking.
4. Bacon and the fat in meat.

The amount of fat in the normal diet varies a good deal, usually according to the type of work done. Heavy manual workers require a lot of fat to give them sufficient energy.

The fats after digestion by the intestinal and pancreatic juices are absorbed into the body, which they supply with energy and heat. Fat is stored in the subcutaneous tissues, which are almost all fat, thus providing a large reserve for future energy requirements.

Factors Affecting Control of Fat Metabolism.

1. Bile is necessary for the digestion and absorption of fat, and in obstructive jaundice (in which bile is absent from the intestinal tract) there is improper absorption of fat. The fæces then become bulky and pale from excess of fat.

2. If the intestinal juices, especially the pancreatic juices, are absent the fat will not be split up into a form suitable for absorption and an excess of fat will therefore be excreted in the fæces. Absence

of the pancreatic juice is sometimes seen in infants with disease of the pancreas.

3. In some diseases, such as sprue and cœliac disease of infants, there is a deficient absorption of fat. Here again, the result is an excess of fat in the stools, which are pale and bulky. In these diseases, due to lack of proper absorption of fats, wasting and deficient growth are present.

4. In a normal diet carbohydrates and fats are the chief foods supplying energy. If the carbohydrates are not being utilised properly, e.g., as in the disease diabetes mellitus, an excessive use is made of the fats instead. Some of the final end-products of fat metabolism are, however, the poisonous acids **diacetic acid** and **acetone,** which normally are burnt down very rapidly. When, however, an excess of fats is being burnt (as in diabetes) diacetic acid and acetone accumulate in the body and the condition known as *acidosis* develops. (These acids are also known as ketone bodies, so the term *ketosis* is also used.) Ketosis (or acidosis) is commonly seen in diabetes and is the cause of diabetic coma. Ketosis is discussed further under Diabetes.

PROTEINS

Protein foods are primarily of value for the replacement of the normal wear and tear of tissues and for the growth of new tissues. Apart from this first essential function they can also be utilised, like carbohydrates and fats, as a source of energy. The main sources of proteins in a normal diet are :—

1. Meat and fish. ⎫
2. Cheese and milk. ⎬ Animal proteins.
3. Eggs. ⎭
4. Peas, beans and flour.   Vegetable proteins.

Proteins are made up of many different types of amino-acids, many of which are essential for the proper building up of the tissues of the body.

Proteins are broken down into the constituent amino-acids in the process of digestion by the pepsin and hydrochloric acid of the stomach and by the intestinal juices. The various amino-acids are then absorbed into the blood stream and distributed to the tissues.

The amino-acids which are not used for repair and building up of tissues are broken down by the liver into urea, which is excreted in the urine. The proteins, unlike the carbohydrates and fats, cannot be stored for future use.

MINERAL SALTS

To maintain good health many different minerals are essential, of which the following are some of the more important :—

1. Sodium and Chlorine.
2. Potassium.
3. Calcium.
4. Iodine.
5. Iron.

1. Sodium and Chlorine.

Salt contains sodium and chlorine, which are essential constituents of all the fluids of the body. Water is not retained in the body without salt. This is clearly seen in the case of heavy manual workers who sweat a good deal, *e.g.*, miners, stokers, and as a result lose both salt and water in the sweat. Drinking ordinary water does not, without salt, replace the lost fluid and they consequently suffer from cramps caused by the lack of fluid. Taking extra salt with water, however, overcomes the cramps.

Again, cutting out salt in the diet is one of the main steps in treating the œdema or accumulation of water in the tissues that occurs in congestive heart failure. If the body is deprived of salt the water cannot be retained and is therefore excreted. The œdema caused by the kidney disease, nephritis, is also treated by salt restriction.

In the disease of the adrenal glands known as *Addison's disease* salt metabolism is upset so that a deficiency of salt develops in the blood. This deficiency leads to a diminished amount of fluid in the body—dehydration. The dehydration can be partially corrected by giving large doses of salt.

Excessive vomiting, such as may occur in *pyloric stenosis* or *intestinal obstruction*, leads to a loss of chlorides in the vomit (gastric juice contains a large amount of chlorides), and in these conditions it is usually necessary to replace the lost chlorides as well as the fluid. In these cases saline is usually given.

Salt Depletion Syndrome.—As mentioned earlier, salt restriction is most important in the treatment of œdema, especially in cardiac and renal œdema. The present-day therapy of œdema with strict salt restriction combined with intensive use of potent diuretics can, however, lead to a severe fall in the body salt with serious results. The early recognition of salt depletion in all patients on a rigid salt-free diet, especially where diuretics and ion-exchange resins are also used, is most important. The signs are :—

(a) The patient becomes lethargic and drowsy and complains of marked weakness.

(b) Appetite is lost and nausea and vomiting may be present.

(c) There is severe reduction in urinary output and in the excretion of urinary chlorides.

(d) Abdominal and muscular cramps are sometimes present.

(e) Œdema may be, and often is, present.

(f) The blood pressure falls.

(g) The blood sodium is severely reduced. The blood urea is raised.

2. Potassium.

Potassium is an important constituent of all tissue cells. Disturbances in potassium metabolism have been increasingly recognised in recent years. Excess of potassium in the blood (hyperkalæmia) occurs to any significant degree only in conditions associated with severe oliguria or anuria (see p. 422) and in the crises of Addison's disease. Symptoms of potassium excess include marked weakness and mental confusion, numbness and tingling of the extremities. Heart block develops with a slow and irregular pulse and finally cardiac arrest occurs.

Potassium depletion (hypokalæmia) is more commonly met with than potassium excess. The causes of potassium depletion are :—

(a) With the prolonged use of diuretics in large doses.

(b) It may develop in any disease or condition with a prolonged low food intake and especially when there is, in addition, excessive intake of sodium. Thus, after major operations, prolonged intravenous saline therapy combined with diminished food intake, is very liable to cause potassium deficiency. Similarly, this deficiency may arise in the recovery stage of diabetic coma, owing to the diminished food intake, intravenous saline therapy and, in addition, the excessive loss of potassium in the urine.

(c) Excessive vomiting and diarrhœa, especially where there is an inadequate diet.

(d) Ion-exchange therapy, by absorbing the potassium in the intestines, can lead to severe potassium depletion.

The symptoms of potassium depletion include severe lethargy and weakness, mental confusion, abdominal distension and finally respiratory and cardiac failure. Potassium depletion is corrected by giving potassium chloride, 8 gm. in divided doses by mouth. In very severe cases intravenous potassium may be necessary.

In prolonged treatment with such potent oral diuretics as the chlorothiazide group of drugs, especially when large doses are given, potassium supplements may be prescribed as a routine to prevent potassium depletion. A most careful watch must be kept on all patients, particularly elderly patients, who are on prolonged therapy with chlorothiazide or similar diuretics and are not eating, as it is in these circumstances that potassium (and sodium) depletion may easily develop.

Potassium deficiency greatly enhances the action of digitalis. Digitalis overdosage is therefore very liable to occur in patients being treated with digitalis and chlorothiazide at the same time. Particular care must therefore be taken to note any signs of digitalis overdosage, and if seen, the dose of digitalis must be reduced.

3. Calcium.

Calcium, which is mainly present in milk and cheese, is essential for health, especially for :—

> (a) Formation of the bones.
> (b) Formation of the teeth.
> (c) Proper functioning of nerves and muscles.

It can be seen, therefore, that the requirements for calcium are likely to be greatest in childhood (the period of growth), and for adults during pregnancy and lactation. For this reason disturbances in calcium metabolism are most often seen during these times of extra need.

Control of Calcium Metabolism.

(a) VITAMIN D.—Vitamin D is necessary for the proper absorption of calcium from the bowel, so that lack of this vitamin causes a deficiency of calcium in the body with consequential effects on the bones. In infancy and early childhood, when there is a great demand for vitamin D, a lack of this vitamin causes the disease known as **rickets,** of which predominant signs are changes and deformities of the bones. In adults a lack of vitamin D is seldom seen except in pregnant women in tropical countries. Here the poor diet and social customs may cause a marked deficiency of vitamin D leading to the disease *osteomalacia*. Osteomalacia causes bone changes similar to those seen in rickets.

In some cases of rickets the lack of calcium may be so great as to lead to a fall in the level of calcium in the blood. Low blood calcium causes the condition known as **tetany** with its irritability of the nerves and muscles.

(*b*) PARATHYROID GLANDS.—Disturbances of the normal hormone secreted by the parathyroid glands (parathormone) have a marked effect on calcium metabolism. Excess of parathyroid hormone, which occurs in tumours of the glands, causes the calcium to leave the bones. The calcium in the blood rises and an excess of calcium is excreted in the urine.

On the other hand, lack of parathyroid hormone causes a fall in blood calcium and is therefore another cause of tetany. Lack of parathormone leading to tetany is occasionally seen after thyroidectomy if the parathyroid glands have been accidentally damaged or removed during the operation.

4. Iodine.

Iodine is essential for the formation of the hormone of the thyroid gland. It is normally found in many foodstuffs, but the amount depends on the soil and water. Soil and water in areas far from the sea, especially hilly areas, may lack iodine, and thus the inhabitants of such areas often suffer from iodine deficiency. Iodine deficiency causes one form of **goitre.**

5. Iron.

Hæmoglobin, which is present in the red blood cells and which is essential for the carriage of oxygen throughout the body, is mainly made up of iron. Therefore, in the absence of sufficient iron there is a deficiency of hæmoglobin resulting in an iron-deficiency anæmia.

Deficiency of iron is usually due to insufficient intake, excessive bleeding or inadequate absorption. Iron is mainly found in meat, liver, eggs, peas and beans, and a diet which does not contain enough of these foods will lead to an iron-deficiency anæmia.

In infants whose sole diet is milk, which has a poor iron content, anæmia is common. In women continued heavy loss of blood in the menstrual flow frequently results in an iron-deficiency anæmia.

The absorption of iron depends on, amongst other things, the presence of hydrochloric acid in the stomach. If there is no acid in the gastrtc juice (achlorhydria) this predisposes to an iron-deficiency anæmia. There is in fact a common anæmia called simple achlorhydric anæmia which is seen in women, where the additional factor of blood loss from menstruation is present.

In addition to the above mineral salts many others are essential for health, but as these others are very rarely lacking, and therefore are not associated with disease, they will not be discussed here.

VITAMINS

These important factors, present in various foods, are fully discussed elsewhere (p. 496).

HORMONES

Hormones, the secretions of the ductless glands, are described under diseases of these glands. Many of these hormones have a profound effect on the body metabolism :—

1. Thyroid Hormone. Deficiency causes stunted growth and sluggish metabolism (cretinism and myxœdema).
2. Pituitary Hormones. Deficiency of the growth hormone causes lack of growth (dwarfism). Excess of the growth hormone causes gigantism and acromegaly.
3. Adrenal Cortical Hormones. Deficiency causes upset in salt and carbohydrate metabolism (Addison's disease).
4. Parathyroid Hormone. Regulates the flow of calcium to and from the bones.

The remaining hormone which plays a most important part in metabolism is the secretion of the islet cells of the pancreas, known as insulin. As this is so important it is discussed at length under Diabetes Mellitus.

WATER

Water makes up nearly 70 per cent. of the total body-weight. It is taken into the body either as fluid or in the solid foods, which themselves contain a considerable amount of water. The amount of water needed in twenty-four hours is approximately 5 pints (2,500 ml. approximately).

Water leaves the body in the following ways :—

1. Through the lungs in the expired air.
2. Through the fæces, which contain a small amount of water.
3. Through the skin, in the sweat.
4. Through the kidneys, in the urine.

The amount of water which leaves the body via the skin and kidneys varies ; the greater the loss through the skin (as seen in very hot conditions) the smaller the excretion by the kidneys. This is part of the body's mechanism to save water. The excessive loss by the skin in high temperatures is a reaction to cool the body and so prevent a rise in body temperature. In very hot conditions, *e.g.*, stoking in an engine room, as much as 15 pints of water can be lost in the sweat in a day.

The body also makes use of the above methods of excretion of water (especially by the kidneys) to get rid of waste products. If, therefore, excretion through the kidneys is very severely diminished these waste products can accumulate in the blood stream with serious effects. This is discussed below under Dehydration.

THIRST.—This is one of the ways in which the body shows that it requires more fluid. The essential mechanism operates by decreasing the flow of saliva thus causing dryness in the mouth. This sets up the sensation of thirst in the nerves on the back of the tongue. Certain drugs, such as atropine, by producing a diminished flow of saliva cause thirst. Excess of salt in the food also causes a dryness in the mouth and consequent thirst.

DISTURBANCE OF WATER BALANCE

1. Deficiency of Water in the Body—Dehydration.
2. Excess of Water in the Body—Œdema.

1. Deficiency in the Body—Dehydration.

Dehydration can be caused by an insufficient intake of water or, more often, by excessive loss of water. Excessive loss of water is seen in the following conditions :—

(*a*) Excessive heat resulting in marked sweating. Dehydration caused through excessive loss of water by sweating is usually seen in stokers or miners, who have to carry out heavy manual work in extremely hot conditions. The loss of water and also of salt (which is present in the sweat) causes stokers' or miners' cramps. Other more serious effects of dehydration are also seen.

(*b*) In diseases which cause excessive loss of fluid from the body, such as :—

    (i) Diseases causing severe vomiting and diarrhœa.

    (ii) Very high fevers, especially in hot climates.

    (iii) Diabetes mellitus (owing to the excessive polyuria).

    (iv) Severe hæmorrhage and burns.

    (v) In prolonged coma, owing to the lack of fluid intake, dehydration may also develop.

Effects of Dehydration.—In the early stages fluid is withdrawn from the skin and tissues in order to maintain the blood volume, whilst to conserve water the kidneys excrete less urine. If the dehydration is not corrected more serious effects follow. The blood volume is reduced and this leads to deficient circulation, especially through the kidneys, which therefore fail to excrete waste products from the body. Acute renal failure (uræmia) then develops, which if not quickly relieved will prove fatal.

Clinical Recognition of Dehydration.

    (*a*) The patient is lethargic and dull. Thirst is often, but not always, present.

    (*b*) The tongue is very dry and leathery in appearance.

    (*c*) The skin loses its normal elasticity and if pinched remains in a fold.

    (*d*) The output of urine is markedly decreased and any urine passed is highly concentrated. The specific gravity of a twenty-four hour specimen is often 1,030 or more.

    (*e*) The blood urea is raised.

The best clinical indications of an *adequate* fluid balance are the twenty-four hour output of urine, which should never fall below 1,000 ml. ($1\frac{3}{4}$ pints), and the condition of the tongue, which should always be moist.

In most cases of dehydration there is a loss of salt as well as of water, so that often in treating the dehydration salt plus water is given in the form of saline by intravenous infusion. In a case of severe dehydration 3,000 to 4,000 ml. a day are often necessary; in less severe cases approximately 2,500 ml.

2. Excess of Water in the Body—Œdema.

Fluid in the body flows from the blood into the tissues or vice versa. There are four main factors which control this flow :—

(*a*) The pressure in the small capillaries and veins tends to force fluid out from the circulation into the tissues. Anything, therefore, that increases the venous pressure tends to force fluid into the tissues. Owing to the force of gravity, increases in the venous pressure are most marked in the lowest parts of the body; as a result the flow of fluid into the tissues is greatest in the most dependent parts. In addition, fluid also quickly collects in the large serous sacs of the body, such as the pleural and peritoneal cavities.

(*b*) Counteracting this venous pressure, which forces fluid out into the tissues, is the opposite action of the proteins in the blood (albumin and globulin). These proteins have the power, often called the *osmotic power* of proteins, of attracting fluid, with the result that they keep fluid in the blood and out of the tissues.

Normally, these two opposing factors, the venous pressure and the osmotic power of the blood proteins, keep a steady balance of fluid within the body. Any upset in either leads, however, to changes in the water balance.

(*c*) A third factor which can affect the amount of fluid in the tissues is damage to the walls of the capillaries, in consequence of which fluid may leak through the walls.

(*d*) Salt is another most important factor in œdema. Retention of salt in the body causes retention of water.

Types of Œdema caused by the above Factors.

(*a*) CARDIAC ŒDEMA.—In congestive heart failure there are two fundamental causes of œdema. First there is an increase in the venous pressure which tends, when the pressure is great enough to overcome the opposing power of the blood proteins, to force fluid into the tissues. The œdema, as explained above, forms in the most dependent parts of the body, as the venous pressure is greatest in these areas. If there is gross œdema, fluid also collects in the pleural and peritoneal cavities.

Secondly, the kidneys in congestive heart failure fail to excrete salt properly so that salt accumulates in the body. This causes retention of water which in turn causes œdema.

(*b*) RENAL ŒDEMA.—In chronic nephritis, owing to the continued loss of protein in the urine (albuminuria) and the consequential diminished power of the proteins in the blood to keep fluid out of the tissues, renal œdema develops. In renal œdema the face is characteristically affected, especially around the eyelids. Œdema of the face is hardly ever seen in congestive heart failure, as the increased venous pressure causing the œdema is most marked in the lower parts of the body.

Œdema is also a feature of the acute stage of nephritis. Here, however, the œdema is not caused by the lowered level of blood proteins, but possibly by damage to the lining walls of the capillaries allowing fluid to leak out into the tissues.

(c) ŒDEMA OF LOCAL VENOUS OBSTRUCTION.—Obstruction to a large vein will cause increased venous pressure behind the vein, resulting in a localised œdema of the area being drained by the affected vein.

Pressure by a tumour in the lungs can cause venous obstruction, resulting particularly in œdema of the face and arms.

A large thrombus in a main vein of a limb commonly causes œdema of the affected limb.

Recognition of Œdema.—This is usually simple. The affected parts are swollen, and pressure on the swollen area causes " pitting " of the area owing to the displacement of the fluid. This pitting on pressure distinguishes the solid swelling of a tumour, or just pure fat in the tissues, from the swelling due to fluid.

Difference between Œdema Fluid and Inflammatory Fluid.—One of the most important changes which occurs in acute inflammation is an increased flow of fluid (exudation) in the inflamed area. When inflammation affects the great lining sacs of the body, such as the pleura and peritoneum, exudation may be very copious, causing a large accumulation of fluid in the chest or peritoneal cavities.

The fluid which collects as a result of inflammation is called an **exudate,** whilst the fluid in œdema is called a **transudate.**

NORMAL GASTRO-INTESTINAL TRACT

For the proper absorption of food and the correct functioning of the body's metabolism it is essential that the intestinal tract should function normally. In many long-standing and chronic diseases of the gastro-intestinal tract there may be deficient absorption of essential foods, vitamins, etc.

1. In *chronic ulcerative colitis* with prolonged diarrhœa severe wasting may occur. Several vitamin deficiencies due to lack of absorption of vitamins and also an anæmia due to lack of iron absorption are often seen too.

2. In *major operations* on the gastro-intestinal tract severe

anæmia can occur owing to lack of absorption of iron. In addition, in the absence of the intrinsic factor in the stomach which is necessary for proper formation of the red blood cells a pernicious form of anæmia may occasionally arise.

3. In certain diseases, such as *cœliac disease* or *sprue*, there is inadequate absorption of fats so that there is severe wasting and lack of growth. Calcium and vitamin D are also poorly absorbed in cœliac disease so that bone changes similar to those of rickets may develop. Tetany, as a result of the low blood calcium, may occur too.

NORMAL LIVER FUNCTION AND BILE CIRCULATION

The liver has many important functions in connection with metabolism. Breakdown of proteins, storage of sugar, formation and storage of the essential factor in the development of the red cells and also the formation and storage of prothrombin (necessary for blood clotting) are all functions of the liver.

Liver diseases may thus severely disturb the normal nutrition of the body and lead to wasting, severe anæmias and deficient blood clotting with hæmorrhages. It should be noted, however, that the liver has such great reserves that it is only when diseases of the liver are very advanced that any serious interferences with body metabolism are met with.

Bile is essential for the proper absorption of vitamin K, which is required for the formation of prothrombin, which is needed for blood clotting. In obstructive jaundice, where no bile is present in the intestines, a lack of vitamin K develops in the body, which in turn causes a deficiency of prothrombin.

COMPOSITION OF A NORMAL DIET

The essential constituents of a normal diet and the other factors necessary for the utilisation of food and water have been outlined. It remains to state how much of these different foods, etc., is needed to maintain health. Naturally, the requirements vary with different people according to the amount of energy they expend.

Fundamentally, all food and other essential factors are needed :—

1. To repair the normal wear and tear of the tissues and to supply the energy to make the tissues and organs perform their work.

2. To supply sufficient energy to enable the individual to lead a normally active life.

The **basal metabolic rate** is the amount of energy expended by a person lying down at complete rest, several hours after a meal, as measured in terms of heat production.

For convenience in calculating the food requirements of the body the amount of energy needed can be expressed in the terms of *calories*. All foods have a calorific value :—

1. One gramme of carbohydrate produces 4 calories (or 1 oz.= 112 calories).
2. One gramme of protein produces 4 calories (or 1 oz.= 112 calories).
3. One gramme of fat produces 9 calories (or 1 oz.=252 calories).

Total Calorific Requirements in Adults per Day.

1. Light or sedentary workers . . 2,500-3,000 calories.
2. Moderately heavy workers . . 3,000-3,500 ,,
3. Very heavy workers . . . 4,000 and upwards.

In converting these calorific requirements into food it is important that certain amounts of each of the individual foods be eaten to secure a balanced diet. A minimum of 70 gm. of protein foods a day is needed to replace wear and tear in the tissues. During times of stress this may have to be increased.

The amount of fat and carbohydrate in a normal diet varies according to the individual taste for much or little fat and also with the economic status. A high fat diet is more expensive than a high carbohydrate one. In an average diet the fats usually supply from 90 to 150 gm. and the carbohydrates 300 to 500 gm.

A balanced diet must include, however, not only the protein necessary for repairing wear and tear of tissues and enough fats and carbohydrates for energy purposes, but also all the mineral salts mentioned earlier. These will be automatically supplied if all the ordinary foods are eaten, especially milk, eggs, butter, meat, fish, cereals, fruit and vegetables. These foods will also supply sufficient vitamins.

At certain periods, especially in childhood and during pregnancy and lactation, the diet may need supplementing. For children a higher proportion of proteins is needed to allow for growth. For this reason the diet should contain plenty of milk, at least 1½ pints a day being required.   Milk also supplies the much needed calcium for growth of bones.

Ample quantities of green vegetables, fruit and cereals are important, both for their vitamin content and for their nutritional value.   In infants extra supplies of vitamins A, D and C are essential.

During pregnancy a full diet is essential as the energy requirements increase with the growth of the fœtus.   Vitamins A, B, C and D are especially important and should be added to the diet. Iron may also be required.

SOME IMPORTANT FOODS

1. **Milk.**—Milk is of particular value because it contains most of the main items necessary for a normal diet, such as carbohydrates, proteins and fats, minerals and vitamins.   The proteins in milk are of high biological value.   In addition, milk is extremely easily digested, as is shown by the fact that it forms the staple article of diet for infants.

The vitamins contained in milk are A, B and D.   Small amounts of vitamin C are present, but most of this vitamin is destroyed in pasteurisation.   This is the only adverse effect of pasteurisation on milk.

The content of minerals in milk is very high, especially of calcium. The iron content is, however, low.   The amount of milk recommended for daily consumption is 1 pint for adults and $1\frac{1}{2}$ to 2 pints for children.

Milk Foods.

BUTTER is formed from sour milk in churning, and being almost pure fat has a very high calorific value.   Butter contains vitamins A and D.   Margarine is a cheaper and artificial substitute for butter, but with added vitamins is of similar value.

CHEESE.—Cheese, formed from curded milk, contains a high percentage of protein and fat, and also of vitamins A and B_2.   It is a very valuable food in an easily digestible form.

2. **Eggs.**—Eggs have a very high nutritional value, particularly for their proteins and fat.   They also contain a high proportion of minerals and vitamins A, B and D.

Eggs are a very valuable food as they are so easily digested, and are particularly useful in illness.

3. **Meat.**—Meat is of especial value because of the important

proteins it contains. Properly frozen meat has the same nutritional value as fresh meat. White meat (poultry and game) is more easily digested than red meat, but there is no appreciable difference between the protein content of red and white meats.

Liver, kidney and heart also contain valuable proteins, and, in addition, very high quantities of vitamins B and A.

4. **Fish.**—Fish contains almost as much protein as meat, and also a plentiful supply of vitamins A and D. Herrings particularly supply valuable protein, a large amount of fat, abundant vitamins A and D and also iodine relatively cheaply.

5. **Cereals.**—Mainly because of their cheapness, cereals are the commonest foods eaten throughout the world. They are also very valuable foods, supplying abundant carbohydrate and a fair amount of protein. The drawbacks of a diet consisting mainly of cereals are that the vitamin content is low; minerals, such as calcium, are insufficient, and the quality of the protein supplied is not of very high value, being inferior to that of meat, eggs and fish.

Commonest Cereals Consumed.

(*a*) Wheat. The commonest grain in Great Britain.
(*b*) Rice. The staple cereal of eastern countries.
(*c*) Barley. Similar to wheat in value; grows in a drier climate.
(*d*) Oats. Higher nutritive value than wheat; grows in harder climates.

In milling wheat to produce white flour some of the value of the wheat is lost. The main advantage of white over darker flour is that it is more easily digested and the calcium is more easily absorbed.

6. **Vegetables.**

(*a*) GREEN VEGETABLES (spinach, cabbage, brussels sprouts, lettuce, etc.).—These are of value in providing roughage in the diet and so preventing constipation. They are also of value in providing bulk in the diet with little calorific value and are therefore used in diets for obesity.

Green vegetables are, in addition, a useful source of vitamins A and C. However, the practice of cooking vegetables for prolonged periods and then discarding the water results in most of the valuable vitamins present being lost.

(*b*) ROOT VEGETABLES (potatoes, carrots, turnips, parsnips).— Potatoes provide much energy at low cost and they also contain vitamin C. Carrots contain much less carbohydrate than potatoes, but contain a large amount of vitamin A. Parsnips have a lot of carbohydrate, whilst turnips and swedes are of little nutritive value except for vitamin C.

(*c*) PEAS, BEANS AND LENTILS.—These vegetables have a large content of both protein and carbohydrate. They also contain iron and vitamin B complex.

7. Fruits.

These supply much-needed roughage and in many cases vitamin C. Oranges and black currants in particular contain a large amount of vitamin C. Fruits are mainly composed of carbohydrates.

TINNED FRUITS AND VEGETABLES.—With modern methods of canning, tinned fruits and vegetables retain their natural properties, and especially their content of vitamin C, for many months at least. Tinned fruits are preserved in syrup so that their carbohydrate value is very high. For this reason they must be avoided in cases of obesity and diabetes.

DIABETES MELLITUS

Diabetes mellitus, a disease primarily affecting the metabolism of carbohydrates, is the commonest metabolic disease. Diabetes is so important it is discussed at length.

Cause.—The pancreas has certain specialised cells which are present in the islets of Langerhans. These cells secrete insulin, a hormone, which is then poured direct into the blood stream like the hormones of the ductless glands.

The cause of the deficiency in insulin is unknown. It is also not known why it is commoner in some people, especially Jews, than in others. Other factors which play a role are obesity and heredity, *i.e.*, there is a tendency for the disease to run in families.

Action of Insulin.—Insulin is essential for the proper utilisation of the carbohydrate or sugar foods, and in its absence sugar cannot be used up. As a result the sugar accumulates in the blood and is excreted by the kidneys (glycosuria).

Consequently the carbohydrates are not available for energy purposes and the body makes use, instead, of the fats, which are burnt up to excess. As seen under the discussion of the fats, the end-products of fat metabolism are, however, certain poisonous acids, acetone and diacetic acid, which, normally, are rapidly burnt down in the body.

In diabetes these acids (or ketone bodies, as they are often called) are produced so fast (owing to the abnormal and excessive burning of fats) that they, too, may accumulate in the blood and be present in excess in the urine. An excess of these ketone bodies (ketosis) may cause diabetic coma.

Symptoms and Signs.

1. The onset is gradual, and in mild cases there may be few symptoms. In such cases the disease may be first diagnosed as the result of a routine examination of the urine for sugar, *e.g.*, in the course of some illness or for insurance purposes.

2. Thirst, associated with a large output of urine (polyuria), is characteristic.

3. Hunger. The patient usually says that his appetite is very good.

4. Loss of weight, especially in young people.

5. Loss of energy.

6. The skin is often dry, with itching (pruritus). Itching, especially around the vulva owing to the action of the sugar in the urine, is common. Boils frequently recur.

7. URINE.—The characteristic and highly important changes in the urine are :—

(*a*) It is large in amount and pale in colour.

(*b*) It has a high specific gravity (due to the sugar), 1,030 to 1,040.

(*c*) Glycosuria (sugar in the urine) is present.

(*d*) Acetone and diacetic acid (ketone bodies) may be present in severe cases and in all cases of diabetic coma.

Diagnosis.—The presence of glycosuria with some of the above symptoms is usually sufficient for the diagnosis of diabetes. A history of loss of weight in spite of a good appetite is also very suggestive of diabetes as most diseases in medicine which cause a loss of weight are also associated with a diminished appetite. Diabetes and thyrotoxicosis are the two exceptions.

If, in the course of a routine examination, sugar is found in the urine with no definite accompanying symptoms, a blood sugar estimation or a series of such in a *glucose tolerance test* is necessary. If the case is one of diabetes then a raised blood sugar will be present.

The tests for sugar in the urine are the Clinitest, Clinistix and Benedict's. The details are given under urine testing in Diseases of the Urinary System (p. 406).

Diabetes in the Young and Old.

Diabetes in young people differs in many respects from the disease in older people. In young patients the disease tends to be much more acute, with severe loss of weight and great liability to coma. In elderly people the disease runs a much less acute course, and loss of weight, although it may be present, is not so severe, most of the patients being actually obese.

The main differences between diabetes in the young and old are summarised in Table IX.

TABLE IX

	YOUNG PATIENTS.	MIDDLE AGED AND ELDERLY PATIENTS.
Onset . . .	Acute, with severe loss of energy.	Gradual; often first detected on routine examination of the urine undertaken for some other purpose.
Weight . . .	A severe loss in weight; patients usually thin.	Loss of weight not a feature; patients usually obese.
Coma . . .	Great liability to coma.	Coma may occur.
Vascular complications	Not common.	Very common.
Sensitivity to insulin .	Liable to have severe insulin reactions if the disease is not strictly controlled.	Often controlled by dietary restriction or tablets.

Complications of Diabetes. These may affect :—

1. The skin. Boils, carbuncles, pruritus and ulcers of the feet.

2. The eyes. Cataract and retinitis.

3. The nerves. Peripheral neuritis.

4. The arteries. Arteriosclerosis, leading to deficient circulation, particularly in the legs, and often to gangrene. Coronary arteriosclerosis, with its danger of coronary thrombosis, is also common in diabetes.

5. The kidneys. Degeneration with marked albuminuria, œdema and, in some cases, renal failure (Kimmelstiel-Wilson syndrome).

In addition to the above, there is also the important complication of **diabetic coma.** Coma is usually precipitated by some infection or other disease or by not keeping to the diet and treatment.

SYMPTOMS AND SIGNS OF DIABETIC COMA

1. Gradual drowsiness going on to a deep coma.
2. Abdominal pain, often with vomiting.
3. Respirations are deep and sighing.
4. Smell of acetone from the breath.
5. Urine contains a lot of sugar and ketone bodies.

Diabetic patients also often suffer from another type of coma, namely, insulin or hypoglycæmic coma. (Hypoglycæmia means too little sugar in the blood as in insulin coma. Hyperglycæmic or diabetic coma is a coma due to too much sugar.) It is therefore very important to be able to distinguish between these two forms of coma since they require directly opposite forms of treatment.

Table X lists the distinguishing symptoms and signs between diabetic and insulin coma.

TABLE X

SYMPTOMS AND SIGNS.	DIABETIC COMA.	INSULIN COMA.
1. Onset . . .	Usually gradual ; may be acute in children.	Sudden, perhaps with convulsions.
2. Breath . .	Smell of acetone.	No acetone.
3. Respirations .	Deep.	Quiet and shallow.
4. Skin . . .	Dry and inelastic from dehydration.	Always moist, and sweating is usually a feature.
5. Tongue . .	Dry and furred.	Moist.
6. Eyes . . .	Sunken.	Not sunken.
7. Urine . . .	Orange or red precipitate in Benedict's test. Acetone and diacetic acid in excess.	If sugar is present it is only a trace. No acetone or diacetic acid.
8. Other signs—		
(a) Abdominal .	History of abdominal pain and vomiting is common.	Nil.
(b) Reflexes .	May be absent.	Present.
(c) Plantar reflex	Often absent or normal.	May be extensor.
(d) Blood sugar	Very high.	Low.
(e) Blood pressure .	Very low.	Normal.

TREATMENT OF DIABETES

1. In all cases, except the very mildest, patients are best treated in hospital as the education of the patient in matters affecting his diet and, when needed, insulin is best undertaken where he is under continuous supervision.

2. Their illness must be fully explained to the patients, who must be told the reactions likely to occur as a result of neglect of their treatment or of an overdose of insulin. They must be fully aware of all the problems of the diet and in what way they can alter the menus without changing the carbohydrate content.

3. They have to be instructed how to test the urine for sugar.

4. The exact technique of the injection of insulin, where necessary, has to be shown, and the significance of the different strengths and varieties of insulin explained.

The Aim of Treatment.—The aim of treatment is to reduce the carbohydrate in the diet to a level which, whilst still being adequate for nutrition, will abolish the sugar in the urine for most of the day. This can be done by diet alone in many mild cases, but in severe diabetes insulin will be needed. In many of these severe cases it will be found impossible always to keep the urine completely sugar free, and indeed in these cases this is not always even desirable as, if the urine is always sugar free, the danger of insulin reactions and insulin coma is very great.

Steps in Treatment.—The exact dietary regimes used in the treatment of diabetes vary according to the views of the individual doctors. The nurse should therefore acquaint herself with the diets available in her hospital. The dietary stages described indicate the usual principles followed in regulating the diet and, if necessary, the insulin, but the details vary according to individual choice.

1. The patient is put on a low calorie diet which is especially low in carbohydrate, of which usually approximately 100 to 120 gm. are allowed a day. This diet is inadequate to maintain proper nutrition, but for a short period it does no harm and reduces the high sugar level in the blood.

2. On this low calorie diet many of the mild cases will become sugar free or almost so. The next step is therefore gradually to increase the diet till it reaches the level required for adequate nutrition. The exact diet needed for a particular patient is calculated on the basis of the standard weight for a person of that age and height. This average weight is found from a standard table. Having obtained the correct weight, 12 to 15 (say 14) calories are allowed for each pound in weight.

EXAMPLE.—The patient's correct standard weight according to the table should be 144 lb. Then total calories needed per day= 144×14 or 2,016 calories.

This total calorific requirement must now be divided up amongst the carbohydrates, proteins and fats in the following way :—

(a) Half a gramme of protein is allowed for each pound of weight. (In children this amount of protein must be increased to allow for growth.)

(b) The amount of carbohydrates is usually fixed between 130 to 230 gm., the exact amount varying according to the type of work performed, whether the patient is obese or not and the individual choice of the doctor. Some doctors prefer low and others high carbohydrate diets.

(c) The remainder of the calories is supplied by the fats.

NOTE.

(a) The allowance of 14 calories for each pound of correct body-weight is the approximate weight needed by the average person. For those engaged on light indoor work, however, 12 calories would probably be sufficient, whilst for heavy manual workers 20 or more calories would be needed.

(b) Most diabetics engaged in sedentary occupations maintain good health on a diet in the region of 2,000 calories a day, whilst diabetics engaged on heavier manual work seldom require more than 3,000 calories.

(c) In many cases (but never with children) the doctors in charge will fix the carbohydrate content of the diet and allow the patient to take average helpings of protein and fat. This is done because some patients (especially the elderly) find it very difficult in practice to regulate exactly all three types of food.

With this more liberal dietary regime a very careful check must be kept on the weight. If the patient is obese the amount of fat in the diet is reduced. On the other hand, if he is underweight more protein and fat should be taken. In diabetic children the diet must be strictly regulated in order to ensure proper growth and development.

3. If the diabetes is not too severe the dietary control (starting with a low calorie diet and gradually increasing the diet as outlined above) will be sufficient to keep the urine sugar free for most of the day. In severe cases, however, dietary control alone is insufficient and insulin will be needed.

4. Insulin Treatment.

There are three main types of insulin :—

(a) Soluble—Quick-acting insulin (clear solution).
(b) Insulin-zinc Suspensions (Lente Insulins).
(c) Protamine-zinc—Slow-acting insulin (cloudy solution).

Insulin is made up in solutions of 40 or 80 units per ml., and the standard insulin syringe has 20 marks per ml. Hence, if 40 strength insulin is used, each mark is worth 2 units. If 80 strength insulin is used, each mark is worth 4 units. Unfortunately, many syringes with different marking systems are available and can lead to considerable confusion.

(a) SOLUBLE (QUICK-ACTING) INSULIN.—Soluble insulin has its greatest effect three to five hours after the injection. When used alone it is usually given by means of one or two injections a day, the meals being arranged so that most of the carbohydrate is given in the meals following the insulin injections. Soluble insulin is given by subcutaneous injection fifteen to twenty minutes before the meal, as it takes that time before it begins to have effect.

(b) INSULIN-ZINC SUSPENSIONS (LENTE INSULINS).—There are three varieties of insulin-zinc suspensions :—

(i) Insulin-zinc Suspensions (amorphous)—Semilente. Effect lasts for twelve hours.
(ii) Insulin-zinc Suspension (crystalline)—Ultralente. Effect lasts for thirty hours or more.
(iii) Insulin-zinc Suspension—Lente. This preparation is a mixture of semilente and ultralente to give an effect lasting approximately twenty-four hours.

Insulin-zinc suspensions must *not* be mixed with unmodified soluble insulin or with protamine-zinc insulin. They may, however, be mixed with each other to vary the action as required to meet the individual needs of the patient.

The majority of the less severe cases of diabetes, and about 80 per cent. of all patients needing insulin, can be satisfactorily controlled on one injection of insulin-zinc suspension (lente) daily. The lente insulins seem to cause fewer hypoglycæmic reactions than does protamine-zinc insulin and, in addition, less local (allergic) reaction at the site of the injection. Insulin-zinc suspension is the most widely used insulin to-day.

(c) PROTAMINE-ZINC (SLOW-ACTING) INSULIN.— Protamine-zinc insulin (P.Z.I.) has its greatest effect in twelve to eighteen hours.

Before the introduction of the lente insulins it was the insulin most commonly used, either alone or combined with soluble insulin. To the severe diabetics who cannot be satisfactorily controlled on one injection a day of lente insulin, an injection is given before breakfast of protamine-zinc insulin and soluble insulin. The soluble insulin is given to control the rise in the blood sugar after breakfast when slower acting protamine-zinc insulin has not yet come into action.

When both types of insulin are used on the same patient some doctors give the insulin in two separate injections, whilst others mix the two insulins together in the same syringe so that only one injection is necessary. If the insulins are mixed, care must be taken not to contaminate the bottle of soluble insulin with the protamine insulin. This is because when protamine-zinc insulin comes in contact with soluble insulin it can slowly convert the soluble insulin into protamine-zinc insulin. Therefore, if repeated small amounts of protamine-zinc insulin are injected into the bottle of soluble insulin, the soluble insulin eventually becomes mostly protamine-zinc insulin.

Special insulin syringes are available, graduated in units as well as millilitres.

INSTRUCTIONS FOR PATIENTS ON INSULIN

All patients on insulin must be fully instructed in all the following points :—

(a) The actual dose of insulin needed in terms of units and millilitres.

(b) The actual strength of the insulin to be used, 40 or 80 units per ml.

(c) The type of insulin or insulins to be used.

(d) The exact manner and technique of giving a subcutaneous injection. (The patients should be told to vary the site of the injections and not to use the same site for successive injections.)

(e) The proper care and sterilisation of the syringe and needles.

(f) The importance of taking a meal after an insulin injection. (If for some reason a meal cannot be taken after insulin has been injected then a glucose drink or sugar must be taken.)

(g) If, for example, through some acute illness, the patient is prevented from taking his normal diet, he must not omit his insulin but must consult his doctor, who will regulate the insulin and the diet.

16

(h) The importance of carrying two lumps of sugar at all times so that at the first sign of an insulin reaction the sugar can be taken. The patients must be able to recognise the early signs of an insulin reaction—faintness, giddiness and sweating. As violent exercise lowers the blood sugar, it may therefore precipitate an insulin reaction. Extra sugar may then have to be taken during periods of strenuous exercise.

5. Oral Hypoglycæmic Drugs.

It has been found that certain drugs can lower the blood sugar. They have the great advantage over insulin that they can be given by mouth, but on the other hand they have only a moderate hypoglycæmic action. These drugs are therefore of no value for patients with severe diabetes, particularly young diabetics. They have, however, proved of value in less severe cases, e.g., with middle-aged or elderly patients whose diabetes cannot be controlled by diet alone.

At present, the two most widely used and satisfactory oral hypoglycæmic drugs are tolbutamide (rastinon) and chlorpropamide (diabinese). Tolbutamide is usually given in 0·5 to 1 gm. doses twice a day; the average dose of chlorpropamide is 100 to 250 mgm. once a day.

Toxic effects which may occur with either drug include nausea, skin rashes and, more rarely, blood dyscrasias.

6. After-control.

The patients can be considered stabilised as soon as they cease to have anything but minimal amounts of sugar in the urine or, better, are sugar free for most of the day, and are also free from insulin reactions.

(a) DIET.—By this time, too, the patients should have been instructed how to give variety to their basic diet by substituting different articles of food of the same calorific value. Suitable diabetic cookery books are available and should be used by all diabetics.

All food must be weighed at first until the patient has gained by experience an accurate idea of the amounts needed. Suitable weighing scales, weighing in fractions of an ounce, are therefore necessary.

(b) URINE TESTING.—All patients should be instructed how to test the urine for sugar. The Clinitest is the most convenient test for sugar in the urine.

(c) HYGIENE.—In view of the great danger of gangrene, especially in elderly diabetics, special care of the feet is necessary. The feet should be washed daily, particularly in hot weather, and dried carefully; powder should be used. Wet socks must be changed as

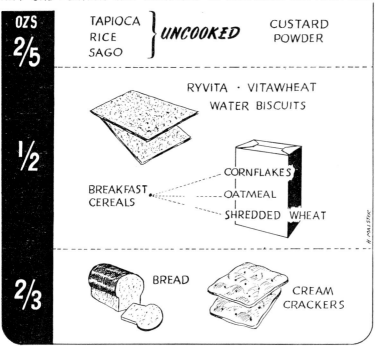

CEREALS
(CARBOHYDRATE CONTENT)

EACH OF THE FOLLOWING PORTIONS CONTAINS **10** GRAMS OF CARBOHYDRATE
ANY ONE PORTION CAN THEREFORE BE EXCHANGED FOR ANOTHER.

OZS

2/5

TAPIOCA
RICE } UNCOOKED
SAGO

CUSTARD
POWDER

RYVITA · VITAWHEAT
WATER BISCUITS

1/2

BREAKFAST
CEREALS

CORNFLAKES
OATMEAL
SHREDDED WHEAT

2/3

BREAD

CREAM
CRACKERS

FIG. 164

soon as possible. The toe nails must be cut short and proper attention paid to corns.

Septic spots must not be neglected as diabetics frequently suffer from boils or carbuncles which if not properly treated may precipitate diabetic coma.

(d) All diabetics should attend their doctor or diabetic clinic at regular intervals to maintain control of their diabetes.

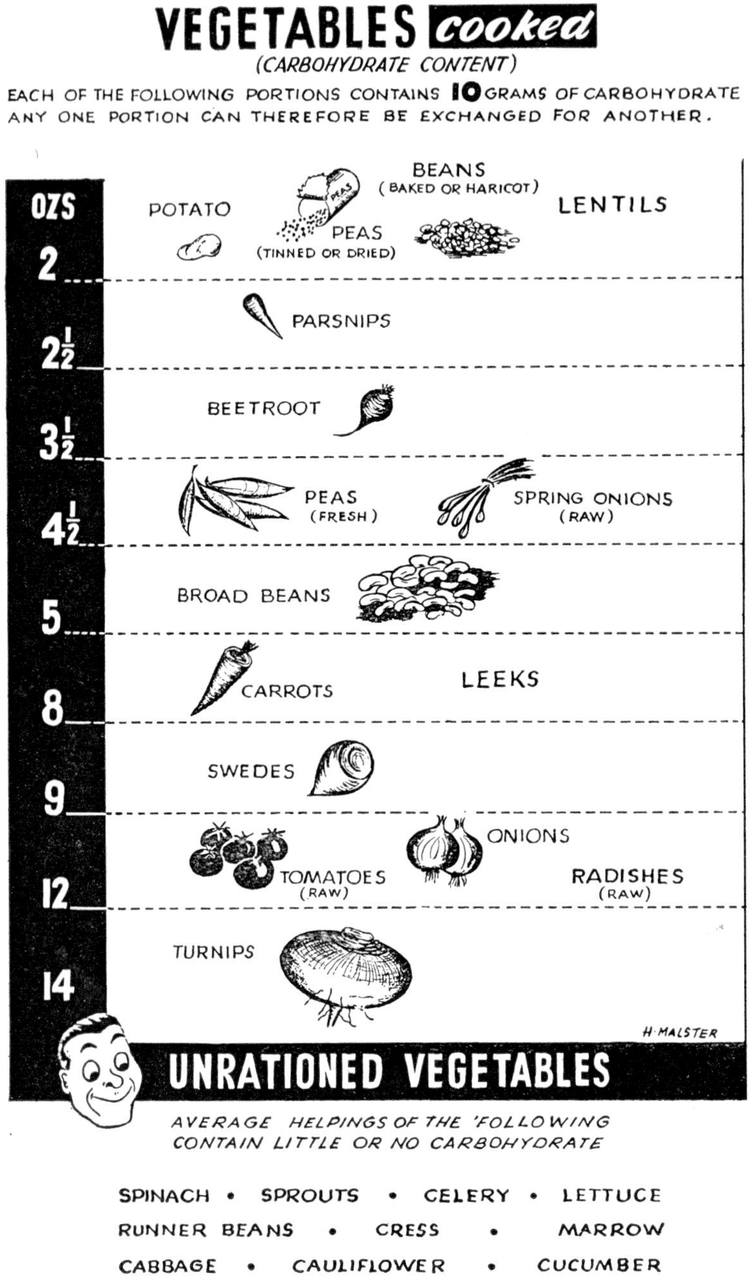
VEGETABLES cooked
(CARBOHYDRATE CONTENT)
EACH OF THE FOLLOWING PORTIONS CONTAINS 10 GRAMS OF CARBOHYDRATE
ANY ONE PORTION CAN THEREFORE BE EXCHANGED FOR ANOTHER.
OZS
2
POTATO
PEAS (TINNED OR DRIED)
BEANS (BAKED OR HARICOT)
LENTILS
2½
PARSNIPS
3½
BEETROOT
4½
PEAS (FRESH)
SPRING ONIONS (RAW)
5
BROAD BEANS
8
CARROTS
LEEKS
9
SWEDES
12
TOMATOES (RAW)
ONIONS
RADISHES (RAW)
14
TURNIPS
H. MALSTER
UNRATIONED VEGETABLES
AVERAGE HELPINGS OF THE FOLLOWING CONTAIN LITTLE OR NO CARBOHYDRATE
SPINACH • SPROUTS • CELERY • LETTUCE
RUNNER BEANS • CRESS • MARROW
CABBAGE • CAULIFLOWER • CUCUMBER

FIG. 165

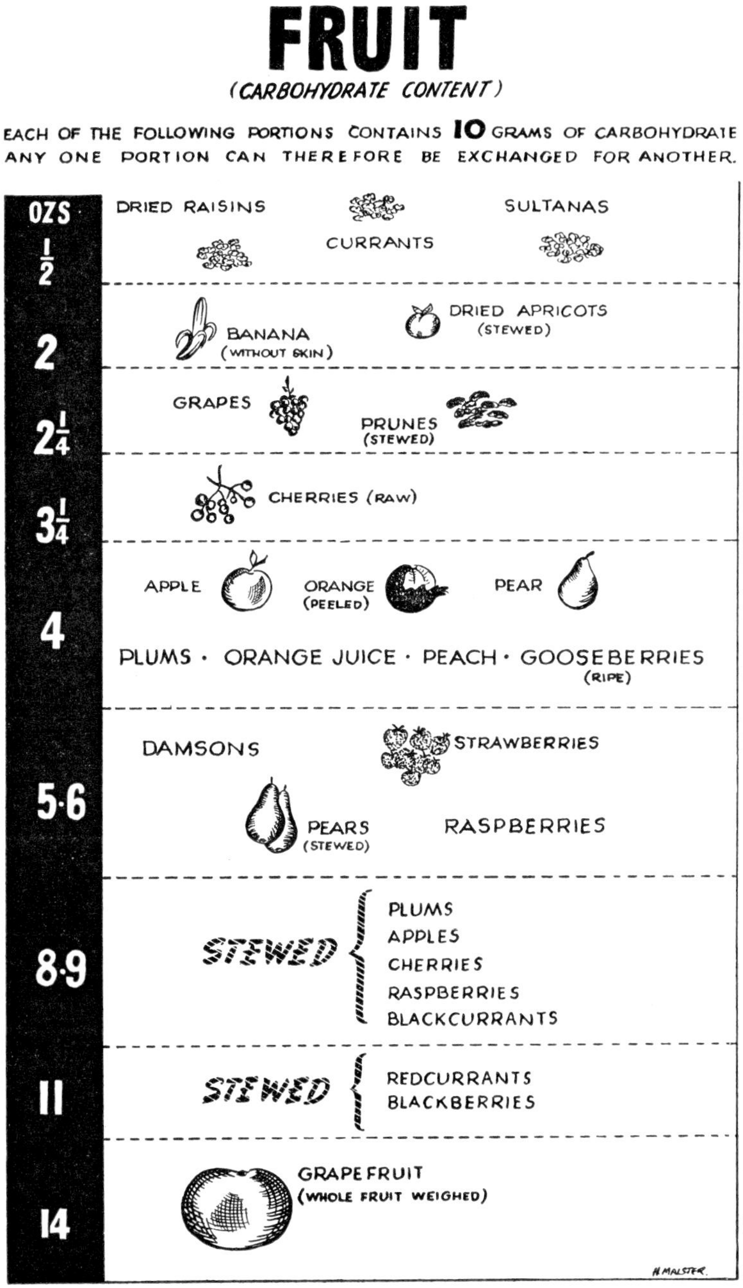

FRUIT

(CARBOHYDRATE CONTENT)

EACH OF THE FOLLOWING PORTIONS CONTAINS **10** GRAMS OF CARBOHYDRATE
ANY ONE PORTION CAN THEREFORE BE EXCHANGED FOR ANOTHER.

OZS	
$\frac{1}{2}$	DRIED RAISINS CURRANTS SULTANAS
2	BANANA (WITHOUT SKIN) DRIED APRICOTS (STEWED)
$2\frac{1}{4}$	GRAPES PRUNES (STEWED)
$3\frac{1}{4}$	CHERRIES (RAW)
4	APPLE ORANGE (PEELED) PEAR PLUMS · ORANGE JUICE · PEACH · GOOSEBERRIES (RIPE)
5·6	DAMSONS STRAWBERRIES PEARS (STEWED) RASPBERRIES
8·9	STEWED { PLUMS APPLES CHERRIES RASPBERRIES BLACKCURRANTS
11	STEWED { REDCURRANTS BLACKBERRIES
14	GRAPEFRUIT (WHOLE FRUIT WEIGHED)

H MALSTER.

FIG. 166

BEVERAGES · PRESERVES & SWEETMEATS
(CARBOHYDRATE CONTENT)

EACH OF THE FOLLOWING PORTIONS CONTAINS **10** GRAMS OF CARBOHYDRATE.
ANY ONE PORTION CAN THEREFORE BE EXCHANGED FOR ANOTHER

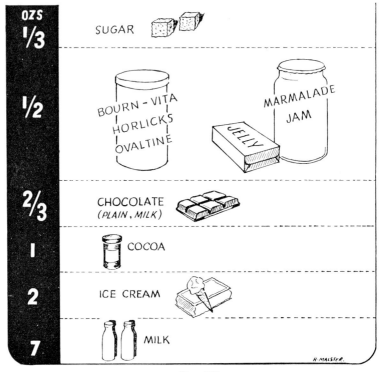

OZS	
1/3	SUGAR
1/2	BOURN-VITA / HORLICKS / OVALTINE — MARMALADE JAM — JELLY
2/3	CHOCOLATE *(PLAIN, MILK)*
1	COCOA
2	ICE CREAM
7	MILK

H. MALSTER.

FIG. 167

TREATMENT OF DIABETIC COMA

Diabetic coma is a medical emergency and it is essential that all steps be taken as quickly as possible to restore the patient to consciousness.

1. INSULIN.—This must be given in large doses and at frequent intervals. The first dose is usually about 100 units of soluble insulin, and of this 40 units or so will be given intravenously to ensure rapid action. In coma there is circulatory failure so that there is poor absorption from the subcutaneous route.

2. An intravenous saline drip is set up and 1,000 ml. are given rapidly within about an hour to overcome the severe dehydration.

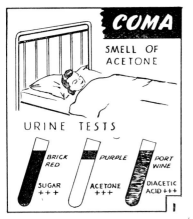

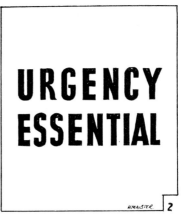

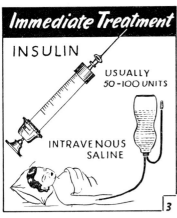

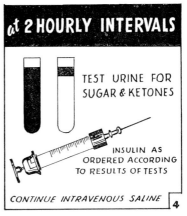

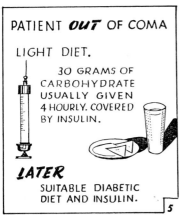

FIG. 168

The treatment of
diabetic coma.

After this the drip may be slowed and continued at this slower rate till the patient is aroused and able to take fluids by mouth.

3. Urine is obtained every two hours, a retention catheter being useful for this purpose. The urine is tested for sugar and ketone bodies. As long as there are any ketone bodies present the patient is in serious danger.

4. A blood sugar test is usually taken at the outset. The level of the blood sugar is a guide to treatment, as if the initial blood sugar is very high (500 mgm. per cent. or over) the first dose of insulin may have to be quickly supplemented by another large dose.

5. The above measures are taken immediately, and in two hours' time the case is reviewed. If the urine examination then shows no reduction in the ketone bodies a further large dose of 100 to 200 units of insulin will be needed. In most cases, however, the patient should respond to prompt treatment and show a reduction in the ketone bodies. If so a smaller dose of insulin, 50 units or less, depending on progress, will be given.

Until the patient recovers consciousness soluble insulin is given every two to three hours.

6. Glucose. In the initial stages, when a deep coma is present, giving glucose with the insulin is not necessary. When, however, the urine begins to show a reduction in the sugar content, glucose (1 gm. for every unit of insulin) is then given. This is to prevent any danger of the large doses of insulin causing the patient to swing over into an insulin coma.

7. Gastric lavage and enemas. Once the immediate measures outlined above have been carried out, a stomach washout, to relieve the abdominal distension, is sometimes ordered. Also, as there is usually obstinate constipation, an enema often helps.

8. Circulatory failure and shock. These are always present in diabetic coma, and are treated by raising the foot of the bed and by giving intravenous saline to overcome the dehydration which causes the shock. It should be stressed that intravenous fluids are second in importance only to large doses of insulin in the treatment of diabetic coma.

9. When the patient regains consciousness, four-hourly feeds are given of 25 to 30 gm. of carbohydrate in the form of glucose, fruit juices, milk or any suitable equivalent food the patient is able to take. Insulin will be ordered with each feed or less often, according to how much is needed to keep the urine sugar free. When the

patient can swallow, potassium chloride or potassium citrate 2 gm. six-hourly, is given by mouth. Potassium is needed during the recovery stage of diabetic coma because there is a severe fall in the blood potassium (see p. 462).

As soon as the patient is fit the ordinary treatment for diabetes is started.

10. In most cases of coma the onset is precipitated by some infection or septic focus, and so in all such cases any such sepsis must be treated from the start with penicillin or any other appropriate measure.

TREATMENT OF HYPOGLYCÆMIC (INSULIN) COMA

In the early stages of an insulin reaction, in which only the initial symptoms of giddiness, faintness and slight sweating may be present, giving two lumps of sugar (approximately 10 gm. of carbohydrate) may be sufficient to counteract the overdosage of insulin. For this reason all patients taking insulin are advised to carry some sugar with them at all times to take at the slightest signs of any insulin reaction.

If the patient is already in coma, $\frac{1}{2}$ to 1 ml. of adrenaline or pituitrin, subcutaneously, may raise the blood sugar level enough to make the patient conscious, whereupon sugar by mouth can be given. In more severe coma intravenous injection of 25 gm. of glucose will be necessary.

Finally, it is important to remember that protamine-zinc insulin causes very insidious reactions, usually in the early hours of the morning when its effect is greatest. In these cases severe headache and nausea may be the only evidence for some time of the imminence of a severe insulin coma. Coma due to protamine-zinc insulin may require energetic treatment as the patient, after responding to the first injection of glucose, may collapse later and go once more into coma.

GOUT

Gout, like diabetes, is a disorder of metabolism. It is an upset of the metabolism of certain types of protein called purines, which are present in the tissue cells. Normally the waste product of purines, *uric acid*, is excreted in the urine. In gout, however, for some unknown reason the uric acid is instead retained in the blood and becomes deposited in the joints.

16 A

Symptoms and Signs.

1. Gout is usually seen in people who have taken alcohol in excess and have lived on rich foods.

2. Acute attacks of severe pain in the joints occur. The big toe joint is characteristically affected, becoming swollen, red and extremely tender.

3. The patient is very irritable and restless from the severe pain.

4. In between the acute attacks lesser degrees of pain and discomfort in the joints occur, and a chronic arthritis of the affected joints develops.

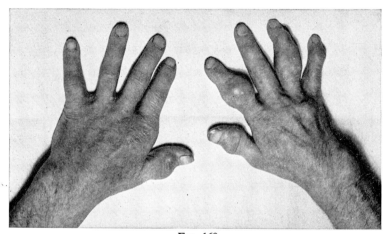

FIG. 169

Chronic gout showing the appearance of the hands with swelling and deformity of the joints.

5. Characteristic tophi occur in the lobes of the ears and around the finger joints. These are nodules of soft cheesy material which often ulcerate.

Treatment.

1. IN THE ACUTE STAGE.—Colchicum is the best drug for relieving the pain of acute gout. It can be given either as a tincture in 15 minim doses or in tablet form ($\frac{1}{120}$ gr.) every four hours. It can also be combined with salicylates to advantage. Phenylbutazone (butazolidin) has also proved effective in the treatment of acute gout in 400 to 600 mgm. doses daily. The danger with phenylbutazone is its toxic effects, particularly agranulocytosis (see p. 391).

In very severe attacks of gout, cortisone and allied drugs have proved very effective.

The affected joint should be protected from injury by a bed cradle and by wrapping in warm wool.

2. IN THE CHRONIC STAGE.—Salicylates (about 90 gr. daily) or probenecid (benemid, 1 to 2 gm. daily) are the two drugs most often used. Recently a new and much more potent drug for the treatment of chronic gout has become available, namely anturan, given in 100 mgm. doses three or four times a day.

All foods rich in uric acid—liver, sweetbreads, roe, kidneys, sprats, sardines, herrings and game—are best restricted. Alcohol should be taken in moderation.

ACIDOSIS AND ALKALOSIS

The reaction of the blood normally remains constant and is always alkaline. It never becomes acid or death would be the result. Even a slight change in the reaction of the blood leads to profound and serious changes in the body.

Normally there is a complicated mechanism by which the reaction of the blood is kept constant, for although in the process of normal metabolism acids are formed, the body continues to get rid of them in several ways, e.g., carbon dioxide, which is an acid, is washed out in the lungs whilst the kidneys also excrete any excess acid.

ACIDOSIS

Acidosis means the accumulation of excess acids so that the reaction of the blood becomes less alkaline. It arises chiefly in the following conditions :—

(a) Diabetes mellitus. In this disease excessive combustion of fats occurs owing to the disturbance of carbohydrate metabolism. As the final result of fat metabolism is the formation of the acid ketone bodies, these may then accumulate in the body (see p. 459).

(b) Renal failure. Here the kidneys fail to excrete the acids formed during normal metabolism.

(c) Prolonged diarrhœa, especially the severe acute forms in children. A large quantity of alkali may be lost in the fæces with resultant acidosis.

(d) Severe prolonged illnesses or major operations.

Treatment.—It is, of course, essential that the disease causing the acidosis should be treated wherever possible. In addition, however, to any such specific treatment, abundant fluids with salt must be given. This is because in any case of acidosis the body, in an effort to get rid of the excess acids, also depletes itself in various ways of a great deal of fluid and salt.

Excess carbon dioxide causes an increased respiration rate and thus an increased loss of water in the respirations. The kidneys in excreting more acids excrete more urine (fluid) too. Severe illnesses with prolonged pyrexia and the associated sweating also lead to an excessive loss of fluid, whilst the marked dehydration associated with the ketosis of diabetes has already been noted. It is therefore necessary to give abundant fluids, often by the intravenous route. Glucose is also of great value in acidosis.

ALKALOSIS

The opposite to acidosis, alkalosis, is most usually seen as a result of :—

(a) Prolonged vomiting. Here the alkalosis is due to the excessive loss of the hydrochloric acid in the gastric juice. Pyloric stenosis with its persistent vomiting is often accompanied by alkalosis.

(b) Hysterical overbreathing, where the alkalosis is caused by the loss of acid, carbon dioxide.

(c) Ingestion of alkalis, as used in the treatment of peptic ulcer. Nowadays, however, the alkalis in common use (magnesium trisilicate, aluminium hydroxide) are not absorbed into the blood and there is therefore no risk of alkalosis. Sodium bicarbonate in large quantities is the alkali most likely to cause alkalosis.

The main chemical result of alkalosis is tetany, which is discussed elsewhere. The treatment of alkalosis is to remove the cause and to give calcium for the tetany.

SUMMARY

NORMAL METABOLISM

1. The body continuously uses up energy, not only whilst working, but even when at rest, as the various functions of the body go on all the time, e.g., the heart never stops pumping blood, the lungs never cease to expand to supply the vital oxygen, etc.

2. To provide this energy, fuel is needed ; this is supplied in the form of foods and other vital factors.

(a) Carbohydrates, the sugar foods, are the main source of energy and form the main constituent of most normal diets.

(b) Fats (butter, margarine, oils) are next in importance to the carbohydrates in supplying fuel to the body. The last main type of food, the

(c) Proteins, are responsible for growth and for rebuilding the tissues which have become " worn out " through wear and tear.

3. In addition to the three main foods the body must have several other items if it is to function properly.

Mineral Salts.—Sodium is necessary to maintain a proper fluid balance in the tissues and the blood. Calcium is mainly required to build up the bones, but it also controls the functioning of the nerves and muscles. Iodine is essential for the thyroid gland to work properly, and iron is necessary for the building up of the hæmoglobin in the red blood cells. These salts are some of the many required by the body for its daily function.

4. In addition to the above there are certain other essential factors (present in various foods) which control different forms of bodily activity. These are called " vitamins," of which the following are the most important :—

(a) Vitamin A necessary for the proper growth of certain tissues such as the skin and mucous membranes.

(b) Vitamin B complex. This includes various essential factors which are mainly concerned with the function of the nerves, blood, skin, tongue and eyes.

(c) Vitamin C is essential for the normal development of the lining endothelial cells of the small blood vessels (capillaries).

(d) Vitamin D is required for the proper growth and development of the bones and the nerves.

(e) Vitamin K manufactures an essential constituent of the blood called " prothrombin," which is necessary for the clotting of blood.

5. These are the main foods, minerals and vitamins which must be taken into the body for it to work properly. Once, however, these foods and other essentials have been ingested it is vital that they should be properly utilised. For this purpose there exist various glands called the " ductless glands," which produce secretions called " hormones." Many of these play a direct part in normal metabolism :—

(a) The pituitary gland secretions are responsible amongst other functions for the growth of the body.

(b) The parathyroid glands control calcium metabolism, neuro-muscular irritability and the development of the bones.

(c) The adrenal glands control salt metabolism.

(d) The pancreas is most vital in the proper control of carbohydrate metabolism.

6. Other organs in the body, apart from the ductless glands and their hormones, are also primarily concerned in metabolism. The liver plays a large part by storing the carbohydrates, preparing the proteins for proper use and by the formation of the bile salts which are essential for the absorption of fat and vitamin K from the bowel. If the liver is removed death rapidly occurs.

7. To ensure that all the above foods and vital factors are properly absorbed the gastro-intestinal tract must be normal. Diseases affecting this tract may cause disorders and upsets of metabolism.

8. The foods, minerals and vitamins mentioned above are all required for normal metabolism. It is, however, also important to realise that 70 per cent. of the body is composed of water. Deficiency of water leads to dehydration ; excess of water in the body leads to œdema. Either may be fatal.

COMMON DISORDERS OF METABOLISM AND RELATED DISEASES

1. Carbohydrate Metabolism.—Here, diabetes mellitus, due to deficiency of the insulin secretion of the pancreas, is the commonest upset.

2. Fat Metabolism.—Disturbance of fat metabolism is a secondary factor in diabetes, leading to the production of poisonous acids (ketosis) and so to diabetic coma.

In obstructive jaundice the absence of bile salts from the intestinal tract prevents the fats from being absorbed.

Chronic diseases of the intestines, such as sprue and cœliac disease, also lead to deficient fat absorption.

3. Protein Metabolism.—Disorders of protein metabolism are not common but do occur in certain rare congenital diseases. In addition, continued loss of protein in the urine, leading to severe œdema, is seen in one form of chronic nephritis. Gout is also a form of protein upset.

4. Minerals.

    (a) Sodium (salt) metabolism is disordered in Addison's disease of the adrenal glands.

    (b) Calcium metabolism is upset in rickets, of which the cause is lack of vitamin D. Disease of the parathyroid glands also leads to disorders of calcium metabolism. Tetany is one manifestation of disturbance of calcium metabolism.

    (c) Lack of iodine causes a disease of the thyroid gland known as goitre.

    (d) Iron.—Many forms of anæmia occur owing to a deficiency of iron in the diet or to excessive loss in hæmorrhage.

5. Vitamin Deficiencies.—These are discussed at length under the vitamins. It is sufficient to say here that the most important deficiencies are :—

Beriberi, pellagra, peripheral neuritis (vitamin B complex) ; scurvy (vitamin C) ; rickets (vitamin D) ; hæmorrhagic disease of the newborn and hæmorrhage in jaundice (vitamin K).

6. Ductless Glands.—Disorders of the ductless glands leading to disturbance of metabolism are very common, and are discussed under diseases of the ductless glands. Gigantism, acromegaly, dwarfism and Simmonds' disease, due to pituitary disease ; cretinism, myxœdema and thyrotoxicosis, due to thyroid disorders ; and Addison's disease, due to adrenal disease, are the commonest disorders seen.

7. Water Balance.—Water is continually being lost in the respirations, sweat, fæces and urine. Water is taken in with the food and as fluid. Normally a fairly constant balance is maintained in the body, e.g., if an excess amount of water

is lost in sweat then there is diminished output of urine, and vice versa. If too much water is lost from the body (as can happen with excessive sweating, severe vomiting, diarrhœa and polyuria) then dehydration results. This may lead to serious changes in the body, e.g., fall in blood pressure, rise in blood urea and eventually circulatory failure.

On the other hand, if too much water is retained in the body the condition of œdema results. There are two main types of œdema :—

(a) Cardiac œdema, due partly to the excessive congestion and pressure in the capillaries forcing fluid into the tissues and partly to retention of salt. This form of œdema is especially marked in the most dependent tissues, i.e., the legs, lower half of the body and the large serous sacs.

(b) Renal œdema, due to loss of albumin in the urine. Albumin exerts a force within the blood which keeps fluid in the circulation and out of the tissues. Loss of albumin leads to a reduction of this force and a consequent accumulation of excessive fluid in the tissues. In renal œdema fluid collects in the most lax and easily distensible tissues, especially the face, legs and serous sacs.

CHAPTER XV

DISEASES DUE TO VITAMIN DEFICIENCY

VITAMINS are certain factors present in various foods which are essential for the proper maintenance of health. There are many different vitamins, all of which tend to have some specific action on some part of the body's metabolism. Lack of a vitamin usually leads to certain well-recognised changes in the body.

Deficiency of a vitamin may arise in several ways. *Inadequate diet* is a frequent cause of vitamin deficiency. Again, even if the diet is entirely adequate, *deficient absorption* from the gastro-intestinal tract, because of some disease in the tract, may lead to vitamin deficiency. Finally, at certain times there may be an *increased demand* for vitamins, which if not met may give rise to vitamin deficiency. It is for this reason that vitamin deficiencies are most frequent during the periods of active growth, during pregnancy, in the course of severe prolonged illnesses and after major operations.

VITAMIN A

Action.—Vitamin A is necessary for the proper growth of certain epithelial cells of the body, especially those of the eyes, respiratory tract and skin.

Sources.—Animal fats, butter, cream, eggs, milk and cod-liver oil.

DISEASES DUE TO LACK OF VITAMIN A

1. EYE DISEASES.

> (*a*) Conjunctivitis and corneal ulceration, due to improper development of the epithelium of the eye.
>
> (*b*) Night blindness, *i.e.*, great difficulty in seeing in the dark. Here the pigment in the eyes (visual purple) which is necessary for proper vision is not adequately formed.

2. RESPIRATORY INFECTIONS.—The absence of vitamin A leads to a lowering of the resistance of the mucous membranes, with the result that infections of the respiratory tract tend to develop. Hence, vitamin A is often called the anti-infective vitamin.

VITAMIN B COMPLEX

Action.—Vitamin B is not a single vitamin but is made up of several factors, many—though not all—of which are known to have a specific action.

The more important factors in the vitamin B complex are :—

1. B_1 FACTOR (also called *thiamine* or *aneurine*). Richest sources are yeast, cereals, peas, beans and eggs.

2. NICOTINIC ACID (*niacin*), mainly found in yeast, meat, liver and fish.

3. RIBOFLAVINE, chiefly found in milk, eggs, liver and kidney.

4. VITAMIN B_{12} (see p. 363).

5. FOLIC ACID (see p. 364).

DISEASES DUE TO LACK OF THE VITAMIN B COMPLEX

In practice, although diseases may result from a deficiency of any one of the separate vitamins of the vitamin B complex, it is nevertheless more common for diseases to arise when several of the vitamins in this group are lacking at the same time.

1. Beriberi.

The disease known as beriberi is supposed to be caused by a deficiency of the B_1 factor (aneurine). It is probable, however, that other factors are involved as well, because pure vitamin B_1 will not always cure the disease whereas an adequate diet, especially in protein, usually does.

Beriberi is very common in such Eastern countries as China, Japan and India where the staple food is polished rice, as the polishing of the rice removes most of the vitamin B and especially the B_1 factor.

The disease is seen in two forms : wet beriberi, which causes a marked œdema with congestive heart failure, and dry beriberi, which causes a peripheral neuritis.

2. Pellagra.

Pellagra is common in America and certain parts of Europe, and occasionally occurs in this country. The specific deficiency which causes pellagra is not known, but it is clear that a lack of the nicotinic acid factor plays a large part. Pellagra is often seen in people living on an inadequate diet who have, in addition, a history of chronic alcoholism. Alcoholism increases the metabolism of the body, which in turn increases the body's requirements of food and vitamins. At the same time, however, in chronic alcoholism the amount of food eaten is usually much reduced. This combination of increased need for and decreased intake of the necessary food and vitamins is very prone to cause nutritional and vitamin deficiencies, of which pellagra is one.

The main symptoms of pellagra can be divided into the following groups :—

(a) Gastro-intestinal. Severe glossitis, stomatitis and diarrhœa.
(b) Skin changes. Symmetrical dermatitis of the face and hands, with characteristic dark pigmentation in the later stages.
(c) Mental. Dementia.

Treatment of pellagra mainly consists of the provision of an adequate diet, supplemented by large doses of nicotinic acid and, if necessary, by the other vitamin B factors. Beriberi is treated by giving a properly balanced diet and aneurine.

VITAMIN C (Ascorbic Acid)

Action.—Vitamin C is necessary for the proper growth of the capillary endothelium and for the repair of tissues. The main result of deficiency of this vitamin is hæmorrhage from the capillaries.

Sources.—Oranges, tomatoes, blackcurrant juice, lemons, potatoes and green vegetables.

DISEASES DUE TO LACK OF VITAMIN C

Scurvy is the only disease known to be due to lack of vitamin C, which is often therefore called the antiscorbutic vitamin. Scurvy was at one time a very common disease, especially amongst sailors and infants. Sailors on long voyages used to have to live on a diet lacking in fresh foods, especially fruits and vegetables. Infants fed on the bottle with heated milk also commonly developed scurvy as heating milk destroys all its vitamin C content.

As a result of the recognition of the cause of scurvy the disease is now very rare, especially in the infantile form.

There are two main types of scurvy :—

1. INFANTILE SCURVY.—This, as just mentioned, is now rare owing to the widespread preventive use of orange juice or other source of vitamin C. Breast-fed babies do not develop scurvy

because there is sufficient vitamin C present in human milk to prevent the disease. The necessary boiling or pasteurisation of cow's milk, however, destroys practically all the small amount of vitamin C present; as milk is the main if not the sole diet of infants, scurvy will develop in bottle-fed babies unless vitamin C is specially given.

Symptoms and Signs.—The underlying specific lesion which accounts for most of the symptoms is *hæmorrhage.*

(*a*) Symptoms usually appear about the age of 8 to 10 months and never before 6 months. Scurvy never, as already explained, develops in breast-fed babies.

(*b*) The commonest complaint is of severe fretfulness in the infant, especially if the limbs, which may be swollen, are touched. The child if old enough to walk is often said to " go off its feet." The pain and swelling of the limbs is caused by hæmorrhages under the periosteum of the bones.

(*c*) The gums are swollen, red and spongy. The teeth if present decay and fall out.

(*d*) Hæmorrhages may also occur from the kidneys, bowel or nose. Anæmia is common.

2. ADULT SCURVY.—In adult scurvy the main symptoms are hæmorrhages from the nose or into the skin (purpura). Swelling and bleeding of the gums with general debility and anæmia are all also commonly present. There is also pronounced delay in the healing of any wound or ulcers that may be present. The bone changes characteristic of the infantile form are not a marked feature of adult scurvy.

Treatment.—For adults, as for infants, preventive treatment is important in certain conditions. In chronic gastro-intestinal diseases necessitating a strict and prolonged dietary regime, care should be taken to ensure that a sufficiency of vitamin C (and, of course, of all other vitamins, too) is given. Extra supplies of the vitamin in the form of ascorbic acid, 100 to 200 mgm. daily, are often advisable. The treatment of an established case of scurvy is to give large doses of ascorbic acid, 200 to 500 mgm. daily.

VITAMIN D

Action.—Vitamin D is responsible for the proper absorption of the calcium present in the diet. In its absence calcium is not absorbed from the bowel, and the resultant lack of calcium impedes both the normal growth of bone and the normal activity of nerves and muscles.

Sources.—The same foods as supply vitamin A, *i.e.*, animal fats, butter, cream, eggs, milk and fish-liver oils. In addition, however, to these food sources of the vitamin, sunlight (or ultra-violet light) has the peculiar property of being able to manufacture vitamin D by its action on the skin.

DISEASES DUE TO LACK OF VITAMIN D

1. Rickets.

Before the widespread prophylactic use of cod-liver oil or similar preparations for infants made rickets so much less common

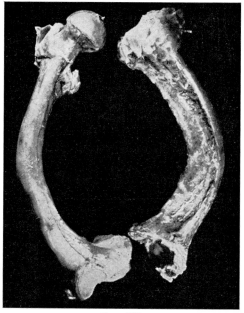

FIG. 170
Rickets showing the bowing and curving of the
bones.

in this country, the disease was usually seen in infants brought up in bad hygienic conditions. Here the lack of sunlight combined with a poor diet caused active rickets. It is interesting to note, however, that infants in the tropics, because of the continuous sunlight, even if brought up on a poor diet, rarely develop rickets.

Rickets is also seen in infants as a complication of chronic gastro-intestinal disease. In this type of disease vitamin D is not properly absorbed from the bowel and this accounts, for example, for the rickets of cœliac disease.

The main changes in rickets are those of disordered bone development caused by the lack of the vitamin, which is essential for normal growth of bone.

Symptoms and Signs.

(*a*) These are first noticed, as a rule, at about the age of 6 months; the infant sweats a good deal, especially around the head, whilst respiratory infections are also common.

(*b*) The wrists and ankles become enlarged at an early stage. The legs become bowed or, alternatively, knock-kneed when the child begins to walk owing to the weight of the body on the softened calcium-deficient bones. The arms, as they are not weight-bearing, are less likely to show such signs.

(*c*) The skull is softened and enlarged, and the typical appearance is one of a square head with a widely patent fontanelle. The spine may be bowed (kyphosis) or twisted (scoliosis).

(*d*) The ribs show a characteristic beading ("rickety rosary") owing to the enlarged epiphyseal margins.

(*e*) All the muscles and ligaments are very flabby and lax.

(*f*) There may be signs of tetany owing to the low blood calcium. Carpopedal spasms and spasm of the larynx with dyspnœa and cyanosis (laryngismus stridulus) are commonly seen in the tetany of infantile rickets.

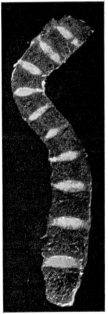

Fig. 171

Rickets showing the curving of the spine.

Treatment.—Vitamin D in the form of cod-liver oil or similar preparations (adexolin, radiostoleum) completely restores the bones to normal in early cases. In more advanced cases corrective active exercises may be necessary. If the bony deformities do not disappear under treatment, splints and operations may be employed to try to correct them.

2. Osteomalacia.

Osteomalacia causes bony changes identical to those of rickets, but the disease is seen in women living in certain areas in the tropics. Here the combination of leading an indoor life lacking in sunlight with an inadequate diet leads to the disease. In addition, the prevalence of frequent early pregnancies is an aggravating factor.

3. Tetany.

Tetany is due to a lowering of the blood calcium. One cause of this is lack of vitamin D, and in these cases tetany accompanies rickets. As, however, other factors—apart from vitamin D—are also involved in the control of the blood calcium (especially some of the ductless glands), tetany has a variety of causes and can therefore occur unassociated with rickets.

Tetany is fully described under Diseases of the Ductless Glands (see p. 454).

VITAMIN E

This vitamin appears to play no definite major role in man. It prevents sterility in rats and it is believed by some that it may possibly have a similar effect in human beings. It is therefore often called the anti-sterility vitamin.

VITAMIN K

Action.—Vitamin K is necessary for the formation of pro-thrombin, which is normally present in the blood and is one of the essential factors in blood clotting.

Sources.—Spinach, cabbage, cauliflower and oats. In addition, the bacteria normally present in the bowel can manufacture vitamin K.

CONDITIONS ASSOCIATED WITH A LACK OF VITAMIN K

1. Hæmorrhagic Disease of the Newborn.

In the first few days of life, owing to deficient storage of vitamin K in the fœtus, there is a low content of prothrombin in the blood. This can lead to hæmorrhage if the deficiency is sufficiently severe (see p. 384).

2. Obstructive Jaundice.

Bile salts are essential for the proper absorption of vitamin K, and so in obstructive jaundice there is deficient absorption of this vitamin. In consequence, in prolonged cases of obstructive jaundice a low prothrombin level with resulting hæmorrhages may arise.

3. Gastro-intestinal and Liver Diseases.

In such chronic diseases of the gastro-intestinal tract as sprue and chronic ulcerative colitis, or after extensive removal of the bowel, the resultant deficient absorption of vitamin K from the intestines may lead to prothrombin deficiency and hæmorrhages.

Severe liver damage, such as may arise in cirrhosis of the liver or severe cases of hepatitis, can prevent the formation and storage of prothrombin in the liver

4. Anticoagulant Drugs.

Certain drugs can destroy the prothrombin in the blood and so lead to a prolonged clotting time. Phenindione, dicoumarol, tromexan and other allied anticoagulant drugs are very potent in this respect and in medicine are used for the sole purpose of producing a prolonged clotting time in the treatment of venous and coronary thrombosis.

Salicylates have an effect which is similar to but much less powerful than that of the anticoagulant drugs.

SOME COMMON VITAMIN PREPARATIONS

1. Vitamins A and D.

Liq. Vitamin A and D conc. (B.P.).
Capsules Vitamin A and D (National Formulary).

PROPRIETARY PREPARATIONS.

Adexolin.
Davitamon.
Radiostoleum.
Ostelin (Vitamin D only).

2. **Vitamin B Complex.**

(*a*) **B$_1$ (Aneurine).**

Tab. Aneurin Hydrochlor (B.P.).
Inj. Aneurin Hydrochlor (B.P.).

PROPRIETARY PREPARATIONS.

Benerva.
Betaxan.
Davitamon B$_1$.

(*b*) **Riboflavine (Vitamin B$_2$).**

PROPRIETARY PREPARATIONS.

Beflavit.
Ribovel.

(*c*) **Nicotinic Acid.**

Tab. Acid Nicotinic (B.P.).

PROPRIETARY PREPARATION.

Nicovel.

3. **Vitamin C.**

Tab. Acid Ascorbic (B.P.).

PROPRIETARY PREPARATIONS.

Ascorvel.
Davitamon C.
Redoxon.

4. **Vitamin K.**

Tab. Acetomenaphthone (B.P.).
Inj. Menaphthone (B.P.).

PROPRIETARY PREPARATIONS.

Prokayvit.
Synkavit.
Vitavel K.

CHAPTER XVI

DISEASES OF THE JOINTS AND BONES

JOINTS

ARTHRITIS

INFLAMMATION of a joint, or joints, is known as arthritis and is due to many different causes. The term *arthritis* is also often used to include disease of the joints which is not, strictly speaking, due to inflammation.

Causes.

1. Traumatic Arthritis.

Injury to a joint is one of the commonest causes of arthritis, and this form is fully described in surgical textbooks. Trauma, even of a trivial nature, may also cause a predisposition to other forms of arthritis as will be seen when osteo-arthritis is discussed.

2. Specific Infective Arthritis.

Arthritis caused by known specific organisms is usually classed as infective arthritis. There are many different forms of this type of arthritis, and as some of them are rare only the more common forms will be mentioned.

(*a*) ACUTE SEPTIC ARTHRITIS.—Pyogenic organisms such as streptococci, staphylococci and pneumococci may gain entrance to a joint either by direct invasion or by blood stream infection. Usually one joint only is affected; the result is acute severe inflammation with swelling, tenderness and pain in the joint. Pus may be present.

The general condition is, in most cases, that of a severely ill toxic person with high fever and often with rigors. The treatment is an intensive course of one of the antibiotic drugs such as penicillin, tetracycline or chloromycetin. If the condition does not rapidly improve surgical drainage by aspiration or incision into the joint is necessary.

(*b*) TUBERCULOUS ARTHRITIS.—This form of arthritis is usually seen in young adults and tends to affect one joint only, such as the hip or elbow joint. The tuberculous infection may spread into the surrounding muscles and tissues to form an abscess. This abscess has several special features in that it travels to the surface to break down and form a chronic sinus. Because it is unlike the abscess due to a pyogenic infection, of which increased local heat is always a feature, a tuberculous abscess is often called a " **cold abscess.**"

The diagnosis of tuberculosis as the infective agent is most important as for this form prolonged rest with streptomycin is necessary. X-ray examination of the joint is very valuable in determining the diagnosis.

(*c*) GONOCOCCAL ARTHRITIS.—The gonococcus often causes a generalised arthritis affecting several joints, including the knee, elbow and temporo-mandibular. Generally there is a history of a recent attack of gonorrhœa, and blood tests may be positive for the gonococcal infection. General constitutional symptoms, including fever, are present. Penicillin is given, which has a very good effect. Later, active massage and heat treatment are given.

(*d*) SYPHILITIC ARTHRITIS.—Syphilis does not often cause a direct infection of the joints, any involvement of the latter usually being due to spread from syphilitic disease of bones or a result of syphilitic neurological diseases (see Charcot's Joints).

Congenital syphilis, however, often causes a chronic swelling in both knee-joints (Clutton's joints).

3. Osteo-arthritis.

This is an extremely common form of arthritis mainly seen in people over 40 years of age. It is often called a degenerative, as opposed to an infectious, joint disease. The exact cause is unknown, but there are several factors which may play a part in producing the disease. Trauma, often only trivial, may initiate the arthritis, and strain from obesity, which is commonly present with this disease, is also important. The weight-bearing joints of the lower limbs are most frequently affected, especially the knees and hips. In these patients degenerative changes in the terminal finger joints may also cause the nodular swellings (*Heberden's nodes*) which are so often seen.

This form of arthritis differs from the other type common in adults (rheumatoid arthritis) in that the disease remains a local affection of the joint and causes little general constitutional disturbance. The patients complain of pain and swelling of the joint with limitation of movement, so that getting about may be difficult.

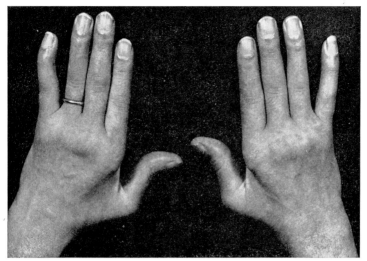

FIG. 172

Early rheumatoid arthritis of the hands, showing the characteristic
swelling and deformity of the joints.

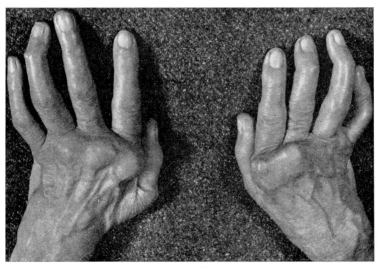

FIG. 173

Advanced rheumatoid arthritis of the hands, showing the gross
deformity and the typical position of the hands.

Treatment consists mainly of heat and active movements to prevent the joints becoming fixed. Reduction of weight in the obese patient is very important. There are various surgical operations (arthroplasty and prosthesis) which may be performed in some cases of osteo-arthritis of the hip joint to relieve pain and give greater mobility. Intra-articular injections of hydrocortisone often give rapid relief of pain with increased mobility, but it is as yet too early to assess the value of hydrocortisone in the treatment of osteo-arthritis.

4. Rheumatoid Arthritis.

Rheumatoid arthritis is one of the most important types of arthritis because it is very common and can be so severe that many patients become severely disabled or even bed-ridden.

Cause.—The disease is of a chronic inflammatory nature, but so far no specific organism or known infection has been established as its cause.

Symptoms and Signs.

(*a*) The disease occurs more frequently in women, and is especially common around the menopause. It tends to run a chronic progressive course, despite remissions during which the symptoms subside.

(*b*) The main effect of the disease is on the joints, several of which, especially the hands, wrists, shoulders, ankles and knees, are usually affected. The joints become swollen, thickened, painful and limited in their movements and eventually fixed and deformed. At this stage the patient finds great difficulty in carrying on a normal life, and if enough joints are affected becomes bed-ridden.

(*c*) General constitutional symptoms such as fever, anæmia, loss of energy and weight are present in the active stage of the disease.

Diagnosis.—Diagnosis is usually easy; characteristic features are swelling and pain affecting several joints (particularly the hands and feet), general ill-health and a chronic course with remissions. Osteo-arthritis, the other common form of arthritis, tends to affect only single joints whilst the general health is not seriously disturbed.

Treatment of Rheumatoid Arthritis.—It is important to realise that, as yet, no specific cure exists and so treatment has to be prolonged and intensive. In the acute stages, especially in early cases, bed rest is necessary. The affected joints must be kept at rest in their optimum positions, if necessary by the aid of light splints. Cradles must be used to take the weight of the bed clothes off the affected limbs.

Physiotherapy is an essential part of the treatment. Heat applied by means of radiant heat cradles, infra-red lamps or short-wave diathermy is most useful in relieving pain. The joints should be put through a full range of movements daily to prevent their becoming fixed. Active movements are undertaken as soon as the acute pain subsides. As movements are easier to perform under water, special baths are very helpful in the treatment of these cases.

Aspirin is probably the best available drug for most patients with rheumatoid arthritis. It should be given in daily doses of approximately 90 gr. until signs of overdosage (tinnitus, slight deafness) appear, when the dose is reduced.

Gold injections (usually in the form of myocrisin) have been found useful in some cases when weekly intramuscular injections of 0·01 to 0·05 gm. are given. Gold is a toxic drug and may cause toxic reactions, such as damage to the kidneys, dermatitis and agranulocytosis. The urine should be tested for albumin before each injection and frequent blood counts taken.

Cortisone and its allied steroids (see p. 597) sometimes have the effect of relieving the pain and stiffness of the joints in rheumatoid arthritis. Unfortunately, this form of treatment does not remove the cause of rheumatoid arthritis, which is unknown. As a result, since it only offers relief of symptoms, when this treatment is discontinued the patient tends to get worse again. On the other hand, the longer these steroids are administered, and the higher the dose, the greater the dangers of toxic effects. These include obesity, thinning of the bones, liability to infection, high blood pressure, peptic ulcer and œdema. Hence it is clear that cortisone and other steroids must be administered with great caution and in small doses. These tablets should never be discontinued suddenly, since the normal secretion of the adrenal cortex is suppressed when cortisone is given and the gland lies dormant for a long time after it has been stopped. If cortisone is discontinued gradually, the gland has time to recover.

Cortisone itself leads to œdema too easily, so that prednisolone is commonly used in the treatment of rheumatoid arthritis. It is best not to exceed 9 mgm. daily and to use it only in certain of the patients who do not respond to aspirin or phenylbutazone. Other forms of cortisone sometimes used in the treatment of rheumatoid arthritis include dexamethasone, betamethasone and triamcinolone.

Phenylbutazone (butazolidin) is very effective in relieving the pain in rheumatoid arthritis, thus enabling the patient to do more for himself. Unfortunately, phenylbutazone is a toxic drug and blood disorders (agranulocytosis and aplastic anæmia) and œdema may result from its use. The use of this drug is best limited to patients who have failed to respond to physiotherapy and aspirin and to patients with spondylitis. The average dose is 100 to 200 mgm. two or three times a day.

Recently the drug chloroquine and its derivative (plaquenil) have been used in the treatment of rheumatoid arthritis but it is too early to say with what result. An initial dosage of 200 to 600 mgm. of plaquenil is used.

5. Rheumatoid Spondylitis.

Arthritis may affect the joints in the spinal column, causing changes very similar to those seen in the ordinary form of rheumatoid arthritis. Arthritis which affects the spine is usually called a spondylitis, and as the cause is commonly believed to be similar to the cause of rheumatoid arthritis the disease is often known as rheumatoid spondylitis. Other names given to this or similar lesions are *ankylosing spondylitis* or *spondylitis ankylopoietica*.

The main result of this type of progressive arthritis is fixation of the spine which causes a rigid or " poker " back. The spine becomes fused into one rigid bony column. The X-ray is characteristic, showing the " bamboo spine." The patients, usually younger than those affected by the ordinary form of rheumatoid arthritis, complain of severe pain and limitation of movement of the spine. Eventually, if the disease is not arrested the patients become bed-ridden.

Treatment is as outlined under rheumatoid arthritis. Deep X-ray therapy in the early stages has proved most useful. Cortisone may also be of benefit in these cases and, in addition, phenylbutazone is said to be of particular value in reducing the pain.

6. Joint Neuropathies.

In some diseases of the central nervous system the sensory nerves from the joints and muscles are affected, leading to loss of the sensation of pain. Because they cause no pain, repeated trivial injuries or strain may then be incurred without being noticed, with consequent extensive damage to the joints. The arthritis produced is a form of osteo-arthritis, except that it is much more severe, resulting in almost complete destruction of the joint. This is grossly swollen and can be moved into many abnormal positions without any pain.

Charcot was the first to describe this form of arthritis in neurological disease and so it is usually called " Charcot's joint." Generally Charcot's joints occur in tabes dorsalis, due to syphilis. In the less common disease, syringomyelia, Charcot's joints are also seen.

7. Deficiency Diseases and Arthritis.

In scurvy hæmorrhages occur around the joints, causing swelling and pain. In rickets arthritis is not common, the ligaments and bones being primarily affected.

DISEASES OF THE CONNECTIVE TISSUE

FIBROSITIS

(Non-articular Rheumatism, Muscular Rheumatism)

Recurring pains in the muscles are often called fibrositis or " non-articular rheumatism." The exact cause and nature of the disease is unknown. Some people are particularly liable to recurrent attacks of fibrositis and they often refer to themselves as being subject to " rheumatism." Why the disease attacks some people again and again in acute or subacute form and does not affect others is unknown. Factors which appear to be of some importance are damp weather, change in temperature and physical fatigue, which often precipitate an attack. It is now thought that in many cases of fibrositis there is an underlying emotional strain or anxiety neurosis.

Symptoms and Signs.—These depend on the areas affected, some sites being involved very often. Acute fibrositis of the lumbar muscles causes the well-known syndrome of *lumbago*, with severe pain in the back and extreme stiffness of the lumbar muscles. Acute " stiff neck " is commonly due to fibrositis of the cervical area. After the acute attack subsides movement and power are fully regained.

There are also more subacute forms which cause pain, stiffness and limitation of movement of the affected area (which may be any muscle group). The symptoms may last for weeks, especially in wet weather, and recur over years. Even in these cases there is practically full recovery in between the attacks so that these patients do not become bed-ridden.

Treatment.—Massage, heat and active exercises are the mainstay of treatment. The heat relieves the pain and allows freer movement. Massage helps to break down the nodules and relieves the spasm and stiffness of the muscles. Rubbing in a liniment such as methyl salicylate (oil of wintergreen) acts as a massage and also as a counter-irritant which relieves pain. Sedatives such as aspirin or codeine are also most useful for the pain. Active exercises are undertaken as soon as the acute stage is over to prevent continuing stiffness of the muscles.

DISEASES OF THE BONES

Diseases of the bones are of much greater importance in surgery than in medicine. This is because the most common bone lesions are injuries, tumours and infections, all of which come under the scope of surgical diseases. Many of the diseases of the bones which are seen in medicine are rare and only a brief mention of the more important and interesting of these diseases will be made.

1. The changes in the bones in acromegaly, gigantism, rickets, osteomalacia and in the rare but interesting disease of the parathyroid glands known as osteitis fibrosa cystica have all already been described.

2. In **achondroplasia** abnormality of the bones in fœtal life leads to short limbs, normal trunk and large head. These people are usually dwarfs and are characteristically very good humoured. Most of the dwarf clowns seen in a circus are examples of achondroplasia.

3. In the rare bone disease known as **fragilitas ossium (osteogenesis imperfecta),** the extraordinary fragility of the bones results in recurrent fractures, leading to gross deformities. This disease occurs in infancy and is due to a heredity defect in bone development. Many of these patients have characteristic blue sclerotics of the eyes.

4. In any long-standing chronic illness, especially in elderly people, marked softening of the bones may develop (**osteoporosis**) which, in extreme cases, may cause fractures. Fracture of a bone resulting not from an injury but from disease in the bone is known as a *pathological* fracture. The commonest cause of pathological fractures is malignant secondary deposits (*metastases*) which have spread from a primary malignant growth in some organ or tissue to the bones by way of the blood stream. Carcinomas of the prostate, breast and thyroid gland are particularly liable to give rise to secondary deposits in the bones with consequential necrosis (destruction) of the bone.

5. Softening of the bones is very commonly met with in ageing and senile people and is then called *senile osteoporosis*. It is usually seen in women, generally after the menopause, and hence is also

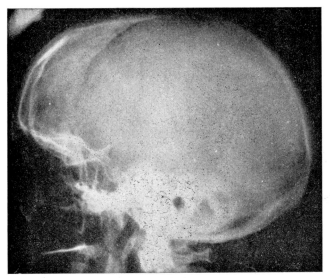

FIG. 174
X-ray of a normal skull.

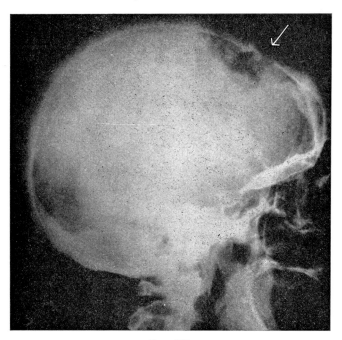

FIG. 175
Secondary deposits in the skull from a primary carcinoma of the thyroid. The bone is being eaten away by the malignant tissue.

17

often called post-menopausal osteoporosis. Treatment with calcium gluconate and œstrogen hormones is frequently very effective.

6. In **multiple myelomatosis** there is widespread invasion of the bones by deposits of myeloma cells. The condition is progressive and fatal. The patient usually complains of severe pains in the bones and a profound degree of anæmia is often present. Spontaneous fractures are common.

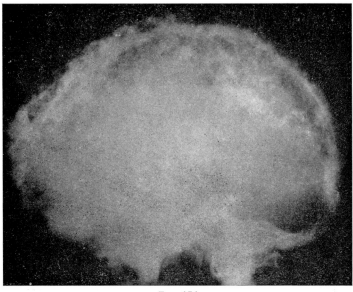

FIG. 176

X-ray of the skull in Paget's disease, showing the marked thickening and sclerosis of the bone.

Osteitis Deformans, otherwise known as *Paget's disease* of the bones, is perhaps one of the more common bone diseases. The cause is unknown, but it leads to progressive thickening and deformities of the bones, especially the skull, tibia, femur, spine and pelvis. The disease occurs after the age of 40, and men are more frequently affected than women. The head becomes enlarged so that an increasing size in hats is needed. The legs become bowed and thickened and the spine curved so that the height is reduced. X-ray examination reveals the typical thickening of the bones. So far no treatment has been found effective, but most patients live to a fairly good age, especially in those cases in which the disease remains localised in one bone.

CHAPTER XVII

DISEASES OF THE SKIN

IN a general textbook of medicine it is impossible to give a comprehensive account of all skin diseases. It is therefore intended to mention here only the commoner of the diseases of the skin that the nurse is likely to meet with in a general hospital.

Before dealing with the individual skin diseases a brief word on the general terms used in describing different types of skin lesion is perhaps useful :—

1. *Macules* are flat spots which are not raised above the skin and are usually red or brown in colour.
2. *Papules* are small raised skin lesions.
3. *Vesicles* are very small blisters filled with clear serous fluid.
4. *Bullæ* are large vesicles.
5. *Pustules* are vesicles filled with pus instead of serous fluid.
6. *Wheals* are areas of skin swollen by œdema so that they are a white colour with a red margin.
7. *Scaling* is caused by dead epithelium of the skin flaking off, usually as a result of inflammation of the skin.
8. *Weeping* in skin lesions arises when there is marked exudation of serum or lymph from the skin. It is usually the result of acute or subacute inflammatory lesions.
9. *Crusts* or *scabs* usually result from the drying up of the serum in weeping lesions.

Many other terms are also used in skin diseases, but these are generally self-explanatory.

GENERAL PRINCIPLES OF TREATMENT

In addition to the various specific treatments used in diseases of the skin there are certain general principles applicable to most skin lesions.

1. It is essential to **remove the cause** of the skin disease if possible, *e.g.*, stop any drug which may be causing the skin eruption, remove

any offending articles either in the diet or coming in contact with the skin, or kill any parasite.

2. **External Applications.**—External applications play a large part in the treatment of skin diseases. The following are the applications most commonly used :—

(*a*) POWDERS.—These are used on slightly moist areas to dry the skin. They are also useful in preventing friction on the skin. Talc and zinc oxide are powders in frequent use.

(*b*) LOTIONS.—Lotions are widely used, particularly for weeping lesions. Calamine lotion is a very commonly used preparation. Lotions are best applied by dabbing them on with lint. Sedatives, *e.g.*, phenol, to allay itching may be combined with the lotion, as also may antiseptic preparations, *e.g.*, ichthyol.

(*c*) CREAMS AND LINIMENTS.—These are mainly used in weeping and inflamed areas of skin. They should be smeared on or applied on gauze.

(*d*) OINTMENTS AND PASTES.—These preparations are applied when there is no excessive weeping. Pastes are most useful for subacute slightly moist lesions, whilst ointments are preferred for the more chronic scaling lesions. When ointments or pastes are applied, the removal of the old application should be effected by swabbing with cotton wool soaked in oil in order to prevent damage to the underlying skin. Ointments and pastes should be thickly applied and as little covering as possible used. Lassar's paste is a most effective and frequently used paste.

(*e*) POULTICES.—Boric and starch poultices are mostly used in skin diseases for removing thick crusts. Fomentations are used for septic skin lesions.

3. **Cold, Heat and Radiation.**—These are all frequently used in the treatment of diseases of the skin. Cold, usually in the form of carbon dioxide snow, is used in the removal of warts and nævi; heat, often in the form of a cautery, is also used to remove warts and nævi, whilst radiation in various forms, such as ultra-violet light, thorium X, superficial X-rays and radium, is used in a wide variety of skin diseases.

4. **Antibiotics.**—Antibiotics, *e.g.*, the tetracyclines and neomycin are used in the treatment of skin diseases due to infection. Streptomycin is given for tuberculosis of the skin. Because sensitisation is very likely to develop, penicillin and chloramphenicol are not used for local application.

5. **Cortisone and allied Drugs** (hydrocortisone, prednisone,

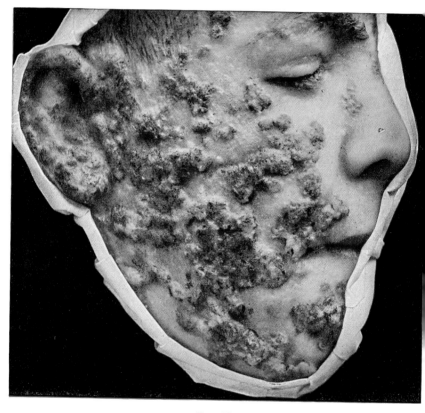

FIG. 177
Impetigo.

[To face page 517

prednisolone and triamcinolone).—These drugs are given with very good effect in several severe and uncommon diseases such as disseminated lupus erythematosus, pemphigus and exfoliative dermatitis. Local application of 1 per cent. hydrocortisone is also used in some resistant cases of eczema, erythema multiforme and allergic skin conditions.

SKIN DISEASES DUE TO STREPTOCOCCAL AND STAPHYLOCOCCAL INFECTION

IMPETIGO

Impetigo is a very common skin disease, which is most frequently met with in infants and young children. It is caused by infection of the skin by staphylococci or streptococci.

Features of the Eruption.

1. The eruption usually starts on the face, especially around the mouth and behind the ears, and may spread to the scalp.

2. Vesicles form in the first stage, which later develop into crusts of a yellowish colour. These crusts are typically described as having a " stuck-on " appearance.

Treatment.—Impetigo is very contagious and can spread rapidly. This characteristic is particularly important when treating impetigo in infants in a nursery or ward. Every care must be taken to isolate a case occurring in a nursery, and a careful search must be made in order to trace and isolate the source of the staphylococcal or streptococcal infection.

In the treatment of impetigo thick crusts must first be removed by bathing or by the use of starch poultices. Local applications include paints, *e.g.*, 1 per cent. brilliant green and crystal violet, and mercury ointment (unguentum hydrarg. ammon. dil.).

Antibiotic ointments have proved of value in impetigo and are often used in severe and resistant cases. Oxytetracycline (terramycin), chlortetracycline (aureomycin), neomycin and neomycin combined with bacitracin are all very effective. Penicillin and chloramphenicol should not be used for local application as sensitisation is very liable to develop. This will then debar all future use, either external or internal, of these antibiotics for these patients. Sensitivity to neomycin is said to occur only on rare occasions. Even if it does occur, however, the fact that the patient has become sensitive to the antibiotic is of little importance because neomycin is in any case not usually given internally owing to its toxic effects by this route.

SYCOSIS

Sycosis is an infection of the hair follicles of the beard region by the staphylococcus. Sycosis is, with impetigo, often included in the term *barber's rash* because infection is often acquired at the barber's.

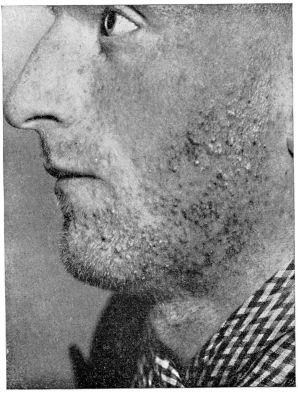

FIG. 178
Sycosis.

Features of the Eruption.

1. The common sites are the upper lip and chin, but in severe cases the lesions rapidly spread all over the beard region.

2. There is generalised redness of the area with small pustules surrounding each hair follicle. A weeping pustular rash soon develops.

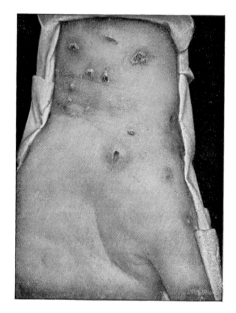

Fig. 179
Scabies.

[*To face page* 519

3. The condition is very liable to become chronic and resistant to treatment.

Treatment.—Sycosis is very resistant to treatment and relapses are very prone to occur necessitating prolonged therapy. During the active stage shaving is stopped, the hair being kept short by clipping. As many as possible of the pustular hair follicles are removed.

Quinolor and vioform ointments have been used with benefit in many cases.

Antibiotics by local application are often given with good effect. Oxytetracycline, chlortetracycline and neomycin are most commonly used at present.

FURUNCULOSIS (BOILS)

Furunculosis, caused by infection of the hair follicles with staphylococci, is usually seen in debilitated people. Furunculosis is particularly prone to be found together with diabetes. Areas subject to irritation such as the back of the neck are frequent sites. The typical lesion is the presence of multiple boils. In severe cases the boils may become carbuncles.

Penicillin usually clears up the condition. The general health of the patient must be attended to, and the urine should always be examined for the presence of sugar.

SKIN DISEASES DUE TO ANIMAL PARASITES

SCABIES

Scabies is a very common contagious skin disease caused by the female parasite the *Acarus scabiei* (itch mite). This parasite burrows into the skin where it lays its eggs. The eggs hatch out, and then the small mites in their turn burrow through the skin, causing the typical eruption.

Close contact with an infected person is necessary to spread infection. Furthermore, the acarus usually burrows at night. Infection is therefore usually contracted by sleeping with an infected person.

Features of the Eruption (Fig. 179).

1. The typical eruption is the burrow which is commonest in the webs of the fingers, and on the wrists, axillæ and buttocks. The

acarus may often be seen, with the aid of a hand lens, as a tiny white speck at the end of the burrow. In some cases, if the point of a needle is inserted into the burrow, the acarus will adhere to the needle and the mite can then be identified under the microscope.

2. Owing to the severe itching, at night especially, a red papular eruption with scratch marks is always present. Secondary infection is also very liable to occur, with the result that impetigo is often present too.

3. Scabies is very liable to affect several people in the same household as it is a contagious disease.

Treatment.—The usual treatment is with benzyl benzoate emulsion, which is applied all over the body from the neck downwards, the patient having first had a hot bath and thoroughly scrubbed all the lesions to lay open the burrows. The benzyl benzoate emulsion dries in about ten minutes. A second application is often applied on the next day.

PEDICULOSIS

Three kinds of lice infect man—the head, the body and the crab lice. Infestation with lice occurs through lack of cleanliness.

(*a*) PEDICULUS CAPITIS (head louse).—Infestation with head lice is particularly common in children, especially girls. The eggs of the louse, the nits, become firmly attached to the hairs. The lice feed on blood, and the bites of the lice cause severe persistent itching; the consequent scratching generally results in infected lesions, such as impetigo. The cervical glands of the neck are usually enlarged.

There are many effective forms of treatment for head lice. A 2 per cent. D.D.T. emulsion and lethane are both in frequent use.

(*b*) PEDICULUS CORPORIS (body louse).—Infection with body lice is usually confined to people who neglect proper cleanliness, and is particularly common in tramps or in overcrowded conditions with a lack of proper hygiene, *e.g.*, in camps in time of war. The body louse lives in the seams of the underclothes and feeds by biting the person. The itching leads to severe scratch marks, particularly on the shoulders. The bites of the lice are seen as small red macules.

Apart from the severe irritation and secondary skin infections caused by body lice, these parasites transmit such important diseases as typhus and relapsing fever.

The treatment consists of the application of 10 per cent. D.D.T. powder to the underclothes. Hot ironing of the seams of the clothes will kill off all the lice. The provision of adequate water supplies for washing and laundering in all camps is an essential preventive measure.

(c) PEDICULUS PUBIS (crab louse).—*Pediculus pubis* generally affects the pubic region and anus, but also affects the axillæ. Infestation is most frequently acquired during sexual intercourse or from an infected lavatory seat. Severe irritation, with scratch marks, occurs as a result of the bites of the lice.

D.D.T. powder or emulsion thoroughly applied to the affected parts is usually very efficacious ; so also is benzyl benzoate, applied as in scabies.

DISEASES DUE TO FUNGI

Fungus infections of the skin are very common. The stomatitis seen in infants and known as *thrush* is due to a fungus infection.

INTERTRIGO

A fungus (monilia) is often responsible for the condition known as intertrigo. This is a moist papular red eruption commonly seen in areas of friction, *e.g.*, under the breasts in women, and in the groins, axillæ and natal cleft.

Salicylic and benzoic acid ointment or a paint such as brilliant green and crystal violet usually clears up the monilia infection. In prevention, frequent bathing and keeping the areas as dry as possible by the use of powder are important.

RINGWORM

Ringworm or tinea is due to various fungi, which may affect the skin, hair or nails.

1. Ringworm of the Skin.

Ringworm usually affects such sites as the feet, groins, beard region and hands.

(a) *Ringworm of the feet* is extremely common and causes a sodden white maceration of the skin between the toes. Infection is probably spread through bath mats or wet floors in bathrooms. The commonly seen thickened skin (hyperkeratosis) of the heel is also due to ringworm infection.

17 A

(*b*) *Ringworm of the groins* (*Tinea cruris*) is usually referred to as " dhobie itch." It causes a red inflamed irritating eruption in the groins, which often spreads to the natal cleft. Like all ringworm infections it usually flares up in hot weather owing to the increased sweating.

(*c*) *Ringworm of the beard* (*Tinea barbæ*) is usually contracted at the barber's and is the third type of " barber's rash " (the other two being impetigo and sycosis). The lesions may be dry, red, scaly and ringed in appearance, or suppurative, with purplish nodules. In both types the hairs break off, leaving stumps.

(*d*) *Ringworm of the hands and the body* is usually in the form of red scaling lesions which heal in the centre, thus giving the characteristic ringed or circular outline from which the disease gets its name.

Ringworm of the feet and groins is treated by the application of salicylic and benzoic acid ointment (Whitfield's) or any of the many preparations available for the purpose (mersagel, mycozol, tineafax). Every care must be taken to keep the parts as dry as possible. Underclothes and socks must be thoroughly boiled, and care should be taken to prevent reinfection in swimming baths and from wet floors.

Ringworm of the body and hands is similarly treated with Whitfield's ointment or such preparations as mersagel or tineafax. In resistant cases dithranol (cignolin) ointment is used, but this preparation is irritating and also stains the clothes.

Ringworm of the beard may be treated by X-rays, which remove all the affected hairs, and by the use of salicylic and benzoic acid ointment.

2. Ringworm of the Scalp.

Ringworm of the scalp is usually seen in children. It causes a scaling bald patch on the scalp, the hairs in the affected patch breaking off just above the level of the scalp and leaving well-marked stumps. The affected hairs when examined in a dark room with Wood's light show a characteristic green fluorescence.

There is also another variety of ringworm infection of the hair which does not cause the scaling bald patches just described, namely " black-dot " ringworm. Here a circular bald patch is seen in which the hairs are broken off close to the scalp, giving rise to the " black-dot " appearance. In some cases of ringworm, suppuration may occur, resulting in swollen inflamed areas in which pus is present.

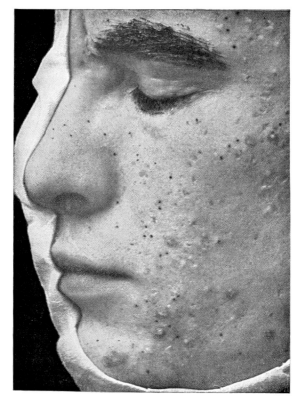

Fig. 180
Acne vulgaris.

[*To face page* 523

Ringworm of the scalp is treated by X-rays or by the antibiotic griseofulvin.

3. Ringworm of the Nails.

Ringworm of the nails is a very resistant infection causing rough cracked nails and scaling. There is also another type of fungus infection which causes chronic paronychia of the nails in women who constantly have their hands in water. In this form of fungus infection the nail folds become red, swollen and septic.

More recently all forms of ringworm have been successfully treated by giving the antibiotic griseofulvin (grisovin, fulcin) in daily doses of 1 to 2 gm. Treatment may have to be continued for months till all the infected hairs or nails have been shed.

OTHER COMMON SKIN DISEASES

ACNE VULGARIS

Acne vulgaris is a skin disease which is extremely common about the age of puberty, but rarely arises after the age of 30.

Features of the Eruption.—The face, chest and back are the sites usually affected. The typical lesions are *blackheads* (comedones), red papules and pustules. In severe cases with much pustule formation scars may develop with consequential permanent damage.

Acne occurs most frequently in people with greasy skins (seborrhœa), and dandruff (scurf, seborrhœa sicca) of the scalp is also usually present. In some cases diet may aggravate the condition, especially overindulgence in carbohydrates.

Treatment.—Patients with a tendency to acne suffer from greasy skin and must therefore be discouraged from using greasy preparations on the skin. In the treatment frequent washing of the affected parts to remove the excessive grease is necessary. The application most commonly used is a sulphur lotion (often combined with calamine lotion), which must be applied for a long period. It is also essential to express as many blackheads as possible, either by hand or by the use of a special comedo extractor.

The diet should be regulated where necessary and any dandruff present must also be treated.

In severe cases which do not respond to the above treatment X-rays are extremely useful and widely employed.

ACNE ROSACEA

Acne rosacea is another very common form of acne, but here the condition usually occurs after the age of 30 and is particularly common in women or in people continually exposed to the weather.

Features of the Eruption.

1. In acne rosacea, in contrast to acne vulgaris, there are no blackheads. The eruption characteristically starts as a redness and flushing of the nose and cheeks, which occurs particularly after hot meals or drinks. A history of dyspepsia is very common in acne rosacea, and strong tea and alcohol are predominant factors.

2. The redness and flushing of the face become permanent and dilated vessels can clearly be seen. Red papules are also frequently present, and secondary infection may lead to pustular formation.

3. In very chronic cases in men, marked enlargement and hypertrophy of the nose (*rhinophyma*) result.

Treatment.—The dyspepsia must be treated and the diet adjusted. Strong tea and alcohol especially must be avoided. In some cases the dyspepsia is associated with a lack of hydrochloric acid in the gastric juice (achlorhydria), and here dilute hydrochloric acid (30 minims before meals) is useful.

Calamine lotion with the addition of 2 per cent. sulphur is a very effective local application. Other useful applications include lead or ichthyol combined with calamine lotion.

PSORIASIS

The very common skin disease known as psoriasis usually starts about the age of 10 and is very chronic, recurring over a period of many years at irregular intervals. The cause of the condition is unknown, but in many cases there is a strong familial factor.

Features of the Eruption.

1. The sites characteristically affected are the extensor aspects of the elbows and knees, the scalp and the trunk. The hands, particularly the nails, may also be affected, but rarely the face.

2. The typical lesion is a red papular eruption surrounded by scales which when scraped off have a silvery colour. The lesions are dry and infection rarely develops. Itching is not a feature.

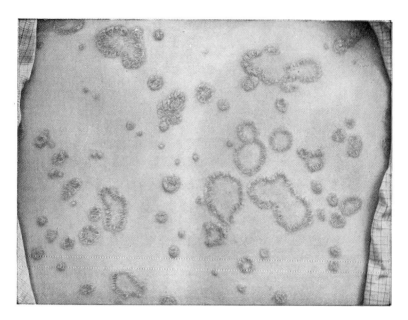

Fig. 181
Psoriasis.

[*To face page* 524

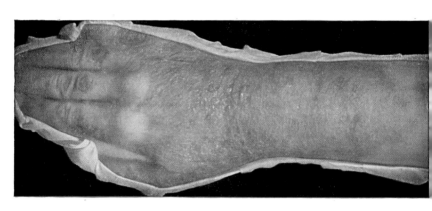

FIG. 182
Eczema.

3. The extent of the lesions varies considerably, from a small patch on a knee or elbow to large confluent patches covering large areas. The patches often have a circular ringed outline.

4. Psoriasis of the nails causes deep pitting in some cases, whilst in others it causes separation of the nails from the nail beds, the nail ultimately breaking off.

Treatment.—Individual attacks usually clear up with intensive treatment, but it is impossible to prevent further attacks. In the acute stage, with extensive spreading lesions, the patient is treated in bed, and at this point only a sedative soothing lotion such as calamine or a zinc cream is used. When the lesions cease to spread mercury ointment or a weak preparation of tar is applied.

In the more chronic cases dithranol is a very effective local application; it is rubbed into the lesions daily until eventually each patch becomes red, after which the dithranol is stopped and a sedative zinc cream applied. Before using dithranol the scales should be removed by means of soap and a hot bath. Dithranol must be used with care as it can cause a severe inflammation of the skin; in particular, it must be prevented from coming in contact with the eyes as a severe conjunctivitis results. Dithranol has also the disadvantage that it stains linen.

In psoriasis of the scalp scabs must be removed by frequent shampooing and a salicylic and tar ointment rubbed in daily.

X-rays are occasionally used in the treatment of very chronic and localised patches of psoriasis. Some patients may be treated with the steroid triamcinolone, which is the only steroid to have any effect in psoriasis.

ECZEMA

The term *eczema*, or *eczematous dermatitis*, is used to describe several varieties of skin condition which have, however, a number of common features. The exact cause or causes of eczema are imperfectly understood. In many cases eczema can be attributed to external irritants, *e.g.*, soaps, dyes, polishes, chemicals, plants, food-stuffs, etc. Why eczema should develop in some people from contact with such substances is unknown, and it appears that there must be some other internal factor present which renders eczematous patients very sensitive to mild irritants. In support of this theory is the fact that various forms of eczema are associated with the allergic diseases like asthma and hay fever.

Features of the Eruption.—The many and various types of eczema have different individual features, but in most cases the skin lesions have the following general characteristics :—

1. The lesion usually starts as a diffuse reddening or erythema of the skin.
2. Vesicles form on this erythema.
3. Weeping usually occurs owing to serum exuding from the vesicles, and crusts may form.
4. The condition usually becomes chronic, and in this stage dry scaling lesions with thickening and pigmentation of the skin (lichenification) develop.
5. Eczematous lesions usually itch.

Types of Eczema.—It is impossible in the space available to give more than a few of the commoner types of eczema.

1. INFANTILE ECZEMA.—This form is very common in infants, particularly males under the age of 2. The face is especially affected, the eczema being weeping and crusted. Itching is usually severe.

2. FLEXURAL ECZEMA (Besnier's prurigo).—Besnier's prurigo usually follows infantile eczema and is associated with asthma. The flexures of the elbows and knees are particularly prone to be affected, hence the term *flexural eczema*. The face and neck may also be affected. The lesions are usually of the chronic, thickened, lichenified type. Most but by no means all cases tend to improve after puberty.

3. VARICOSE ECZEMA.—This form is extremely common, occurring in elderly people with varicose veins and ulcers.

4. ECZEMA OF THE HANDS AND FEET.—Eczema of the hands and feet produces a vesicular eruption which is commonly likened to sago grains in the skin. Chronic forms are very frequent in which the skin, owing to its inelasticity, becomes cracked and deep fissures form. Eczema is one cause of a vesicular dermatitis of the hands which often goes under the name of *cheiropompholyx*. Cheiro-pompholyx may also be caused by external irritants (soap detergents used in cleaning, polishes, dyes, chemicals, etc.) and by fungus infections (ringworm).

Treatment of Eczema.—The first essential is to remove any irritant which may possibly be causing the eczema. In prevention the use of barrier creams or glycerin preparations by people who continually use strong soaps or cleansing powders is very valuable.

The patient's resistance must be built up and any septic focus or disease must be treated.

Local treatment is most important and the particular application depends on the stage of the eczema. In the acute weeping stage a lotion is used such as calamine or lead lotion. These should be applied on gauze or lint and as little covering as possible used. Sedatives, *e.g.*, 1 per cent. phenol or 2 per cent. tar, may be added to the lotion to allay the itching. In the less acute stage an oily liniment is preferred, *e.g.*, calamine liniment, to which 2 per cent. ichthyol may be added. In the chronic stages pastes are the most useful applications, and zinc paste with the addition of tar as a stimulant, or crude coal tar itself, is commonly used.

In infantile eczema it may be necessary to prevent the child scratching the lesions by means of cardboard splints. White's tar paste is a useful application for infantile eczema and is best applied on a mask of butter muslin.

In all cases of eczema soap and water usually aggravate the skin so that their use must be forbidden as far as possible.

In severe cases of eczema which do not respond to the above measures hydrocortisone by local application in a 1 per cent. ointment is often given with dramatic effects. Local application of hydrocortisone has the great advantage that it does not cause any of the side effects seen when hydrocortisone and allied drugs are given systemically. Unfortunately, in some cases after cessation of treatment, the condition may relapse.

SEBORRHŒIC DERMATITIS

Seborrhœic dermatitis is a very common inflammation of the skin which particularly affects the scalp, backs of the ears and flexures.

Features of the Eruption.

1. Seborrhœic dermatitis of the scalp in the mildest form causes the well-known condition of a scurfy head (*dandruff*). In more acute cases red weeping crusted lesions develop. The scales and crusts in seborrhœic lesions have a typical greasy appearance.

2. Seborrhœic dermatitis of the face produces red or yellow greasy scaling patches; it particularly affects the eyebrows, sides of the nose and ears.

3. Seborrhœic dermatitis of the flexures mainly arises in the

axillæ, groins and front of the chest under the breasts. Red follicular papules are usually seen at the edge of the weeping erythematous dermatitis.

Treatment.—Frequent shampooing of the scalp to remove all the scales is necessary, and a lotion containing salicylic acid is applied. In acute cases with much crusting starch and boric poultices are first used to remove the crusts.

The preparation selenium sulphide (selsun) has also proved very effective in the treatment of seborrhœic dermatitis of the scalp. One or two teaspoonfuls are applied to the scalp and warm water added to make a lather. The lotion is allowed to remain in contact with the scalp for five minutes, after which the hair is thoroughly rinsed. Selsun is applied twice weekly for two weeks.

For seborrhœic dermatitis of the face and body, crusts are first removed and a soothing calamine lotion applied. In the subacute and chronic stages when the lesions are comparatively dry a sulphur and salicylic ointment is used.

URTICARIA (Nettle-rash)

The characteristic lesion in urticaria is the wheal, with pale œdematous centre and red margin similar to that caused by the sting of a nettle, hence the name " nettle-rash " (Fig. 183).

Causes.—Urticaria can be caused by a wide variety of different agents :—

1. Following injection of serum.
2. By food, particularly shell fish, strawberries, eggs, etc.
3. By drugs, *e.g.*, phenobarbitone, quinine, penicillin, etc.
4. By bites of insects.

In some cases the direct cause of the urticaria is unknown, and in many of these cases the urticaria is an allergic manifestation in a sensitised person. In the chronic recurring attacks of urticaria it is particularly difficult to ascertain the exciting cause.

In addition to the ordinary form of urticaria known as simple urticaria, another type called angioneurotic œdema or giant urticaria is not uncommonly seen. Here there is gross swelling of the mucous membranes, especially those of the eyes, lips and mouth, in addition to the ordinary skin lesions.

Treatment.—A careful search must be made for any exciting factors. In the recurring cases which have no obvious cause a

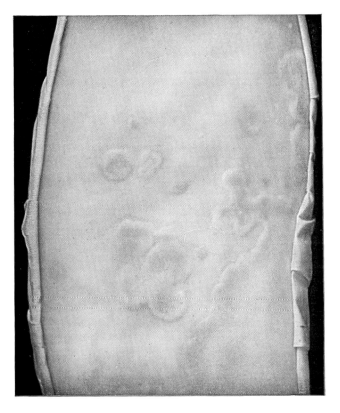

FIG. 183
Urticaria.

[*To face page* 528

prolonged investigation may be required ; nevertheless, even then in many cases, despite a diligent search, it may not be possible to find the exciting factor. Antihistamine drugs (antistin, anthisan, benadryl and phenergan) are very useful in relieving individual attacks. In angioneurotic œdema, adrenaline injections have a dramatic effect in relieving the gross swellings. In very severe attacks (particularly in angioneurotic œdema) which have not responded to the above treatment, cortisone and allied drugs (prednisone, prednisolone, dexamethazone) are usually given with a very beneficial effect in most cases.

ERYTHEMA NODOSUM

Erythema nodosum consists of a localised eruption with general constitutional symptoms.

Cause.—The exact cause of erythema nodosum is still in doubt, and it is probable that the disease is either a specific fever or a manifestation of sensitisation to various organisms, particularly streptococci and tubercle bacilli. In some cases active tuberculosis or rheumatic fever have followed attacks of erythema nodosum.

Symptoms and Signs.

1. The onset is acute with the general constitutional symptoms of fever, including headaches, malaise and, particularly, joint pains.

2. The localised eruption is usually on the front of the legs and consists of raised, indurated, red, tender nodes.

3. The red swellings gradually change colour like a bruise, becoming purple and yellow.

Treatment.—The patient should be nursed in bed till all symptoms and signs have disappeared. This usually takes about fourteen days. No specific treatment is required as the condition subsides of its own accord. Signs of streptococcal infection or tuberculosis are carefully looked for and an X-ray of the chest is usually taken.

ERYTHEMA MULTIFORME

Cause.—Unknown. The disease affects males much more often than females.

Symptoms and Signs.

1. The onset is often sudden with general constitutional upset including fever, headache, malaise and sore throat.

2. Skin eruption. Characteristic circular lesions develop especially on the hands and feet.

3. Eye and mouth lesions particularly conjunctivitis and stomatitis.

4. Inflammation of the genital area with ulceration is usually present.

Course and Treatment.—The disease has a tendency to recur from time to time. It is believed that erythema multiforme may sometimes occur as a toxic reaction to certain drugs or as an allergic condition. Severe forms of erythema multiforme are often known as Steven-Johnson's syndrome. There is no specific treatment.

TUBERCULOSIS OF THE SKIN

There are very many different types of tuberculous skin lesion, and it is possible here to mention only the more important forms.

Lupus Vulgaris.

Lupus vulgaris is the main type of skin tuberculosis. It is a chronic and slowly progressive lesion which usually starts on the face and neck. The characteristic lesion is the " apple-jelly " nodule, which is composed of miliary tubercles. As the skin lesion spreads it causes severe ulceration of the skin. The mucous membranes of the nose and mouth are frequently affected, and in these cases the ultimate effect of severe lupus is serious deformity of the nose and mouth with ulceration and scarring.

Syphilis in the tertiary stage may cause severe deformity of the face with ulceration similar to that caused by lupus vulgaris. In syphilitic cases, however, the common deformity is destruction of the bridge of the nose, producing the well-described " saddle-nose," whereas in tuberculous lesions the tip of the nose is mainly affected.

Another type of skin disease which has to be distinguished from lupus vulgaris is **lupus erythematosus.** Lupus erythematosus is also a chronic and progressive disease, commonest on the face and causing fine scarring. In these cases, however, no deep ulceration is present, and the characteristic lesion is a red scaling patch which leaves a fine scar in the centre when the lesion heals. Lupus erythematosus may affect the hair, causing baldness, and also the hands, causing changes resembling severe chilblains.

Lupus vulgaris is treated by a prolonged course of chemotherapy with streptomycin, isoniazid and para-aminosalicylic acid, as for all forms of active tuberculosis (see p. 93).

Bazin's Disease (Erythema Induratum).

Bazin's disease is another form, most frequently seen in young women, of tuberculosis of the skin. Hard subcutaneous nodules develop on the back of the lower half of the legs. The nodules, which are purple in colour, may break down, forming ulcers which leave deep scars when they heal. In many of these cases there are signs of tuberculosis elsewhere, particularly tuberculous glands.

ALOPECIA AREATA

Alopecia means loss of hair, and may be caused by a variety of conditions. The common form of senile baldness which affects, men particularly, is well known. Loss of hair may also occur in young men where there is a strong hereditary factor. Seborrhœa capitis (dandruff) too is an important factor in causing early loss of hair. Ringworm of the scalp causes bald scaly patches, but this variety is usually met with in children.

Alopecia areata is a common form of baldness which occurs in young people and is rare after the age of 40. The cause is unknown, although endocrine disturbances or anxiety states are supposed to play a part. In many cases the onset is abrupt, with a bald patch developing overnight. The skin in these patches is completely smooth, with no scaling or inflammation. In some cases complete loss of hair may result, affecting all parts of the body.

Most cases of alopecia areata recover completely after varying lengths of time. Any possible causative factor must be investigated and the general health built up. Regrowth of the hair may be hastened in many cases by the use of ultra-violet light.

CHAPTER XVIII

ON PAIN AND VOMITING

PAIN

PAIN is such a common and important symptom in diseases of practically all systems that a general approach to the problem of pain is perhaps justifiable.

Pain is a sensation which travels from the fine nerve endings present in practically all tissues of the body via the peripheral nerves, posterior roots and sensory tracts up to the brain. Pain arising in such tissues as the skin, muscles, tendons, joints and main serous linings is a fairly simple mechanism in that the pain originating in these places is usually felt locally in the affected area.

Pain which has its origin or cause in certain of the viscera or internal organs, however, may not be felt directly over the affected organ but in a more distant site. For instance, disease affecting the gall-bladder may cause pain over the tip of the right shoulder, whilst in renal colic the pain is often felt down the inner aspect of the thigh. This type of pain felt at a distance from the affected organ is known as **referred** pain.

How does this pain occur ? It is a complex mechanism which is not yet fully explained. Put simply, one theory is that the pain impulses from the affected viscera travel along the nerve fibres into the spinal cord, where these fibres are intimately associated with fibres from other areas entering the same segment of the cord. In the example quoted above, the impulses from the gall-bladder enter the spinal cord at the same segment as the pain fibres from the tip of the right shoulder. When pain therefore arises in the gall-bladder it may spread to these shoulder tip fibres with which the nerve fibres from the gall-bladder are in close contact.

Referred pain is very important in medicine, as many important examples occur which must be understood if a correct diagnosis of disease is to be made.

Certain of the internal organs are insensitive to touch, cutting or tearing. This explains why operations without a general anæsthetic can be performed on the gastro-intestinal tract as long as all the abdominal muscles and tissues and the peritoneum are adequately anæsthetised with a local anæsthetic. (The peritoneum, like the pleura and pericardium, is very sensitive to all the ordinary forms of pain.) Stretching or contraction of the gastro-intestinal tract, however, as of most of the other hollow viscera, can give rise to severe pain. Spasm of the muscle wall of the hollow viscera is a common cause of such severe pain.

COMMON TYPES AND SITES OF PAIN

1. Heart Pains.

Pain in the heart usually arises from the pericardium (pain in pericarditis) or from disease of the heart muscle or arteries, as seen in coronary artery disease. Disease of the coronary arteries gives rise to the characteristic syndrome of pain known as angina pectoris. A thrombus, or clot, in the coronary arteries also gives rise to pain similar to but more severe than angina.

The radiation of the pain in angina and coronary thrombosis to the left arm, neck, right arm or abdomen is an example of referred pain.

2. Chest Pains.

(a) The pain which is most common in chest diseases is that due to an acute pleurisy, when the inflamed layers of pleura rub together during respiration. For this reason pleuritic pain is felt most on breathing, and characteristically " catches the breath." The same explanation also accounts for the short suppressed cough typical of pleurisy.

Abdominal pain occurs in chest diseases when the diaphragmatic pleura is inflamed, because the nerves supplying the diaphragm also supply the abdominal wall (referred pain).

(b) In any disease which causes pressure on any of the nerves in the thorax, pain is usually present, and is usually referred around the chest wall along the distribution of the intercostal nerves— " girdle pain." Such pain can be due to aneurysm of the aorta and tumours of the lungs and mediastinum.

(c) Severe chest pain occurs in the disease herpes zoster when the posterior sensory root of an intercostal nerve is affected. After a few days the typical eruption of herpes develops along the area of the pain.

3. Abdominal Pains.

Abdominal pain is a feature of many diseases of the abdominal organs, and it is intended to give only a brief general review of the subject here. More detailed descriptions of the different types of pain are given under the causative diseases.

(a) Diseases of the stomach and duodenum (peptic ulcer,

carcinoma) cause pain in the epigastrium. The pain is of a steady boring type, but there are periods of complete remission. This pain is usually related to meals, and vomiting often occurs with it.

(b) Acute appendicitis and diseases of the cæcum cause pain in the right iliac fossa, and they also cause referred pain to the umbilicus or epigastrium, especially in the initial stages.

(c) Pain from disease of the hepatic flexure of the colon is felt in the right hypochondrium, and from the splenic flexure in the left hypochondrium.

The nature of the pain in disease of the small and large intestines is characteristically " colicky," that is, it comes and goes in repeated sharp bouts which often, if severe, double the patient up.

(d) Biliary colic due to diseases of the gall-bladder and the bile ducts, e.g., cholecystitis and gall-stones, is felt in the right hypochondrium. The pain radiates around the right lower intercostal margin and also to the tip of the right shoulder. As mentioned earlier, the latter is a referred pain of great value in diagnosis.

(e) Renal colic, usually due to inflammation or stones in the renal tract, is felt in the loin and is referred to the front of the abdomen and downwards to the inner side of the thigh.

The pain in biliary or renal colic typically makes the patient very restless so that he tosses and turns. This restlessness in colic is the direct opposite to the attitude of the patient with acute appendicitis, peritonitis or perforation. Here the patient remains still, as any movement aggravates the pain.

4. Vascular Pain.

Very severe pain arises when the blood supply to tissues, especially muscles, is cut off. In cases of thrombosis or embolism of a peripheral artery the pain is often agonising. It is situated in the affected limb. The severe pain in coronary thrombosis is another example of vascular pain.

5. Headache.

Headache, or pain in the head, is an extremely common symptom and arises both from local diseases of the head and general illnesses, such as any acute fever.

To account for the headache in acute general diseases, increased pulsation of the cerebral arteries, causing a throbbing headache, has been suggested. The headache of migraine is also considered to be due to changes in the arteries.

Inflammation of the meninges, as in meningitis, gives rise to a severe persistent headache. Any stretching of the arteries or dura, such as may occur in cases of brain tumour, also gives rise to severe headaches.

A headache is such a common symptom in so many diseases that it would be valueless to list all the causes. Certain diseases, however, have headaches as a *presenting* feature of the disease and these include :—

    (*a*) All forms of meningitis and encephalitis.

    (*b*) Cerebral tumours, abscesses and aneurysms.

    (*c*) Diseases of the nasal and paranasal sinuses.

    (*d*) Hypertension (in some cases the headache may be slight).

    (*e*) Migraine.

TREATMENT OF PAIN—GENERAL OBSERVATIONS

First and foremost in any consideration of treatment of pain it must be realised that pain is only a symptom of an underlying disease, and therefore the first essential is to treat the disease. In most diseases which give rise to pain, especially acute diseases, the general measures undertaken to cure the underlying disease are normally sufficient to relieve the pain. For instance, in most cases of acute pleurisy due to an underlying pneumonia the treatment of the latter (with penicillin or other antibiotics) will clear up the pleurisy and with it the associated pain.

1. Rest.

In most cases pain is aggravated by movement of the affected part since, obviously, movement of an inflamed tissue is bound to irritate further the nerve endings. Again, a common cause of pain (as mentioned earlier) is a diminished oxygen supply resulting from disease or obstruction in the arteries cutting off the blood to the affected area. Rest, which diminishes the requirements of oxygen, is therefore a vital measure in treating such causes of pain.

Local rest for the affected part can in appropriate cases be ensured by means of splints, sandbags or strapping, and is a common means of relieving pain.

2. Heat.

Heat, because it reduces sensitivity to pain, is very commonly used in various forms to relieve pain.

The common ways in which heat may be applied include :—

    (*a*) Hot-water bottles, suitably covered to prevent burns.

(b) Poultices, such as antiphlogistine, which are useful in that they retain their heat properties for some time.

(c) Hot packs, which are sometimes useful and have been employed with success in relieving the muscle pains in poliomyelitis.

(d) Radiant heat cradles, which are a valuable means to supply heat over a wide superficial area.

(e) Infra-red lamps, mainly used to produce a more penetrating heat over a localised area.

(f) Short-wave diathermy, which produces the most penetrating heat of all and is widely used for deep-seated muscle and joint lesions.

A word of caution must, however, be said about the application of heat for the relief of pain or, for that matter, for any other purpose. Every care must be taken to avoid burning the patient. Hot-water bottles are notorious for losing their protective covers when patients are restless. As these are the very cases who are likely to be seriously ill and so may have their mental perceptions dulled, they are thus very liable to be burned by hot-water bottles.

3. Cold.

For the relief of pain in some diseases cold is often very effective. Cold compresses or ice-bags are often used for the relief of headache. In thrombosis or embolism of a peripheral artery keeping the affected limb cool by exposure to the air is most important. Applying heat to a limb which has had its blood supply cut off only increases the predisposition to gangrene and therefore local heat must be avoided.

4. Drugs.

Drugs which relieve pain are known as *analgesics*. These drugs vary a good deal in their action, some being capable of relieving only mild degrees of pain whilst others are far more potent. The following analgesics are in frequent use in medicine :—

(a) *Aspirin and Phenacetin.*—These drugs are widely used for the relief of headache, muscular pains (fibrositis) and neuralgia. They are safe and not habit-forming. Aspirin and phenacetin are, however, capable of relieving only relatively mild degrees of pain.

(b) *Codeine.*—This drug is slightly more powerful than aspirin or phenacetin and is often combined with them. Codeine is mainly used for the same purposes as are aspirin or phenacetin. It is not habit-forming to any degree.

(*c*) *Paracetamol* (panadol) is a useful analgesic which is safe and not habit-forming. It is given in average doses of one to two 0·5 gm. tablets.

(*d*) *Morphine and Opium.*—Morphine and its allied preparations (omnopon, nepenthe, opium) are called *narcotics* because they produce a deep sleep with the abolition of pain. Morphine is the drug which is most widely used to secure sleep when pain is present. The main drawback to morphine is that its use is very liable to form a habit, so that larger and larger doses become necessary. Therefore it must *not* be used in any chronic painful condition unless this is incurable. Nor should it be used in infants because they tolerate morphine very badly. In chest diseases associated with sputum or hæmoptysis, morphine is also contraindicated as it depresses the cough reflex and respirations. The specific antidote for morphine poisoning is nalorphine (lethidrone) which can be injected intravenously in 5 to 10 mgm. doses.

(*e*) *Pethidine* (dolantal, demerol).—Pethidine too is a potent analgesic which also has the advantage of being an antispasmodic. It is used in midwifery during labour. It is also useful in the relief of pain due to renal and biliary colic, where morphine is inclined to cause spasm.

The dose of pethidine is 25 to 100 mgm. ($\frac{2}{5}$ to $1\frac{1}{2}$ gr.) given by mouth or intramuscularly. Pethidine is, like morphine, a habit-forming drug and should therefore not be used in the treatment of chronic pain. To counteract the depressant effect of pethidine on the respirations, the antagonist levallorphan tartrate (lorfan) is sometimes given with pethidine especially if large doses are being used. Pethilorphan is a combined preparation of 100 mgm. pethidine and 1·25 mgm. of levallorphan.

(*f*) *Methadone* (physeptone, adanon).—Methadone is a powerful analgesic drug resembling morphine but with a less sedative (hypnotic) action. It has a markedly depressant action on the cough reflex. The dose of methadone is 5 to 15 mgm. orally or by intramuscular injection. Addiction to methadone can occur but is less difficult to cure than morphine addiction.

(*g*) *Phenadoxone* (heptalgin).—This potent analgesic resembles methadone and it too has little hypnotic or sedative action. Addiction does not readily occur. The dose of phenadoxone is 10 to 30 mgm. orally or by intramuscular injection.

(*h*) *Levorphanol* (dromoran, methorphinan).—This is a recently introduced analgesic. It resembles morphine, but has a much less sedative action and the risk of addiction is said to be less. Levor-phanol has little depressant action on the cough reflex. It is likely to cause nausea and vomiting. Levorphanol is given in 2 mgm. doses by mouth or by subcutaneous injection.

(*i*) *Anæsthetic Drugs.*—Anæsthetic drugs abolish the conduction of sensory impulses. General anæsthetics produce a total loss of consciousness with loss of sensation and reflex action. General anæsthetics are used to enable painless operations to be performed. Ether, nitrous oxide, chloroform, trilene and cyclopropane are given by inhalation, while pentothal and hexobarbitone are given by intravenous injection.

Local anæsthetic drugs produce a localised area of loss of pain sensation and are widely used for the performance of minor operations. In addition, local anæsthetics are used to relieve deep-seated and severe muscular pain. The most common local anæsthetic is procaine in 1 or 2 per cent. solution.

(*j*) *Chlorpromazine* (largactil).—This drug has little analgesic action when used alone but it enhances the action of the other analgesic drugs mentioned above. Chlorpromazine appears to create a conscious indifference to pain with a consequential alleviation of anxiety and tension. Chlorpromazine has been used with success in the treatment of severe intractable pain caused by malignant disease.

In addition to its use in the treatment of pain, chlorpromazine is remarkably beneficial in relieving such conditions as persistent hiccough, nausea and vomiting (*e.g.*, post-operative and during pregnancy) and anxiety states.

Chlorpromazine is given by mouth or by intramuscular injection in 25 to 100 mgm. doses three times a day. It occasionally gives rise to an obstructive type of jaundice, especially if given at the higher dose.

Promazine (sparine) and trifluoperazine (stelazine) have very much the same effect as chlorpromazine and are used for similar purposes.

5. Massage.

In the various forms of fibrositis where there is muscular pain, massage, especially if combined with heat, is most beneficial in relieving the pain.

VOMITING

Vomiting, like pain, is a very common feature of many diseases and it is important to understand how it occurs. The actual act of vomiting is very complex: in brief, it consists of a contraction of stomach, abdominal and diaphragmatic muscles and a relaxation of the cardiac opening of the stomach. There is a centre, the vomiting centre, in the medulla of the brain, which controls this complicated act. This centre is closely connected with the vagus nerve, especially with the branches from the abdominal viscera.

Vomiting can be divided into three well-recognised groups :—

1. Reflex Vomiting.

This, the commonest type, is due to stimulation of the vagus nerve. The usual causes of reflex vomiting are :—

(a) *Diseases in the Stomach.*

Acute gastritis.	Pyloric stenosis.
Peptic ulcer.	Carcinoma of the stomach.

(b) *Diseases in other Abdominal Organs.*

Renal and biliary colic.

Inflammations such as appendicitis and peritonitis.

Tumours and obstruction of the intestinal tract.

(c) *Drugs (Emetics).*—Certain drugs irritate the stomach or stimulate the vomiting centre, thus causing vomiting, and are often used for this purpose, *e.g.*, in cases of poisoning when it is desirable to get rid of any poison in the stomach. These drugs are called emetics and common examples are :—

(i) Salt, a tablespoonful in a tumbler of warm water (repeated if necessary).

(ii) Mustard, two teaspoonfuls in warm water.

(iii) Powdered ipecacuanha, 30 gr. in water.

(iv) Apomorphine, $\frac{1}{10}$ gr. subcutaneously.

(d) *Diseases of the Ear.*—The vestibular part of the ear deals with posture and equilibrium and is closely associated with the vomiting centre. Conditions affecting the vestibular apparatus often cause severe vomiting. Travel sickness and the disease known as *Ménière's syndrome* are two examples of this type of vomiting.

2. Vomiting due to Direct Stimulation of the Vomiting Centre.

Various cerebral diseases can cause direct pressure on the vomiting centre. Vomiting is therefore a feature of such diseases of the nervous system as cerebral tumour, abscess and meningitis, in which increased intracranial pressure is present.

3. Vomiting due to Stimulation from the Higher Cerebral Centres.

This class covers the vomiting resulting from emotional disorders, such as nervous tension, anxiety, fear and hysteria. This vomiting is often successfully controlled by chlorpromazine or allied drugs.

Finally, it should be remembered that any severe illness can by reflex toxic action give rise to vomiting.

CHARACTERISTICS OF VOMITING IN THE MORE COMMON DISEASES

Vomiting tends to be more predominant and severe in diseases of the stomach and abdominal organs. Vomiting is a feature of peptic ulcer and usually relieves the pain which is present. The vomiting is, however, not as severe as in pyloric stenosis, in which vomiting is a cardinal feature. In these cases the copious vomiting, often of food eaten the previous day, is diagnostic of stenosis. In the pyloric stenosis of infants the vomiting, apart from being copious, is typically projectile in character.

In gastric carcinoma vomiting is common, the vomit often being bloodstained and looking like coffee grounds. A more profuse hæmatemesis may occur, but it is not as common as in peptic ulcer ; peptic ulcer is the commonest cause of hæmatemesis. Obstruction of the portal vein, leading to vomiting of blood, is usually the result of cirrhosis of the liver.

Acute dilatation of the stomach, which may complicate abdominal operations, is attended by most severe and copious vomiting. In acute inflammatory abdominal diseases, such as acute appendicitis, vomiting is usually associated with abdominal pain and occurs early at the onset of the illness.

In acute intestinal obstruction vomiting is persistent, and the vomit may be fæcal in character. Fæcal vomit is dark brown or black in colour and has a typically fæcal smell.

In cerebral diseases associated with increased intracranial pressure, vomiting usually occurs with a severe headache. Vomiting is more predominant in the acute diseases causing intracranial pressure (such as meningitis) than in the more subacute diseases like cerebral tumour.

EFFECTS OF VOMITING

Vomiting is likely to have serious effects only if it is persistent and copious, as in cases of pyloric stenosis, intestinal obstruction and acute dilatation of the stomach. The main result of continued vomiting is loss of fluid and acid. The loss of fluid leads to dehydration, which causes collapse (p. 467) and in some cases acute renal failure (p. 418). The loss of hydrochloric acid in the vomit causes an alkalosis, which can lead to tetany (p. 454).

CHAPTER XIX

ON ACUTE POISONING AND COMA

ACUTE POISONING

POISONING is usually the result of swallowing or inhaling poison, although very occasionally poisons may enter the body by injection.

GENERAL OUTLINE OF TREATMENT

1. The poison must be removed from the body as quickly as possible.

In most cases in which the poison has been swallowed **gastric lavage** is best. If this is not available emetic drugs to cause vomiting are used, but they are not as effective as gastric lavage. Cases of poisoning by corrosive acids or alkalis must not, however, be treated by gastric lavage or emetics owing to the consequential danger of perforation of the stomach or œsophagus.

2. **Asphyxia.**—Cyanosis and failure of the respiratory movements will denote the presence of asphyxia. This calls for prompt measures as a clear air passage must be maintained, if necessary by the use of a tongue forceps or airway. Oxygen is given by a B.L.B. mask. If these measures do not rapidly restore respiratory movement then artificial respiration is necessary.

3. **Shock.**—Usually with severe poisoning shock is present, recognised by the cold, clammy and pale skin and the rapid feeble pulse. The patient must be kept warm with adequate coverings and hot-water bottles, but it must be realised that it is dangerous to overheat the patient. Radiant heat cradles are therefore best avoided, whilst good care is also necessary to prevent burns from hot-water bottles; such burns are particularly likely to arise with unconscious patients.

In most cases of poisoning, copious fluids should be given, and hot strong coffee, which also acts as a stimulant, is useful. Intravenous glucose saline will be needed in some cases. The foot of the bed should be raised in cases of shock.

4. **Coma.**—Coma is a feature of many common types of poisoning, especially in cases due to barbiturates, alcohol, aspirin and morphine. If coma is present the utmost skill is necessary in nursing the patient

to prevent obstruction of the air passages. The patient must never be allowed to become cyanosed. Suction to prevent the mouth secretions from obstructing the airway must be carried out at regular intervals. The patient is best nursed in the prone or semi-prone position with the foot of the bed elevated as this helps to keep the air passages clear. The patient must be turned frequently from side to side to prevent pressure sores. Oxygen will be given.

For some patients stimulants may be administered and those often used include :—

(a) Nikethamide (coramine) administered intravenously and subcutaneously in 2 to 5 ml. doses.

(b) Strychnine, $\frac{1}{20}$ to $\frac{1}{10}$ gr. subcutaneously.

(c) Bemegride (megimide), 50 mgm., and amiphenazole, (daptozole), 15 mgm., intravenously.

(d) Picrotoxin, 2 to 6 ml. intravenously or intramuscularly.

(e) Hot strong coffee.

5. **Specific Antidotes.**—In general, the use of specific antidotes in poisoning is of secondary value to the general measures outlined above as in many cases it may be difficult at first to ascertain what poison has been taken. However, in corrosive acid and alkali poisoning and also in morphine, methadone and pethidine poisoning, the appropriate neutralising antidote is of value.

(a) *For corrosive acids* (hydrochloric, nitric, acetic, spirits of salts) weak alkalis, such as milk of magnesia, 4 to 10 oz. ; lime water (calcium hydroxide solution), 6 oz., or aluminium hydroxide, 3 oz., are given. In an emergency wall plaster crushed in water or dilute soap solution may be used.

(b) *For corrosive alkalis* (caustic soda or potash, ammonia, weed-killer) large quantities of dilute vinegar, lemon juice or orange juice are given.

The appropriate weak alkali or acid should then be followed by demulcents such as olive oil, milk or white of egg.

Gastric lavage and emetics must not be used in corrosive poisoning.

(c) For morphine, methadone and pethidine poisoning, the specific antidote is nalorphine, which is very effective (see p. 609).

POISONING DUE TO INHALATION

The poison which is most usually inhaled is carbon monoxide gas from gas stoves, the exhausts of motor cars or in badly ventilated mines. In gas poisoning the essential task is to eliminate the poison from the lungs as rapidly as possible. The patient must be brought into the fresh air and oxygen given. If breathing has stopped and does not rapidly respond to oxygen, then artificial respiration must at once be carried out.

In the commonest form of gas poisoning—carbon monoxide poisoning—the skin has a characteristic pink colour.

GASTRIC LAVAGE IN POISONING

As mentioned above, gastric lavage is carried out in most cases of swallowed poisons except those of corrosive poisoning. To be effective, however, it must be performed within four to six hours

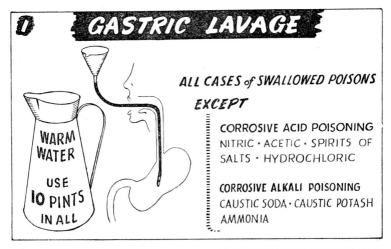

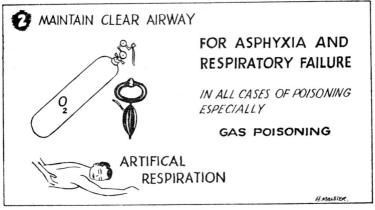

Fig. 184

The treatment of acute poisoning.

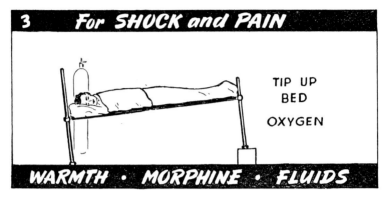

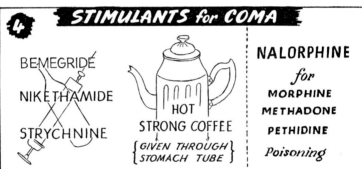

For CORROSIVE ACID POISONING	For CORROSIVE ALKALI POISONING
ALKALIS by mouth	**WEAK ACIDS** by mouth
ALUMINIUM HYDROXIDE	DILUTED VINEGAR
MILK OF MAGNESIA	ORANGE JUICE
SOAP SOLUTION	
LIME WATER	LEMON JUICE

H. MALSTER.

FIG. 184—*continued*
The treatment of acute poisoning.

after the poison was taken and it must be carried out properly. Thorough knowledge of all the essential details is therefore necessary. The patient is placed in the prone position on a table or bed; a large stiff, rubber stomach tube is lubricated with liquid paraffin or glycerine and, after any false teeth have been removed from the patient, the tube is passed gently but firmly into the stomach. The average distance from the mouth to the stomach in an adult is 20 in., and in children under 2 years is approximately 10 in.

One pint of warm water is introduced into the stomach via the stomach tube, and is then immediately syphoned back by quickly inverting and lowering the funnel attached to the end of the tube. This first washout is most likely to contain the maximum amount of poison and should be at once set aside and kept *separate* from all further washings. The washout is then continued using 1 pint of water at a time, until at least 10 pints have been used. It is useless to try to wash out the stomach with a few pints of fluid only.

All the stomach washings, with the first washout kept separately, are properly labelled with the name of the patient, date and time, and sent to the laboratory for analysis. On no account should any of the stomach washings be thrown away.

COMA

When an individual is unconscious for any length of time he is said to be in coma. Coma can be caused by very many different conditions, most of which are both extremely important in medicine and of common occurrence.

COMMON CAUSES OF COMA

1. **Injury,** especially head injury. In most severe cases there is a fracture of the skull and laceration of the brain (contusion). The term *concussion* is often used to describe a transitory loss of consciousness due to head injury.

2. **Apoplexy,** due to cerebral thrombosis, hæmorrhage or embolism.

3. **Acute alcoholic coma** (the " dead drunk "). This is a very common cause of coma, but may not appear so to the nurse as the majority of cases are not admitted to hospital.

4. **Poisoning.** Overdosage with certain drugs, especially the hypnotics, is a common cause of coma. The overdosage may be

18

accidental or deliberate. The drugs which most commonly cause coma are :—

  (a) The *barbiturate* group of hypnotic drugs (medinal, pheno-barbitone, amytal, etc.).

  (b) *Aspirin.*

  (c) *Morphine* or opium.

Apart from poisoning with drugs, coma is frequently seen as a result of *carbon monoxide poisoning.* Again, the poisoning may be either accidental or deliberate—an attempt at suicide. Miners working in badly ventilated mines are often affected with carbon monoxide poisoning.

  5. **Diabetes** (hyperglycæmic coma).

  6. **Insulin** (hypoglycæmic coma).

  7. **Uræmia.**

  8. **Hysteria.**

DIAGNOSIS AND MANAGEMENT OF A CASE OF COMA

When a patient is admitted to hospital in coma certain routine examinations and investigations are carried out in all cases. The nurse should be fully aware of the importance of all the following points, as when she is undressing the patient she will be able to verify the presence or absence of important details which can help to indicate the treatment of the patient.

  1. The history of the case leading up to the coma is most important. The presence or otherwise of any *injury*, any past history of disease, such as hypertension, diabetes or kidney disease, and whether or not the patient has been taking drugs, especially sleeping drugs, are all significant factors.

  2. Careful examination of the head to find any scalp wounds or *bleeding* from the ears or nose is necessary. A fractured base of the skull often causes bleeding from the ear, which can be missed unless the ears are carefully looked at.

  3. The size and shape of the *pupils* are important, especially any inequality of the pupils. The latter immediately points to local damage in the brain, as from injury or apoplexy. The very small pin-point pupils of morphine poisoning should be looked for. The pupils in hysteria are often widely dilated.

  4. The *breath* should be smelt, the typical sour smell of the alcoholic being easily recognised. The diagnosis of alcoholic coma,

however, solely on the evidence of the smell of alcohol from the breath is most dangerous. A drunken person is very liable to sustain an injury which may well be the real cause of the coma. Indeed, the combination of alcohol and head injury is most common. Therefore in all cases of seemingly alcoholic coma the scalp and ears must be carefully examined for signs of injury and bleeding.

A sweet sickly smell, often likened to sweet pears or apples, is due to acetone in the breath and is characteristic, in particular, of diabetic coma.

5. The character of the *respirations* is important in diagnosis. Deep stertorous respirations are common in apoplexy and in diabetic coma. In insulin coma and in cases of severe injury and hæmorrhage the respirations are shallow. In morphine poisoning the respiration rate is markedly depressed and may be as slow as 8 to 10 a minute. The peculiar waxing and waning respirations of Cheyne-Stokes frequently occur in apoplexy.

6. The *skin* is cold and clammy in shock, which would be present in coma due to severe injuries. A moist skin, often with marked sweating, is met with in insulin coma whilst, on the other hand, in diabetic coma the skin is extremely dry. The skin in diabetic coma remains in a fold when it is pinched owing to the dehydration which is always present.

7. The limbs and trunk will be examined by the doctor for any injury, and the utmost care and gentleness used to ensure that any injury present is not made worse by handling the patient. Apart from locating an injury, it is also possible sometimes, even with the patient in coma, to discern a *paralysis* of one side of the body. This would of course lead to a diagnosis of hemiplegia, probably due to apoplexy.

8. Examination of the *urine* is done as a routine in all cases of coma. If the cause of the coma is obvious, *e.g.*, a head injury or carbon monoxide poisoning, then the examination of the urine can be delayed till the first convenient moment. In cases of suspected diabetes or poisoning, such as barbiturate or aspirin, or in uræmia, and in all cases where the diagnosis of the coma is not immediately obvious, examination of the urine is carried out immediately, and for this catheterisation will be necessary.

The urine is tested at once for sugar, acetone and albumin, and the remainder is saved and sent to the laboratory for further detailed examination. This will include tests for barbiturates and aspirin.

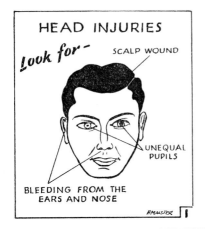

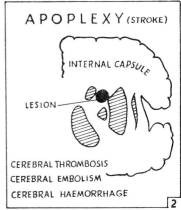

HEAD INJURIES

Look for –

SCALP WOUND

UNEQUAL PUPILS

BLEEDING FROM THE EARS AND NOSE

H. MALSTER   1

APOPLEXY (STROKE)

INTERNAL CAPSULE

LESION

CEREBRAL THROMBOSIS
CEREBRAL EMBOLISM
CEREBRAL HAEMORRHAGE   2

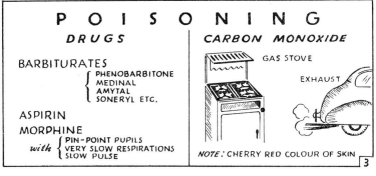

P O I S O N I N G

DRUGS

BARBITURATES
  { PHENOBARBITONE
    MEDINAL
    AMYTAL
    SONERYL ETC.

ASPIRIN

MORPHINE
  with { PIN-POINT PUPILS
          VERY SLOW RESPIRATIONS
          SLOW PULSE

CARBON MONOXIDE

GAS STOVE

EXHAUST

NOTE: CHERRY RED COLOUR OF SKIN   3

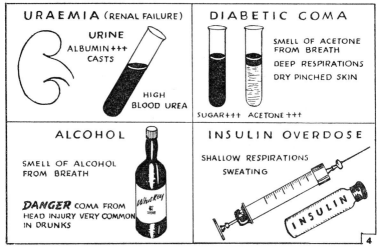

URAEMIA (RENAL FAILURE)

URINE
ALBUMIN +++
CASTS

HIGH BLOOD UREA

DIABETIC COMA

SMELL OF ACETONE FROM BREATH
DEEP RESPIRATIONS
DRY PINCHED SKIN

SUGAR+++   ACETONE +++

ALCOHOL

SMELL OF ALCOHOL FROM BREATH

DANGER COMA FROM HEAD INJURY VERY COMMON IN DRUNKS

Whisky

INSULIN OVERDOSE

SHALLOW RESPIRATIONS
SWEATING

INSULIN   4

FIG. 185

Some common causes of coma.

The importance of saving all the urine for laboratory examination cannot be too forcibly stressed.

The presence of a heavy glycosuria and acetone immediately gives a diagnosis of diabetic coma in nearly all cases. A urine loaded with albumin would point to a possible uræmia.

By this stage the cause of the coma will be apparent in most cases. In a small number of cases, however, further immediate examinations, such as a lumbar puncture (to reveal blood in the cerebrospinal fluid or a possible meningitis) and blood urea and blood-sugar estimations, may be necessary to establish the diagnosis of the cause of the coma.

Treatment.—The treatment of coma varies according to the cause and is therefore dealt with in the sections devoted to the causative conditions. The nursing of a patient in coma, whatever the cause, is of particular importance, and the general nursing care of a comatose patient is described in full under Apoplexy (p. 312).

CHAPTER XX

PSYCHOLOGICAL MEDICINE

By Henry R. Rollin

IF the complicated history of psychological medicine is studied two threads can be seen weaving their way through the story. Firstly, there is the alternating acceptance and denial of the importance of emotional factors in the understanding and treatment of disease. Secondly, there is the ever-changing attitude of the medical profession and, in turn, the public in general, towards mental illness. These threads run somewhat parallel courses and could indeed be somehow connected.

It was Plato in ancient times who deplored the separation by physicians of the soul from the body. In modern times it was Virchow (1821-1902), a German pathologist, who by his brilliant discoveries in cell-structure was indirectly responsible for again separating the mind from sickness and the consequent study of sickness as a disorder affecting cells and organs only. His work heralded the onset of the " machine age " in medicine, a period which, it must be pointed out, coincides with one of the blackest ages in the treatment of the mentally afflicted.

Today, the wheel has gone almost full circle : there is now a heightened awareness of the indivisibility of mind and body in the total picture of any disease process. It may be, incidentally, not entirely by chance that at this very moment, in England at any rate, an infinitely more liberal and humane policy towards the mentally ill is being pursued as exemplified by the Mental Health Act of 1959 which will begin to come into effect in 1960.

It is the purpose then of this chapter to bring the history of psychological medicine up to date. In so doing it is hoped to give not so much a glimpse of what happens on the psychological side of the fence which, as far as teaching is concerned, artificially divides the field of medicine into its physical and mental components, but to tear the fence down and show the essential unity of the two.

For purposes of descriptive convenience the chapter is divided into six sections. The last section which gives a brief summary of the provisions of the new Mental Health Act is included because from now on it is likely that a knowledge of nursing of those suffering primarily from mental illness will be of more than academic importance to those nurses undergoing " general " training.

The sections are :—

1. The psychological development of the individual.
2. The neuroses.
3. Psychosomatic medicine.
4. The psychological effects of illness.
5. The psychological role of the nurse.
6. The Mental Health Act (1959).

THE PSYCHOLOGICAL DEVELOPMENT OF
THE INDIVIDUAL

The Infant.

The infant is born into the world utterly dependent on others for his nourishment and well-being and this state of dependency continues for a period far in excess of that necessary in the offspring of any other species. It is said with considerable justification that the foundations of mental health are laid during this period and that the very stuff of these foundations is the infant's feeling of security in a relationship with his mother, or an adequate substitute, which must be warm, continuous and rewarding to both. It is a truism that a child in a ducal nursery enjoying all the material benefits of the situation into which he is born may yet be " maternally deprived," whereas the child in the workman's cottage with very scant resources may luxuriate in maternal riches.

Despite the fact that artificial feeding meets almost all the physiological needs of the infant, the vast benefit which accrues to the one which is breast-fed is in the loving, intimate relationship which exists between mother and child, so that his emotional needs are satisfied at the same time as his hunger. Thus it follows that if the child comes to accept his mother's milk as a symbol of her love then a sudden cessation of breast-feeding can be interpreted as a denial of love. Weaning is, therefore, a critical stage in the emotional development of the child and it is essential that when the cup or bottle comes to be substituted for the breast the greatest care is taken to see that time and devotion are spent on the feeds so that the child's love and trust in his mother are re-established.

There comes a time in the life of the child when training and discipline must begin.   Usually the first discipline to be imposed is in relation to the control of the bladder and bowels.   There can be no doubt that until quite recently too much was expected of the child and that excretory control was sought before the physiological mechanisms were ready, *i.e.*, before roughly the first year.   The psychological importance of too much emphasis being placed on soiling or wetting at too early an age must be stressed.   Because of the association of reproof in the child's mind with fæces and urine he may come to adopt a fear or phobia of dirt to which he relates his excreta, and acquire thereby pathological standards of cleanliness, tidiness and exactness in his personal conduct.   It is alleged that the obsessive-compulsive personality, or taken a stage further, the obsessive-compulsive neurosis to which reference is made later (see p. 561) may result from a too early and slavish insistence on toilet training.   Alternatively, the constant changing and fussing over dirty napkins may lead to an unhealthy preoccupation with the genitalia and in turn, later, to an unhealthy attitude to sex.

When further discipline is insisted on as part of the business of growing up the parents have to steer a difficult course between over-indulgence and over-authority.   Of late, there has been a swing away from the complete indiscipline once recommended.   What can be stated quite categorically is that a child must have some discipline. He is too inexperienced and naïve to form his own standards of conduct and they must, therefore, be laid down by others.   However, the effects of too much or too little authority will depend on the psychological make-up of the child.   The tough, aggressive child will seize on parental weakness as a means of manipulating the environment to his own advantage and the tendency to bully his way through life will tend to ensue.   The same child faced with over-discipline will tend to resent parental authority and in later life resent the discipline of others who stand in authority over him and rebel against them.   On the other hand, the weaker, more compliant child will react to parental weakness by whining and crying for what he needs, or to over-discipline, partly because of fear of the consequences, by unquestioning obedience.   In either case the result may be to produce an adult who is inadequate and incapable of making decisions or accepting responsibility.

Although the ideal is midway between discipline and indulgence, a vacillating course between one and the other is disastrous.   It must result in confusion and anxiety in the child's mind as he attempts to decide with his inadequate mental equipment whether he is rejected or loved by his parents.

Particularly in his first year, the child is very much the property, concern and joy of his mother. The father by virtue of his masculinity and his preoccupation with providing for his family is precluded from that constant intimacy with his offspring which the mother enjoys, although his pride by remote control may be no less. As the child becomes more and more independent of his mother the opportunities for love and companionship by the father increase.

Emotionally the role of the father in the development of the child will depend on its sex. In the case of a boy, according to the Freudian psychoanalysts, the father may be construed as a rival for his mother's love and resented or even hated. In this triangular drama is seen the " Œdipus situation " on the unsatisfactory resolution of which, it is claimed, so much mental ill-health may result. With a girl the roles of mother and father are reversed, *i.e.*, the mother is the rival for the father's love.

Sooner or later the child will have to learn that the world is populated by people other than his parents on whom he can make demands, and who will in turn make demands on him. Those who will most likely erupt into his environment are brothers and sisters, the arrival of each bringing new problems in family and social adaptation. The birth of a younger child must be an unmitigated disaster to an older one. In it he sees a competitor for the love of his mother and a threat to his erstwhile omnipotence. The " sibling rivalry " which is created is easily understood. In an attempt to compete with this rival and regain the love which he fears he may have lost, the older child may " regress " or adopt earlier patterns of behaviour, such as bed-wetting, thumb-sucking and general indiscipline, in order to again focus his mother's attention on him. Later, however, as he begins to appreciate that he is not excluded but only asked to share in his mother's love, a real companionship between the two children begins. With the arrival of other children further upsets are inevitable, but they should settle themselves so that later all the peculiarly intimate ties which constitute the emotional life of the family are established.

The birth position of the child is psychologically important. The only child—and each first child is for a time an " only child "— is at a disadvantage. With all the will in the world adults cannot enter into a child's world and, without the companionship of children of roughly his own age in his world, he must suffer from some defects in his capacity to form social relations. The oldest child in a family usually has thrust upon him, or assumes, some of the responsibility for the care of the younger ones, and according to his psychological make-up, becomes anxious because of it, or falls easily into the role of a leader. The youngest child is and may remain the " baby of the family," spoilt and over-indulged by his parents and older siblings.

The School Child.

The next psychological hurdle which has to be cleared by the child is that of attending his first school. He is in every sense the " new boy " and the attendant anxiety in meeting the situation in which he finds himself may, and very often is, reactivated at various stages of his career—at each change of school, on going to the university or his first job, on enlistment into the armed forces, for example. The apron strings which tie mother and child are beginning to be cut and for guidance and perhaps comfort he must look, not to his mother only, but to his teachers. The psychological damage which can be done by unsympathetic, or frankly cruel teachers at this or any stage cannot be over-emphasised. In the same way that social adjustments had to be made to the arrival of other children in the family so adjustments, but on a much greater scale, have to be made to this body of strangers which surround him.

With the beginning of his formal education there begins an entirely new orientation to the world at large. His exploratory activities, before confined to toys and things, are directed now into ideas and the symbols of letters, words, pictures and maps.

His capacity to learn in the academic sense will depend on two factors, his emotional stability and his intelligence. It is obvious that the child who has failed to adjust to the emotional problems which going to school presents, and is as a result anxious and unhappy, will not be able to give his lessons the attention and concentration they require.

The question of intelligence requires more careful study. There is no one satisfactory definition of intelligence, but for our purposes it may be considered as an innate endowment whereby the individual is able to learn by experience. Inherent in this definition is the fact that a high or low intelligence is a faculty with which a person is born, and that it can only be modified by education and the cultural environment in which that person is raised. No amount of education or coaching can, therefore, make a dull child bright, although they may make the best of his intellectual potential. Further, to attempt to force a dull child to keep pace academically with his brighter colleagues will only lead to anxiety, frustration, or rebellion and truancy.

Let it be made quite clear that the vast majority of children clear the psychological hurdle of going to school satisfactorily. But in those who fail there may be seen symptoms of psychological illness or regression as, for example, bed-wetting, nightmares, thumb-sucking, temper tantrums, truancy, etc., which may, of course, clear up later, or may persist into adulthood.

The Adolescent.

Puberty, which heralds the onset of adolescence, is a period of major development in both the physical and psychological sense. All the endocrine glands working through the sex glands exert their influence and bring about the emergence of the so-called " secondary sexual characters." Physiologically the child becomes an adult, that is, parenthood becomes possible. Psychologically, in our culture at any rate, it is only a period of transition and the responsibility of marriage and mating must be delayed for some years. Because of this paradox many of the problems and emotional difficulties of adolescence arise.

Resulting from his sexual maturation a greater interest in sexual matters must arise. A variety of sexual experiments may be indulged in, such as masturbation, and depending on what preparation he has had from parents or teachers, anxiety and guilt may ensue. Interest in girls, or " crushes " begins and the more imaginative boy feels the impact of romanticism as expressed in poetry or music. There is a greater attention paid to personal cleanliness and tidiness with the obvious, yet always denied, object of making himself attractive to girls.

Because of the half-way house between childhood and adulthood in which he finds himself, coupled with his sexual urges and the taboos imposed on them, the perplexity which results may be expressed in moodiness, awkwardness and other manifestations of maladaptation. He feels really at home only amongst boys of his own age and thus " the gang " becomes important, either in the shape of Boy Scouts or Youth Clubs, or in a less concrete way but with the same emotional ties, as in a crowd of boys who " hang around together." With the transfer of interests and sources of emotional satisfaction from the home to foci outside it the last of the maternal apron strings is ready to be cut.

Although, as in the previous stages, most adolescents will weather the storms of this difficult period perfectly well there are some who will never grow up, either because of inherent personality difficulties, probably carried over from earlier stages, or because of the refusal of parents, almost always at a subconscious level, to allow them to reach psychological maturity. Peter Pan may be delightful as a dramatic concept, but in real life he must be accepted as a psychologically sick person.

The Young Adult.

The young man in his teens, or early twenties, is a person who ideally, although perhaps still economically dependent on his parents, is psychologically capable of standing on his own two feet, making his own decisions and shaping his own career. Either at the university, in his job, or in the armed forces he can make a satisfactory adjustment to the social and intellectual buffetings he will receive and will be able to participate in the give and take which will eventually equip him for full citizenship.

Again ideally, he will abandon his furtive sexual pursuits and be ready for a permanent emotional relationship with the one girl of his choice leading to courtship and marriage. A successful marriage is perhaps the greatest proof of psychological maturity, only exceeded perhaps by the successful adaptation to the trials and tribulations of parenthood. The ideal marriage is not necessarily the rule. If it were the newspapers would be deprived of most of their sensationalism and plays and novels robbed of their plots.

The Period of Middle Age.

The onset of middle age is the end of an epoch. In women " the change " as it is colloquially called, or the menopause, is much more dramatic in its manifestations and occurs much earlier than is the case with men. It is for women the end of the child-bearing period and is brought about, as is the onset of puberty, by the endocrine glands working through the sex glands.

Some physiological reaction to the upheaval which takes place at the menopause is the rule rather than the exception, as manifested, in addition to the cessation of menstruation, by hot flushes, a gain in weight, coarsening of skin and features, etc. There are often, too, symptoms of a more psychological nature such as irritability and emotional instability which in some cases deepens into a serious depression called involutional melancholia. This serious psychological illness may occur in men too, but usually at a much later age, *i.e.*, 60 or so.

Although most of the changes seen in middle age are due to endocrinological influences, some are undoubtedly psychologically determined. The fact that youth has gone and that age has set limitations on physical activities and sexual attractiveness are sad and sobering thoughts whose effects will depend largely on the store set previously on these assets. Again, by this time the children will have grown up and, if they have not already left the parental home, will normally be leading independent lives. The parents feel that their job is just about done. As a form of compensation at this stage other activities, such as hobbies and devotion to causes and good works in the community, take the place of parenthood.

The Period of Old Age.

Old age, the " last scene of all that ends this strange eventful history," is heralded by a further decline in the physical and intellectual abilities of the individual. Psychologically, the memory becomes impaired, particularly for recent events, resulting in a tendency to live in the past; there is a decrease in flexibility so that interests become narrowed and an exact routine insisted on. Although lifelong preparation for retirement may have been made, its actual advent may come as a bitter disillusionment. For one who has enjoyed power and prestige, the realisation that one is no longer needed—and the " need to be needed " is a fundamental human prerequisite—is a sad blow from which some never recover.

THE NEUROSES

In the final analysis, a neurosis is an abnormal mental state resulting from an unresolved mental conflict. This conflict may be due to a faulty adaptation to difficulties arising from without, *i.e.*, environmental hazards of a contemporary nature, or from within the personality itself.

Amongst the contemporary hazards to which the neurotic may have been subjected mention can be made of financial stress, domestic difficulties, including bad housing and marital disharmony, occupational maladjustment and the strain of war or insecure peace. These difficulties are obvious and unfortunately commonplace.

The personality defects, on the other hand, are of a more subtle order and require specialised knowledge and a specialised technique for their elucidation. This is due to the complexity of the evolution and structure of the human personality even in health.

As with certain physical aspects of an individual, for instance, height, weight and muscular development, there are in the total personality elements which are inborn, that is, genetically determined, and others which are due to environment, but an environment more complex and more remote than the one already mentioned. It is the age-old problem of nature and nurture.

The genetics of mental illness, particularly of the neuroses, are so involved, and for the moment so speculative, that there is little point in going further into the subject here. The problem of the environmental setting of the neuroses deserves further mention. It is inconceivable, for instance, that a person, particularly an impressionable child or adolescent, cannot be adversely affected by an unhappy home, a " broken home " (that is, one where a child has sustained the loss of one or other or both parents at an early age), gross economic privations, or what is more important psychologically, an unsatisfactory parent-child relationship. In other words, any conditions bringing about emotional disharmony or insecurity in the environment may result in flaws in the personality. Further, it cannot be over-emphasised that life is a continuum and that traumatic experiences or faulty attitudes acquired at any stage in an individual's psychological development may produce repercussions at any time and may result, in certain circumstances, in mental illness.

In the assessment of personality, or rather, what most concerns the psychiatrist, the defects in the personality, use is made of clinical interviews and of psychological tests. By these means an estimate—admittedly arbitrary—is made of what is known as neurotic predisposition, i.e., the degree to which a person is liable under conditions of stress to develop a neurotic illness, or what is popularly known as " a nervous breakdown." It is pertinent, perhaps consoling, to add that, despite the enormous differences in the thresholds of nervous stability in different individuals, given sufficient stress anyone may break down. More than ample proof of this was afforded in the recent war when both combatants and civilians were treated for nervous illness who, under normal peace-time conditions, would have gone through life proud, even smugly so, of their apparent 100 per cent. stability.

THE UNCONSCIOUS MIND

To discuss psychiatry to-day without some mention of the unconscious mind and, in turn, the principles and practice of psychoanalysis, would be like describing recent advances in physics without including a note on the influence of the discovery of atomic energy. The parallel is by no means overdrawn. There are many psychiatrists who doubt the value of psychoanalysis as a therapeutic procedure, but there must be singularly few who do not appreciate the enormous contribution to psychiatry of psychoanalysis as a psychological theory.

It is mainly to Sigmund Freud (1856-1939) that the credit for the elaboration of psychoanalytic principles is due. He it was who evolved the concept of the unconscious mind as it is understood to-day.

There are many quite homely examples of the workings of the unconscious mind. For instance, everyone at some time forgets to do something and then by means of some incident during the day which gives a clue to the thing forgotten is brought up sharply with an embarrassing, " Oh, dear, I've just remembered ! " It cannot be a mere coincidence that the thing forgotten is so often something which the individual would prefer not to have remembered ; for instance, paying a bill, an appointment with the dentist, or more pointedly, at one stage during treatment, an appointment with a psychoanalyst. Again, how frequently has one wrestled unsuccessfully with a problem—the crossword addict experiences it often—when suddenly there is a Eureka-like whoop of joy and the problem seemingly solves itself. The only possible explanation of such a phenomenon is that although the problem has been consciously set aside, unconsciously the mind continues the struggle. Recently on the music-hall stage there have been innumerable bona fide examples of mass and individual hypnotism. A popular feature of these acts is to command a person in a state of hypnotic suggestibility to perform some absurd act at a given time. Of this command, when he is brought out of his trance, the individual has no conscious knowledge, yet when the appointed time arrives the command will be obeyed to the amusement of onlookers but to the consternation of the individual who will advance all sorts of specious reasons for his behaviour. In his intriguing book, " Psychopathology of Everyday Life," Freud has shown that slips of the tongue and of memory are not accidents but are determined by the workings of the unconscious,

It is, however, in relation to the unconscious mind in neurotics that Freud's work has assumed its present importance. He maintained that as the human being passes through its various stages of psychological development, its primitive desires come more and more into conflict with the requirements of the society in which it lives and are thrust back into the unconscious, or *repressed*. As a result of his researches he went further and laid it down that the repressed desires were predominantly of a sexual nature—using the term " sexual " in its broadest possible sense. Furthermore, using the same mechanism of repression, unpleasant memories, again often of a sexual kind, are withheld from consciousness. Although, Freud went on, this elaborate system of repressing desires and memories goes on in everyone, in the neurotic repression is not entirely successful and these same desires or memories reappear in consciousness, but only in disguise, that is, as neurotic symptoms. In the same way as the Lord Chamberlain protects public morality by the censorship of plays, films, etc., so there is a personal censor which safeguards personal morality by keeping from consciousness that which is incompatible with the dictates of society. To continue the analogy: the censorship of indelicate situations or obscene words by the Lord Chamberlain is evaded by the use of subterfuges in the form of innuendoes or by a play on words—said with a broad wink (a visit to any music-hall will convince the most pure in heart), so the personal censor is side-stepped by the emergence of these repressed desires and memories as symptoms.

Freud's theory of the unconscious may well seem fanciful, but he has produced a wealth of evidence in support of it. He claims, with considerable justification, that the delusions and hallucinations of the insane are the products of the workings of the unconscious mind as are, in the sane, the slips of the tongue and memory already referred to.

It is, however, in his analysis of dreams that Freud makes his most brilliant exposé of his theory. The analysis of dreams, he says, is the royal road to the study of the unconscious. The dreams of children in which a simple wish is gratified are the most elementary types. Thus, some much coveted toy or sweetmeat denied him in reality is supplied, usually in plenty, in his dreams. In adults, though there may be also the gratification of a wish in their dreams, both the wish and its gratification may be disguised in a variety of subtle and varyingly complex ways. In " The Interpretation of Dreams " Freud gives a guide to the inner meaning, or latent content of dreams —in accordance with his own theories.

TYPES OF NEUROTIC ILLNESS

For our present purpose the actual types of neurotic illness are of secondary importance. Furthermore, no classification is satisfactory and almost every writer on this subject has evolved one of his own and has added to the confusion.

Broadly speaking, the neuroses fall into four groups, although it is more the rule than the exception to find elements of any or all of the groups in any particular case. They are :—

1. **Anxiety States.**—In psychological medicine " anxiety " implies something over and above the usually accepted implications of the term. It is essentially a *feeling*—a feeling of disquiet, of apprehension, of foreboding which may grow in intensity to produce a state of panic. What is even more tragic is that, as opposed to the anxiety caused by fear-producing situations which everyone has experienced, the anxiety neurotic may be consciously unaware of what produces this unpleasant feeling. In other words the cause lies in his *unconscious.* He may, for instance, be seized with panic for no apparent reason while sitting quietly in a cinema or theatre, in a bus or a tube, in a drawing-room or even while walking along a country lane.

2. **Hysteria.**—The term " hysteria " is overworked and much abused, so much so that it has come to mean anything or nothing. To the psychiatrist it implies a negative reaction to, or a retreat from, a state of mental conflict which the individual is unable to resolve at a conscious level. Thus the soldier in action, torn between his sense of duty and the instinct to preserve his life, develops a paralysis of a limb. As a combatant he is of no further immediate use. He is carried off the field away from danger. Here again the genuine hysteric, in contrast to the malingerer, is unaware of what has brought about his paralysis, *i.e.*, it has occurred as the result of unconscious mechanisms.

3. **Obsessive-Compulsive States.**—Although perhaps the least common form of neurosis, it is always serious and difficult to treat. The essential symptoms are irrational and irresistible urges to think along certain lines or to behave according to certain patterns. The psychopathology is difficult (one possible cause has been mentioned, see p. 552), but fundamentally these strange thoughts or practices are used to protect the individual, once more unconsciously, from prohibited thoughts or actions. There is a great similarity in these compulsions and obsessions to the ritualistic practices or magic

rites of primitive communities. Even in our own sophisticated culture remnants of this behaviour are seen as, for example, touching wood or not walking under ladders, to prevent disaster.

4. **Depressive States.**—Depression is essentially a feeling-tone of sadness and in its milder form is varyingly described as " feeling low," " feeling down in the dumps," " feeling browned-off," etc.

A state of depression may occur in response to environmental upsets such as bereavement, disappointment or frustration and is known then as reactive, or exogenous depression. Depression may arise, however, from within the personality itself, that is, for unconscious reasons, and have no bearing on external events. This type is known as endogenous depression, one variety of which, involutional melancholia, has already been referred to (see p. 557). This is a serious illness requiring urgent and specialised treatment because of the real danger of suicidal attempts.

THE TREATMENT OF THE NEUROSES

Before any form of treatment, that is, one of a variety of psycho-therapeutic procedures, is undertaken it is essential that the complaint as a neurosis, or as a psychosomatic expression thereof, is established. This nowadays is not done in a negative way, that is, by the exclusion of organic disease, but in a positive way by analysing the symptoms in relation to the patients' past and present life situations, heredity, their personalities and their usual pattern of response to emotional stresses. If, as so very often happens, the illness as it presents itself is rooted partly in an organic disease and partly in a mental elaboration of its symptoms, then it must be determined how much is due to one and how much to the other and rational attention given to both in appropriate measure.

1. **Explanation and Reassurance.**—This is by far the most common procedure used in psychiatric out-patient work. In it, it is impossible to overestimate the importance of the first interview, always a long one. In this the psychiatrist attempts to gain the confidence of the patient; this is known as " establishing rapport." Although apparently exploratory in that an estimate is obtained of what has already been described as " neurotic predisposition," and the factors in the environment which may have precipitated a " nervous breakdown," it is also curative in so far as the patient, perhaps for the first time, is permitted to talk about himself to someone who is prepared to listen sympathetically.

Subsequent interviews build a therapeutic edifice on the foundations laid during the first interview.

If as a result of one or several interviews the cause and effect of the nervous illness can be established then an explanation of how the body and mind are interrelated is given, using illustrations from " organ language " (see p. 566) or by showing how the symptoms of which they complain are exaggerations or caricatures of the normal responses of the body to emotional stress. Obviously, if adverse environmental factors are brought to light, such as unsatisfactory marital relations, difficulties with children and a host of others, technical advice is opportune and often produces gratifying results. Further, if disharmony is due to unsatisfactory housing, occupational maladjustment, economic privation, or threatening dissolution of a marriage, much can be done by goading the local housing authorities into action, an explanatory letter to the Labour Exchange, or by putting the patient in touch with charitable or social organisations such as the Marriage Guidance Council, etc. The psychiatrist is by his training the patient's guide, mentor and friend, but it would be churlish not to mention the invaluable assistance he so often receives from the Lady Almoner's Department and the psychiatric social worker in the execution of his multiple duties.

2. **Abreaction.**—Frequently, particularly in war time, a painful memory is repressed together with the emotion associated with it. Hysterical or " conversion " symptoms, such as have been described, result. If the patient is reduced to a drowsy state by means usually of an intravenous anæsthetic such as pentothal, the resistance to the recovery of the now unconscious memory is reduced and the patient can be encouraged to relive the traumatic episode. The emotional release is often violent during which the patient indulges in an orgy of abuse and recrimination, often against himself for having failed in his duty, or against his superiors for having brought about the situation in which he found himself. With the bringing to consciousness of these tremendously emotionally saturated episodes, the " mental energy " which has been " converted " into symptoms, is discharged and the symptoms evaporate.

The use of this treatment is limited, but there can be no doubt that because of it the great numbers of so-called " shell-shock " cases in the 1914-18 War were avoided or reduced in the recent conflict.

3. **Continuous Narcosis.**—There are large numbers of neurotics

who mainly because of loss of sleep and appetite have been reduced to nervous wrecks. By continued sedation over a period of days the patient is kept continuously asleep and the nerve-racked body given a chance to recuperate.

4. **Modified Insulin.**—Loss of appetite, and as a result, loss of weight are common neurotic symptoms. Carefully graduated doses of insulin can be given to stimulate appetite and increase weight so that the improved sense of physical well-being may in turn improve the mental outlook.

With the last three therapeutic procedures, it is always essential to follow them up with more intensive psychotherapy of the sort already outlined. They are all essentially first-aid measures.

5. **Psychoanalysis.**—It is a popular misconception that all psychiatric treatment is psychoanalytical. Nothing could be further from the truth. What is not generally appreciated is that a psychoanalysis is time-consuming and expensive and that the number of recognised analysts is very limited. Even if these factors did not obtain it would be fatuous to suppose that every neurotic would benefit from an analysis. A sledge-hammer is not necessary to drive in a tack.

This is not to suppose that psychoanalysis has not got a place in psychiatric practice. There are cases, unfortunately not inconsiderable in number, which resist the procedures sketched above. By means of psychoanalysis the depths of the patient's unconscious can be explored. In so doing the root cause of his present emotional difficulties can be related to difficulties in his past which have been forgotten or repressed. He can thus theoretically and often in practice be re-educated and, with the help of the analyst, led into healthier ways of life.

PSYCHOSOMATIC MEDICINE

Progress in medicine is a two-edged weapon. In the rush for improved scientific and mechanical diagnostic and therapeutic aids, man as a thinking and feeling being has tended to be forgotten. There has grown up the practice of studying a patient as a complicated automaton in whom the machinery either functions normally or abnormally. If, after being passed through the infinite number of tests, electrical, biochemical, radiological, etc., no abnormality is found, then the patient is assured that he is physically fit and is sent on his way nursing his headache, stomach-ache, heartache and a grievance against and scepticism about the modern physician. Had that physician the time and training to explore the *emotional* life of his patient, he might not have been so ready with his bland reassurances.

Fortunately, not all doctors have been blinded by the brilliance of modern scientific discoveries and in recent years the idea of human illness as a *psychosomatic* derangement has been growing in importance. Now the term psychosomatic, although new in itself, is a concept as old as the practice of healing. It means merely that the mind and the body must inevitably and invariably function together and that a disorder in one is more than likely to give rise to a disorder in the other. To take examples almost at random : it is scarcely conceivable that the thinking and feeling of an individual will not be coloured by the knowledge that he has tuberculosis ; on the other hand, for reasons which will be explained later, it is equally unlikely that a person suffering from anxiety-neurosis will not suffer some upset in the normal working of one or more organs of the body. But it must not be thought that on analysing a particular symptom-complex it is necessarily a matter of deciding if the fault lies in the psyche, that is, the mind, or in the soma, that is, the body. In a high proportion of cases, the decision to be made is how much is it the fault of one and how much of the other. Further, in the rational treatment of a case due attention must be paid to both.

MIND-BODY RELATIONSHIPS

Experimental Evidence.

Criticism has been levelled at the upholders of the psychosomatic approach on the grounds that their evidence of the interrelationship of mind and body was too speculative and nebulous. Of late, experimental evidence, sufficient to satisfy the most sceptical, has been forthcoming.

A few years ago, Wolf and Wolff, in America, brilliantly exploited the opportunity of observing a patient, " Tom," who had a gastric fistula. They were able to note the reactions of the stomach to a variety of emotional situations. They describe how, for example, in conditions of fatigue, depression, and the " alarm reaction," the gastric mucosa blanched and how there was a reduction in both the movements of the stomach and in the amount of secretion. It is easy to see that under these emotional conditions, with the resulting interference in gastric function, meals eaten are likely to be ill-digested or not to be digested at all.

Much more recently Grace, Wolf and Wolff (1951) have published their observations on the human colon. They studied four subjects in whom segments of the colon have become accidentally evaginated and repose on the abdominal wall. As in the experiments on the stomach, the alterations in the mucosa, motor contractions and mucus output of the colon could be noted in response to day-to-day life situations evoking emotions of one sort or another. Here again it was shown that there was a distinct variation in the behaviour of the colon according to the prevailing emotional state of the individual concerned. Thus, when the patient's mood was one of anger and resentment the secretion of the colon was thick, tenacious and profuse; when he was cheerful the mucus was thin, watery and scanty. With these findings in mind it is understandable how easy it is to produce colonic dysfunction, e.g., constipation or diarrhœa, as the result of emotional disharmony.

Organ Language.

Although not as acceptable to the scientist as the experimental evidence illustrated above, " organ language " is of extreme importance in showing how, in an intuitive way, an appreciation of psychosomatic relationships has come to be expressed in everyday speech and in the verbal imagery of poets and writers. Examples abound and relate to every organ in the body.

The head or brain : " muddle-headed " as an expression of mental confusion. " There's a headache on every page," to denote a particularly difficult book.

The heart : " a broken heart," or " a heavy heart " ; " light-hearted," " brave heart," " warm-hearted," " an overflowing heart," etc., are in such common use and have such accepted connotations that explanations are superfluous.

The stomach : " sick with excitement," " sick with fear," " unable to stomach " (a situation), " no stomach to this fight," " a weak stomach," or " a strong stomach," are again all self-explanatory.

The liver : " chicken-livered " or " lily-livered " to denote cowardice.

The bowels : " Have you no bowels, no compassion ? " (John Gay), " . . . and shutteth up his bowels of compassion . . . " (First Epistle General of John). Both these quotations exemplify the acceptance since time immemorial of the influence of the emotions on the bowels. It is only recently (see above) that experimental validation has been forthcoming.

To these few examples—scores of others come to mind—could be added such expressions as " paralysed with fear," " trembling with emotion," " black with rage," " eyes popping with excitement," etc. These are all graphic uses of organ language to express psychosomatic experiences.

PSYCHOSOMATIC SYMPTOMS

It requires only a moment's reflection to convince one that all have at one time or another experienced the physical symptoms of emotional upset. Who, for example, has not fainted at the sight of something repugnant, or experienced tachycardia as the result of anticipating an event, pleasurable or unpleasurable ? The child dressing for a party or the pantomime is often sick with excitement. The candidate, before the doors of the examination hall open, is smitten with urgency or frequency of micturition. The runner before the start of a race feels his mouth dry up. A restless, disturbed night often anticipates a day in which some difficulty has to be dealt with. The list is limitless : every emotion can interfere with the normal working of any organ of the body.

Bearing in mind these emotional reactions, which are accepted by all as normal occurrences, it is easy to understand how they can be precipitated and perpetuated in a person whose emotional life is chronically upset. It is no exaggeration to say, in fact, that every symptom of every known organic disease can be mimicked in nervous disorders of one sort or another.

Why in these illnesses one organ is selected rather than another to manifest symptoms is another problem. It may be that, for instance, an anxiety neurotic, whose entire life is fogged with anxiety, misinterprets the tachycardia or palpitations which, as has been shown, are a normal concomitant of anxiety, and convinces himself that he has heart disease. The resulting hypochondriacal preoccupation produces a vicious circle ; the more he worries about himself the more persistent the symptoms become. On the other hand, he may have at one time suffered from an organic illness, but his anxiety produces symptoms similar to those he has previously experienced and convinces him that the organic complaint has recurred. Or he may have lived in a household where a member has had a disease, the symptoms of which he himself is now experiencing. He must, he argues illogically, be therefore suffering from the same complaint.

Previously it has been stated that there is no clear line of

2. No "designated hospitals".—Any kind of hospital may receive any type of mental patient on an informal basis or under detention. This implies that the "general" nurse may well be called upon to nurse psychiatric cases. From now on, therefore, it will be essential for every nurse to have at least a working knowledge of the principles and practice of psychological medicine.

3. **Appeal Tribunals.**—These tribunals, which are shortly to be set up, will consider applications from patients (and relatives) for release from hospital. They will have the power to discharge patients.

4. **Detention Safeguards.**—Compulsory powers of detention will be exercisable only when no other appropriate methods of dealing with a mentally-ill patient are available.

5. **Powers of Discharge.**—The general rule will be that the nearest relative of all patients admitted under the new procedures will hold the power of discharge.

6. **Administration.**—The mental-health services will be integrated with other health and welfare services under the Ministry of Health. The Board of Control (the body at present responsible for the administration of the lunacy laws in England) will cease to exist for it will have no function.

Further recommendations written into the new Act emphasise that, "the division of functions between the hospitals, local authorities and the other official bodies should be broadly the same in relation to mentally disordered patients as in relation to others." Implicit in these recommendations is the obligation of the local authority to prevent admission of the mentally ill to hospital by comprehensive out-patient and prophylactic services. For those who do not, or who no longer, need in-patient treatment, all types of care within the community are advocated, such as, Day Hospitals, Night Hostels, Social Clubs and in this context special emphasis is placed on the care of the aged.

The new Act is at the moment a piece of legal machinery of tremendous potential which has as yet not been set into motion. Whether or not it will work depends on the efforts not only of psychiatrists and mental nurses, but on the goodwill of all physicians and nurses who will be called upon to play their part, not to mention the tolerance of the general public amongst whom so many mentally-sick people will be expected to live.

CHAPTER XXI

IMPORTANT DRUGS

CHEMOTHERAPY AND ANTIBIOTICS

THE discovery of the sulphonamide group of drugs has brought forth tremendous changes in the control and treatment of infectious diseases. Sulphonamides exert their effect mainly through preventing the growth of susceptible organisms; they thus allow the defensive mechanisms of the body to rapidly overcome the invading organisms.

The sulphonamides have effect only on a limited range of organisms, so that continuous research has gone on to discover other drugs which would have a lethal effect on a wider range. Penicillin, which was the next great advance after the sulphonamides, has this greatly increased range of action, although there are, nevertheless, many organisms which are resistant to its action.

Following the introduction of penicillin, rapid strides were made in the discovery of many new antibiotics, such as streptomycin, chloramphenicol and the tetracyclines (aureomycin, terramycin and achromycin) with still greater possibilities in the inhibition of the growth of organisms.

Penicillin, streptomycin and the tetracyclines are not chemical drugs but are products of living organisms such as moulds and fungi; the name *antibiotics* has been introduced to describe these valuable agents. As the developments in the discovery of new antibiotics are so rapid it is impossible to keep up to date in the best use of the different antibiotics in the different diseases.

THE SULPHONAMIDES

The sulphonamide group of drugs were the first major advance in chemotherapy and they are now widely used in medicine, although the use of many of the original drugs of this group has been discontinued because of their toxicity. These drugs have been replaced by other less toxic preparations.

It is impossible in a short space to mention all the different sulphonamides which may currently be in use. Therefore the more commonly used preparations only will be given.

1. Sulphadimidine (Sulphamezathine).

Sulphadimidine is at present widely used and is one of the least toxic of the sulphonamide drugs, particularly in respect of renal complications. Sulphadimidine is relatively slowly excreted with the result that it can be given at six-hourly intervals.

2. Sulphafurazole (Gantrisin).

Sulphafurazole is one of the newer sulphonamides and has low toxicity. It has to be given at four or six-hourly intervals to maintain an adequate blood concentration.

3. Sulphadiazine.

This preparation is widely used in America and is a very potent drug. It also has the great advantage of being rapidly absorbed into the cerebrospinal fluid. It has to be given at four-hourly intervals.

4. Sulphamethoxypyridazine (Lederkyn, Midicel).

This sulphonamide is very slowly excreted so that only one dose a day is said to be effective.

Sulphaphenazole (orisulf) and sulphadimethoxine (madribon) are two long-acting sulphonamides which have been more recently introduced. One or two doses a day are sufficient.

5. Sulphonamide Mixtures—Sulphatriad and Tresamide.

In recent years the tendency has been to combine several of the sulphonamides together in one tablet. This causes fewer toxic reactions, especially in the kidneys, and also produces a potent preparation which is given at four to six-hourly intervals.

Sulphatriad is a combination of sulphamerazine, sulphathiazole and sulphadiazine.

6. Sulphamethizole (Urolucosil).

This preparation of sulphonamide is useful in treating infections of the renal tract as it does not form crystals in the urine (and so block the renal tubules). A high fluid intake is not therefore necessary.

7. Low Absorption Group of Sulphonamides.

- (*a*) Sulphaguanidine.
- (*b*) Succinylsulphathiazole.
- (*c*) Phthalylsulphathiazole.

8. Sulphasalazine (Salazopyrin).

This is a combination of a sulphonamide and a salicylate, used particularly in the treatment of ulcerative colitis.

These drugs are all poorly absorbed from the intestinal tract and so exert their effect locally in the bowel. For this reason they are used entirely for their local action in disease of the intestinal tract.

Before operations on the bowel this group of low absorption sulphonamides are usually given so as to render the intestinal tract as sterile as possible. In bacillary dysentery and some chronic localised intestinal diseases, such as colitis, these drugs are often beneficial.

MAIN USES OF THE SULPHONAMIDES

Since the introduction of penicillin and the other antibiotics capable of replacing the sulphonamides in their actions against many organisms, the use of sulphonamides has become more limited. Sulphonamides are more toxic than penicillin. The choice between sulphonamides and antibiotics (penicillin, tetracycline, chloramphenicol, etc.) depends on many factors, such as the individual doctor's preference, whether it is possible to give injections as opposed to oral therapy or vice versa and also on the availability of the preparation. For these reasons it is impossible to compile a complete or useful list of all the diseases in which sulphonamides should or should not be given. The following are, however, among the commonest conditions for which the sulphonamides are frequently given :—

1. Acute tonsillitis.
2. Urinary tract infections by *B. coli* organisms.
3. Bacillary dysentery.
4. Before operations on the bowel, to render it as sterile as possible.
5. Bacterial pneumonias.
6. Meningococcal meningitis. Sulphonamides remain the drug of choice for this form of pyogenic meningitis.

DOSES AND ADMINISTRATION OF THE SULPHONAMIDES

The aim in treatment with all sulphonamides (except the low absorption group) is to obtain a rapid high concentration of the drug in the blood, and to maintain this level so that the organisms will be destroyed. To achieve a high level rapidly a large initial dose of 2 to 3 gm. (four to six tablets) is given. To maintain an adequate blood level the initial dose must be followed by smaller doses varying from 1 to $1\frac{1}{2}$ gm. four to eight-hourly, according to the preparation used and also the severity of the infection. It is essential that the drug be given at the prescribed times if effective treatment is to be achieved. With the newer long-acting sulphonamide (lederkyn, midicel) two tablets (1 gm.) are given as an initial dose, followed by one daily dose of 0·5 gm.

The drug is continued until all signs of the infection have gone. The termination of the infection is usually denoted by the presence of a normal temperature for two or three days, after which the drug is stopped. To continue for a longer period than is necessary is only to invite serious toxic reactions from the drug. Again, as a working rule, it can be assumed that if the temperature has *not* fallen to normal after two or three days on sulphonamides then little is to be gained by continuing with the drug. This is because failure of the temperature to fall to normal after several days on sulphona-mides usually means that the causative organism is insensitive to the drug, and in that case one of the antibiotics should be given instead.

It should be noted that children tolerate sulphonamides very well and relatively large doses, considering their age, can be given.

The use and dosage of the low absorption group of sulphona-mides are different, however, from the above, which apply to the absorbable group. The low absorption sulphonamides (succinyl-sulphathiazole, phthalylsulphathiazole, etc.) are used where only a local effect in the bowel is required. As the drugs in this group are almost wholly unabsorbed into the blood stream and are therefore unlikely to cause toxic reactions, large doses of these sulphonamides are given, *e.g.*, 2 gm. four to six-hourly.

TOXIC EFFECTS OF THE SULPHONAMIDES

Different sulphonamides have varying degrees of toxicity, and it is probable that the combinations of several preparations as in sulphatriad are the least toxic. The following are the main toxic effects of the sulphonamides :—

1. **Renal.**—The drugs may form crystals in the kidneys as they are being excreted, which may in some cases cause blocking of the kidney tubules. This leads to hæmaturia, diminished output of urine (oliguria) and, in severe cases, to complete stoppage of urine (anuria). The longer the drug is given, the heavier the dose and the more concentrated the urine, the more likely is it that renal complications will develop.

It is essential, therefore, to give all patients on any of the sulphona-mides a large amount of fluids (at least 4 pints in the twenty-four hours). This fact must be stressed and the nurse must see that the

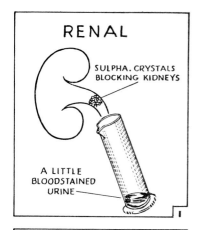

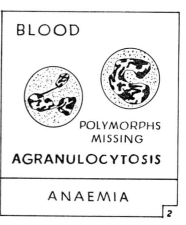

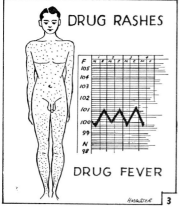

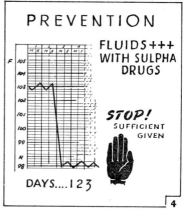

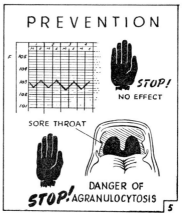

Fig. 186
Toxic effects
of the
sulphonamides.

patient is taking an adequate amount of fluid and also passing a normal output of urine (that is, about 40 oz. in the twenty-four hours).

Sulphonamides should be immediately stopped with any patient who develops hæmaturia or whose urinary output suddenly drops.

2. **Agranulocytosis.**—This is a most serious complication wherein the polymorphonuclear or granular white blood cells become markedly diminished in number or, in the most severe cases, may be almost completely absent. Like most of the other serious toxic reactions from sulphonamides, agranulocytosis is more likely to develop the longer the drug is used and the heavier the dosage. The patient usually complains of a sore throat and the temperature rises to 102° to 104° F. or, if already raised, goes higher still. These signs are of the utmost importance, and with any patient who develops a sore throat while on sulphonamides the drug must be stopped at once and a white blood count taken. This will reveal the urgency of the condition.

In order to forestall the development of agranulocytosis all patients who have been on sulphonamides for over a week should have a white cell count taken as a routine check. In addition, the importance of stopping the drug as soon as it is clear that the infection has been halted or is not responding must again be stressed.

3. **Rashes.**—Morbilliform or scarlatinaform rashes may occur, and in these cases the drug is usually stopped.

4. **Nausea and Vomiting.**—The complications nausea and vomiting vary with different preparations and with different people. The drug should not be stopped unless the vomiting is persistent. Sulphonamide tablets are best given crushed up in milk or fruit juices if they cause nausea.

5. **Drug Fever.**—A raised temperature due to the drug itself may occur and is often associated with drug rashes. The drug must then be stopped.

6. **Anæmia.**—Severe anæmia is a rare but serious toxic reaction.

PENICILLIN

Penicillin is the commonest of the antibiotics in current use. It was the first to be discovered, but since then many other antibiotics have been and are continuing to be introduced.

Penicillin acts by preventing the organisms from growing and also by actually destroying the organisms. Its action varies with different bacteria, being highly effective against some while having little or no effect against others.

MAIN USES OF PENICILLIN

Table XI gives the main diseases and their causative organisms for which penicillin is used.

TABLE XI

DISEASES.	CAUSATIVE ORGANISMS.
Septic infections (wounds, abscesses)	Streptococci and Staphylococci.
Osteomyelitis	,, ,,
Septicæmia	,, ,,
Acute tonsillitis . . .	Streptococci.
Bacterial endocarditis . .	,,
Eye infections (conjunctivitis) .	,,
Pneumonia	Pneumococci, streptococci, staphylococci.
Syphilis	*Treponema pallidum.*
Gonorrhœa	Gonococci.

Penicillin has little or no effect on such organisms as :—

1. The enteric, dysentery and food poisoning group.
2. The *B. coli* group, which are frequently responsible for urinary tract infections (pyelitis, cystitis) and also for some cases of septic peritonitis.
3. The tubercle bacillus.
4. The whooping-cough bacillus.
5. Any of the viruses which are the causative organisms of so many acute infectious fevers (measles, poliomyelitis, chickenpox, smallpox, etc.).

DOSES AND ADMINISTRATION OF PENICILLIN

There are several preparations of penicillin in use, the following being those most widely used :—

1. **Phenoxymethylpenicillin (Penicillin V).**—This preparation of penicillin is fully effective when given by mouth, unlike most other forms of penicillin, which are largely destroyed by the acid gastric juice. Except for severe general infections, oral therapy with penicillin V is usually sufficient and obviates the need to give frequent intramuscular injections. This is of particular value when treating children.

Phenoxymethylpenicillin (distaquaine V) is given in 60 to 125 mgm. doses four-hourly to six-hourly. The last daily dose may be doubled to avoid waking the patient at night.

2. **Crystalline Benzylpenicillin.**—This is the ordinary soluble sodium (or potassium) salt which is usually referred to as " penicillin." This form of penicillin is very rapidly absorbed into the blood stream but is also quickly excreted by the kidneys. The larger the dose of penicillin given, the longer the therapeutic effect lasts, but up to a definite limit only. It is probable that even the largest doses are all excreted within eight hours. The dose of penicillin given depends both on the severity of the infection and the frequency of the injections. The tendency nowadays is to give very large doses of penicillin, at longer intervals.

For moderately severe systemic infections, six-hourly to eight-hourly injections of 100,000 to 250,000 units are usually given, although injections of 500,000 units, twelve-hourly, have also been used with a good therapeutic response. In very severe infections, and particularly where it is known that the causative organism is not highly sensitive to penicillin, as much as 500,000 or 1,000,000 units, six-hourly or eight-hourly, may be given.

In addition to the above administration, crystalline penicillin is also used locally in eye infections and injected into the pleural cavity in cases of empyema.

3. **Procaine Benzylpenicillin.** — (This preparation is usually referred to as procaine penicillin.) Combining procaine with crystalline soluble penicillin delays its absorption so that an effective blood concentration can be maintained for a much longer time. This means that less frequent injections can be given, usually at twelve-hourly or twenty-four-hourly intervals. Owing to its slow absorption, however, a high concentration of penicillin is not usually achieved with procaine penicillin and therefore severe systemic infections are usually treated, not with procaine penicillin, but with soluble crystalline penicillin.

Procaine penicillin is thus mainly used for treating localised infections or the less severe general systemic infections. The usual dose is 300,000 to 600,000 units at twelve-hourly or twenty-four-hourly intervals. For an immediate effect soluble crystalline penicillin (100,000 units) is often combined with procaine penicillin.

Abbocillin, avloprocil, distaquaine and seclopen are some procaine penicillin preparations.

4. **Benzathine Penicillin.**—This form of penicillin was the most effective preparation for oral use before penicillin V was introduced. It is also given by injection when it has a very prolonged action lasting for several weeks.

TOXIC EFFECTS OF PENICILLIN

Penicillin is one of the least toxic drugs even in extremely high doses of many millions of units. This makes penicillin a most valuable antibiotic and explains why it is the most commonly used of all antibiotics. Nevertheless, some patients develop hyper-sensitive (allergic) reactions, such as urticaria, fever, or, even more serious, an anaphylactic state which may be fatal. Great care therefore should be taken to ascertain whether the patient is sensitive to penicillin. Patients who are known to suffer from allergic diseases such as asthma, hay fever or eczema, are particularly likely to develop severe reactions to penicillin injections if they are sensitive to the antibiotic.

External contact with penicillin may give rise to dermatitis. Nurses and doctors who are repeatedly preparing penicillin injections are especially liable to develop a contact dermatitis.

STREPTOMYCIN

Streptomycin is one of the most effective drugs at present in use against the tubercle bacillus. It has, however, two great disadvantages :—

1. It is a toxic drug which in large doses over a prolonged period affects the auditory nerve causing *deafness* and *giddiness* (vertigo).

2. In some cases the tubercle bacillus becomes resistant to the drug so that the drug loses its effect. As tuberculosis in most of its forms is a chronic disease requiring prolonged treatment this is a great drawback. However, if para-aminosalicylic acid (P.A.S.) or isoniazid is given with the streptomycin the development of resistance by the organisms to streptomycin is considerably lessened.

Streptomycin is given by intramuscular injection, 1 gm. daily. For further details on the use of this drug in tuberculosis see page 189.

In addition to its use in the various forms of tuberculosis, streptomycin is frequently used in the following conditions :—

(a) Infections of the urinary tract (pyelitis, cystitis) which have not responded to sulphonamide or other therapy.

(b) In cases of subacute bacterial endocarditis which have not cleared up with penicillin, streptomycin is often combined with penicillin to good effect.

(c) In the severe tropical disease plague, streptomycin has been given with very beneficial results in both the bubonic and pneumonic forms.

(d) Before operations on the bowel and also in cases of septic peritonitis.

THE TETRACYCLINES

The tetracyclines are three antibiotics with very similar actions. They are :—

    1. **Tetracycline** (Achromycin, Tetracyn).
    2. **Demethylchlortetracycline** (Ledermycin).
    3. **Oxytetracycline** (Terramycin).

These antibiotics have a very wide range of activity—they are often referred to as " broad spectrum antibiotics "—being effective in streptococcal, staphylococcal, pneumococcal, meningococcal, gonococcal and *Bacillus coli* infections. In addition they are effective in rickettsial and certain virus infections.

Tetracycline and oxytetracycline are usually given by mouth in 250 mgm. doses six-hourly. The more recently introduced demethyl-chlortetracycline (ledermycin) is more potent and more long acting so that 300 mgm. twice daily are usually sufficient. In those very severe infections where the patient, for whatever reason, cannot take oral therapy, tetracycline and oxytetracycline may be given by intravenous or intramuscular injection. Local irritation and pain are likely to occur, however, with parenteral therapy, so that as soon as possible oral therapy is started.

The tetracycline antibiotics are also used for local application in a 1 per cent. ointment for bacterial skin diseases such as impetigo and sycosis.

TOXIC EFFECTS.—Nausea, vomiting and diarrhœa are not infrequently seen, particularly after intensive and prolonged therapy. Tetracycline causes the least gastro-intestinal upset. With prolonged therapy, excessive growth of insensitive organisms, such as fungi and staphylococci, may occur in the bowel with resultant infection of the gastro-intestinal tract. This infection may cause severe inflammation of the bowel (ileocolitis) with severe diarrhœa and fever and in some few cases has proved fatal.

Another adverse effect very likely to arise with prolonged therapy or with heavy dosage is vitamin deficiency, particularly of vitamins B and K. This is due to the alteration of the normal intestinal bacterial flora. When the tetracyclines are given for more than a few days, vitamin B complex should be given.

CHLORAMPHENICOL (Chloromycetin)

Chloramphenicol (the proprietary preparation is called chloromycetin) is similar in its action to the tetracyclines but in addition it is the one antibiotic effective in the treatment of typhoid fever. Chloramphenicol is given in oral doses of 500 mgm. six-hourly.

The toxic effects of chloramphenicol are similar to those of the tetracyclines, whilst, in addition, chloramphenicol may give rise to the more serious danger of severe aplastic anæmia. Aplastic anæmia, which is often fatal, has most often occurred in children on prolonged and heavy dosage. The use of chloramphenicol is best restricted to the treatment of typhoid fever and to infections not responding to penicillin or the tetracyclines.

ERYTHROMYCIN

Erythromycin is an antibiotic effective against staphylococci, streptococci and pneumococci. Its action is in many ways similar to that of penicillin. The chief use of erythromycin is in the treatment of staphylococcal infections resistant to penicillin and the other antibiotics. Staphylococci, probably more than any other organisms, are very likely to become resistant to penicillin or other antibiotics, and for these infections erythromycin has proved very valuable.

Erythromycin is given by mouth in tablets, in 200 to 300 mgm. doses six-hourly. No serious side effects have so far been noted and it is said that erythromycin does not materially alter the normal intestinal flora, with the result that it rarely causes gastro-intestinal upset or vitamin deficiency.

Ilotycin and erythrocin are proprietary preparations of erythromycin.

NOVOBIOCIN

Novobiocin (albamycin biotexin, cathomycin) is effective against streptococcal, staphylococcal and pneumococcal infections. The usual dose is 250 mgm. six-hourly by mouth. Skin rashes have been noted and patients treated with novobiocin.

The main indication at present for the use of novobiocin is in staphylococcal infections resistant to penicillin, erythromycin and other antibiotics.

NEOMYCIN

Neomycin is an antibiotic with a very wide range of activity. It is never given by injection as it is too toxic, causing severe kidney damage and deafness.

Uses.

1. Neomycin is mainly used for local application in bacterial skin infections such as impetigo, sycosis and infected eczema. Unlike penicillin, bacterial resistance to neomycin rarely develops.

2. In bacterial infections of the eye, neomycin in ointment form is often very effective.

3. Neomycin is not readily absorbed when given by mouth, so severe toxic effects are not likely to develop when it is given in this way. Neomycin is therefore used orally in the treatment of gastro-enteritis of infants.

4. Oral neomycin is also given before operations on the intestinal tract.

5. In severe cirrhosis of the liver when the patient shows mental changes neomycin is given to sterilise the bowel and reduce toxic absorption.

NYSTATIN

As has already been mentioned, one of the most serious disadvantages of the use of broad spectrum antibiotics, such as the tetracycline antibiotics, is " superinfection," *i.e.*, the undue growth of insensitive organisms, particularly staphylococci and fungi such as candida albicans (monilia). Candida albicans can cause thrush, vaginitis, pruritus and generalised systemic infection.

Nystatin is believed to be effective in monilial infections and is given orally in doses of two tablets (500,000 units) six-hourly for systemic infections. Nystatin is also available in ointment form for fungal skin infections and as vaginal tablets for vaginitis.

SOME OTHER ANTIBIOTICS

Many other antibiotics are being used but as they are as yet used to a more limited extent, only a brief mention will be made of them.

1. **Oleandomycin** (matromycin romicil) is effective against streptococcal, staphylococcal and pneumococcal infections. It is therefore a useful alternative for the treatment of staphylococcal infections which have become resistant to other antibiotics. The combination of oleandomycin and tetracycline (sigmamycin) is

believed to enhance the action of both antibiotics and, more important, to delay the emergence of resistant strains of organisms, particularly drug-resistant staphylococci. The usual dose is 250 mgm. six-hourly by mouth.

2. **Spiramycin** (rovamycin) is an antibiotic with a narrow range of activity and is used in streptococcal and pneumococcal infections of the respiratory tract and middle ear. It is given by mouth in 500 mgm. doses six-hourly. It does not cause serious side effects.

3. **Bacitracin** is sometimes combined with neomycin for use locally in skin diseases (neobacrin), or is occasionally given by mouth. It is too toxic for parenteral use.

4. **Cycloserine** (seromycin) is at present undergoing trial for the treatment of tuberculosis. It is used only for those patients who have developed resistance to the other more commonly used antibiotics such as streptomycin. Cycloserine is usually given combined with isoniazid in 0·5 to 1 gm. doses daily. It is a toxic drug and can cause convulsions.

In addition to its use in tuberculosis, cycloserine has also proved effective in treating chronic urinary infections resistant to other antibiotics.

5. **Viomycin** (viocin) is used only in tuberculosis. If resistance to streptomycin or isoniazid develops viomycin is an alternative drug. It is, however, a very toxic drug, especially if given in large doses; therefore the drug is usually given not more often than twice weekly in 2 gm. doses intramuscularly for limited periods.

6. **Kanamycin** (kannasyn) is a new antibiotic similar in action to neomycin but given by intramuscular injection (1 gm. in two equal doses daily). Kanamycin is effective in staphylococcal, genito-urinary and respiratory tract infections. The main toxic effect is severe deafness if large doses and prolonged therapy are given, so that the drug must be stopped after one week.

CHOICE OF CHEMOTHERAPEUTIC AGENT

It will be seen that there are several different antimicrobial agents at present available which may be given with good therapeutic effect in the treatment of many of the infective diseases. Ideally, the first essential would be to isolate the causative organism and then, by means of sensitivity tests, determine to which antibiotic or sulphonamide preparation the organism is most sensitive. In practice, however, especially with all acute and serious illnesses, the delay involved in isolating the organism and in doing sensitivity

19 A

tests would react to the detriment of the patient. Also, in many of the infective diseases it is not always possible to isolate the causative organisms.

In acute and serious illnesses, where in any case the probable causative agent is often known, chemotherapy is usually started at once. Where applicable, the sulphonamides or penicillin are usually given as a first choice. If these drugs fail to have effect (*i.e.*, if the temperature fails to fall and there is no improvement in the patient's condition) a different antimicrobial agent must be given. By this time, in many cases, it will have been possible to isolate the causative organism and sensitivity tests can then be done to find out to which antibiotic the organism is most sensitive.

In the more chronic, and particularly in recurring infections, such as urinary tract infections and staphylococcal infections, this determination of the sensitivity of the organism to the various antibiotics is, whenever possible, essential; otherwise the organism may very rapidly develop resistance to the antibiotics.

SENSITIVITY TESTS

The importance of finding out to which antibiotic or sulphonamide preparation the organism is most sensitive, particularly in the more chronic and recurring infections, has been stressed. The appropriate bacteriological specimen (sputum, urine, throat swab, pus, blood culture, cerebrospinal fluid, etc.) is sent to the laboratory and the organism is cultured by incubation in a suitable medium (see p. 22). On the culture plate are placed small discs of filter paper impregnated with the various antibiotics or sulphonamide. If the organism is sensitive to an antibiotic or sulphonamide preparation, it will not grow in the immediate vicinity of the disc impregnated with that antibiotic or sulphonamide preparation. On the other hand, if the organism is resistant to an antibiotic, growth of the organism will not be affected in the immediate vicinity of the disc.

It is important to realise that sensitivity tests take time (as does the culture of all organisms) as the organisms must be incubated in a proper medium for many hours, usually twenty-four.

SOME COMMON IMPORTANT DRUGS

ADRENALINE (Epinephrine) AND NORADRENALINE

Adrenaline and noradrenaline are the two secretions of the medulla of the adrenal gland.

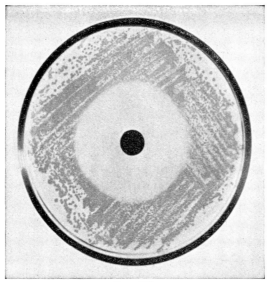

FIG. 187

Penicillin-sensitive staphylococci. The organisms have failed to grow in the immediate vicinity of the penicillin-impregnated paper disc.

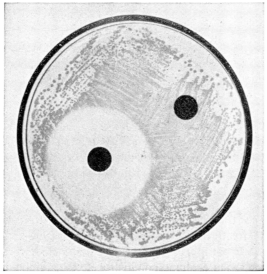

FIG. 188

Staphylococci resistant to penicillin, but sensitive to erythromycin. The paper disc on the right was impregnated with penicillin which failed to inhibit growth of the organisms, but around the erythromycin-impregnated disc on the left is a clear area where the organisms have failed to grow.

Actions of Adrenaline.

1. Constricts the arterioles of the skin and mucous membranes.
2. Relaxes the smooth muscle of the bronchioles of the lungs.
3. Raises the blood sugar by releasing glucose from the liver into the blood stream.
4. Increases the rate and force of the heart.

Uses of Adrenaline.

1. To stop bleeding from mucous membranes, as in epistaxis; gauze plugs soaked in adrenaline are used. Adrenaline is also used in local anæsthetic solutions to constrict the vessels and so reduce the amount of bleeding.

2. In asthma it is one of the most valuable drugs available and is usually given by subcutaneous injection in 3 to 8 minim doses. A more recent preparation of adrenaline, isoprenaline (neo-epinine, neodrenal) is available in tablets which are allowed to dissolve under the tongue. A spray solution is also effective.

3. In anaphylaxis, serum sickness, urticaria and other hyper-sensitive reactions subcutaneous injections of 0·5 ml. of adrenaline are of great value.

4. In insulin coma adrenaline injections may revive the patient sufficiently for him to take glucose by mouth.

5. In Stokes-Adams syndrome, where convulsions occur owing to severe heart block with cardiac arrest, adrenaline injected directly into the heart may start the heart beating again.

Action and Use of Noradrenaline.

Noradrenaline is used only to raise the blood pressure in cases of severe shock. It is given by slow intravenous drip, 4 mgm. to each litre. Levophed is a proprietary preparation of noradrenaline.

ALKALIS (Antacids)

Alkalis are drugs which are used to neutralise the acid gastric juice in the treatment of peptic ulcer and dyspepsia. There are very many different alkalis at present in use, including calcium and magnesium carbonate, aluminium hydroxide gel, aluminium glycinate and magnesium trisilicate. Sodium bicarbonate, which is a very potent alkali, is not nowadays used in the treatment of peptic ulcer because of the danger of alkalosis (see p. 492). Alkalis are further discussed on page 238.

AMINOPHYLLINE

Actions.

1. Relaxes the smooth muscles of the bronchioles.
2. Increases the output of urine (and is therefore a diuretic).
3. Dilates the coronary arteries.

Uses.

1. In bronchial asthma intravenous injection (0·25 gm. in 10 ml. of sterile distilled water) is of great value in severe attacks which have not responded to other measures.

2. In cardiac asthma.

3. To enhance the effect of the mercurial diuretics in cardiac œdema.

4. In angina pectoris.

Aminophylline is given in tablet form by mouth (0·1 gm.), by intramuscular injection (0·5 gm. in 2 ml.) or intravenously (0·25 gm. in 10 ml.).

AMPHETAMINE (Benzedrine)

Amphetamine has a markedly stimulating effect on the central nervous system resulting in temporarily increased energy and mental alertness. Amphetamine, or benzedrine as it is often called, is used in the treatment of mental depression and alcoholism and to overcome the hypnotic action of such drugs as the barbiturates. Amphetamine is given by mouth in 5 mgm. tablets. It should not be given late in the day, otherwise it may cause insomnia.

Dexamphetamine (dexedrine) has a similar effect to amphetamine but is also used to suppress the appetite in obese patients trying to reduce weight.

ANALGESICS

Analgesics are drugs which relieve pain and are fully discussed on page 536. Morphine, which was the first of these drugs to be used and is still the most important, is discussed in detail on page 607.

ANTHELMINTICS

Anthelmintics (vermifuges) are drugs used in the treatment of intestinal worms (helminths). The anthelmintic drugs in common use at present include piperazine (antepar, entacyl), dichlorophen (anthiphen) and mepacrine. All these drugs are fully discussed on page 267 *et seq.*

ANTICOAGULANT DRUGS

Anticoagulant drugs are used in the prevention and treatment of vascular thrombosis and embolism. These drugs, by prolonging the clotting time of the blood, may prevent a clot forming in a blood vessel. Also, when a clot has already formed, they may prevent further extension of the clot and so lessen the risk of embolism. Anticoagulant drugs are now widely used in the treatment of deep venous thrombosis to prevent pulmonary embolism, and also in coronary thrombosis to prevent further thrombotic and embolic episodes.

The anticoagulant drugs most frequently used at the present time include :—

(a) Orally—

    (i) Phenindione (dindevan, indema).

    (ii) Phenprocoumon (marcoumar).

    (iii) Warfarin sodium (marevan).

    (iv) Nicoumalone (sinthrome).

    (v) Dicoumarol (dicoumarin).

    (vi) Ethyl biscoumacetate (tromexan).

(b) By injection—

Heparin (liquemin, pularin).

Phenindione, warfarin and similar drugs act by destroying the prothrombin in the blood, thereby prolonging the clotting time. Heparin, which takes immediate effect when injected, differs in its action from the other anticoagulant drugs (see pp. 126 and 127).

Anticoagulant drugs must be administered with great caution and their use must be carefully controlled by frequent estimation of the prothrombin clotting time in the case of phenindione and similar drugs. Overdosage with anticoagulant drugs can lead to severe hæmorrhage. In addition, phenindione may on rare occasions cause a skin rash, when the drug should be stopped.

Anticoagulant drugs are fully discussed under coronary thrombosis (pp. 126 and 127).

ANTICONVULSANTS

Anticonvulsants are drugs used in the prevention and treatment of convulsions or fits, particularly epileptic fits. The most commonly used (and oldest) anticonvulsants are phenobarbitone and phenytoin sodium (epanutin, dilantin). Newer anticonvulsants, such as troxidone, primidone, methoin and phenurone, have recently come into use and are fully discussed on page 339.

ANTIHISTAMINE DRUGS

In certain diseases the toxic substance histamine is liberated in the body. Such diseases are the allergic or hypersensitive diseases like urticaria, hay fever, angioneurotic œdema, certain forms of dermatitis and eczema, serum sickness, sensitivity reactions, etc. Antihistamine drugs, which antagonise the action of histamine, are very effective in relieving the symptoms in the various allergic diseases mentioned above. The effect of the antihistamines varies in the different allergic diseases : urticaria, serum sickness, angioneurotic œdema and sensitivity reactions (due to penicillin, sulphonamides or other drugs) respond best. The antihistamine drugs are also effective in preventing motion (travel) sickness.

There are very many different preparations of antihistamine drugs available, some being more powerful than others. Overdosage with these drugs can cause toxic reactions, especially drowsiness, so that hypnotic drugs (e.g., barbiturates) must not be given at the same time as the antihistamines. Other toxic effects include giddiness, weakness and nervousness.

There are so many different antihistamine preparations available that it is impracticable to list them all. Antihistamines are best known under their trade names. The following are some of the more commonly used preparations with their official names, where given, in brackets :—

Ancolan (meclozine), 25 mgm. tablets.
Anthisan (mepyramine maleate), 50 and 100 mgm. tablets.
Antistin (antazoline), 100 mgm. tablets.
Avomine, 25 mgm. tablets.
Benadryl, 25 and 50 mgm. capsules.
Di-paralene (chlorcyclizine), 50 mgm. tablets.
Dramamine, 50 mgm. tablets.
Histantin (chlorcyclizine), 50 mgm. tablets.
Phenergan (promethazine), 10 and 25 mgm. tablets
Sandosten (thenalidine), 25 mgm. tablets.
Thephorin (phenindamine), 25 mgm. tablets.
Vallergan (trimeprazine), 10 mgm. tablets.

The usual dose is one to three tablets daily,

ANTITHYROID DRUGS

Antithyroid drugs depress the activity of the thyroid gland and are used solely in the treatment of thyrotoxicosis. The antithyroid drugs at present in use are carbimazole (neo-mercazole), thiouracil and potassium perchlorate. These drugs are discussed in detail on page 439.

ARSENIC

Uses.

1. In certain skin diseases, such as psoriasis and pemphigus, arsenic in the form of liquor arsenicalis, 2 to 8 minims, is often used.

2. In the treatment of vaginitis caused by the parasite *Trichomonas vaginalis* tablets of acetarsol are inserted locally into the vagina.

3. In certain tropical diseases like amœbic dysentery and sleeping sickness arsenic is often given.

4. It is also used, because of its poisonous effect, as a rat poison and a weed-killer.

Toxic Effects.—Arsenic is very poisonous if used in large doses. It can cause both acute and chronic poisoning.

1. ACUTE POISONING.—The main effect of the drug is to cause severe gastro-enteritis and collapse. The treatment consists in washing out the stomach and leaving in peroxide of iron or magnesia. Morphine is useful to combat the shock and collapse in doses of $\frac{1}{6}$ to $\frac{1}{4}$ gr. Fluids may have to be given intravenously when the vomiting and diarrhœa are very severe.

2. CHRONIC POISONING.—Taking arsenic for a prolonged period can cause :—

    (*a*) Peripheral neuritis.

    (*b*) Dermatitis (often very severe in the form of an exfoliative dermatitis where large areas of the skin are shed). Pigmentation of the skin is also common.

    (*c*) Chronic gastro-enteritis with vomiting and diarrhœa.

    (*d*) Jaundice from liver damage.

In the chronic form of poisoning injections of dimercaprol (B.A.L.) intramuscularly are an effective antidote, especially for the dermatitis.

ATROPINE

Atropine is similar in its action to belladonna, stramonium and hyoscine.

Actions.

1. It depresses the parasympathetic nerve-endings in cardiac and smooth muscle.

2. Reduces the secretions of the salivary glands, sweat glands and the gastric mucous membrane.

3. Dilates the pupil of the eye.

Uses.

1. To relieve spasm of smooth muscle in cases of biliary or renal colic. It is also very valuable in relieving pylorospasm and the pain in peptic ulcer.

2. In paralysis agitans and post-encephalitic Parkinsonism, to reduce the excessive salivation and lessen the muscular rigidity.

3. In eye diseases, such as iritis and corneal ulcers, to dilate the pupil and prevent adhesions forming. Atropine also rests the eye.

4. Pre-operatively, combined with morphine, to diminish the bronchial secretions and also to prevent vagal inhibition of the heart under the anæsthetic.

5. In infants with congenital hypertrophic pyloric stenosis, to relieve the pylorospasm. In early or mild cases atropine may cure the condition, thus obviating operation. It is given in the form of drops (eumydrin) or as lamellæ placed on the tongue and allowed to dissolve (pylostropin).

Toxic Effects.—Atropine can produce the following toxic effects :—

1. Dryness of the mouth owing to decreased saliva.

2. A dry hot skin often accompanied by rashes and a raised temperature.

3. Delirium, with widely dilated pupils.

4. Respiratory failure, with death from asphyxia.

Treatment of Atropine Poisoning.

1. The stomach is washed out with saline or a dilute solution of tannic acid.

2. General warmth is important and fluids should be given freely.

3. Oxygen and artificial respiration may be necessary.

Dose and Preparations.

1. $\frac{1}{240}$ to $\frac{1}{60}$ gr. by subcutaneous injection.

2. $\frac{1}{100}$ gr. tablets by mouth.

3. Lamellæ, drops and ointment for ophthalmic use.

4. Lamellæ and drops for use in congenital pyloric stenosis.

One lamella (or 1 to 3 minims of the alcoholic solution) is given before each feed.

BARBITURATES

The barbiturate drugs are very many in number and widely used in medicine. They are hypnotics and so induce sleep. They also act as sedatives. Some of the barbiturate drugs are very quick in their action while others take much longer to have effect.

Uses.

1. To induce sleep (*i.e.*, as hypnotics).

2. As sedatives to depress the nervous system. For this purpose they are used in anxiety states and to lessen any stress factor in some diseases.

3. In epilepsy, as sedatives to prevent fits.

4. As anæsthetics, by intravenous injection.

Preparations and Doses.

1. As HYPNOTICS.

Allobarbitone (dial), $\frac{3}{4}$ to 3 gr.
Amylobarbitone (amytal), $1\frac{1}{2}$ to 3 gr.
Barbitone, 5 to 10 gr.
Barbitone Sodium (medinal), 5 to 10 gr.
Butobarbitone (soneryl), $1\frac{1}{2}$ to 3 gr.
Pentobarbitone Sodium (nembutal), $1\frac{1}{2}$ to 3 gr.
Quinalbarbitone Sodium (seconal), $\frac{3}{4}$ to 3 gr.

2. As SEDATIVES AND IN EPILEPSY.

Phenobarbitone (luminal, gardenal), $\frac{1}{2}$ to $1\frac{1}{2}$ gr. tablets; 1 to 3 gr. by intramuscular injection.

3. As AN ANÆSTHETIC.

Thiopentone (pentothal), 0·5 to 1 gm. intravenously.

Toxic Effects.—The main toxic effect is depression of the central nervous system, causing drowsiness and coma. Death is usually due to respiratory failure or to pneumonia resulting from the prolonged coma.

Treatment of Barbiturate Coma.

The stomach is washed out thoroughly (the stomach contents being saved for examination) and hot strong coffee then put in. The patient is best nursed in the prone or semi-prone position, with the foot of the bed slightly elevated. This is to allow the maximum drainage of the mouth secretions and so prevent blocking of the air passages. Care must be taken to ensure that a clear airway is at all times maintained and the patient must never be allowed to become cyanosed. In deep coma it may be necessary to insert an endotracheal tube.

Suction of mucus from the mouth and upper respiratory tract is necessary at frequent intervals to prevent pulmonary collapse and blocking of the airway. A suction apparatus must at all times therefore be available at the bedside. If the coma lasts more than twelve hours an intravenous glucose saline drip is set up to give sufficient fluid intake. Penicillin is given as a prophylactic measure against the great danger of pneumonia.

The measures outlined above are undoubtedly the most important part of the treatment of barbiturate poisoning. Recently the drugs bemegride (megimide) and amiphenazole (daptazole) have been tried and may prove useful in overcoming severe respiratory depression. Fifty milligrams of megimide are given in an intravenous saline infusion every five minutes till the respirations improve and the reflexes return. If too much is given, however, convulsions may occur, which may deepen the coma.

BELLADONNA

Belladonna has a similar action to that of atropine. The usual preparation is tincture of belladonna given in 5 to 15 minim doses.

BISMUTH

Uses.

Bismuth has an astringent action in diminishing secretions and is used for this effect in the treatment of diarrhœa. Bismuth carbonate in 10 to 30 gr. doses given by mouth in a mixture is the preparation usually used. Bismuth is also used in the treatment of dyspepsia.

Toxic Effects.—Toxic effects from bismuth are seen only after intramuscular injection. Stomatitis, excessive salivation and a black line on the gums are the usual signs of bismuth poisoning. Dimercaprol (B.A.L.) is a valuable antidote in bismuth poisoning.

CAFFEINE

Caffeine is found in tea and coffee, and the stimulating effect of these drinks is due to their caffeine content.

Uses.

1. As a stimulant (in the form of strong black coffee) in cases of poisoning due to morphine, alcohol and other cerebral depressants.

2. Combined with aspirin and phenacetin in tablet form to relieve headaches and pain.

CALCIUM

Calcium is an essential component of blood and tissues, and is usually prescribed during pregnancy to supply the extra demands of the fœtus. Calcium is also given in cases of tetany due to such diseases as parathyroid deficiency, cœliac disease and sprue. In the tetany of rickets, which is, however, seldom seen nowadays, calcium is also prescribed.

Calcium is given intramuscularly or intravenously as calcium gluconate in 5 to 20 ml. doses. By mouth calcium is given as calcium chloride in a mixture or in tablet form (calcium lactate or gluconate in 10 to 15 gr. doses).

CHLORPROMAZINE (Largactil)

Chlorpromazine is used at present in many different conditions, the principal being :—

1. To enhance the action of analgesic drugs for the relief of severe pain, particularly where this is due to malignant disease (see p. 538).
2. To relieve persistent nausea and vomiting associated with uræmia, toxic drugs and pregnancy and following operations.
3. To control persistent hiccups.
4. To enhance the action of hypnotics and anæsthetic drugs.
5. In anxiety neurosis.

Side Effects.—Chlorpromazine is a toxic drug and jaundice, agranulocytosis and skin rashes have been noted during treatment with it.

Chlorpromazine is given by mouth in doses of about 75 to 150 mgm. daily and by injection in 25 to 50 mgm. doses. Larger doses may be needed in treating psychiatric disorders.

Promazine (sparine) has actions and uses similar to those of chlorpromazine. The average dose is 25 to 200 mgm.

Chlorpromazine and promazine enhance the effect of anti-coagulant drugs so that extra care must be taken if these drugs are given together with anticoagulants.

COCAINE AND ITS SUBSTITUTES

Actions.

1. Cocaine has a most powerful local action on the fine nerve-endings of the pain and touch fibres, causing complete local anæsthesia. It is effective when applied to the surface of mucous membranes; it has *no* action when applied to the unbroken skin.

2. Taken internally cocaine is a stimulant to the higher centres in the brain. Overdosage causes delirium and convulsions.

Uses.—Cocaine is used (applied to the surface of the mucous membranes) as a local anæsthetic in operations on the nose, throat and eyes. It is *not* used by subcutaneous injection as it is too toxic, and where such injections are necessary it has been replaced by other less toxic cocaine substitutes.

Procaine is the cocaine substitute most widely used as a local anæsthetic and is administered by infiltration of the subcutaneous tissues with a 1 or 2 per cent. solution. It is the least toxic of all the local anæsthetics. It has, however, very little action when applied to the surface of such mucous membranes as those of the eye, nose or throat and so is not used in these areas. Procaine is also widely known under the trade name of Novocain.

Cinchocaine (Nupercaine) is another cocaine substitute used for local infiltration anæsthesia and is perhaps most valuable as a spinal anæsthetic. For use in spinal anæsthesia it is made up in two different solutions known as light and heavy nupercaine.

Amethocaine, in 1 or 2 per cent. solution, is chiefly used as a surface anæsthetic in operations on the nose and throat. It is safer for this purpose than cocaine. Amethocaine is also known under the trade names Decicain and Anethaine.

Lignocaine (Xylocaine) is a long-acting local anæsthetic which can be used for both surface and infiltration anæsthesia.

CORTISONE AND ALLIED CORTICOSTEROIDS

Cortisone is one of several hormones isolated from the adrenal cortex and at present being used in a wide variety of diseases. These hormones (known as corticosteroids or simply steroids) have many functions and in particular control the metabolism of such minerals as sodium and potassium. They also play a part in protein and carbohydrate metabolism (see p. 447).

Cortisone and allied corticosteroids have two great disadvantages which greatly limit their use. Firstly, in most diseases where the drugs are used, when they are stopped the symptoms usually recur. Secondly these drugs, when given in doses large enough to be of value, often cause serious side effects. The dose has therefore to be reduced as rapidly as possible to the lowest maintenance dose which will relieve the symptoms.

Since the isolation of cortisone many further hormones have been isolated from the adrenal cortex and other steroids have been synthesised which have a similar action and are available for clinical use. The following are the principal corticosteroids at present in use :—

1. **Cortisone.**—This is usually given by mouth or by intramuscular injection. The dose of cortisone varies according to the severity of the disease. In severe conditions initial doses of 200 to 300 mgm. daily may be necessary for a few days, after which the dose must be reduced in order to avoid side effects. The maintenance daily dose of cortisone is usually 50 to 75 mgm. and hould rarely exceed 100 mgm. daily if side effects are not to develop.

Cortisone is also used locally in diseases of the eye.

2. **Hydrocortisone** (cortisol).—Hydrocortisone is very similar in action to cortisone and is given by mouth, intramuscular injection and locally in eye diseases. In addition hydrocortisone is given intravenously, particularly in an acute adrenal crisis, and by local injection into joints in arthritis. Hydrocortisone in a 1 per cent. ointment is the steroid preparation of choice for the treatment of skin diseases.

Hydrocortisone is more potent than cortisone and only four-fifths as big a dose is needed.

3. **Prednisone and Prednisolone.**—These are synthetic forms of, respectively, cortisone and hydrocortisone, but are four times as potent, so that much smaller doses are needed. Prednisone and prednisolone have actions similar to those of cortisone and hydrocortisone and can therefore be used instead of these drugs. Moreover, prednisone and prednisolone (unlike cortisone and hydrocortisone) have the very important advantage of not causing salt and water retention ; œdema therefore does not usually develop when they are

used, and salt restriction is not normally necessary with patients on prednisone and prednisolone. The average maintenance dose of prednisone is 5 to 20 mgm. daily.

Methylprednisolone (medrone) is similar in its action to prednisolone but, being much more potent, the average maintenance dose is only 4 to 12 mgm. daily.

4. **Triamcinolone.**—Triamcinolone (ledercort, adcortyl) is a recently introduced synthetic steroid similar in action to prednisone but even more potent. Very small doses are therefore sufficient. As with prednisone, salt and water retention does not occur. The average maintenance dose is 2 to 8 mgm. daily. Triamcinolone may however cause severe anorexia, marked muscular wasting and weakness.

5. **Fluorohydrocortisone** (florinef).—This steroid has a very potent sodium retaining action so that œdema is very likely to occur. Fluorohydrocortisone is at present used only in certain cases of Addison's disease.

6. **Dexamethasone** (decadron, dextelan) is the most recently introduced steroid and is the most potent anti-inflamatory steroid now available, being almost thirty times as effective as cortisone. Sodium retention does not usually occur. The average maintenance dose is 0·75 mgm. to 1·25 mgm. daily. Betamethasone (betnelan) is a similar compound.

7. **Corticotrophin (ACTH).**—ACTH is the pituitary adrenocorticotrophic hormone which stimulates the adrenals to produce cortisone. ACTH has actions similar to those of cortisone but it has to be given by intramuscular injection, which limits its use. ACTH is usually given in initial doses of 25 mgm. six-hourly and in maintenance doses of 10 mgm.

8. **Aldosterone.**—This is believed to be the chief natural adrenal cortical hormone regulating the metabolism of sodium and potassium. It is as yet not available for general clinical use.

TOXIC EFFECTS OF CORTICOSTEROIDS.

1. Œdema and increase in body weight. This is due to corticosteroids causing retention of salt and water in the body. For this reason patients on large doses of corticosteroids are best kept on a low salt diet.

2. Hypertension.

3. Glycosuria and aggravation of diabetes mellitus. Because corticosteroids inhibit the utilisation of carbohydrate and also

increase the conversion of protein to carbohydrate, corticosteroids must be given with great caution to all diabetics. Frequent routine examination of the urine for sugar is necessary and, if glycosuria occurs, repeated blood sugar tests will be needed. Diabetic patients on corticosteroids will probably require larger doses of insulin than previously.

4. Lessens resistance to infection when given in large doses. Patients on corticosteroids may show delayed healing of wounds and quicker spread of any infective process. Tuberculosis, if present, is very liable to spread rapidly. Patients with active peptic ulcer should likewise be given corticosteroids with great caution as healing of the ulcer may be delayed and perforation has also been known to occur.

5. Mental disturbance including severe agitation and mania.

6. Acne and excessive growth of hair on the face is a distressing feature often seen in women.

7. Triamcinolone may cause severe flushing, anorexia, marked muscular wasting and weakness.

8. Potassium loss. The retention of sodium (salt) is accompanied by increased excretion of potassium in the urine. Severe muscular weakness, lethargy and sometimes paralysis may occur.

All the above toxic effects are more likely to develop when large doses are used. Therefore it is essential to reduce the dose as rapidly as the progress of the patient will allow. Patients on corticosteroids should be examined carefully (and weighed if possible) for the development of œdema. The blood pressure should be recorded at regular intervals and the urine tested for sugar. The presence of severe muscular weakness and lethargy will call for immediate cessation of therapy.

USES OF CORTICOSTEROIDS.

1. Addison's disease. Cortisone and hydrocortisone are usually used, with intravenous injections of hydrocortisone in an acute adrenal crisis. Fluorohydrocortisone may be necessary in a few patients (see p. 449).

2. After total adrenalectomy for Cushing's syndrome, malignant disease or severe hypertension. These patients require maintenance doses of cortisone for life.

3. Adrenal cortical hyperplasia. Cortisone and hydrocortisone are given to children with adrenal hyperplasia to suppress the overactivity of the gland (see p. 451).

4. Simmonds' disease. Cortisone is usually given with good effect.

5. Severe skin diseases. Certain serious skin diseases which may be fatal often dramatically improve with corticosteroids. These include pemphigus, exfoliative dermatitis, severe eczema and disseminated lupus erythematosus.

For local application in skin diseases, *e.g.*, eczema, 1 per cent. hydrocortisone is the preparation of choice.

6. Eye diseases. Local applications of cortisone and hydrocortisone have proved of great value in such serious inflammatory eye conditions as iritis, keratitis, sympathetic ophthalmia, uveitis, etc.

7. Allergic states. In severe status asthmaticus, drug allergy and angioneurotic œdema which have not responded to other measures, corticosteroids are usually given, often with very good effect. In hay fever, local application of hydrocortisone snuff or spray has been of benefit.

8. Blood diseases. Corticosteroids have produced relief in hæmolytic anæmia and purpura. Temporary remissions have also been brought about in acute leukæmia.

9. Rheumatoid arthritis. The use of corticosteroids in this disease is nowadays limited to the very severe cases which have not responded to other treatment (see p. 509).

10. Rheumatic fever. In severe attacks of rheumatic fever corticosteroids may be used as it is believed that they have some beneficial effect on this disease.

11. Ulcerative colitis. Temporary remissions have sometimes been induced by corticosteroid therapy and it is therefore used in patients not improving on other treatment.

12. Nephrotic syndrome. In certain cases of chronic nephritis severe œdema is most disabling and persistent. Corticosteroid therapy sometimes causes a marked diuresis with relief of the œdema.

CYANOCOBALAMIN (Vitamin B$_{12}$)

Cyanocobalamin is the specific drug for the treatment of pernicious anæmia and is fully discussed on page 372.

Proprietary preparations of cyanocobalamin include anacobin, cytamen, bitevan, distivit, megalovel and rubramin.

DIGITALIS AND DIGOXIN

The action and uses of these most valuable drugs are fully described under Auricular Fibrillation (see pp. 148 and 149).

DIMERCAPROL (B.A.L.)

Dimercaprol (British Anti-Lewisite) is used in the treatment of poisoning by heavy metals, such as arsenic, mercury, bismuth and gold. It is given by intramuscular injection in 2 ml. doses.

DIURETICS

Diuretics are drugs which increase the output of urine and are used in the treatment of œdema. The diuretics most commonly used at present include :—

1. **Mercurial diuretics,** especially mersalyl given by intramuscular injection. Mercurial diuretics may cause renal damage so their use is usually confined to the treatment of cardiac œdema.

2. **Chlorothiazide** group. These diuretics have the great advantage of being fully effective when given by mouth: they can also be used in the treatment of renal œdema as they do not cause renal damage. They are the best and most potent diuretics at present available and are in widespread use.

Chlorothiazide (saluric) is given in 0·5 to 1 gm. doses twice daily for three to five days a week. Hydrochlorothiazide (hydrosaluric, esidrex) and hydroflumethiazide (naclex, hydrenox) are much more potent so that the usual dose is 25 to 50 mgm. twice daily.

3. **Spironolactone** (aldactone) counteracts the effect of aldosterone and hence leads to a loss of salt and fluid. It is prescribed at a dose of 200 mgm. t.d.s. but is too expensive at present for wide use.

Diuretics are more fully discussed on page 140 *et seq.*

EPHEDRINE

Ephedrine is similar in action to adrenaline but is effective when given by mouth.

Main Uses.

1. To relieve the bronchial spasm in asthma, $\frac{1}{2}$ to 1 gr. doses in tablets by mouth two or three times a day being the average dose.
2. In the form of nasal drops to relieve the nasal congestion in rhinitis and hay fever.

3. To prevent the fall in blood pressure which often follows spinal anæsthesia.

4. In cases of bed wetting in children (nocturnal enuresis), when ephedrine is sometimes valuable.

GOLD

Gold salts (myocrisin) were at one time much more widely used in medicine, but to-day their use is mostly confined to the treatment of some cases of rheumatoid arthritis. Gold is usually given in a course of weekly intramuscular injections of 0·01 to 0·05 gm.

Toxic Effects.—Gold is a toxic drug to which some people are very sensitive, so that great caution has to be used in its administration. Gold can cause renal damage, dermatitis and agranulocytosis (see p. 391).

In the treatment of a toxic gold reaction, injections of dimercaprol (B.A.L.) have proved very useful. Once gold has caused a toxic reaction the drug must never be given again to the same patient.

HEROIN

Heroin is described under Morphine on page 608.

HYOSCINE

Hyoscine has a similar action to that of belladonna, stramonium and atropine.

Uses.

1. Injections of hyoscine (scopolamine) are a powerful depressant (narcotic) of the higher nerve centres and are used for this effect in cases of delirium and acute mania. Hyoscine is also often combined with morphine for use as a sedative before a general anæsthetic. The dose of hysocine is $\frac{1}{200}$ to $\frac{1}{100}$ gr. subcutaneously.

2. Hyoscine is also used to reduce the salivation and muscular rigidity in paralysis agitans.

3. Hyoscyamine, which contains hyoscine, is used to relieve the pylorospasm of peptic ulcer and also the spasm of the bladder in cases of cystitis and prostatitis.

4. Hyoscine dilates the pupil and is used in inflammatory eye conditions (iritis, corneal ulceration) to rest the eye.

HYPNOTICS

Hypnotics are drugs which induce sleep and are very widely used in medicine. The following hypnotics are in common use :—

1. Morphine and Opium Derivatives. Morphine and allied preparations are among the most valuable drugs used to induce sleep and allay anxiety. Unlike the other hypnotic drugs mentioned below they also have an analgesic effect and so are particularly useful to induce sleep when pain is present. Morphine and allied preparations are described in detail on pages 607 to 610.

2. Chloral Hydrate. Chloral hydrate is a safe and useful hypnotic for both children and elderly patients. The usual adult dose is 15 gr. and for a child of one year $2\frac{1}{2}$ gr. Recently the combination of chloral and phenazone (welldorm) has been introduced with success in the treatment of insomnia. The usual dose is one to two 10 gr. tablets for an adult and one $2\frac{1}{2}$ gr. tablet for a child.

3. The Barbiturates. These are by far the most frequently used hypnotics. The barbiturates are fully discussed on page 594.

4. Paraldehyde. This is a very useful hypnotic and has the advantage that it rarely causes addiction, probably because it tastes so bad. It is best given with some orange or lemon in a syrup to disguise the taste. It is useful in insomnia due to heart disease, anxiety and febrile states. It does not relieve pain and so is useless for insomnia associated with pain.

Paraldehyde is usually given orally in 30 to 120 minim doses. In some cases, however, especially with delirium or in maniacal states, paraldehyde is given intramuscularly in 5 ml. doses.

5. Glutethimide (doriden). Doriden is a useful and effective hypnotic. The average adult dose is 500 mgm. (two tablets). It is said to be particularly useful for elderly patients.

6. Carbromal (adalin). This is a mild hypnotic which is sometimes combined with a barbiturate (carbrital). An average dose for an adult is 5 to 15 gr.

7. Methylpentynol (oblivon, atempol, somnesin). A mild hypnotic used in 500 mgm. doses. It is doubtful if this drug is a very effective hypnotic.

8. Methyprylone (noludar). A mild hypnotic with no side effects, which is given in doses of 200 to 400 mgm.

9. Thalidomide (distaval). A new hypnotic said to have practically no side effects and to be particularly useful for children. The average adult dose is 100 mgm. and for a child 25 to 50 mgm. Prolonged use leads to peripheral neuritis.

For children, aspirin ($2\frac{1}{2}$ to 5 gr.) is also a very useful and safe hypnotic.

HYPOTENSIVE DRUGS

Drugs which reduce blood pressure are known as hypotensive drugs, and are at present widely used in the treatment of the more severe forms of hypertension. The various hypotensive drugs and their administration are described on page 132.

In addition to their use in hypertension, hypotensive drugs are sometimes used to reduce the blood pressure below normal at operations in order to obtain a bloodless field.

INSULIN

Insulin is used mainly in diabetes mellitus and is fully dealt with under this disease (see p. 480).

IPECACUANHA

Actions and Uses.

1. Ipecacuanha is a strong emetic causing instant vomiting when given in large doses of 15 to 30 gr.

2. In smaller doses ipecacuanha acts as a reflex expectorant and is used in diseases of the lungs to ease the coughing up of a sticky sputum. Ipecacuanha forms one of the main constituents of most expectorant mixtures.

3. In the preparation known as *emetine* it is used in the tropical form of dysentery caused by the entamœba parasite—amœbic dseyntery. In the treatment of amœbic dysentery emetine is given in 1 gr. injections intramuscularly.

IRON

Action.—Iron is present in such foods as spinach, green beans, liver and, in small amounts, in milk. Human milk contains far more than cow's milk. Iron is essential for the formation of the hæmoglobin of the red blood cells, which are the means by which oxygen is carried throughout the body. Iron is absorbed from the stomach and intestines; the hydrochloric acid in the gastric juice helps in the absorption of iron.

Uses.—Iron is essential for the treatment of the iron-deficiency anæmias, which include the following types :—

1. Simple achlorhydric anæmia as seen in middle-aged women owing to the absence of hydrochloric acid in the stomach, a poor diet and menorrhagia.
2. Nutritional anæmia of infants. This anæmia is very common in infants, especially when artificially fed, as an exclusive diet of cow's milk contains very little iron. Premature infants are particularly liable to suffer from an iron-deficiency anæmia.
3. Iron-deficiency anæmia of pregnancy.
4. Chronic hæmorrhagic anæmias (*e.g.*, in cases of hæmorrhoids, menorrhagia, bleeding peptic ulcer, etc.), wherein the iron is required to replace the lost hæmoglobin.
5. An iron-deficiency anæmia is sometimes seen in sprue and cœliac disease.

Preparations and Dosage.

1. ORAL.

   (*a*) Ferrous gluconate.
   (*b*) Ferrous sulphate.
   (*c*) Ferrous succinate.

These three preparations are given in tablet form (3 to 5 gr.), one tablet three times a day. Ferrous succinate is said to cause the least gastro-intestinal upset.

2. INTRAVENOUS.

   Saccharated iron oxide (ferrivenin, iviron), 2 to 5 ml. (50 to 100 mgm.) on alternate days.

ISONIAZID AND PARA-AMINOSALICYLIC ACID (P.A.S.)

These two drugs are used only in the treatment of tuberculosis and are fully discussed on pages 193 and 194.

KAOLIN

Kaolin is an aluminium powder which has a marked astringent action and is used in doses of $\frac{1}{2}$ to 2 oz. to relieve persistent diarrhœa. Kaolin is also used extensively in the form of a poultice (antiphlogistine) to relieve pain.

MEPHENTERMINE

Mephentermine (mephine) is a vasopressor drug used to raise the blood pressure in cases of severe shock not caused by hæmorrhage. It is often given to combat the shock in severe coronary thrombosis as an alternative to noradrenaline (see p. 127).

Mephentermine is given intravenously or intramuscularly in 15 to 30 mgm. doses at repeated intervals until the blood pressure is maintained at 100 mm. Hg.

MORPHINE AND ALLIED PREPARATIONS OF OPIUM

1. Morphine.

Morphine is the principal substance found in opium, which is derived from the poppy. Codeine and papaverine are other substances found in opium. Morphine is one of the most widely used and valuable drugs in medicine.

Actions.

    (*a*) Diminishes sensitivity to pain and also induces a deep sleep.

    (*b*) Depresses the respirations and cough reflex.

    (*c*) Stimulates, at first, the vomiting centre.

    (*d*) Causes spasm of the pylorus and bile ducts.

    (*e*) Diminishes intestinal peristalsis.

    (*f*) Slows the heart rate.

Uses.

    (*a*) For relief of pain. Morphine is one of the best drugs available for this purpose, but it has the great drawback that addiction to the drug rapidly develops. For this reason it is used for the relief of pain only in acute diseases or in chronic incurable conditions.

(b) As a hypnotic. Morphine should be used only where sleeplessness is due to severe pain, otherwise other hypnotics (barbiturates, chloral hydrate, paraldehyde) which are not so habit-forming should be used. Morphine is never used as a hypnotic in chronic illnesses except when the condition is incurable. Morphine is of marked benefit for the first night or so in the treatment of congestive heart failure as it enables the patient to rest and sleep. After the patient has had a good night's rest other hypnotics must be used.

(c) To relieve acute pulmonary œdema (cardiac asthma) in cases of left heart failure.

(d) As a sedative to allay anxiety and restlessness in all cases of shock associated with severe injuries or hæmorrhage.

(e) As a pre-operative sedative, when it is usually combined with atropine which reduces the bronchial secretions.

Contraindications.—Morphine must *not* be used :—

(a) In infancy, as infants tolerate morphine very badly.

(b) In any case of pneumonia or bronchitis, as depression of the cough reflex as a result of the morphine would cause difficulty in bringing up the sputum.

(c) In the treatment of pain of any duration, except in incurable diseases.

Dose.—Morphine is usually given by subcutaneous injections in $\frac{1}{8}$ to $\frac{1}{3}$ gr. doses. It is also given by mouth to depress a severe cough due to malignant disease.

2. Heroin (diamorphine).

Heroin has a similar action to that of morphine, but has a much more depressant effect on the respiratory centre. It is chiefly used in medicine to suppress an irritating cough due to malignant disease of the lungs. Heroin, like morphine, is very habit-forming.

3. Opium.

Opium, as distinct from morphine, is mainly used in the form of a tincture or powder to control persistent diarrhœa usually due to carcinoma of the bowel. Opium combined with ipecacuanha as *Dover's powders* is often used to induce sweating and relieve pain in acute febrile conditions.

4. Papaveretum (omnopon).

Papaveretum, most often used in the preparation known as omnopon, has the same sedative and pain-relieving properties as morphine but is said to cause less depression of the cough reflex and to be less likely to cause constipation and vomiting. Papaveretum is used extensively as an alternative to morphine in $\frac{1}{6}$ to $\frac{1}{3}$ gr. doses, given subcutaneously.

5. Papaverine.

Papaverine is obtained from opium and has a narcotic action stronger than that of codeine but weaker than that of morphine. Papaverine has a marked effect in relieving spasm of smooth muscle and, for this reason, is chiefly used to relieve the pain of biliary and renal colic. It is also used in peripheral vascular disease and sometimes, instead of morphine, to relieve the pain in coronary thrombosis.

The dose of papaverine is 2 to 4 gr. orally or $\frac{1}{2}$ to $1\frac{1}{2}$ gr. subcutaneously.

6. Nepenthe.

Nepenthe is a frequently used liquid preparation of morphine containing 1 gr. of morphine in approximately 2 drachms. It is a useful preparation for children, for whom the usual dose is 1 minim for each year of age. As already mentioned, however, morphine should not be used for infants.

TOXIC EFFECTS OF MORPHINE AND ALLIED PREPARATIONS

As morphine is used so extensively in medicine it is important for the nurse to be able to recognise the main symptoms of morphine poisoning.

ACUTE POISONING.

Symptoms and Signs.

1. Drowsiness proceeding to coma.

2. The respirations become progressively slower, irregular and finally stertorous. The patient dies of asphyxia.

3. The face and lips are blue, the skin cold and clammy.

4. The pupils are very small—the " pin-point " pupils of morphine poisoning.

Acute morphine poisoning is diagnosed by differentiating it from the other causes of coma, which are discussed elsewhere (p. 545).

Treatment.

1. The stomach is at once washed out with large quantities (10 to 12 pints) of potassium permanganate solution. Hot strong coffee should be left in the stomach after the lavage as a stimulant.

2. Oxygen is usually necessary to stimulate the depressed respirations, and in severe cases with respiratory failure artificial respiration may be required.

3. The specific antidote for morphine poisoning is nalorphine (lethidrone). Nalorphine is injected intravenously in 5 to 10 mgm. doses and usually within a few minutes a marked increase in the rate and depth of respiration takes place. Nalorphine is also very effective in cases of overdosage with pethidine, levorphanol (dromoran), methadone (physeptone) and phenadoxone (heptalgin) but has no effect in barbiturate poisoning.

4. Penicillin or other antibiotics are usually given to prevent or control broncho-pneumonia.

CHRONIC POISONING—MORPHINE OR OPIUM ADDICTION.

Morphine addiction may arise through the long-continued administration of the drug for the relief of pain. Alternatively, the morphine or opium habit may have been acquired through taking the drug for its exhilarating effect, *e.g.*, in China and India many people take opium. If morphine addicts stop taking the drug various symptoms develop, including severe mental depression, lassitude, severe abdominal cramps, vomiting and diarrhœa. In addition, severe insomnia leading to marked deterioration in the general health supervenes. The craving for the drug becomes intense.

The *treatment* of morphine or opium addiction must be carried out in an institution. The usual procedure is to reduce the drug very gradually over a period of six weeks. In the early stages, codeine is usually given to reduce the effects of the withdrawal of morphine.

NIKETHAMIDE

Nikethamide (coramine, anacardone) is a respiratory stimulant and is frequently used in cases of coma and poisoning due to barbiturates, morphine and chloral hydrate. Nikethamide is given in 2 to 5 ml. doses intravenously or subcutaneously.

NITROFURANTOIN

Nitrofurantoin (furadantin) is a synthetic antibacterial substance used exclusively in urinary tract infections such as pyelitis and cystitis, when it is a useful alternative drug in cases where these infections are resistant to sulphonamides and antibiotics. The usual dose is 100 mgm. four times a day. Side effects include nausea and skin rashes. When skin eruptions develop the drug should be stopped.

More recently an antibacterial agent called furaltadone (altafur), similar to furadantin, has been introduced for the treatment of staphylococcal infections resistant to penicillin and other antibiotics. The usual dose is one 250 mgm. tablet four times a day. Side-effects include nausea and skin rashes.

PHENYLBUTAZONE (BUTAZOLIDIN)

Phenylbutazone is chiefly used in the treatment of rheumatoid arthritis, particularly in rheumatoid spondylitis (ankylosing spondylitis) and in gout. It is, however, a toxic drug and has to be used with caution. Its main side effects are :—

(a) Sodium retention causing œdema.
(b) Gastro-intestinal symptoms such as nausea, abdominal pain and hæmatemesis.
(c) Blood dyscrasias, such as agranulocytosis and purpura. It should not be given at the same time as anticoagulant drugs.

The use of phenylbutazone in rheumatoid arthritis is described on page 509.

PURGATIVES

Purgatives (also known as aperients or laxatives) help evacuation of the bowel and are used in the treatment of constipation. The following purgatives are commonly used :—

1. Saline purges. Magnesium sulphate (Epsom salts) is given in 30 to 240 gr. doses. Sodium sulphate (Glauber's salt) is given in the same dosage.
2. Senna. This is a useful purgative, usually taking six to eight hours to have effect. Senokot is a most effective preparation of senna. One to two teaspoonfuls of the granules is the normal adult dose.

3. Cascara Sagrada. A safe purgative similar in action to senna. Common preparations are the extract and the elixir, given in 25 to 50 minim doses.
4. Phenolphthalein. A mild purgative given in 1 to 5 gr. doses. It may cause a drug rash in some patients.
5. Liquid paraffin. This is an oil which acts by its lubricating effect. The usual dose is 2 to 8 drachms.
6. Magnesium hydroxide (cream of magnesia) is a useful mild purgative, especially valuable for young children. Half a drachm is the usual dose for a child of one year.

QUINIDINE

Quinidine is used in the treatment of auricular fibrillation, where by its slowing effect on the conducting mechanism of the heart it frequently converts the heart rhythm back to normal. Quinidine therefore differs from digitalis in that the action of digitalis is to slow the heart rate in auricular fibrillation but not to change the abnormal rhythm back to normal.

Quinidine is mainly used in cases of auricular fibrillation due to thyrotoxicosis. In many cases of thyrotoxicosis, auricular fibrillation, if present, may still persist even after the thyrotoxicosis has been treated. In these cases quinidine is very useful in restoring a normal heart rhythm. Quinidine is *not* used in cases of auricular fibrillation associated with heart failure.

Quinidine is usually given in 3 to 5 gr. doses by mouth.

QUININE

Uses.

1. Quinine is used in the treatment of the tropical disease malaria. It is very effective, although in recent years it is tending to be replaced by other drugs, such as paludrine and chloroquine.
2. It is also used in the treatment of varicose veins, as a local sclerosing agent to cause thrombosis.
3. In some types of the rare muscular disorders known as the myopathies, quinine relieves the muscular spasm, if present.

Dose.—Quinine is usually given by mouth in 5 to 10 gr. doses. It can cause toxic effects such as ringing in the ears (tinnitus), slight deafness and in severe cases delirium. Quinine may cause purpura whereupon the drug must be stopped.

RADIOACTIVE ISOTOPES

Radioactive isotopes (elements which are radioactive) are frequently used in medicine both for diagnosis and treatment. At present the following radioactive isotopes are most commonly used :—

1. **Radioactive Iodine (I^{131}).**—Radioactive iodine has proved most successful in the treatment of thyroid disorders. It is an alternative method of treatment for thyrotoxic goitre and is given where surgery is contraindicated or when medical treatment has not produced the desired effect. It is most often used for older patients, especially those who also have heart disease and therefore would not tolerate operation. Because there is still some slight doubt whether malignant change may not develop many years after the administration of radioactive substances, radioactive iodine is not usually given to patients under 45 years.

Radioactive iodine is also used in the treatment of carcinoma of the thyroid gland.

For the diagnosis of thyrotoxic goitre radioactive iodine has proved useful. A test dose of radioactive iodine is given and the amount subsequently passed in the urine is measured. In thyrotoxic goitre this amount is low because the overactive gland takes up an abnormally large amount of radioactive iodine. Alternatively, the actual amount of iodine taken up by the thyroid gland can be measured by scanning the neck with a suitable counter.

2. **Radioactive Phosphorus (P^{32}).**—Radioactive phosphorus is the therapy of choice in the disease **polycythæmia vera.** In this disease there is a marked increase in the number of red blood cells. P^{32} destroys red cells and thus reduces the number to normal.

P^{32} is also used with good results in the treatment of chronic leukæmia as an alternative to deep X-ray therapy and in the treatment of superficial skin lesions such as carcinoma of the skin. This isotope (along with several others) is also used to find the position of brain tumours. After giving the radioactive isotope, the radiation emerging from the head is measured by a suitable counter. The pattern of the radiation given off is then often a reliable guide to the position of the tumour.

3. **Radioactive Gold (Au^{198}).**—Radioactive gold is at present mainly used as a palliative measure to prolong life and relieve symptoms in inoperable carcinomas. It has proved useful in this way in advanced inoperable carcinoma of the prostate. Radioactive

gold is also instilled into the pleural and peritoneal cavities in cases of malignant pleural effusions and malignant ascites; the isotope often reduces the need for repeated paracenteses and relieves the pain. It can also be inserted into the pituitary fossa to destroy an adenoma in acromegaly.

4. **Radioactive Iron (Fe^{59}).**—This isotope is used for investigation of the absorption of iron, both in normal people and in some patients with iron-deficiency anæmias.

5. **Radioactive Chromium (Cr^{51}).**—Radioactive chromium is used to study the survival of red cells and to measure the volume of blood.

6. **Radioactive Cobalt (Co^{60}).**—Radioactive cobalt has properties similar to those of radium and is therefore an alternative treatment for certain forms of carcinoma. This isotope is also used to study the absorption of vitamin B$_{12}$.

SALICYLATES

The salicylates, of which aspirin is one form, are valuable drugs and used in several diseases.

Actions.

1. They lower the temperature in disease owing to their direct action on the heat regulating centre. They therefore belong to the group of drugs known as antipyretics.

2. They relieve pain, especially in the muscles and joints.

3. In strong concentrated solutions they are irritants.

Uses.

1. The most specific effect of the salicylates is on the temperature and joint pains of acute rheumatic fever. So specific is this action that if full doses of salicylates do not lower the temperature and relieve the joint pains, the disease is unlikely to be acute rheumatic fever. Doses of 15 to 30 gr. four or six-hourly are given.

2. Aspirin (60 to 90 gr. daily) is also the most useful drug available for relieving the pain in rheumatoid arthritis.

3. Aspirin is very commonly used in 5 to 15 gr. doses to relieve headache and also the pains associated with fibrositis.

4. They are also given in the treatment of varicose veins by local intravenous injections.

Toxic Effects.—Salicylates and aspirin in full doses cause tinnitus, slight deafness and fullness in the head. They can also irritate the gastric mucous membrane so as to cause bleeding and therefore should be avoided in gastric lesions. For these cases a soluble form of aspirin (soluble aspirin-disprin) is available which does not cause irritation to the stomach.

Acute aspirin poisoning (causing drowsiness proceeding to coma) is mainly seen as a result of deliberate overdosage in cases of attempted suicide. The treatment of aspirin poisoning is to wash out the stomach, if the drug has been taken within the previous six hours, and then in all cases to carry out the routine nursing measures as outlined under barbiturate poisoning (p. 594). Intravenous alkali (sodium lactate) is given to combat the acidosis and penicillin to prevent pneumonia.

STRAMONIUM

Stramonium has a similar action to that of belladonna and atropine. It is chiefly used in the treatment of paralysis agitans and bronchial asthma, and is usually given in the form of a tincture in 5 to 30 minim doses.

THYROID EXTRACT

Thyroid extract is used in the treatment of cretinism and myxœdema, where the normal secretion of the thyroid is lacking. The dose of thyroid extract needed varies with the individual patient and must be regulated according to the response. One-fifth grain at 6 months of age and $\frac{3}{4}$ to 1 gr. at 1 to 4 years are average doses. In adults the initial dose is usually 1 gr. daily and increasing to a maximum of 2 to 3 gr. as necessary.

Thyroxin is the active principle of thyroid and is a more precise method of prescribing. 0·1 mgm. tablet of thyroxin is equivalent to about 1 gr. thyroid.

VASODILATOR DRUGS

Vasodilator drugs are used to improve the blood supply to tissues and organs. They relax the smooth muscle of the small blood vessels and so dilate them.

Vasodilator drugs include amyl nitrite, pentaerythritol tetranitrate (peritrate, mycardol) and trinitrin (glyceryl trinitrate), used in the treatment of angina pectoris (see p. 123), and phenoxybenzamine (dibenyline), tolazoline (priscol), ronicol, cyclospasmol and hydergine, used in peripheral vascular diseases (see p. 160).

SOME OTHER COMMON DESCRIPTIVE TERMS
USED FOR GROUPS OF DRUGS

Antiseptics.—Iodine, Spirit, Proflavine, Cetrimide.

Substances which inhibit the growth of organisms and are extensively used to procure sterility in operative procedures.

Antipyretics.—Salicylates, Aspirin, Phenacetin.

Drugs which lower the temperature.

Carminatives.—Peppermint, Charcoal.

Drugs which relieve gas in the stomach.

Cough Depressants.—Codeine, Opiate Squill Linctus, Morphine.

Drugs which depress the cough reflex and are used to suppress a persistent irritating cough. Usually given in the form of a linctus.

Disinfectants.—Cresol (Lysol, Izal, Jeyes' Fluid), Phenol (Carbolic Acid), Dettol.

Substances which destroy organisms. They are mainly used to sterilise instruments, and render excreta safe from spreading infection. They are too poisonous to be used on the human body. Some disinfectants when suitably diluted act as antiseptics and may then be used on the body.

Emetics.—Mustard, Salt, Apomorphine, Ipecacuanha.

Substances which cause vomiting and which are chiefly used in medicine to get rid of poisonous substances which have been swallowed.

Enemas.—Soap, Olive Oil, Turpentine.

Fluid preparations used for rectal injection. If used to procure a bowel action, as is usual, then a copious amount of fluid is given. If they are meant to be retained so that absorption can take place (retention enema) a small amount of fluid is used.

Expectorants.—Ammonia, Ipecacuanha Pot. Iodide, Saline Mixture.

Drugs which facilitate the production of sputum.

Muscle Relaxants.—Tubocurarine, Suxamethonium (Scoline), Gallamine Triethiodide (Flaxedil).

Drugs which produce complete relaxation of muscles.

Respiratory Antispasmodics.—Adrenaline, Ephedrine, Isoprenaline (Neo-epinine, Neodrenal), Aminophylline, Atropine.

Drugs which relax the muscles of the respiratory bronchioles.

Respiratory Stimulants.—Nikethamide, Picrotoxin, Strychnine, Nalorphine, Megimide, Daptazole.

Drugs used to stimulate the respirations. Most frequently used in respiratory failure due to poisoning.

DANGEROUS DRUGS ACT

The use and administration of certain drugs come under the control of the Dangerous Drugs Act. These drugs are :—

1. Morphine.
2. Diamorphine (heroin).
3. Cocaine.
4. Indian Hemp.
5. Pethidine.
6. Methadone (physeptone).
7. Phenadoxone (heptalgin).
8. Levorphanol (dromoran).

All D.D.A. prescriptions must be signed by the doctor with his full signature, the date and the number of doses to be given. One of the persons concerned in the administration of these drugs must be a State Registered Nurse and each dose must be checked before administration by a second nurse. A record of each dose given is made in a special register. The entry must state the name of the patient, the date on which the drug was given, the name of the drug, the dose and the time at which it was administered. Both the person giving the drug and the witness must sign the register. D.D.A. registers must be kept for two years after the date of the last entry.

Dangerous drugs must be stored in a special cupboard marked D.D.A. The cupboard must be kept locked and the key kept by a State Registered Nurse. The drugs must be checked at frequent intervals. Fresh supplies can be obtained only on a signed medical order, and the pharmacist supplying the drugs is given a receipt after checking the drugs with the nurse.

THE POISONS ACT

The following drugs come under the First Schedule of the Poisons List :—

1. All preparations containing more than 0·15 per cent. of atropine and belladonna.

20 A

2. All barbiturate drugs, *e.g.*, phenobarbitone, medinal, soneryl, amytal, nembutal, etc.
3. All sulphonamides.
4. Digitalis and digoxin.
5. Codeine.
6. Mercurial preparations, *e.g.*, mersalyl.
7. Antihistamine drugs, *e.g.*, anthisan, antistin, benadryl, phenergan, etc., except ancolan (meclozine).
8. Dover's powders.
9. Hexamethonium, *e.g.*, vegolysen, hexathide.
10. Veratrum viride, *e.g.*, veriloid.
11. The muscle relaxant drugs, curare, gallamine triethiodide (flaxedil) and suxamethonium (scoline, anectine).
12. Nalorphine.
13. The anticonvulsant drugs, paramethadione, phenylacetylurea (phenurone) and troxidone.
14. Phenylbutazone (butazolidin).
15. Amphetamine (benzedrine and dexedrine).
16. Picrotoxin.
17. All preparations containing more than 0·2 per cent. strychnine.
18. Chlorpromazine (largactil).
19. Papaverine.
20. Emetine.
21. Arsenical preparations.
22. Ergot preparations.
23. Carbachol.
24. Methylpentynol (oblivon).

The Act requires that drugs coming under the First Schedule of the Poisons List must be kept in a cupboard apart from all other drugs and must be given only on the written order of a doctor.

CHAPTER XXII

POINTS TO REMEMBER

1. Patient as an Individual.

It is all too easy when working in a hospital or institution to forget that the patient is an individual—to regard him not as Mr Charles Smith but as " the heart failure case in bed 4." Patients soon realise when they are not being treated as individuals and then rapidly lose confidence in their treatment. There is, perhaps, nothing that will get a patient better more quickly than to make him feel he is having the individual care and attention of his nurse and doctor.

It is essential for nurses to appreciate that a patient who is ill is suffering from a double anxiety: firstly, the worry over his illness and its outcome and, secondly, the fact that he has probably had to give up his work, with all the financial loss that this may mean. Similarly, a mother will worry about the care of her children while she is in hospital. The longer the illness the greater will be these anxieties. It will take all the sympathy, tact and understanding of the nurse to allay these anxieties in her patients. They will need constant reassurance, particularly if the illness is severe and prolonged, and the nurse must never forget to treat her patients as individuals.

The Lady Almoner's department can usually help to overcome many of the social difficulties the patient may have as a result of illness and, therefore, if there is any evidence of such anxieties, an interview between the almoner and the patient should be arranged.

2. Rest.

Rest is one of the fundamental treatments in all acute and subacute illnesses, and during some stage or other in severe chronic illnesses. It is not enough, however, just to put all patients to bed under the same fixed, rigid routine. The amount and nature of the rest may well have to be varied to suit different patients. Too rigid a routine for certain patients may only increase their anxieties. Treatment should be dovetailed so as to disturb the patient as little as possible, especially in any serious illness. Remember that one of the best ways of ensuring adequate rest is by means of a good night's sleep. This may be particularly important, for instance, in patients with heart failure.

It may sometimes be easier to rest sitting up in a chair than lying in bed, *e.g.*, in many cases of severe heart failure. In many illnesses, especially respiratory illness, adequate rest is dependent upon the patient's position in bed.

3. Clothes.

Tight-fitting clothes are difficult to remove; unsuitable clothing may therefore cause patients a good deal of disturbance when they have to be washed or examined by the doctor. Attire must therefore be loose and pyjamas are usually more convenient than nightdresses.

Bed-clothes must not be too tightly tucked in as this restricts movements of the legs especially in frail, elderly people and in the seriously ill. Such restriction of movement predisposes to pressure sores and venous thrombosis.

4. The Problem of the Bed-pan.

Many patients find it extremely difficult to use a bed-pan. If the doctor agrees, the lavatory chair should be used instead. Much more use should also be made of the bed-side commode than is normal practice in hospitals to-day. There is often far less strain in using a commode or lavatory chair than in using a bed-pan.

5. Nursing of Elderly Patients.

Elderly patients are particularly prone to develop pressure sores, especially on the buttocks and heels. These patients are most reluctant to move about in bed and must be encouraged to undertake active movements as much as possible. Passive movements, especially of the legs, are essential to prevent venous thrombosis and its serious complication, pulmonary embolism. Patients with paralysis are particularly liable to pressure sores and also to respiratory and urinary infections. It is essential to get all patients up as soon as their condition allows.

When nursing elderly, seriously ill patients, the nurse may have special difficulty in inducing them to take sufficient fluids and food. Care is therefore needed to ensure that such patients do in fact take an adequate diet.

6. Diet.

Special diets are becoming of increasing importance in the treatment of many diseases, and it is essential for the nurse to fully understand the principles of all special dietary regimes and be able to carry them out; big meals must not be given to seriously ill patients as these may cause abdominal distension and consequential distress.

Apart from any special dietary regime, it is important that all meals should be served in an attractive manner and that the food should not be lukewarm. Loss of appetite is a usual accompaniment of many illnesses and for a full and speedy recovery an adequate diet is important. With many patients, especially those who are elderly or seriously ill, in order to induce them to take adequate nourishment it is essential to serve meals that are varied and attractive both to the eye and to the palate.

The maintenance of an adequate fluid balance is always a prime consideration and will call for special attention in such circumstances as frequent vomiting, severe diarrhœa, persistent and severe sweating, particularly if accompanied by a high temperature, and in all comatose patients. Signs of dehydration must be carefully watched for—dry, leathery tongue, pinched skin and a low output of urine. Particular care will also be required to ensure an adequate fluid intake in the case of infants and elderly people.

7. General Observations of the Patient and his Demeanour.

Very often, in the assessment of a patient's progress, too much reliance is placed on the results of various tests, and far too little on a close and intelligent observation of the patient's attitude and general demeanour. These can reveal a great deal. A patient who is lying quiet and relaxed in bed is probably progressing favourably. Restlessness often indicates an underlying anxiety, or a more serious complication such as internal hæmorrhage—hæmatemesis, melæna, etc. Any sudden change in the patient's general behaviour is important. This change may be in his demeanour, or in his colour or breathing. Sudden pallor may indicate hæmorrhage; cold, clammy skin—shock or hæmorrhage; cyanosis—perhaps a serious respiratory or cardiac complication. If the colour of a patient suddenly becomes cyanosed, it may mean that the airway is blocked and needs urgent attention. Patients with paralysis of the respiratory muscles, as in poliomyelitis, are particularly prone to develop an alteration in their breathing or cyanosis.

8. Dyspnœa.

The sudden onset of difficulty in breathing often means the onset of a respiratory or cardiac complication. Pulmonary embolism may be first detected by the sudden onset of dyspnœa. The onset of cardiac failure is usually associated with breathlessness, especially nocturnal dyspnœa. In a patient being treated for coronary thrombosis the development of dyspnœa often means a recurrence of his thrombosis or the onset of cardiac failure, either of which is serious. Severe dyspnœa is always an important symptom demanding urgent attention.

9. Sweating.

Severe sweating is always an important sign. Sweating is a common accompaniment of a high temperature. The sudden onset of severe sweating may mean the occurrence of a coronary thrombosis. It may also indicate a sudden perforation in a patient with a peptic ulcer. Sweating is a sign of overdosage of insulin and is also common in severe aspirin poisoning. It is important to realise that with severe and persistent sweating the amount of fluid loss can be considerable and should be replaced.

10. Coma.

The importance of laboured respirations and cyanosis as signs of a blocked airway has already been pointed out. Such blockage must always be guarded against. Pressure sores and respiratory complications are especially likely to develop with comatose patients. Such patients must therefore be nursed in the prone position and turned frequently, if necessary every two hours, from side to side.

Care must be taken to see that at all times the limbs are in the optimum position of muscular relaxation to avoid undue stretching of the muscles, which may cause permanent damage. Keeping the limbs in the optimum position of muscular relaxation is, of course, also essential in all patients with paralysis, *e.g.*, hemiplegia, paraplegia, poliomyelitis, polyneuritis, etc. Foot-boards, pillows under the calves, thighs and in the axillæ ; handrolls and pillows or sandbags to prevent external rotation of the leg must be used where indicated.

With all patients in prolonged coma the question of providing an adequate fluid intake will arise and call for special care. This is particularly so if there is also a fever and severe sweating. Signs of dehydration must, therefore, be carefully watched for.

11. The Pulse.

Any change in the pulse rate, whether the rhythm becomes slower, faster, or in particular irregular, is extremely important. Changes in the pulse are to be particularly looked for in heart disease, especially in coronary thrombosis and rheumatic fever. The onset of hæmorrhage is usually associated with a rise in the pulse rate whilst a falling pulse rate in a patient with hæmorrhage usually means the bleeding is subsiding. The slow pulse of digitalis overdosage must be recognised. With rapid auricular fibrillation, owing to the large pulse deficit the pulse is not a true estimate of the rate of the heart and in these circumstances an apex chart must be kept.

12. Testing of Urine.

The routine testing of urine for albumin and sugar in all patients is, of course, essential. The daily volume of urine passed is also of considerable importance. If the volume of urine is normal it is a good indication that the patient is having enough fluid. Any sudden diminution in output may mean the development of anuria, which is liable to occur when the patient is in such conditions as severe shock and hæmorrhage and also when treated with sulphonamide drugs. With severe hæmorrhage there is usually a marked diminution in output of urine and when the patient begins to pass urine in adequate amounts it is always a good sign of the return of normal circulation and blood pressure. Sudden diminution of output in nephritis and congestive heart failure is always serious and to be noted. So is the presence of acetone in the urine, particularly in patients who are being treated for diabetes mellitus, as it may be an indication of impending coma.

13. Inspection of Sputum.

It is always essential to examine the sputum and note its characteristics, particularly whether it contains blood or is purulent. The need to save all specimens of sputum for examination must be stressed, especially if there is any question of pulmonary tuberculosis.

14. Inspection of Vomit.

The characteristics of any material vomited must be noted, particularly for the presence of food contents and blood; the amount passed must be measured. The importance of vomiting in infants must be realised as it is always a serious sign. The copious vomiting of pyloric stenosis must be recognised. Vomiting is often associated with shock; vomiting in diabetes may herald the onset of coma and is a most important sign.

15. Inspection of Stools.

Stools must always be inspected, particularly in patients with gastro-intestinal diseases and diarrhœa. In every case of hæmorrhage from the gastro-intestinal tract—hæmatemesis and melæna—all stools must be saved for examination. In patients suffering from diarrhœa the number of stools passed and their characteristics must be accurately assessed and specimens saved, if necessary, for bacteriological examination. Patients being treated for peptic ulcer usually have regular specimens of stools saved for examination for occult blood. In the nursing of infants the character and number of stools passed are extremely important, especially if the stools are watery or contain blood.

16. Œdema.

The presence of œdema, especially in patients with cardiac and renal diseases, must be constantly looked for. When the patient is in bed, it is usually first noticed as a small sacral pad. In the patient who has been up and about the onset is usually in the lower limbs. The presence of œdema is always of the first importance. Regular weighing whenever possible to assess the amount of œdema is usually a more reliable guide than a fluid balance chart.

17. Pain.

This symptom is always important and the onset for the first time of pain in any patient frequently denotes spread or exacerbation of his illness, or the development of some complication. In a patient with a peptic ulcer or typhoid fever it may mean the onset of a perforation. Pain in the chest may denote pulmonary embolism as the result of a thrombus having become detached from the leg or pelvis. A pain in the leg, however slight, especially in the calf, usually denotes venous thrombosis. Severe pain in the foot especially if accompanied by cold, discoloured skin, usually indicates arterial thrombosis or embolism. The pain of pleurisy is characteristic, also the substernal pain in the chest radiating to the arm in coronary thrombosis. In a patient with coronary thrombosis the recurrence of pain often means a deterioration in his condition.

18. Prevention of Pulmonary Embolism.

Pulmonary embolism is a complication of venous thrombosis; the best way of preventing embolism is therefore to prevent venous thrombosis. This can be done by active and passive movements of the limbs and by early mobilisation. The danger of venous thrombosis and pulmonary embolism is especially great in severe, prolonged illness, and in patients with paralysis and congestive heart failure and in all elderly patients.

Recognition of the early symptoms of deep venous thrombosis— slight pyrexia, slight pain or aching in the leg—is most important as early treatment may prevent an embolism.

19. Blood Transfusions.

The importance must be stressed of carefully checking the name, blood group, etc., on every bottle of blood before it is given to a patient. On first starting a transfusion the patient must be closely watched for signs of incompatibility—restlessness, rigors, pain in the back, etc. All used bottles must be saved and sent to the laboratory without being washed.

20. Drugs.

It is most important for the nurse to recognise the early toxic effects which may occur from practically any drug.

(a) DIGITALIS.—Loss of appetite often precedes nausea and vomiting. The importance of a slow pulse must be noted. The effect of digitalis may be greatly enhanced if prolonged therapy with the chlorothiazide group of diuretics is given at the same time: in these circumstances digitalis overdosage is particularly liable to occur.

(b) DIURETICS.—Mersalyl is a toxic drug. Routine examination of the urine for gross albuminuria must be carried out before the injection of mersalyl. It is important to recognise the early symptoms of a low salt syndrome and also of potassium deficiency in all patients receiving intensive diuretic therapy, especially when this is combined with a low salt diet. This is particularly so when such potent diuretics as mersalyl and chlorothiazide (saluric) are given for long periods and in big doses.

(c) SULPHONAMIDES.—The output of urine must be watched, also the development of hæmaturia. An adequate fluid intake is essential to prevent renal complications. A sudden rise in temperature may be a drug fever. Rashes must be looked for. A sore throat may be the onset of the serious complication agranulocytosis.

(d) ASPIRIN.—Aspirin may cause hæmatemesis, especially in patients with a peptic ulcer and in patients receiving anticoagulant drugs. Aspirin must, therefore, never be given at the same time as anticoagulant drugs. Overdosage of aspirin causes the early symptoms of ringing in the ears and deafness.

(e) ANTIBIOTICS.

(i) *Penicillin.*—It is necessary to find out whether or not a patient is sensitive to penicillin before the drug is given. If the patient is sensitive to it penicillin may cause a serious reaction such as anaphylaxis which is often fatal. Penicillin can also cause rashes.

(ii) *Tetracycline Antibiotics.*—These may cause nausea and, particularly important, diarrhœa. Severe diarrhœa is a most serious complication, as it is usually due to staphylococcal ileo-colitis which may prove fatal.

(iii) *Chloramphenicol.*—This antibiotic may cause severe blood disorders such as agranulocytosis.

(iv) *Streptomycin.*—The onset of giddiness, difficult or staggering gait (ataxia) and deafness must be closely watched for, particularly in elderly patients and those receiving the drug for a long time and in large doses.

(v) *Neomycin and Kanamycin.*—Both these antibiotics may, like streptomycin, cause permanent deafness, especially in elderly patients and those having large doses.

(f) HYPOTENSIVE DRUGS.—Giddiness, especially when the patient first adopts an upright position, is important as it shows that the blood pressure is too low. It is essential for an accurate reading of the blood pressure while the patient is taking hypotensive drugs to take the blood pressure reading with the patient standing and not lying down. Constipation, which is likely to develop with many hypotensive drugs and may enhance their action to the extent of leading to a severe fall in blood pressure, must be guarded against at all costs.

(g) CORTISONE AND ALLIED STEROIDS.—The danger of fluid retention and the development of œdema must be watched for. Patients with diabetes while on steroid therapy may show a deterioration in their diabetes so that a careful watch must be kept on their urine for an increase in glycosuria and the development of acetonuria.

(h) ANTICOAGULANT DRUGS.—The first sign of bleeding, e.g., from the nose or in the urine, etc., must be carefully looked for. The danger of giving at the same time as anticoagulant drugs, certain drugs which may cause hæmorrhage, such as aspirin and phenylbutazone (butazolidin) must be stressed. Broad spectrum antibiotics (tetracycline antibiotics, chloramphenicol) enhance the action of anticoagulant drugs and must be given with care to patients on anticoagulants. Chlorpromazine (largactil) and similar drugs (sparine) also enhance the effect of anticoagulant drugs and it is therefore inadvisable to give these drugs at the same time as anticoagulants.

(i) PHENYLBUTAZONE.—Hæmatemesis may occur, especially in patients with a peptic ulcer, and as just mentioned phenylbutazone must never be given at the same time as anticoagulant drugs because of the danger of bleeding. Phenylbutazone may also cause blood disorders, such as purpura and agranulocytosis.

(j) GENERAL.—The development of a sore throat in a patient receiving such drugs as the sulphonamides, antithyroid drugs, chloramphenicol and phenylbutazone, is most serious, as it may mean the onset of the serious complication agranulocytosis. The development of rashes may be due to drugs such as sulphonamides, salicylates, barbiturates, quinine, etc. A rise of temperature may be due to a drug fever.

It is essential to check all potent drugs and not only those which come under the Dangerous Drugs or Poisons Acts. Especially important in this respect is the checking of the doses of anticoagulant drugs and adrenaline. Many fatal mishaps have occurred through giving the wrong dose and strength of adrenaline. A careful inspection of the label on all containers of drugs is essential; if the label is not clearly written the drug must not be given.

NAMES OF DRUGS

Approved or Chemical Name.	Trade Names.	Action or Diseases in which Used.
1. ACETARSOL	STOVARSOL	Amœbic Dysentery
2. ACETARSOL PESSARIES	DEVEGAN, MONARGAN	Trichomonas
3. ACETAZOLAMIDE	DIAMOX	Diuretic (see p. 143)
4. ACETOMENAPHTHONE	PROKAYVIT ORAL, VITAVEL K	Vitamin K analogue
5. ALLOBARBITONE	DIAL	Barbiturate, Hypnotic (see p. 594)
6. ALOXIDONE	MALIDONE	Anticonvulsant
7. ALUMINIUM GLYCINATE	PRODEXIN, TABNET	Alkali (see p. 238)
8. ALUMINIUM HYDROXIDE	ALGELOX, ALOCOL, ALUDROX, COLLUMINA	Alkali (see p. 238)
9. ALUMINIUM PHOSPHATE	ALUPHOS	Alkali
10. ALUMINIUM SILICATE	NEUTRALON	Alkali
11. AMETHOCAINE	ANETHAINE, DECICAIN	Local anæsthetic
12. AMIDOPYRINE	PYRAMIDON	Analgesic
13. AMINACRINE	ACRAMIDINE, ACRAMINE, MONACRIN	Antiseptic
14. AMINOMETRADINE	MICTINE	Diuretic
15. AMINOPHYLLINE	CARDOPHYLLIN, THEODROX	Asthma
16. 4-AMINOPTEROYLGLUTAMATE	AMINOPTERIN	Leukæmia (see p. 390)
17. AMIPHENAZOLE	DAPTAZOLE	Barbiturate poisoning (see p. 595)
18. AMISOMETRADINE	ROLICTON	Diuretic (see p. 143)
19. AMMONIUM MANDELATE	MANDELIX	Urinary Infections
20. AMODIAQUINE	CAMOQUIN	Malaria
21. AMPHETAMINE SULPHATE	AMPHAMED, BENZEDRINE	Stimulant, Vasoconstrictor
22. AMYLOBARBITONE	AMYTAL	Barbiturate, Hypnotic, Sedative (see p. 594)
23. AMYLOBARBITONE SODIUM	AMYTAL SODIUM, DORMINAL	Barbiturate, Hypnotic
24. ANEURINE	BENERVA, BETALIN S, BETAVEL, BETAXAN, CRYSTO-VIBEX, DAVITAMON B₁	Vitamin B₁ (see p. 497)
25. ANISINDIONE	MIRADON	Oral anticoagulant
26. ANTAZOLINE	ANTISTIN, HISTOSTAB	Antihistamine (see p. 591)
27. ASCORBIC ACID	ASCORVEL, CANTAN, CEVALIN, DAVITAMON C, REDOXON	Vitamin C (see p. 498)
28. ATROPINE METHONITRATE	EUMYDRIN, PYLOSTROPIN	Congenital Pyloric Stenosis (see p. 248)
29. BARBITONE SODIUM	MEDINAL	Barbiturate, Hypnotic (see p. 594)
30. BEMEGRIDE	MEGIMIDE	Barbiturate poisoning (see p. 595)

Approved or Chemical Name.	Trade Names.	Action or Diseases in which Used
31. BENACTYZINE	CEVANOL, LUCIDIL, NUTINAL, SUAVITIL	Sedatives, anxiety states
32. BENETHAMINE PENICILLIN	BENAPEN	Antibiotic
33. BENZALKONIUM CHLORIDE	ROCCAL	Antiseptic
34. BENZATHINE PENICILLIN	DIBENCIL, NEOLIN, PENIDURAL, PERMAPEN	Antibiotic (see p. 580)
35. BENZETHONIUM	PHEMERIDE	Antiseptic
36. BENZHEXOL	ARTANE, PIPANOL	Parkinsonism
37. BENZYL BENZOATE	ASCABIOL, BENZEVAN, PROSCABIN	Scabies (see p. 521)
38. BENZYLPENICILLIN	CRYSTAPEN, PRADUCIL, PRADUPEN, SUGRACILLIN	Antibiotic (see p. 580)
39. BETAMETHASONE	BETNELAN	Corticosteroid (see p. 597)
40. BISMUTH	BISGLUCOL, BISMOSTAB	Syphilis, Lupus Erythematosus
41. BRETYLIUM TOSYLATE	DARENTHIN	Hypertension (see p. 132)
42. BUSULPHAN	MYLERAN	Leukæmia (see p. 390)
43. BUTHALITONE SODIUM	TRANSITHAL, ULBREVAL	Barbiturate intravenous anæsthetic
44. BUTOBARBITONE	SONERYL	Barbiturate, Hypnotic (see p. 594)
45. CALCIFEROL	DITUVITAN, FORTODYL, OSTELIN, RADIOSTOL, STEROGYL, VITAVEL D	Vitamin D (see p. 499)
46. CALCIUM ACETYLSALICYLIC ACID	DISPRIN	Analgesic, Antipyretic
47. CALCIUM BENZAMIDOSALICYLATE	THERAPAS	Tuberculosis
48. CARAMIPHEN	PARPANIT	Parkinsonism
49. CARBACHOL	MORYL	Paralytic Ileus, Postoperative retention of urine
50. CARBARSONE	LEUCARSONE	Amœbic Dysentery (see p. 83)
51. CARBIMAZOLE	NEO-MERCAZOLE	Thyrotoxicosis (see p. 439)
52. CARBROMAL	ADALIN	Hypnotic, Sedative (see p. 604)
53. CETRIMIDE	CETAVLON	Antiseptic
54. CHINIOFON SODIUM	AVLOCHIN	Amœbic Dysentery
55. CHLORAMPHENICOL	ALFICETYN, CHLOROMYCETIN	Antibiotic (see p. 583)
56. CHLORBUTOL	CHLORETONE	Sedative
57. CHLORCYCLIZINE	DI-PARALENE, HISTANTIN	Antihistamine (see p. 591)
58. CHLORMERODRIN	MERCLORAN	Mercurial diuretic (see p. 140)

Approved or Chemical Name.	Trade Names.	Action or Diseases in which Used.
59. CHLOROQUINE	ARALEN, AVLOCLOR, NIVA-QUINE	Malaria, Lupus Erythematosus, Amœbic Hepatitis
60. CHLOROTHIAZIDE	SALURIC	Diuretic (see p. 142)
61. CHLORPROMAZINE	LARGACTIL	Sedative (see p. 596)
62. CINCHOCAINE	NUPERCAINE	Local anæsthetic
63. CORTICOTROPHIN	ACTHAR, CORTROPHIN	Simmonds' Disease, etc. (see p. 599)
64. CORTISONE	CORTELAN, CORTISTAB, CORTISYL	Corticosteroid (see p. 597)
65. CYANOCOBALAMIN	ANACOBIN, BITEVAN, COBALIN, COBASTAB, CYTAMEN, DISTIVIT B_{12}, EUHÆMON, FERMIN, MEGALOVEL, RUBRAMIN	Pernicious Anæmia (see p. 372)
66. CYCLIZINE	MARZINE	Antihistamine
67. CYCLOSERINE	SEROMYCIN	Antibiotic (see p. 585)
68. CYCLOBARBITONE	PHANODORM	Barbiturate, Hypnotic
69. CYLOCUMAROL	CUMOPYRAN	Anticoagulant
70. DAPSONE	AVLOSULFON	Leprosy
71. DEMECOLCINE	COLCEMID	Leukæmia
72. DEMETHYLCHLORTETRA-CYCLINE	LEDERMYCIN	Antibiotic (see p. 582)
73. DEOXYCORTONE ACETATE	CORTIRON, DECORTACETE, DOCA, PERCORTEN, SYNCORTYL	Addison's Disease (see p. 449)
74. DESERPIDINE	HARMONYL	Hypotensive drug
75. DEXAMETHASONE	DECADRON, DEXACORTISYL, DEXTELAN, MILLICORTEN, ORADEXON	Corticosteroid (see p. 599)
76. DEXAMPHETAMINE	DEPHADREN, DEXAMED, DEXEDRINE	Stimulant, Depressive States, Obesity
77. DEXTRAN	DEXTRAVEN, INTRADEX	Burns, Shock
78. DICHLORALPHENAZONE	WELLDORM	Hypnotic (see p. 604)
79. DICHLOROPHEN	ANTHIPHEN	Tapeworms (see p. 269)
80. DICOUMAROL	DICOUMARIN	Anticoagulant (see p. 127)
81. DIETHAZINE	DIPARCOL	Parkinsonism
82. DI-IODOHYDROXYQUINOLINE	DIODOQUIN, EMBEQUIN, FLORAQUIN, SAVORQUIN	Amœbic Dysentery
83. DIMENHYDRINATE	DRAMAMINE	Antihistamine (see p. 591)
84. DIMERCAPROL	B.A.L.	Metallic poisoning
85. DIMETHYLTUBOCURARINE	DIAMETHINE	Muscle relaxant
86. DIODONE	ARTERIODONE, DIODRAST, PERABRODIL, PYELOSIL, PYLUMBRIN, URIODONE, VASIODONE, VISKIOSOL	X-ray Diagnosis, Pyelography, Angiography

Approved or Chemical Name.	Trade Names.	Action or Diseases in which Used.
87. DIPHENHYDRAMINE	BENADRYL	Antihistamine (see p. 591)
88. DISULFIRAM	ANTABUSE, CRONETAL	Chronic Alcoholism
89. DISULPHAMIDE	DISAMIDE	Diuretic
90. DITHRANOL	CIGNOLIN	Psoriasis
91. DOMIPHEN BROMIDE	BRADOSOL	Antiseptic
92. DOXYLAMINE	DECAPRYN	Antihistamine
93. ERGOTAMINE TARTRATE	FEMERGIN	Migraine
94. ERYTHROMYCIN	ERYTHROCIN, ILOTYCIN	Antibiotic (see p. 583)
95. ETHOPROPAZINE	LYSIVANE	Parkinsonism
96. ETHYL BISCOUMACETATE	TROMEXAN	Anticoagulant
97. ETHYL IODOPHENYLUNDE-CANOATE	ETHIODAN, MYODIL, PANTO-PAQUE	X-ray Diagnosis, Myelography
98. FERROUS FUMARATE	FERSAMAL	Iron Deficiency Anæmias
99. FERROUS GLUCONATE	CEREVON, FERGON, FER-LUCON, FERRONICUM, FERRONYL	Iron Deficiency Anæmias (see p. 606)
100. FERROUS SUCCINATE	FERROMYN	Iron Deficiency Anæmias (see p. 606)
101. FERROUS SULPHATE	FERCUMAN, FEROSAN, FER-SOLATE, TONIRON	Iron Deficiency Anæmias (see p. 606)
102. FLUDROCORTISONE	FLORINEF	Addison's disease (see p. 449)
103. FOLIC ACID	FOLVITE	Macrocytic Anæmias (see p. 364)
104. FURALTADONE	ALTAFUR	Antibacterial agent (see p. 611)
105. GALLAMINE	FLAXEDIL	Muscle relaxant
106. GAMMA BENZENE HEXA-CHLORIDE	LOREXANE	Insecticide, Pediculosis
107. GLUTETHIMIDE	DORIDEN	Hypnotic (see p. 604)
108. GRISEOFULVIN	FULCIN, GRISOVIN	Antibiotic. Ringworm (see p. 522)
109. GUANETHIDINE	ISMELIN	Hypertension (see p. 132)
110. HALOPYRAMINE	SYNOPEN	Antihistamine
111. HEPARIN	LIQUEMIN, PULARIN	Anticoagulant (see p. 127)
112. HEXAMINE MANDELATE	MANDELAMINE	Urinary Infections
113. HEXOBARBITONE	CYCLONAL, EVIPAN	Barbiturate, Intra-venous anæsthetic
114. HYALURONIDASE	HYALASE, RONDASE, WYDASE	" Spreading Factor," Subcutaneous Infusions
115. HYDRALLAZINE	APRESOLINE	Hypertension
116. HYDROCHLOROTHIAZIDE	DIREMA, ESIDREX, HYDRIL, HYDROSALURIC	Diuretic (see p. 602)

Approved or Chemical Name.	Trade Names.	Action or Diseases in which Used.
117. HYDROCORTISONE	CORTEF, CORTRIL, EF-CORTELAN, HYDROCORTISTAB, HYDROCORTISYL, HYDROCORTONE, PABRACORT	Corticosteroid (see p. 598)
118. HYDROFLUMETHIAZIDE	DI-ADEMIL, HYDRENOX, NACLEX	Diuretic (see p. 602)
119. HYOSCINE METHOBROMIDE	PAMINE	Antispasmodic
120. IMIPRAMINE	TOFRANIL	Depression
121. INSULIN ZINC SUSPENSION	INSULIN NOVO LENTE	Diabetes Mellitus (see p. 480)
122. INSULIN ZINC SUSPENSION (AMORPHOUS)	INSULIN NOVO SEMILENTE	Diabetes Mellitus (see p. 480)
123. INSULIN ZINC SUSPENSION (CRYSTALLINE)	INSULIN NOVO ULTRALENTE	Diabetes Mellitus (see p. 480)
124. IODIPAMIDE METHYLGLUCAMINE	BILIGRAFIN	X-ray Diagnosis, Cholecystography
125. IODISED OIL	IODATOL, IODIPIN, LIPIODOL, NEO-HYDRIOL	X-ray Diagnosis, Bronchography
126. IODOCHLORHYDROXYQUINOLINE	VIOFORM	Fungicide (see p. 519)
127. ION-EXCHANGE RESINS	CARBO-RESIN, KATONIUM	Cardiac Œdema
128. IOPANOIC ACID	TELEPAQUE	X-ray Diagnosis, Cholecystography
129. ISONIAZID	COTINAZIN, I. N. H., MYBASAN, NEUMANDIN, NYDRAZID, PYCAZIDE. RIMIFON, TUBOMEL, VAZADRINE	Tuberculosis (see p. 193)
130. ISOPRENALINE	ALEUDRIN, ISUPREN, NEODRENAL, NEO-EPININE, NORISODRINE	Asthma (see p. 200)
131. KANAMYCIN	KANNASYN	Antibiotic (see p. 585)
132. KHELLIN	BENECARDIN, KHELLANALS, VISCARDAN	Angina Pectoris
133. LEPTAZOL	CARDIAZOL, CENTRAZOL, PHRENAZOL	Respiratory stimulant
134. LEVALLORPHAN	LORFAN	Antidote to morphine, pethidine
135. LEVORPHANOL	DROMORAN	Analgesic (see p. 537)
136. LIGNOCAINE	XYLOCAINE, XYLOTOX	Local anæsthetic
137. LIVER EXTRACTS	ANAHÆMIN, ANAHEPOL, CAMPOLON, EXAMEN, HEPASTAB, HEPOL, LIVADEX, NEO-HEPATEX, PARENAMPS, PERHEPAR, PERNÆMON, PLEXAN, PRŒTHRON	Macrocytic Anæmias, Sprue
138. MAGNESIUM TRISILICATE	MAGSORBENT, NOVASORB	Alkali (see p. 238)
139. MECAMYLAMINE	INVERSINE	Hypertension (see p. 132

Approved or Chemical Name.	Trade Names.	Action or Diseases in which Used.
140. MECLOZINE	ANCOLAN	Antihistamine (see p. 591)
141. MENAPHTHONE	PROKAYVIT	Vitamin K.
142. MEPACRINE	ATEBRIN, QUINACRINE	Malaria, Tapeworms (see p. 269)
143. MEPHENESIN	MYANESIN, TOLSERAM	Muscle relaxant
144. MEPHENTERMINE	MEPHINE	Circulatory stimulant (see p. 607)
145. MEPROBAMATE	EQUANIL, MEPAVLON, MIL-TOWN	Sedative, anxiety states
146. MEPYRAMINE MALEATE	ANTHISAN	Antihistamine (see p. 591)
147. MERALLURIDE	MERCARDAN	Mercurial diuretic (see p. 140)
148. MERCAPTOMERIN SODIUM	THIOMERIN SODIUM	Mercurial diuretic (see p. 140)
149. MERCAPTOPURINE	PURI-NETHOL	Leukæmia (see p. 390)
150. MESULPHEN	SUDERMO	Scabies
151. METHACHOLINE CHLORIDE	AMECHOL, MECHOLYL	Paralytic Ileus
152. METHADONE	PHYSEPTONE	Analgesic (see p. 537)
153. METHAPHENILENE	DIATRIN	Antihistamine
154. METHOIN	MESONTOIN	Anticonvulsant (see p. 339)
155. METHOXYPHENAMINE	ORTHOXINE	Hay Fever
156. METHYLAMPHETAMINE	DESOXYN, METHEDRINE	Cerebral stimulant
157. METHYLPENTYNOL	ATEMPOL, INSOMNOL, OBLIVON, SOMNESIN	Hypnotic (see p. 605)
158. METHYL PHENIDATE	RITALIN	Mental depression
159. METHYLPHENOBARBITONE	PROMINAL	Barbiturate, Anticonvulsant
160. METHYLPREDNISOLONE	MEDRONE	Corticosteroid (see p. 599)
161. METHYPRYLONE	NOLUDAR	Hypnotic
162. NALORPHINE	LETHIDRONE	Antidote to morphine, etc. (see p. 610)
163. NAPHAZOLINE	PRIVINE	Rhinitis
164. NEOMYCIN	MYCIFRADIN, NEOMIN	Antibiotic (see p. 584)
165. NEOSTIGMINE	PROSTIGMIN	Myasthenia Gravis (see p. 358)
166. NICOTINIC ACID	NICOVEL	Pellagra
167. NICOTINYL ALCOHOL	RONICOL	Peripheral vasodilator (see p. 615)
168. NICOUMALONE	SINTHROME	Anticoagulant
169. NIKETHAMIDE	ANACARDONE, CORAMINE, CORVOTONE, NICAMIDE	Respiratory stimulant (see p. 610)
170. NITROFURANTOIN	FURADANTIN	Urinary infections (see p. 611)
171. NORADRENALINE	LEVOPHED	Shock (see p. 588)
172. NOSCAPINE	COSCOPIN, NICOLANE	Cough Depressant

Approved or Chemical Name.	Trade Names.	Action or Diseases in which Used.
173. NOVOBIOCIN	ALBAMYCIN, BIOTEXIN, CATHOMYCIN	Antibiotic (see p. 583)
174. NYSTATIN	MYCOSTATIN	Antibiotic (see p. 584)
175. OLEANDOMYCIN	MATROMYCIN, ROMICIL	Antibiotic (see p. 584)
176. OXYPHENONIUM BROMIDE	ANTRENYL	Anticholinergic drug
177. OXYTETRACYCLINE	TERRAMYCIN	Antibiotic (see p. 582)
178. PAMAQUIN	PLASMOQUINE, PRÆQUINE	Malaria
179. PARACETAMOL	PANADOL	Analgesic (see p. 537)
180. PARAMETHADIONE	PARADIONE	Anticonvulsant (see p. 339)
181. PENETHAMATE HYDRIODIDE	ESTOPEN	Preparation of Penicillin
182. PENTAERYTHRITOL TETRA-NITRATE	MYCARDOL, PERITRATE	Angina Pectoris (see p. 123)
183. PENTOBARBITONE SODIUM	NEMBUTAL	Barbiturate, Hypnotic, Sedative (see p. 594)
184. PENTOLINIUM TARTRATE	ANSOLYSEN	Hypotensive drug (see p. 133)
185. PETHIDINE	DEMEROL, DOLANTAL	Analgesic (see p. 537)
186. PHENACEMIDE	PHENURONE	Anticonvulsant (see p. 591)
187. PHENADOXONE	HEPTALGIN	Analgesic (see p. 537)
188. PHENINDAMINE	THEPHORIN	Antihistamine (see p. 591)
189. PHENINDIONE	DINDEVAN, INDEMA	Anticoagulant (see p. 127)
190. PHENOBARBITONE	GARDENAL, LUMINAL	Anticonvulsant, Sedative (see p. 594)
191. PHENOXYBENZAMINE	DIBENYLINE	Vasodilator (see p. 615)
192. PHENOXYETHANOL	PHENOXETOL	Antiseptic
193. PHENOXYMETHYLPENICILLIN	CALCIPEN V, COMPOCILLIN V, DISTAQUAINE V, ESKACILLIN V, PENAVLON V, PENICILLIN V, V-CIL-K	Antibiotic (see p. 579)
194. PHENPROCOUMON	MARCOUMAR	Anticoagulant
195. PHENSUXIMIDE	MILONTIN	Epilepsy
196. PHENTOLAMINE	ROGITINE	Phæochromocytoma (see p. 451)
197. PHENYLACETYLUREA	PHENURONE	Anticonvulsant
198. PHENYLBUTAZONE	BUTAZOLIDIN	Rheumatoid Arthritis, Gout (see p. 611)
199. PHENYLEPHRINE	NEOPHRYN	Vasoconstrictor
200. PHENYLMERCURIC ACETATE	MERSAGEL	Fungicide
201. PHENYLMERCURIC NITRATE	MERFENIL	Fungicide
202. PHENYTOIN SODIUM	DILANTIN SODIUM, EPANUTIN, EPTOIN	Anticonvulsant (see p. 339)
203. PHOLEDRINE	PHOLETONE	Circulatory stimulant
204. PHTHALYLSULPHACETAMIDE	ENTEROCID, STERATHAL	Sulphonamide

Approved or Chemical Name.	Trade Names.	Action or Diseases in which Used.
205. PHTHALYLSULPHATHIAZOLE	CREMOTHALIDINE, SULFA-THALIDINE, THALAZOLE, THALISTATYL	Sulphonamide (see p. 574)
206. PIPERAZINE	ANTEPAR, ENTACYL, VEROXIL, HELMEZINE	Threadworms, round-worms (see p. 267)
207. PIPEROCAINE	METYCAINE	Local anæsthetic
208. PIPEROXANE	BENODAINE	Pheochromocytoma
209. PIPRADOL	MERATRAN	Mental depression
210. POLYVIDONE	PLASMOSAN	Burns, Shock
211. PREDNISOLONE	CODELCORTONE, DELTA-CORTEF, DELTA-CORTRIL, DELTA-STAB, HYDELTRA, PRENOLONE	Corticosteroid (see p. 598)
212. PREDNISONE	DECORTISYL, DELTACORTONE, DELTRA, DELTASONE, DELTA-CORTELAN, ULTRA-CORTEN	Corticosteroid (see p. 598)
213. PRIMIDONE	MYSOLINE	Anticonvulsant (see p. 339)
214. PROBENECID	BENEMID	Gout
215. PROCAINAMIDE	PRONESTYL, PROCARDYL	Irregular Heart Action
216. PROCAINE	GENOCAIN, NOVOCAIN, PLANOCAINE	Local anæsthetic (see p. 597)
217. PROCAINE BENZYLPENICILLIN	AVLOPROCIL A.S., DISTA-QUAINE G, DURACILLIN, ESKACILLIN 200, MYLIPEN, PRO-STABILLIN	Antibiotic (see p. 580)
218. PROCHLORPERAZINE	STEMETIL	Migraine, Ménière's disease
219. PROCYCLIDINE	KEMADRIN	Parkinsonism
220. PROGUANIL	PALUDRINE	Malaria
221. PROMAZINE	SPARINE	Sedative (see p. 597)
222. PROMETHAZINE	PHENERGAN	Antihistamine (see p. 591)
223. PROMETHAZINE THEOCLATE	AVOMINE	Travel sickness
224. PROPANTHELINE BROMIDE	PRO-BANTHINE	Anticholinergic drug (see p. 238)
225. PROPYLIODONE	DIONOSIL	X-ray Diagnosis, Bronchography
226. PYRIDOSTIGMIN	MESTINON	Myasthenia Gravis
227. PYRIMETHAMINE	DARAPRIM	Malaria
228. QUINALBARBITONE SODIUM	SECONAL SODIUM	Barbiturate, Hypnotic (see p. 594)
229. RAUWOLFIA SERPENTINA	HYPERTENSAN, RAUDIXIN, RAUWILOID	Hypertension (see p. 132)
230. RESERPINE	QUIESCIN, RESERPAMED, RESERPEX, SERPILOID, SANDRIL, SERPASIL	Hypertension (see p. 132)
231. RIBOFLAVINE	BEFLAVIT, RIBOVEL	Vitamin B_2

Approved or Chemical Name.	Trade Names.	Action or Diseases in which Used.
232. RISTOCETIN	SPONTIN	Antibiotic
233. SACCHARATED IRON OXIDE	COLLIRON I.V., FERRIVENIN, IVIRON, NEO-FERRUM	Iron Deficiency Anæmias (see p. 606)
234. SELENIUM SULPHIDE	SELSUN	Seborrhœic Dermatitis (see p. 528)
235. SENNA	SENOKOT	Laxative (see p. 611)
236. SODIUM ACETRIZOATE	DIAGINOL	X-ray Diagnosis, Angiography, Pyelography
237. SODIUM AMINOSALICYLATE	AMINACYL, BACTYLAN, ENTEPAS, PARAMISAN SODIUM, PAS ENSEALS	Tuberculosis
238. SODIUM AUROTHIOMALATE	MYOCRISIN	Rheumatoid Arthritis (see p. 603)
239. SODIUM DIATRIZOATE	HYPAQUE	X-ray Diagnosis
240. SOLAPSONE	SULPHETRONE	Leprosy
241. SPASMOCYCLONE	CYCLOSPASMOL	Peripheral vasodilator
242. SPIRAMYCIN	ROVAMYCIN	Antibiotic (see p. 585)
243. STREPTODORNASE-STREPTO-KINASE	DORNOKINASE, VARIDASE	To liquefy blood clots and exudate
244. STREPTOMYCIN	STREPTAQUAINE, STREPOLIN	Antibiotic (see p. 581)
245. SUCCINYLSULPHATHIAZOLE	COLISTATIN, CREMOSUXIDINE, SULFASUXIDINE	Sulphonamide (see p. 574)
246. SULPHACETAMIDE	ALBUCID, STERAMIDE	Sulphonamide
247. SULPHADIAZINE	CREMODIAZINE	Sulphonamide (see p. 574)
248. SULPHADIMETHOXINE	MADRIBON	Long-acting sulphonamide
249. SULPHADIMIDINE	SULPHAMEZATHINE	Sulphonamide (see p. 574)
250. SULPHAFURAZOLE	GANTRISIN	Sulphonamide (see p. 574)
251. SULPHAMETHIZOLE	UROLUCOSIL	Sulphonamide (see p. 574)
252. SULPHAMETHOXYPYRIDAZINE	LEDERKYN, MIDICEL	Sulphonamide (see p. 574)
253. SULPHAPHENAZOLE	ORISULF	Long-acting sulphonamide
254. SULPHASALAZINE	SALAZOPYRIN	Ulcerative colitis
255. SULPHASOMIDINE	ELKOSIN	Sulphonamide
256. SULPHATHIAZOLE	CIBAZOL, THIAZAMIDE	Sulphonamide
257. SUXAMETHONIUM BROMIDE	BREVIDIL M	Muscle relaxant
258. SUXAMETHONIUM CHLORIDE	ANECTINE, SCOLINE	Muscle relaxant
259. SUXETHONIUM BROMIDE	BREVIDIL E	Muscle relaxant
260. TETRACYCLINE	ACHROMYCIN, TETRACYN	Antibiotic (see p. 582)
261. THALIDOMIDE	DISTAVAL	Hypnotic (see p. 605)
262. THENALIDINE TARTRATE	SANDOSTEN	Antihistamine (see p. 591)
263. THIALBARBITONE	KEMITHAL	Barbiturate, Intravenous anæsthetics

Approved or Chemical Name.	Trade Names.	Action or Diseases in which used.
264. THIOMERSAL	MERTHIOLATE	Antiseptic, Fungicide
265. THIOPENTONE SODIUM	INTRAVAL SODIUM, PENTOTHAL	Barbiturate, Intravenous anæsthetic (see p. 594)
266. THYROID	ELITYRAN, PROLOID, THYRANON	Myxœdema, Cretinism (see pp. 442, 445)
267. THYROXINE	ELTROXIN	Myxœdema, Cretinism
268. TOLAZOLINE	PRISCOL	Peripheral vasodilator (see p. 615)
269. TOLBUTAMIDE	RASTINON, ORINASE	Diabetes Mellitus (see p. 482)
270. TRIAMCINOLONE	ADCORTYL, LEDERCORT	Corticosteroid (see p. 599)
271. TRIMEPRAZINE TARTRATE	VALLERGAN	Antihistamine
272. TRIMETHAPHAN	ARFONAD	Hypotensive drug
273. TRINITRIN	ANGISED, NITROCENE	Angina Pectoris (see p. 123)
274. TRIPARANOL	MER 29	Lowers cholesterol
275. TRIPELENNAMINE	PYRIBENZAMINE	Antihistamine
276. TROXIDONE	TRIDIONE	Anticonvulsant (see p. 339)
277. TUBOCURARINE CHLORIDE	TUBARINE	Muscle relaxant
278. VASOPRESSIN	PITRESSIN	Diabetcs Insipidus (see p. 434)
279. VERATRUM VIRIDE	VERATRONE, VERILOID	Hypertension
280. VIOMYCIN	VIOCIN	Antibiotic (see p. 585)
281. VITAMIN K_1	KONAKION, MEPHYTON	Antidote to anticoagulants (see p. 126)
282. WARFARIN SODIUM	MAREVAN, COUMADIN	Anticoagulant (see p. 590)

TRADE NAMES OF DRUGS

THE number after each drug refers to the corresponding number in the previous table, *i.e.*, reference to that table will show the approved or chemical name of the drug.

ACHROMYCIN, 260
ACRAMIDINE, 13
ACRAMINE, 13
ACTHAR, 63
ADALIN, 52
ADCORTYL, 270
ALBAMYCIN, 173
ALBUCID, 246
ALEUDRIN, 130
ALFICETYN, 55
ALGELOX, 8
ALOCOL, 8
ALTAFUR, 104
ALUDROX, 8
ALUPHOS, 9
AMECHOL, 151
AMINACYL, 237
AMINOPTERIN, 16
AMPHAMED, 21
AMYTAL, 22
AMYTAL SODIUM, 23
ANACARDONE, 169
ANACOBIN, 65
ANAHÆMIN, 137
ANAHEPOL, 137
ANCOLAN, 140
ANECTINE, 258
ANETHAINE, 11
ANGISED, 273
ANSOLYSEN, 184
ANTABUSE, 88
ANTEPAR, 206
ANTHIPHEN, 79
ANTHISAN, 146
ANTISTIN, 26
ANTRENYL, 176
APRESOLINE, 115
ARALEN, 59
ARFONAD, 272
ARTANE, 36
ARTERIODONE, 86
ASCABIOL, 37
ASCORVEL, 27
ATEBRIN, 142
ATEMPOL, 157

AVLOCHIN, 54
AVLOCLOR, 59
AVLOPROCIL A.S., 217
AVLOSULFON, 70
AVOMINE, 223

BACTYLAN, 237
B.A.L., 84
BEFLAVIT, 231
BENADRYL, 87
BENAPEN, 32
BENECARDIN, 132
BENEMID, 214
BENERVA, 24
BENODAINE, 208
BENZEDRINE, 21
BENZEVAN, 37
BETALIN S, 24
BETAVEL, 24
BETAXAN, 24
BETNELAN, 39
BILIGRAFIN, 124
BIOTEXIN, 173
BISGLUCOL, 40
BISMOSTAB, 40
BITEVAN, 65
BRADOSOL, 91
BREVIDIL E, 259
BREVIDIL M, 257
BUTAZOLIDIN, 198

CALCIPEN V, 193
CAMOQUIN, 20
CAMPOLON, 137
CANTAN, 27
CARBO-RESIN, 127
CARDIAZOL, 133
CARDOPHYLLIN, 15
CATHOMYCIN, 173
CENTRAZOL, 133
CEREVON, 99
CETAVLON, 53
CEVALIN, 27
CEVANOL, 31

CHLORETONE, 56
CHLOROMYCETIN, 55
CIBAZOL, 256
CIGNOLIN, 90
COBALIN, 65
COBASTAB, 65
CODELCORTONE, 211
COLCEMID, 71
COLISTATIN, 245
COLLIRON I. V., 233
COLLUMINA, 8
COMPOCILLIN V, 193
CORAMINE, 169
CORTEF, 117
CORTELAN, 64
CORTIRON, 73
CORTISTAB, 64
CORTISYL, 64
CORTRIL, 117
CORTROPHIN, 63
CORVOTONE, 169
COSCOPIN, 172
COTINAZIN, 129
COUMADIN, 282
CREMODIAZINE, 247
CREMOSUXIDINE, 245
CREMOTHALIDINE, 205
CRONETAL, 88
CRYSTAPEN, 38
CRYSTO-VIBEX, 24
CUMOPYRAN, 69
CYCLONAL, 113
CYCLOSPASMOL, 241
CYTAMEN, 65

DAPTAZOLE, 17
DARAPRIM, 227
DARENTHIN, 41
DAVITAMON C, 27
DAVITAMON B₁, 24
DECADRON, 75
DECAPRYN, 92
DECICAIN, 11
DECORTACETE, 73

21

SODIUM CONTENT OF SOME COMMON FOODS

Approximate values in milligrams per ounce.

CEREALS AND CEREAL FOODS

Bread—ordinary	**112–124**
unsalted	10–30
Matzos	2–5
Biscuits—all kinds	**70–130**
Ryvita, Vitawheat	**175**
Cereals—dry, shredded wheat, puffed wheat, puffed rice	1–4
All other dry cereals	**200–350**
Rice, sago, spaghetti, tapioca, arrowroot . . .	1–2
Flour, plain	0·5–1

DAIRY FOODS

Milk	14
Butter—salted	**65**
unsalted	2
Cheese	**150–350**
Cream cheese (unsalted)	10

MEAT

Fresh meats, poultry, tripe	20–30
Brains and kidney	**30–70**
Salted or smoked bacon, ham, corned beef . . .	**250–850**
Sausages	**250–300**

FISH

Fresh	30–40
Smoked or salted haddock, kippers, bloaters . .	**200–300**
Shellfish	**120–1000**
Tinned	**150–220**

VEGETABLES (RAW)

Celery	**38**
Spinach	**34**
Beetroot	**18**
Watercress	**17**
Carrots	**14**
New Potatoes (cooked)	**12**
Red Cabbage	10
Turnips (cooked)	8
All other cooked vegetables	1–5

FRUITS

Dried fruit (raw)	**18–25**
Passion fruit	8
Avocado pears	5
Melon	4
Dates	1–2
All other fresh fruits	0·5–1
Tinned fruits	0·5–4

MISCELLANEOUS

Chocolate—milk		**80**
plain		40
Ice-cream		20–30
Cocoa powder		**185**
Horlicks, Bournvita, Ovaltine		**70–190**
Marmite—unsalted		65–100
salted		**1750**
Beer	per pint	**75–130**
Wines	per ounce	2–4
Herbs—bay leaf, mint, sage, thyme, parsley, etc.		5–12
Spices—allspice, cinnamon, ginger, mace, nutmeg, etc.		5–15
Spirit vinegar, mustard powder, dry horse-radish		1–2

METRIC DOSES WITH APPROXIMATE IMPERIAL EQUIVALENTS

Weights

Metric.	Approximate Imperial Equivalent.
1 kilogram (kg.) . . .	2·2 pounds (lb.).
30 grammes (gm.) . .	1 ounce (oz.)=8 drachms.
4 grammes	1 drachm (dr.)=60 grains.
1 gramme	15 grains (gr.)
0·1 gramme (100 milligrams) .	1½ grains.
50 milligrams (mgm.) . .	¾ grain.
10 milligrams . . .	⅙ grain.

Liquid Measures

Metric.	Approximate Imperial Equivalent.
1 litre (1,000 millilitres) .	35 fluid ounces.
550 millilitres (ml.) . . .	20 fluid ounces (1 pint).
30 millilitres . . .	1 fluid ounce.
4 millilitres . . .	1 fluid drachm (60 minims).
1 millilitre	15 minims (m.).

Note.—1 millilitre=1 cubic centimetre (c.c.).

Approximate Value of Domestic Measures

1 teaspoon . . .	1 fluid drachm.
1 dessertspoon . .	2 fluid drachms (¼ oz.).
1 tablespoon . .	½ fluid ounce.
1 eggcup . . .	1 fluid ounce.
1 teacup . . .	5 fluid ounces.
1 tumbler . .	10 fluid ounces.

INDEX

A

Abbocillin, 578
Abdominal colic, 250
Abdominal pains, 533
Abdominal reflexes, 298
Abortus bacilli, 17
Abreaction, 563
Abscess, amœbic, 83
cerebral, 331
" cold," 506
of lung, 216
peritonsillar, 173
psoas, 89
Acarus scabiei, 519
Acetest, 407
Acetomenaphthone, 504
Acetone in urine, 407
Achalasia, 227
Achlorhydria, 232
in pernicious anæmia, 372
Acholuric jaundice, 381
Achondroplasia, 512
Achromycin, 582
Acid-fast bacillus, 22
Acidosis, 460, 491
Acne rosacea, 524
Acne vulgaris, 523
Acromegaly, 430
ACTH, 597. See Cortisone
Active immunity, 29
Acute anterior poliomyelitis, 331
Acute hepatic necrosis, 287
Acute infective hepatitis, 284
Acute non-specific pericarditis, 144
Acute yellow atrophy, 287
Adalin, 604
Adcortyl, 599
Addison's disease, 448
Adenoma, 11
Adexolin, 503
Adrenal glands, anatomy and physi-
ology, 445
diseases, 448, 451
hyperplasia, 449
tumours, 449
Adrenaline, 586
Adrenocorticotrophic hormone, 599
Adrenogenital syndrome, 450
Agglutination reactions, 23
Agglutinins, 378
Aggression and resentment in hospital
patients, 569, 570
Agranulocytic angina, 391
Agranulocytosis, 391

Alastrim, 76
Albamycin, 581
Albuminometer, Esbach's, 405
Albuminuria, 406
Albustix test, 405
Alcohol, as a cause of coma, 545, 546
in relation to pellagra, 497
Alcohol test meal, 235
Alcoholic cirrhosis of liver, 288
Alcoholic neuritis, 319
Aldosterone, 447, 599
Aleukæmic leukæmia, 390
Alkalis, 238, 588
Alkalosis, 454, 492
Allergic diseases, 32
Allergy, 31
Allobarbitone, 594
Alopecia, areata, 531
syphilitic, 97
Altafur, 611
Aluminium glycinate, 238
Aluminium hydroxide, 238
Amethocaine, 597
Aminophylline, 201, 589
Aminopterin, 390
Amiphenazole, 595
Ammonium chloride, 140
Amodiaquine, 81
Amœbic abscess, 83
Amœbic dysentery, 82
Amœbic hepatitis, 83
Amphetamine, 589
Amyl nitrite, 123
Amylobarbitone, 594
Amytal, 594
Anacardone, 610
Anæmia, 366
aplastic, 376, 383
classification, 367
congenital hæmolytic, 381
drugs in relation to, 376, 379
dyshæmopoietic, 368
hæmolytic, 376
hæmorrhagic, 368
hyperchromic, 366
hypochromic, 366, 373
idiopathic hypochromic, 373
in diseases of the gastro-intestinal
tract, 375
in infants, 374
in leukæmia, 389
in pregnancy 375
iron in relation to, 364, 373
macrocytic, 366
microcytic, 366

645

22